TRANSLATIONAL ENDOCRINOLOGY OF BONE

Reproduction, Metabolism, and the Central Nervous System

ELSEVIER *science & technology books*

....

· *Companion Web Site:*

http://booksite.elsevier.com/9780124157842

....

Translational Endocrinology of Bone: Reproduction, Metabolism, and the Central Nervous system
Gerard Karsenty, Editor

Resources:

- All figures from the book available as both Power Point slides and .jpeg files

TOOLS FOR ALL YOUR TEACHING NEEDS
textbooks.elsevier.com

ACADEMIC
PRESS

TRANSLATIONAL ENDOCRINOLOGY OF BONE

Reproduction, Metabolism, and the Central Nervous System

Edited by

GERARD KARSENTY, M.D., PH.D.

Professor and Chair,
Department of Genetics and Development,
Columbia University,
New York, NY

AMSTERDAM • BOSTON • HEIDELBERG • LONDON
NEW YORK • OXFORD • PARIS • SAN DIEGO
SAN FRANCISCO • SINGAPORE • SYDNEY • TOKYO

Academic Press is an imprint of Elsevier

Academic Press is an imprint of Elsevier
32 Jamestown Road, London NW1 7BY, UK
225 Wyman Street, Waltham, MA 02451, USA
525 B Street, Suite 1800, San Diego, CA 92101-4495, USA

First edition 2013

Notice
No responsibility is assumed by the publisher for any injury and/or damage to persons or property as a matter of products liability, negligence or otherwise, or from any use or operation of any methods, products, instructions or ideas contained in the material herein. Because of rapid advances in the medical sciences, in particular, independent verification of diagnoses and drug dosages should be made

Medicine is an ever-changing field. Standard safety precautions must be followed, but as new research and clinical experience broaden our knowledge, changes in treatment and drug therapy may become necessary or appropriate. Readers are advised to check the most current product information provided by the manufacturer of each drug to be administered to verify the recommended dose, the method and duration of administrations, and contraindications. It is the responsibility of the treating physician, relying on experience and knowledge of the patient, to determine dosages and the best treatment for each individual patient. Neither the publisher nor the authors assume any liability for any injury and/or damage to persons or property arising from this publication.

British Library Cataloguing-in-Publication Data
A catalogue record for this book is available from the British Library

Library of Congress Cataloging-in-Publication Data
A catalog record for this book is available from the Library of Congress

ISBN : 978-0-12-415784-2

For information on all Academic Press publications visit our website at elsevierdirect.com

Typeset by TNQ Books and Journals Pvt Ltd.
www.tnq.co.in

Printed and bound in United States of America

12 13 14 15 16   10 9 8 7 6 5 4 3 2 1

Working together to grow
libraries in developing countries
www.elsevier.com | www.bookaid.org | www.sabre.org

ELSEVIER   BOOK AID International   Sabre Foundation

Contents

Contributors

Michael Amling, MD, University Medical Center Hamburg-Eppendorf, Hamburg, Germany

Paul A. Baldock, PhD, University of New South Wales, Sydney, Australia

S. Bhatt, PhD, Harvard Medical School, Boston, MA, USA

M. Michael Bliziotes, MD, Oregon Health & Science University, Portland, OR, USA and Portland Veterans Affairs Medical Center, Portland, OR, USA

Chadi Calarge, MD, The University of Iowa, Iowa City, IA, USA

Thomas L. Clemens, PhD, Johns Hopkins University School of Medicine, Baltimore, MD, USA; Baltimore Veterans Administration Medical Center, Baltimore, MD, USA

Michael Densmore, ALM, Harvard School of Dental Medicine, Boston, MA, USA

Patricia Ducy, PhD, Columbia University Medical Center, New York, NY, USA

Ronald M. Evans, PhD, Professor and Director, Gene Expression Laboratory, Howard Hughes Medical Institute, The Salk Institute for Biological Studies, La Jolla, CA, USA

Mathieu Ferron, PhD, Columbia University, New York, NY, USA

Seiji Fukumoto, MD, PhD, University of Tokyo Hospital, Tokyo, Japan

Elizabeth M. Haney, MD, Oregon Health & Science University, Portland, OR, USA

Gerard Karsenty, MD, PhD, Columbia University, New York, NY, USA

Masanobu Kawai, MD, PhD, Osaka Medical Center and Research Institute for Maternal and Child Health, Osaka, Japan

Stavroula Kousteni, PhD, Columbia University, New York, NY, USA

R.N. Kulkarni, MD, PhD, Harvard Medical School, Boston, MA, USA

Beate Lanske, PhD, Harvard School of Dental Medicine, Boston, MA, USA

Itamar Levinger, PhD, Institute for Sport, Exercise and Active Living (ISEAL), Victoria University, Melbourne, Australia

T. John Martin, FRS St. Vincent's Institute of Medical Research, Melbourne, Australia; University of Melbourne Department of Medicine, Melbourne, Australia

Franck Oury, PhD, Columbia University, New York, NY, USA

Mohammed S. Razzaque, MD, PhD, Harvard School of Dental Medicine, Boston, MA, USA

Ryan C. Riddle, PhD, Johns Hopkins University School of Medicine, Baltimore, MD, USA; Baltimore Veterans Administration Medical Center, Baltimore, MD, USA

Clifford J. Rosen, MD, Maine Medical Center Research Institute, Scarborough, ME, USA

Thorsten Schinke, PhD, University Medical Center Hamburg-Eppendorf, Hamburg, Germany

Ego Seeman, MD, University of Melbourne, Melbourne, Australia

Natalie A. Sims, PhD, St. Vincent's Institute of Medical Research, Melbourne, Australia; University of Melbourne Department of Medicine, Melbourne, Australia

Shu Takeda, MD, PhD, Keio University, Tokyo, Japan

Kong Wah Ng, MD, FRACP, St. Vincent's Institute of Medical Research, Melbourne, Australia; University of Melbourne Department of Medicine, Melbourne, Australia

Yihong Wan, PhD, University of Texas Southwestern Medical Center, Dallas, TX, USA

Wei Wei, PhD, University of Texas Southwestern Medical Center, Dallas, TX, USA

Vijay K. Yadav, PhD, Wellcome Trust Sanger Institute, Cambridge, UK

Jeffrey D. Zajac, MD, PhD, University of Melbourne, Melbourne, Australia

Foreword

The word "skeleton" comes from the Greek term *skeletos*, meaning "dried body". As this meaning implies, traditionally the skeleton is considered as the body's largest connective tissue, and after death this structure "survives" because as a largely inorganic scaffold it is seemingly not alone. In molecular biology it is often said that "structure leads to function", and in this light the skeleton touches and communicates with all parts of the body — literally from head to toe. This static view of bone as mechanical support, though partially true, belies its vibrant nature. As a highly dynamic tissue, bone constantly undergoes remodeling by the action of two key cell types, bone-building osteoblasts and bone-destroying osteoclasts, at the expense of substantial and continuous energy expenditure. The balance of these two forces is controlled by many factors, including the sympathetic nervous system, parathyroid hormone, calcitonin, osteocalcin, and various nuclear hormone receptor ligands including vitamins A and D. As 70 per cent of bone is composed of calcium phosphate matrix, by necessity many hormones identified regulate serum calcium and phosphate levels by affecting the kidney, intestine and/or bone itself [1]. Bone also harbors bone marrow, which plays a critical role in whole-body physiology, including the maintenance of the hematopoietic and immune systems. Besides this classical view of bone as a mineral reservoir and structural support, numerous reports point to the link between whole-body physiology and integrity of the bone compartment.

One of the major challenges in bone biology is to understand the interplay of various tissues that can regulate bone physiology. The "ying—yang" nature of homeostasis means that bone is not merely a passive recipient but rather a full-time player in body physiology. The growing emergence of a vast repertory of tissue-specific gene expression profiling has begun to open a door regarding the molecules and pathways that mediate and control this vast network. Concurrently, beyond the individual factor, what is more relevant is understanding how networks between various target tissues become coordinately regulated to produce whole-body physiology and metabolism. Recent progress in mouse genetics allows us to study and decipher this interplay between tissues by spatially and temporally inactivating single target genes in specific tissue/cell types. With this approach, we now know that bone is intricately linked to energy metabolism, insulin secretion, and fertility via neural circuitry and endocrine regulators including leptin, serotonin, NPY, osteocalcin, FGF 23, vitamin D_3 and PPARγ ligands [2,3].

These key advances came from assigning new roles and modes of action for already known regulators. For example, while the adipocyte-derived hormone leptin is known to regulate energy metabolism and appetite [4], more recently it was found to be a central regulator of bone mass. This leads to new ideas as to how bone mass and energy metabolism can be coordinated to achieve true metabolic homeostasis of energy and minerals [5]. Thus, this becomes a critical step in deciphering the economic formula of vertebrate evolution regarding how energy metabolism links with the bone remodeling to minimize nutritional and energy deficits. Bone remodeling consumes a fair amount of energy, and the decision to undergo significant remodeling requires a process to evaluate metabolic and nutritional competence. Owing to recent progress, investigation of these signaling events has uncovered new regulators of the bone mass and energy metabolism equation. For example, the sympathetic nervous system and brain-derived serotonin were identified as downstream effectors of leptin signaling [6]. With a finding of duodenum-derived serotonin, the gastrointestinal tract has now been revisited as a bone-mass regulator [7]. Furthermore, the well-known insulin sensitizer TZD, a PPARγ agonist, has been shown to affect the bone remodeling processes [8,9]. The collective studies help to reveal that osteoblast-derived osteocalcin is actually a hormone targeting pancreatic β cells, helping to define the new field of skeletal endocrinology.

The compilation of cell/tissue-specific transcriptomes offers a wealth of facts, but in reality a plethora of information without a cipher can lead us into unsolvable maze. An understanding as to how hormones are called into action to create complex physiology and disease is the next big step in the field. Achieving this goal is challenging, but whole-organism mouse genetics is the most powerful tool to connect the dots of inter-organ communication. It is the goal of this book to highlight breakthroughs and perspectives to brace us for new era of skeletal endocrinology.

Ronald M. Evans
The Salk Institute for Biological Studies

References

[1] Bilezikian J, Raisz L, Martin TJ. Principles of Bone Biology. New York, NY: Academic Press; 2008.

[2] Karsenty G, Oury F. Biology without walls: the novel endocrinology of bone. Annu. Rev. Physiol. 2012;74:87–105.

[3] Kawai M, Rosen CJ. PPARγ: a circadian transcription factor in adipogenesis and osteogenesis. Nature Rev. Endo 2010;6:629–36.

[4] Ahima RS, Saper CB, Flier JS, Elmquist JK. Leptin regulation of neuroendocrine systems. Front. Neuroendocrinol. 2000;21:263–307.

[5] Elefteriou F, Ahn JD, Takeda S, Starbuck M, Yang X, et al. Leptin regulation of bone resorption by the sympathetic nervous system and CART. Nature 2005;434:514–20.

[6] Yadav VK, Oury F, Suda N, Liu ZW, Gao XB, et al. A serotonin-dependent mechanism explains the leptin regulation of bone mass, appetite, and energy expenditure. Cell 2009;138:976–89.

[7] Yadav VK, Ryu JH, Suda N, Tanaka KF, Gingrich JA, et al. Lrp5 controls bone formation by inhibiting serotonin synthesis in the duodenum. Cell 2008;135:825–37.

[8] Akune T, Ohba S, Kamekura S, Yamaguchi M, Chung UI, et al. PPARgamma insufficiency enhances osteogenesis through osteoblast formation from bone marrow progenitors. J. Clin. Invest. 2004;113:846–55.

[9] Wan Y, Chong LW, Evans RM. PPAR-gamma regulates osteoclastogenesis in mice. Nat. Med. 2007;13:1496–503.

Introduction: The Rational of the Work or the Overarching Hypothesis

Gerard Karsenty

Columbia University, New York, NY, USA

For very good reasons it is customary to be endlessly fascinated by the unexpected degree of sequence conservation that one can find in some transcription factors and signaling molecules between yeast and man. It is indeed quite extraordinary that protein motifs could be conserved over a hundred million years. Not to mention the even higher and tighter degree of conservation that exists between fly and human genes. But then again, yeast are not humans, flies are more sophisticated than yeast but do not have many of the functions or organs that vertebrates have, and bony vertebrates differ from other vertebrates in many functional aspects, as this book proposes to show. One reason for that is that this unexpected and rather high degree of conservation between invertebrates and vertebrates affects mostly intracellular signaling molecules and transcription factors. It is in fact not so surprising that the basic molecular equipment of the cell has not changed too much during evolution.

However, if we now look at extracellular signaling molecules, whether they are neuromediators or hormones, the picture that is emerging is completely different. In those cases differences are staggering and, as a matter of fact, expected. For instance, when looking at most eukaryote model organisms—yeast, *C. elegans*, *Drosophila*, mouse, and humans—that are studied in any given department of genetics, what do we see? *C. elegans* has insulin and serotonin, yeast does not. *Drosophila* has many neuropeptides that are not present in worms. It also has organs and functions that are absent in worms. The same can be said for vertebrates that have hormones such as parathyroid hormone that are not present in invertebrates [1]. At the very end of the spectrum bony vertebrates have hormones such as leptin, osteocalcin, and others that have not, for now, been found in any other animals [2,3]. So if there is a great degree of conservation of intracellular pathways

there is also an equally great degree of variety for extracellular signaling molecules from one general stage of evolution to another. If this were not the case how could one explain the progressive acquisitions of organs and functions throughout evolution? This perspective on what is conserved and what is not serves as a preamble for the topics covered by this volume, namely whole-organism physiology in bony vertebrates and how the study of this emerging discipline helps understanding of the pathogenesis of degenerative diseases affecting several organs.

THE TWO FACES OF PHYSIOLOGY

Physiology is a generic term that applies to two disciplines that, if not totally different, are somewhat distinct. The first discipline tries to identify the molecular signaling and transcriptional events occurring in a particular cell type responsible for or implicated in a given physiological function. In a way this aspect of physiology is another form of expression of the historical evolution of biology that over the last half century has become, rightly so, increasingly molecular. This discipline, which can be referred to as molecular and cellular physiology, has been unbelievably successful in identifying and deciphering to the most detailed level many intracellular pathways. As a result, it has allowed the biomedical community to design new and potent drugs for some degenerative diseases affecting multiple physiological functions. It is more than likely that this molecular revolution of physiology is not finished and that we will continue, through it, to improve the treatment of chronic diseases. As we all know one of the most fertile accomplishments in terms of generating new knowledge of the molecular genetic revolution has been the ability we now have to delete a gene of

Translational Endocrinology of Bone
DOI: http://dx.doi.org/10.1016/B978-0-12-415784-2.00001-4

interest in a single cell type of interest and at a time of our choice in the entire animal. An unexpected and somewhat ironic consequence of this technological advance has been that inadvertently it has revived a totally different form of physiology, one that has been dormant for almost a century.

When biology was a purely descriptive discipline the first purpose of physiology was to describe how organs were talking to each other through what Claude Bernard then described with the fuzzy term *milieu intérieur* [4]. The very fact that the name of Claude Bernard is still known 150 years after his death illustrates how important this aspect of physiology has remained for most biologists. By definition, this particular physiology studies events taking place and molecules working outside the cell and connecting organs. Hence, it could be called whole-organism physiology. Over the last 20 years mouse genetics has revived this discipline by revealing connections between organs that were not known and not even suspected to exist. Specifically in less than 20 years novel hormones were discovered and it was shown that kidney affects erythropoiesis [5]; fat is a direct determinant of appetite, bone mass, and fertility by acting in the brain [2,6,7]; brain controls bone mass [8]; bone promotes male fertility [9]; and bone marrow modulates behavior [10], to cite a few of many striking but medically important examples. That so much has been learned in so little time implies that the field of whole-organism physiology is an unchartered territory and that many paradigm-shifting discoveries remain to be made. It may very well be that whole-organism physiology is the next frontier in biology.

The study of whole-organism physiology relies on a few overarching principles; together they form a conceptual framework that is helpful in trying to understand why some of these inter-organ connections exist and also why diseases develop when they go away. The first principle was forged by W. Cannon. It is the principle of homeostasis [11,12]. This means that several organs exert opposite influences on a given physiological process in order to better control it. Closely related to the concept of homeostasis is the principle of feedback regulation that is central to the field of endocrinology [13]. This concept simply means that a regulated organ talks back to the regulating one in order to limit its influence. The second principle that englobes the notion of milieu intérieur and the concept of homeostasis is the principle of functional dependence that was forged in the 1920s by a remarkably original individual: L.J. Henderson [14]. This concept postulates that the function of a given organ will be affected, to various degrees, by many other organs. Although this concept was implicit in the work of Claude Bernard one has to appreciate that at the time it was proposed we knew so little in endocrinology and neuroscience,

not to mention genetics, that it was impossible to believe in it, much less to test it appropriately. That the existence of functional dependence was demonstrated recently to the extent it has been illustrates the importance of the conceptual framework it provides. The last conceptual tool that helps define whole-organism physiology, and in that respect it is not different from developmental biology, is that regulatory molecules, i.e. hormones and neuropeptides, appear during evolution with the functions they need to regulate, not after. Although this sounds self-evident it is particularly important for the purpose of this volume since several of the hormones that will be presented here appear during evolution with bones. What this observation suggests is that the appearance of bone may have modified the physiology of the entire organism to a greater extent than anticipated. This hypothesis can now be tested genetically in model organisms.

THE UNANTICIPATED INFLUENCE OF BONE ON WHOLE-ORGANISM PHYSIOLOGY

Why would bone affect whole-organism physiology so dramatically in the first place? The answer to this question lies with two features of bone and its biology. However, because they are so well known we tend to forget both their importance and their implications. The first one is that bone covers a bigger surface in our body than most organs. As a result one has to assume that the energetic cost of any event occurring in bone will probably be higher than in most other organs. The second and even more important feature of bone is that it is the only tissue that contains a cell type, the osteoclast, whose only function is to destroy the host tissue [15]. This process, which resembles very much a physiological autoimmune reaction, does not occur at random but in the context of a true homeostatic function that occurs daily and in multiple locations in the skeleton. This function is called bone modeling during childhood and bone remodeling during adulthood. In each case there is a permanent succession or destruction or resorption of bone by the osteoclast followed by *de novo* formation by the osteoblasts [16].

How important are and have been these two unglamorous processes? Bone modeling is required for longitudinal growth of bones without which most vertebrates would not be able to ambulate and therefore could not survive. Thus, by definition, bone modeling has been throughout evolution, and remains today, a survival function. As for bone remodeling, its original purpose is to repair micro and macro damages, i.e. fractures. This is certainly not an efficient means to do so, yet until the 20th century it was probably the most widely used one. The tragedy of bone remodeling is that it is affected by a disease that may not be as attractive as others, namely osteoporosis. However, osteoporosis is a disease of people 50 years and older so at the scale of the general population it probably did not exist before the 20th century. Therefore, one had to look elsewhere to understand why evolution had preserved bone remodeling for so long. Moreover, during evolution, if bone modeling and remodeling have been and for the former continue to be so important then it becomes more understandable why on the one hand the existence of bone affects so many physiological functions, while on the other hand so many genes and functions also influence bone mass accrual.

Both the cellular events entailed by bone modeling and remodeling and the surface covered by bones suggest that the energetic cost of bone modeling and remodeling must be high and therefore there is a need to coordinate energy metabolism and bone (re) modeling. This is one of the premises on which most (but not all) of the endocrinology described in this volume is based. I refer here to the influence made in and exerted by hormones and neuromediators on fat, brain, and gut on bone mass. A second premise comes from the clinical arena, which is that the integrity of gonadal functions, in both genders, is needed to maintain bone mass. Thus, one could propose the following hypothesis: bone growth during childhood, bone mass during adulthood, energy metabolism, and reproduction are coordinately regulated. Many of the chapters of this volume will address this general assumption by studying various hormones and neuromediators ranging from serotonin to osteocalcin while others will review our emerging knowledge about another endocrine function of bone, namely its ability to regulate phosphate metabolism.

More generally this volume has two ambitions. The first one, bone-centric, is to demonstrate, through examples of hormones emerging during evolution with bone and coordinating the regulation of bone mass accrual, energy metabolism and reproduction, that the appearance of bone during evolution has profoundly affected the physiology of the entire organism. The second goal is broader but just as important—to illustrate, through the example of the skeleton, how powerful a genetic-based approach to the study of the physiology of a given organ is in revealing multiple new functions for this organ, multiple connections with other organs, and novel identities for supposedly well-known molecules. This, we hope, should be viewed as a general paradigm as it is more than likely that what is true for bone must be true for many other organs.

References

[1] Poole KE, Reeve J. Parathyroid hormone—a bone anabolic and catabolic agent. Curr Opin Pharmacol 2005;5(6):612–7.
[2] Friedman JM, Halaas JL. Leptin and the regulation of body weight in mammals. Nature 1998;395(6704):763–70.
[3] Hauschka PV, Lian JB, Cole DE, Gundberg CM. Osteocalcin and matrix Gla protein: vitamin K-dependent proteins in bone. Physiol Rev 1989;69(3):990–1047.
[4] Bernard C. An Introduction to the Study of Experimental Medicine. Paris: Flamarion; 1865.
[5] Gurney CW. Erythropoietin, erythropoiesis, and the kidney. JAMA 1960;173:1828–9.
[6] Chehab FF. A broader role for leptin. Nat Med 1996;2(7):723–4.
[7] Takeda S, Elefteriou F, Karsenty G. Common endocrine control of body weight, reproduction, and bone mass. Annu Rev Nutr 2003;23:403–11.
[8] Ducy P, Amling M, Takeda S, Priemel M, Schilling AF, Beil FT, Shen J, Vinson C, Rueger JM, Karsenty G. Leptin inhibits bone formation through a hypothalamic relay: a central control of bone mass. Cell 2000;100(2):197–207.
[9] Oury F, Sumara G, Sumara O, Ferron M, Chang H, Smith CE, Hermo L, Suarez S, Roth BL, Ducy P, Karsenty G. Endocrine Regulation of Male Fertility by the Skeleton. Cell 2011;144(5):796–809.
[10] Chen SK, Tvrdik P, Peden E, Cho S, Wu S, Spangrude G, Capecchi MR. Hematopoietic origin of pathological grooming in Hoxb8 mutant mice. Cell 2010;141(5):775–85.
[11] Cannon WB. The Wisdom of the Body. New York, NY, US: W W Norton & Co; 1932;312.
[12] Cannon WB. Organization for physiological homeostasis. Physiological Reviews 1929;9:399–431.
[13] Monod J, Jacob F. Teleonomic mechanisms in cellular metabolism, growth, and differentiation. Cold Spring Harb Symp Quant Biol 1961;26:389–401.
[14] Henderson LJ. The Fitness of the Environment: An Inquiry into the Biological Significance of the Properties of Matter. New York: The Macmillan Company; 1913.
[15] Teitelbaum SL. Bone resorption by osteoclasts. Science 2000;289(5484):1504–8.
[16] Ducy P, Schinke T, Karsenty G. The osteoblast: a sophisticated fibroblast under central surveillance. Science 2000;289(5484):1501–4.

2

Basic Principles of Bone Cell Biology

T. John Martin[1,2], *Kong Wah Ng*[1,2], *Natalie A. Sims*[1,2]

[1]St. Vincent's Institute of Medical Research, Melbourne, Australia [2]University of
Melbourne Department of Medicine, Melbourne, Australia

INTRODUCTION

Far from being an inert envelope encasing the bone marrow, thereby protecting hemopoiesis and development of the immune system, bone is a complex organ, constantly changing under the control of hormones, cytokines, the central and sympathetic nervous systems, and which itself functions as an endocrine organ. As in other complex organs, the function of bone is controlled by a range of specialized cell types; these reside on the bone surface or within the mineralized matrix. Whereas previous views of the origins and functions of bone cells relied on extrapolations from histologic, histomorphometric, and electron microscopic examination of normal and pathological bone specimens, the study of cells isolated and cultured from bone only began at the end of the 1970s. What has been learned in the last three decades from the study of bone cell biology and mouse and human genetics is that the cells of bone communicate with each other through many signaling processes that require the local generation of effector cytokines, growth factors, and other molecules, with hormonal regulation superimposed on some of these. Furthermore, each cell lineage is influenced by cells of the immune and nervous systems, thereby achieving the very tight control of bone modeling and remodeling that is necessary to preserve the structural integrity of the skeleton.

This chapter will describe the cells of bone, some mechanisms by which they communicate with each other and with neighboring cells in the bone microenvironment, and discuss advances made in bone cell biology that have contributed so much to this current understanding. We have chosen to review findings in older literature since this helps explain how methods for the study of bone cells were developed, and which of those methods and conclusions withstand the test of time. The historical consideration also shows us how some recent discoveries have resurrected old concepts that were formulated using earlier technologies.

THE OSTEOBLAST LINEAGE

Osteoblasts are those cells that form bone matrix, and the view that the osteoblast is concerned with bone formation is reflected in its name. However, cells of the osteoblast lineage have a wide range of functions, and confusion has arisen when "osteoblast" is used to describe cells at other stages of the lineage that are not actively forming bone matrix. Mature osteoblasts are readily recognized histologically as plump, cuboidal, mononuclear cells residing in groups on the matrix that they have synthesized. Gap junctions exist between these cells, helping in their communication with each other and with osteocytes within cortical and trabecular bone through a network of canaliculae [1]. Synthesizing osteoblasts have prominent Golgi apparatus and a basophilic cytoplasm that reflects their capacity for protein synthesis. They are rich in alkaline phosphatase (ALP) and synthesize predominantly type I collagen and non-collagenous proteins including osteocalcin, osteonectin, bone sialoprotein, and bone proteoglycans I (biglycan) and II (decorin). They possess many receptors, including the receptor (PTH1R) for parathyroid hormone (PTH) and PTHrP, allowing them to respond to growth factors and cytokines produced by cells of the osteoblast lineage. Production of these factors and expression of the relevant receptors is undoubtedly modulated depending on the stage of differentiation, and activities of osteoblast lineage cells. Figure 2.1 illustrates schematically the relationships of members of the osteoblast lineage.

Translational Endocrinology of Bone
DOI: http://dx.doi.org/10.1016/B978-0-12-415784-2.00002-6

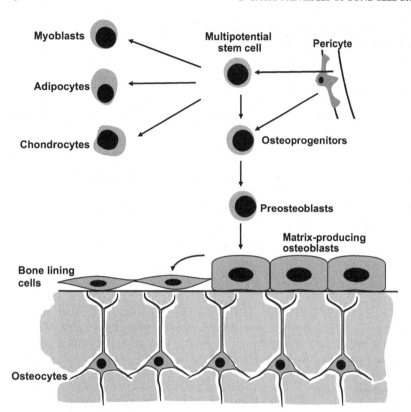

FIGURE 2.1 **The osteoblast lineage.** The mesenchymal stem cell is multipotential, giving rise to muscle (myocytes), fat (adipocytes), and cartilage cells (chondrocytes) as well as to the osteoblast lineage. Osteoblast precursors can also arise from blood-borne stem cells and pericytes. Osteocytes communicate with each other and with surface lining cells and osteoblasts (see text).

Bone lining cells are flattened osteoblast lineage cells resting on endosteal and trabecular surfaces. They have little cytoplasm or endoplasmic reticulum, having largely lost their synthetic function, and have somewhat less cytoplasmic basophilia and alkaline phosphatase activity than matrix-synthesizing osteoblasts. Like the rest of the osteoblast lineage, bone lining cells possess gap junctions with which they communicate with osteocytes and the latter's canalicular system. Regarded as osteoblasts that have completed their synthetic function, they share some properties with synthesizing osteoblasts, including expression of hormone receptors, and possibly the ability to produce some growth factors and cytokines. They are much more abundant than synthesizing osteoblasts, and cover extensive trabecular and endosteal surfaces, where they are thought to serve as a barrier to osteoclasts, to be broached in response to need, and participate in other aspects of intercellular signaling (see below).

Osteocytes are terminally differentiated osteoblasts which have become trapped within the bone matrix, including behind the advancing mineralization front. They become embedded in lacunae within the bone matrix, and connect with each other and with surface cells by their intercellular processes in fluid-containing canaliculae. Osteocytes are the most abundant cell in bone (85–90%) and are very long-lived. They respond to changes in physical forces on bone and to damage,

leading them to transmit signals to surface cells through cell–cell contact, or through production of growth factors and cytokines. In this way they may initiate formation or resorption by surface cells. This will be discussed in detail below.

In the adult skeleton, bone is usually formed in a lamellar arrangement in which collagen fibers are laid in a parallel and orderly fashion. This arrangement is essential to the structure of the Haversian system of cortical bone, in which lamellar fibers are arranged concentrically around the central cavity (Haversian canal), from the center of which there is communication with osteocytes through the canaliculae. During bone development and other states of rapid bone formation, the collagen fiber alignment is more random; this is described as woven bone.

Studying the Osteoblast Lineage

Much of what we understand about the osteoblast lineage has come from the study of cultured cells. When cells were first grown from rodent bone fragments [2], only limited characterization was possible. Some time elapsed before methods were established to extract and culture cells from newborn rodent calvariae using enzymatic digestion [3]. At the same time cells were cultured from osteogenic sarcomata; these were enriched in a number of osteoblastic properties, as were clonal lines derived from these, e.g. UMR106 [4] and ROS17.2/8 [5]. The phenotypic properties of osteoblasts were studied in such rodent cell culture systems, and the observations made in those systems extrapolated to adult bone *in vivo*, leading to concepts of the "osteoblast phenotype." In this way, UMR106 and ROS17.2/8 cells have been very useful in studying mechanisms of hormone or cytokine action. Limitations of both systems were not always realized, in particular the heterogeneity of primary rodent cultures and the fact that osteosarcoma cells are not true osteoblasts, but tumor cells enriched in some osteoblastic features. Careful comparisons between the behavior of primary bone cells with clonal osteosarcoma cells that were enriched in a number of the phenotypic features of osteoblasts allowed general conclusions about osteoblast function to be drawn [6−8].

Cultured cells derived from stromal precursors, or cell lines such as MC3T3-E1 [9] and Kusa subclones [10], have been used extensively to define the pathways of osteoblast differentiation and equate each stage with some function in bone. No single member of the osteoblast lineage would be expected to possess all of the properties of an osteoblast. The proportion of them that a cell possesses depends on its stage of differentiation, its location in bone, and the influence of local and humoral factors. Thus it is not appropriate to claim that a cell is or is not an osteoblast, on the grounds that it expresses or fails to express a particular gene, but rather, gene expression patterns define the different stages of osteoblast lineage differentiation, as illustrated in Fig. 2.1. These findings and those from a great deal of similar data accord with the proposal that osteoblast differentiation can be divided into three phases of a temporal sequence: an initial proliferative phase characterized by synthesis of bone-specific matrix components, a phase of matrix maturation after proliferation is slowed, and a final phase of matrix mineralization [11].

Osteoblasts are derived from stromal mesenchymal stem cells (MSC) present in the bone marrow. These multipotent precursors are capable of differentiating into osteoblasts, chondrocytes, adipocytes, or myocytes (reviewed in 12,13). Our understanding of these pathways owes much to the work of Alexander Friedenstein and Maureen Owen. Friedenstein [14] showed that bone marrow cells, grown to confluence *in vitro*, and subsequently transferred to diffusion chambers and implanted intraperitoneally in rabbits, established a mixture of tissues including bone. The Owen laboratory [15] found that marrow cells close to the endosteum were more osteogenic than those from central marrow, and confirmed Friedenstein's concept of the CFU-F (colony-forming unit-fibroblastic), which he proposed was a self-renewing multipotential stem cell population.

When single stromal cell colonies were transplanted under the renal capsule in mice, the host cells established hemopoiesis and excavated a marrow cavity, providing the first indication of the ability of stromal cells to promote osteoclast generation from hemopoietic precursors [16]. In fact, the skeletal tissues of bone, cartilage, and fat can all be generated from a single bone marrow stromal cell [17], leading Bianco et al. [12] to suggest that the "osteogenic stem cell" of Friedenstein and Owen, should preferably be termed "skeletal stem cell."

In studying rodent bone, cells can be isolated from the organ itself, using enzymatic digestion, but only very limited cell surface markers are available to identify the stages of osteoblast differentiation in bone. Efforts are being made to develop antibodies specific for MSCs and their progeny. In mice, when cells are derived from bone by the necessarily prolonged enzymatic digestion, surface markers are inevitably damaged in ways that hamper FACS analysis, a disadvantage that does not apply to the developmental analysis of hemopoietic cells. Despite this limitation, freshly isolated murine bone cells can be separated broadly into early (Sca-1+CD51−) and relatively mature (Sca-1−CD51+) osteoblast progenitors. This has been done with mice null for the neuropeptide Y2 receptor, in which there was an accumulation of the later cells without an increase in early precursors, indicative of enhanced differentiation [18]. Identification of stages of osteogenic differentiation in mice is being helped by the use of green fluorescent protein (GFP) reporter genes under the control of osteoblast lineage promoters to study lineage progression, and changes in gene expression at mature stages of development [19,20].

Osteoblast progenitors are associated with vascular structures in the marrow, and several studies suggest these progenitors may also give rise to cells forming the blood vessel and pluripotent perivascular cells [21−23] (Figs 2.1 and 2.3). Support for this comes from the use of the smooth muscle alpha-actin (SMAA) promoter to direct GFP to smooth muscle and pericytes, with strong osteogenic differentiation evident in cells positive for SMAA-GFP [24]. This indicates the capacity of SMAA to mark a population of osteoprogenitors, and reinforces the idea that one of the sources of osteoblast progenitors in bone remodeling is the pericyte [23]. Pericytes in different tissues appear to behave in an organ-specific manner, dictated by their anatomy and position. For example, pericytes isolated from muscle generate myocytes *in vitro* [25], consistent with the idea [12] of pericytes in different tissues reflecting a system of organ-specific progenitors with organ-specific potency. Thus the generation of osteoblasts from bone-specific pericytes illustrates the importance of the microenvironment in determining differentiation, likely by the generation and influence of local factors.

When it comes to analyzing mutant mice where osteoblast lineage function has been changed in ways that might influence the distribution of cells throughout the lineage, conclusions are still reached from morphologic assessment, because any relationship between progenitor cells isolated by FACS and their function *in vivo* has yet to be established. Histomorphometry remains the gold standard, combined with appropriate immunohistology, *in situ* hybridization and *ex vivo* studies of cells from such animals. Needed above all else are markers of osteoblast development and methods of visualization that can be applied *in situ* to complement morphologic assessment. The method of laser scanning cytometry is a promising approach, in which image analysis, somewhat like cell sorting, can be carried out on immunostained tissue sections [26].

With human cells, the option to prepare large numbers of cells by enzymatic digestion of bone specimens does not present itself. Most information comes from the study of marrow-derived precursors. The monoclonal antibody, STRO-1, has been used to identify clonogenic precursors in human marrow as CFU-Fs [27]. Combining this with alkaline phosphatase (ALP) in fluorescence-activated cell sorting (FACS) showed that STRO-1+/ALP− cells were able to progress to STRO-1−/ALP+ cells, and these latter cells represented a preosteoblast stage of development expressing the transcription factor cbfa-1 [28,29].

Transcriptional Control of the Osteoblast

Osteoblast differentiation is achieved through the coordinated transcription of a particular sequence of target genes (Table 2.1). Insights into transcriptional control were provided over many years from extensive cell culture approaches that indicated transitional stages in osteoblast differentiation [30−32]. Mouse genetics has advanced understanding of transcriptional regulation, and is summarized in a number of excellent reviews

[33,34]. Detailed aspects of transcriptional control will be discussed by Kousteni (Transcriptional Regulation of the Endocrine Function of Bone—Chapter 9). Runx2 (cbfa1) is an essential transcriptional regulator of the transition from mesenchymal cell to osteoprogenitor; mice rendered null for runx2 die at birth because of complete failure of osteoblast formation [33]. Runx2 also controls bone cell function by maintaining the differentiated mature osteoblast phenotype. Transgenic postnatal overexpression of a dominant negative form of runx2 in mice led to decreased production of endogenous runx2, diminished expression of later genes associated with osteoblast differentiation, and reduced bone formation rate despite normal osteoblast numbers, resulting in osteopenia [35]. Runx2 is central to replenishment of osteoblasts after bone loss, a key requirement in restoring bone; a connection with osteoclast regulation is its ability to activate the osteoprotegerin (OPG) promoter and enhance production of this inhibitor of osteoclast formation [36].

The search for other transcription factors led to the identification of a novel zinc finger-containing transcription factor, osterix (Osx), which is expressed in bone and cartilage. Mice rendered null for the *osx* gene did not develop mineralized bone; like the *runx2−/−* mice they died at birth, with an entirely cartilaginous skeleton [37]. In *osx−/−* mice, runx2 mRNA was expressed at the same level as in wild type. This suggests that Osx is an important transcription factor in osteoblast differentiation that functions downstream from runx2, favoring the transition of progenitors to osteoblasts, a role to which ATF4 [38] and AP-1 [39] also contribute.

Many other transcription factors influence osteoblast differentiation, and their functions form a complex network of overlapping pathways that modify osteoblast differentiation in response to locally acting cytokines or systemic factors. These may act by controlling runx2 expression (upstream factors), such as Msx2 [40] and twist1 [41,42]. Others enhance runx2 action, such as C/EBPβ and C/EBPδ [43] or antagonize runx2, such as ZFP521 [44]. Work on these transcription

TABLE 2.1 Gene Expression at Stages of Osteoblast Differentiation

Early	Intermediate	Late	Osteocytes
Pro-a(1)I collagen	Osteonectin	Osteocalcin	Sclerostin
Growth hormone receptor	Alkaline phosphatase		Matrix extracellular phosphoglycoprotein (MEPE)
Bone sialoprotein	Osteopontin		
Bone proteoglycan I	Matrix gla-protein		
Bone morphogenetic proteins	PTH1R		Dentin matrix protein-1 (DMP-1)
Receptors for retinoic acid			Fibroblast growth factor 23 (FGF-23)

factors has highlighted the close relationship between the osteoblast and adipocyte lineages, with adipocytic differentiation requiring expression of key transcriptional regulators, peroxisome proliferator-activated receptor gamma (PPARγ) [45] and C/EBPα [46]. Since osteoblasts and adipocytes are derived from common progenitors, lineage determination of precursor cells to osteoblasts results in a proportional decrease in adipogenesis. Examples are TAZ, a transcriptional coactivator of runx2 and repressor of PPARγ and ΔFosB [39]; both favor osteogenic differentiation at the expense of adipocytic potential. ZFP467 is a transcriptional cofactor with the reverse effect; its overexpression diverts bipotential precursors to adipocytes at the expense of osteoblasts [47]. This inverse relationship is also observed clinically; an increase in marrow adiposity is associated with age-related osteoporosis [48] and conditions of induced bone loss, such as ovariectomy [48,49] and immobilization [50]. Additionally, reduced osteoblast numbers in genetically altered mice are often associated with increased marrow adipogenesis [51,52], while high bone mass due to increased osteoblast commitment is associated with reduced adipocyte differentiation [39].

One pathway that modifies bone formation by altering, among other steps, the transcriptional control of osteoblasts, is Wnt signaling. In the last decade human genetics has provided the starting point for some major discoveries in osteoblast biology, notably with the discoveries that gain of function, heterozygous mis-sense mutations in low density lipoprotein receptor-related protein 5 (LRP5) are associated with a high bone mass (HBM) phenotype [53], and loss of function mutations of the same protein with an autosomal recessive osteoporosis–pseudoglioma syndrome [54,55], while disruption of *LRP5* in all cells in the mouse resulted in postnatal low bone mass and persistent embryonic eye vascularization, thus recapitulating the osteoporosis–pseudoglioma syndrome [56]. Since Lrp5 has homology to Lrp6 which itself is the vertebrate homologue of Arrow, a co-receptor for the *Drosophila* homologue of the Wnt proteins, these landmark findings brought Wnt signaling into bone biology. Activation of the canonical Wnt signaling pathway leads to stabilization of β-catenin in the cytoplasm through inhibition of glycogen synthase kinase (GSK)-3β-mediated phosphorylation, resulting in accumulation of cytoplasmic β-catenin followed by its translocation to the nucleus and transcriptional activation of specific gene targets. Such activation in mesenchymal cells inhibits chondrocyte differentiation and promotes osteoblast activity [55]. Hence, β-catenin is an obligatory node in canonical Wnt signaling that can be used as a tool to interrogate its biology in osteoblasts using modern genetic techniques.

Using this approach, much evidence emerged that canonical Wnt signaling is a powerful inducer of osteoblast differentiation and inhibitor of chondrogenesis during the early phase of skeletogenesis, a function not shared by Lrp5. Genetically manipulated mouse models were generated, and recapitulated the human mutation syndromes. Transgenic mice engineered to overexpress an HBM-associated mutation in LRP5 showed increased bone mass in one study [57], but not in another [58]. When a single allele of a canonical Wnt signaling inhibitor, *DKK1*, was deleted, mice had increased bone formation and bone mass [59]. Moreover, *in vitro* studies of Wnt signaling in cell culture abound and were consistent with the notion that Wnt signaling enhances osteoblast differentiation and cooperative effects with bone morphogenetic protein [55], and increased bone formation was shown *in vivo* with pharmacological inhibition of GSK-3β [60].

When canonical Wnt signaling was ablated or activated later during development a different picture emerged. That there was no defect in bone formation in mice harboring either an activating or an inactivating mutation of β-catenin in osteoblasts [61] dissociated this pathway at this time point from the one governed by Lrp5. Even more puzzling, these mice showed severe defects of bone resorption, an aspect of bone remodeling not affected by Lrp5 [61]. An identical phenotype and molecular mechanism was observed when deletion of β-catenin in osteocytes resulted in decreased osteocyte production of OPG and increased bone resorption [62]. Taken at face value these cell-specific loss-of-function experiments indicate that the function of canonical Wnt signaling in osteoblast or osteocytes is to promote osteoclast formation, through its regulation of *osteoprotegerin*. Remarkably the same increased bone resorption phenotype was observed in mice lacking Lrp6 [63], in that case due to increased RANKL production. A similar osteopetrotic syndrome due to failed osteoclast development and increased OPG was observed in mice lacking the adenomatous polyposis coli protein (APC) in osteoblasts [64]. APC acts in a complex of proteins with GSK-3β to maintain the normal degradation of β-catenin. Its absence leads to accumulation of β-catenin, resulting in cell-autonomous activation of Wnt signaling in the osteoblast lineage.

As mentioned above and contrasting with these *in vivo*, cell-specific genetic approaches, many cell culture-based experiments indicated that Wnt signaling within the osteoblast lineage is a direct determinant of osteoblast differentiation and bone formation although this was not necessarily linked to Lrp5. At the time of writing this chapter there is some unresolved controversy surrounding this point. Yadav et al. [65] undertook mouse genetic experiments in which they sought to identify other mechanisms by which LRP5 might enhance bone formation. This work will be reviewed in other chapters in this book. What prompted these experiments was their finding that osteoblast-specific loss or gain of function of β-catenin did not appear to affect bone formation [61], and importantly, skeletal effects of LRP5 deficiency in mice only appeared postnatally [56]. Their genetic studies identified tryptophan hydroxylase (Tph1), the rate-limiting enzyme for serotonin synthesis, as a downstream target of LRP5 [65]. Furthermore, although they found that Tph1 is produced in osteoblasts, the intestinal epithelium produces it at much higher levels, and its production in the enterochromaffin cells of the duodenum was regulated by LRP5, which prevented the synthesis and release of serotonin as a circulating hormone. Thus mice with LRP5 deleted specifically in the duodenum had high circulating serotonin levels and decreased bone formation, whereas mice with duodenum targeted expression of an HBM LRP5 mutant developed a high bone mass. These genetic findings, together with other pharmacologic evidence [66,67] were all consistent with a view that LRP5 influenced osteoblast differentiation and bone mass indirectly, and that this was mediated through actions upon intestinal serotonin production, rather than a direct effect of LRP5 in osteoblast lineage cells. These findings have been challenged by work [68] reporting that no bone changes occurred in mice in which LRP5 was deleted, or in which HBM LRP5 mutants were expressed, in serotonin-producing cells of intestine. Further, no changes in circulating serotonin levels were observed in these mice, nor did pharmacological inhibition of Tph1 hydroxylase affect bone formation in ovariectomized mice or rats [68].

Thus, even though it is clear that LRP5 has the ability to affect Wnt signaling in given settings as, for instance, the eye, the question of whether it regulates bone mass as such or through its influence on the synthesis and release of gut-derived serotonin remains to be resolved.

Osteocytes

Osteocytes are terminally differentiated osteoblast lineage cells embedded deep in bone. They comprise by far the most abundant cells of bone, and reside within the calcified bone matrix, with their long processes extending through the matrix to form a communication and sensory network with osteoblasts on the bone surface.

Schematic representation of the links between osteocytes and other cells of bone is provided in Fig. 2.1. A favored view has been that at the end of the remodeling sequence, when matrix synthesis is no longer required, osteoblasts lose their synthetic capacity and either become bone lining cells or become trapped within the bone matrix, becoming embedded in bone as osteocytes.

Osteocytes within individual lacunae communicate with each other and with surface osteoblasts or lining cells by an extensive system of cell microprocesses within canaliculi throughout the bone matrix. Bonewald [69] has summarized evidence suggesting that osteocyte formation is not simply a passive process, but is an active one beginning with embedding of the cells in osteoid, and continuing with the development of dendritic processes into canaliculi under the influence of molecules such as MT1-MMP/MMP-14 [70] and E11/gp38 [71]. As the osteocyte matures, alkaline phosphatase production is decreased, and a number of osteocyte markers appear, including matrix extracellular phosphoglycoprotein (MEPE), dentin matrix protein-1 (DMP-1), fibroblast growth factor 23 (FGF-23) and sclerostin [69].

Osteocyte-derived Sclerostin

Osteocytes have long been thought to function as sensors of pressure changes and microdamage, but only recently have new approaches allowed studies of osteocyte function, largely as a result of discoveries of mutations in genes associated with either osteoporosis or high bone mass syndromes. Indeed, ideas of the control of bone formation have been significantly revised following the discovery of sclerostin, the protein product of the *sost* gene. In bone, it is produced primarily by osteocytes and powerfully inhibits bone formation through inhibition of Wnt signaling (see above), sparking great interest in roles for the osteocyte in bone modeling and remodeling. Sclerostin null mice have very high bone mass, and conversely, severe osteopenia occurs in transgenic mice overexpressing sclerostin in osteocytes [72]. Human *Sost* mutations cause the greatly increased bone mass of sclerosteosis and van Buchem disease [73,74]. Recently, sclerostin antibodies have been shown to stimulate bone formation in rodent models of osteoporosis [75] colitis-induced bone loss [76]. Early clinical trials have also shown that a single injection of anti-sclerostin increased serum markers of bone formation, inhibited markers of bone resorption, and improved bone mass [77]. Physiologically, rapid changes in sclerostin could signal to limit the filling of remodeling spaces by osteoblasts, in addition to maintaining the quiescent state of lining cells on non-remodeling bone surfaces [78].

Sclerostin and Bone Formation

Production of sclerostin by osteocytes *in vivo* and *in vitro* is rapidly decreased by treatment with PTH or PTHrP [79] and by a number of locally acting cytokines that stimulate bone formation, including oncostatin M, cardiotrophin-1 and LIF [52], by prostaglandin E2 [80] and by a hypoxic state [81]. Use of a late osteoblast/ osteocyte-specific cre recombinase to genetically ablate the common receptor for both PTH and PTHR1 resulted in a higher than usual level of sclerostin expression, and ablated the sclerostin response to PTH treatment [82]. Conversely, transgenic mice expressing constitutively active PTHR1 in osteocytes demonstrated a much lower level of sclerostin expression [83].

Mechanical forces experienced by the skeleton, whether through exercise or experimental loading, induce bone formation [84,85]. Cyclical experimental loading dramatically decreased sclerostin mRNA levels, and profoundly decreased the number of sclerostin positive osteocytes in cortical bone 24 hours after mechanical loading [86]. This effect was more pronounced in regions under most strain, and of highest bone formation levels [86]. More recent work established that osteocytes within remodeling trabecular bone also respond to loading with a reduction in sclerostin expression and increase in bone mass in this region [87]. This, and the inhibition of LRP5 signaling by sclerostin, is consistent with earlier data showing an impaired bone formation response to experimental loading in LRP5-deficient mice [85].

While mechanical loading increases bone formation, a lack of mechanical forces due to disuse results in bone loss, in part due to reduced bone formation. This may also involve modification of sclerostin expression. Sclerostin positive osteocytes were significantly increased with sciatic neurectomy, a mouse model of experimental paralysis [87]. In contrast to the region-specific reduction in sclerostin induced by mechanical loading, this effect of disuse on sclerostin expression was uniform throughout the unloaded bone [87]. In murine tail-suspension models of disuse, sclerostin mRNA levels were significantly increased, but this was not detected at the protein level [86,88]. Although circulating sclerostin levels may not reflect only osteocytic changes in sclerostin, serum sclerostin levels were significantly greater in postmenopausal women immobilized by stroke than in a cohort of mobile postmenopausal women [89], consistent with increased osteocytic sclerostin in murine models of disuse. Sclerostin appears to be absolutely required for the bone loss associated with disuse, since sclerostin-null mice demonstrated no bone loss or reduction in bone formation in a tail-suspension model [90], and anti-sclerostin treatment overcame the bone loss associated with tail suspension in rats [91].

Inhibition of sclerostin by mechanical loading provides a mechanism for the much older hypothesis that osteocytes, by virtue of their position within the bone matrix, are well situated to respond to mechanical forces and act as signal transducers to bone-forming osteoblasts on the bone surface. In vitro work also supports this model. In a rat osteosarcoma cell line that expresses high levels of sclerostin (UMR106.01), oscillatory fluid flow, mimicking cyclic bone loading, transiently reduced sclerostin mRNA and protein levels [92]. Reduced sclerostin secretion by osteocytes into the lacuna–canalicular system in loaded bone might release osteoblasts from a sclerostin-imposed tonic inhibition, thereby allowing increased bone formation at sites of highest strain. The mechanism by which sclerostin is targeted to particular sites through the extensive, and multidirectional, lacuna–canalicular system remains obscure. So, too, does the mechanism by which sclerostin is inhibited by mechanical stimulation; this may relate to an influence of paracrine factors such as prostaglandins, nitric oxide, or oncostatin M, all of which rapidly decrease sclerostin expression (see above), and are rapidly modified in response to mechanical stimulation [93–95] (see below).

Sclerostin, Osteocytic Osteolysis and Bone Resorption

Long before the development of the methods in bone cell biology that began only around the end of the 1970s, osteocytes were the subject of much attention from a number of workers, using microradiography, light microscopy, and transmission or electron microscopy. They were considered to be mechanosensory cells, but the concept was also developed of "osteocytic osteolysis." This described a concomitant loss of mineral and organic constituents around osteocytic lacunae, an effect enhanced by parathyroid extract and other agents that promote bone resorption [96–99]. It was argued that osteocytes must be involved in this process, because there were too few osteoclasts, working too slowly, to explain the rapid rise in blood calcium following PTH. The argument for this was advocated especially by Belanger [98], and was the subject of some controversy for a number of years, for example with Boyde [100] strongly opposed, pointing out the acute role of renal conservation in PTH action, as well as the rapid response of osteoclasts to PTH [101]. Decline in support for the idea of osteocytic osteolyis seems to date from a review by Parfitt [102] in which he argued that the mean size of osteocytic lacunae had probably been misinterpreted as evidence of osteocytic osteolysis. The finding that in some circumstances osteocytes also express markers of osteoclasts, particularly acid phosphatase and cathepsin K, e.g. in lactation, gives impetus to the revival of the osteocytic osteolysis concept, including its hormonal control [103,104].

Whatever the outcome of this renewed interest in osteocytic osteolysis as a means by which osteocytes directly influence bone dissolution, there is now very interesting evidence implicating them in bone resorption through RANKL production. It was found in genetically manipulated mice that osteocytes are an abundant source of RANKL [105,106], and indeed were claimed to be the major source of RANKL within the osteoblast lineage [106]. No study was carried out in these papers to explain how osteocyte-derived RANKL could be presented to hemopoietic precursors to promote their differentiation to osteoclasts. It is conceivable that shed RANKL could be generated and pass through the osteocytic canaliculae, but as discussed earlier, there is yet no evidence *in vivo* for the generation of active, shed RANKL. It is also possible that RANKL may be expressed on the surface of osteocyte-derived apoptotic bodies [107]. These findings will be discussed further below with regard to remodeling.

OSTEOCLASTS

The only cell capable of resorbing bone is the osteoclast, named "ostoklast" by Kolliker [108], when he observed these multinucleated cells on bone surfaces and suggested that they were responsible for bone resorption. They became recognized for their unique ultrastructural characteristics which both distinguished them from other cell types and enabled them to be motile and thereby able to efficiently resorb bone [101,109]. Apart from their multinuclearity, a striking feature of the osteoclast is the presence of the "ruffled border," a complex structure of deeply interfolded finger-like projections of the plasma and cytoplasmic membranes adjacent to the bone surface, through which bone-resorbing acids and enzymes are secreted [110–112]. Adjacent to and surrounding the ruffled border is an area of cytoplasm devoid of cellular organelles except for numerous contractile cytoplasmic actin filaments. This is known as the "sealing zone," since the plasma membrane in this region comes into very close apposition with the bone surface to ensure osteoclast attachment via integrins, and to separate the bone-resorbing area beneath the ruffled border from the unresorbed area, thus maintaining a favorable microenvironment for bone resorption. Osteoclasts degrade bone mineral by creating an acid microcompartment under the ruffled border, adjacent to the bone surface [111].

In cellular development, progenitor cells are capable of proliferation but not self-maintenance, and have restricted differentiation capacities, often committing to a single line of differentiation. Osteoclast progenitors are promonocytes or monoblasts, with no readily recognizable characteristics yet identified; they do not express acid phosphatase activity *in vivo* and are very sensitive to irradiation [113]. Osteoclast precursors, or pre-osteoclasts, are mononucleated, post-mitotic cells which may be separated on the basis of enzyme activity into early precursors, which do not express tartrate-resistant acid phosphatase (TRAP), and late precursors, which are TRAP positive [114]. Pre-osteoclasts, alone among the monocyte/macrophage series, also possess increasing numbers of calcitonin receptors (CTR) [115]. In the final step, multinucleated osteoclasts are generated by fusion of mononucleated pre-osteoclasts, fusing either with one another or with existing osteoclasts.

The rich expression of TRAP by osteoclasts provides a convenient marker for *in vitro* generated cells, and this is definitive when combined with multinuclearity, expression of CTRs, and the ability to form resorption pits when grown on thin slices of cortical bone or dentine. Some other properties include possession of vitronectin receptors, cathepsin K, vacuolar ATP-ase, and chloride-7 channels. This combination of properties provides the phenotype that equips osteoclasts uniquely to resorb bone.

Origin of Osteoclasts

Early ideas of osteoclast ontogeny came from autoradiographic evidence of Tonna [116] that they arise from fusion of osteoblasts and can dissociate again into osteogenic precursor cells. Young [117] believed that osteoclasts and osteoblasts originated from a common osteoprogenitor cell, and at a later stage may return to the osteoprogenitor pool. In 1974, Rasmussen and Bordier [118] proposed that endosteal mesenchymal cells differentiate into pre-osteoclasts which may then form an osteoclast by fusion. At a certain time and place the osteoclast then dissociates into pre-osteoblasts, giving rise to osteoblasts and osteocytes. These views of a connective tissue cell origin of osteoclasts were subsequently superseded in the face of compelling evidence for a hemopoietic origin of osteoclasts.

Studies using a variety of model systems including quail-chick chimera experiments, parabiosis experiments, and the restoration of bone resorption in osteopetrosis by bone marrow and spleen cell transplantation showed that osteoclasts are supplied to bone via the circulatory system, and are formed by fusion of mononucleated precursors derived from hemopoietic progenitor cells [119,120]. The important finding common to these experiments was that the precursors of the osteoclast could travel via the blood to an area where osteoclasts were needed, whereas osteoblasts were considered to be recruited from local precursors. This suggested that local precursors could not differentiate into osteoclasts and consequently that the lineages of osteoblasts and osteoclasts are different [120]. Since bone marrow is diverse and contains stromal cells in addition to hemopoietic cells, the above experiments did not show definitively that the osteoclast is derived from the hemopoietic stem cell. Nevertheless, the accumulated evidence strongly suggested that the osteoclast is derived from the fusion of mononucleated precursors of hemopoietic origin.

Osteoclast Development

The lifespan of multinucleated osteoclasts *in vivo* appears to be up to 2 weeks, with a half-life of around 6 to 10 days [121], indicating a need for their continual replenishment to maintain bone resorption. Osteoclast formation is a multistep process involving proliferation and recruitment of osteoclast progenitor cells, differentiation of these progenitors and fusion of mononucleated osteoclast precursors to form multinucleated, mature osteoclasts. This process involves many hormones and cytokines. Since osteoclasts are ultimately derived from hemopoietic stem cells, it is not surprising that the colony-stimulating factors and cytokines known to promote and coordinate hemopoietic progenitor cell proliferation and differentiation also play a very important role in the formation and/or activation of osteoclasts.

Shortly after the development of techniques for culturing bone cells, the observations that isolated osteoblasts of various origins responded to bone-resorbing hormones, and the lack of evidence for receptors or direct responses to these hormones in osteoclasts, led to the concept that bone-resorbing factors must act first on osteoblast lineage cells, most likely bone lining cells. This action was proposed to release factors that influence the formation and bone-resorbing activity of osteoclasts [122,123]. The same hypothesis developed from the argument that since the osteoclast derives from a "wandering" cell supplied by the circulation, it made sense to have its activity programmed by an authentic resident bone cell, i.e. the osteoblast [124]. This was the first time that any concept had emerged that suggested there might be communication among the cells of bone—perhaps this is when bone joined the community of cell biology? The first direct evidence in support of this came when osteoclasts were isolated from newborn rat or mouse bone; to resorb bone, the presence of contaminating osteoblastic cells was required [125].

Work over the next few years established the concept of an osteoblast-derived stimulus of osteoclast-mediated resorption [126–128]. Among the questions raised were whether there exists a single stromal/osteoblastic cell factor responsible for osteoclast activation, and if so, whether it is cell associated or secreted. Would the formation of osteoclasts be at least as important as regulation of their activity? The next real advances came with the development of new methods to study osteoclast formation *in vitro*.

Several *in vitro* systems provided strong evidence that accessory cells are necessary for the generation of osteoclasts from hemopoietic precursors. Burger et al. [113] used a co-culture system in which hemopoietic cells from embryonic mouse liver were co-cultured with fetal long bone rudiments from which the periosteum had been stripped, to show that accompanying cells from the bone are required for osteoclast development. However, it was the development of murine bone marrow cultures and reproducible assays of osteoclast formation that led to major advances [129,130], showing that treatment with bone resorbing agents could promote osteoclast formation in a dose-dependent manner. In the course of these studies, Takahashi [129] noted consistently that more than 90% of the TRAP-positive mononucleated cell clusters and multinucleated cells formed in mouse marrow cultures in response to bone resorbing stimuli were located near colonies of alkaline phosphatase-positive mononucleated cells (possibly osteoblasts). This was a strong indication that osteoblastic lineage cells support osteoclast formation, in addition to the existing evidence of their influence on activity of mature osteoclasts.

The same group then established that osteoclast formation requires a contribution from cells of the osteoblast lineage, and in doing so they provided the concepts and techniques that set the scene for the discovery of osteoclast control by RANKL, RANK, and OPG. When osteoblast-rich cultures from newborn mouse calvariae were co-cultured with mouse spleen cells and treated with $1,25(OH)_2D_3$, osteoclasts were formed. Most importantly, though, direct contact between the two cell types was required for osteoclast formation to occur [131]. Similar results were obtained with the bone marrow-derived stromal cell lines MC3T3-G2/PA6, ST2, and KS-4 [132,133], any of which could be substituted for primary osteoblastic stromal cells in co-cultures with spleen cells, to result in the formation of osteoclast-like cells in the presence of $1,25(OH)_2D_3$.

Regulation of the Pro-osteoclastic Signal from the Osteoblast Lineage

With increasing acceptance of the concept that cells of the osteoblast lineage control osteoclast formation and activity by a contact-dependent mechanism, three distinct signaling mechanisms were all capable of promoting this function. Prostaglandin (PG)-induced osteoclast formation in mouse bone marrow cultures was found to be mediated by a mechanism involving cAMP [126], as were PTH and PTHrP [127], acting through their common receptor. The effect of interleukin-1 (IL-1) resulted from the generation of PGE2 as an intermediate effector [127]. A second signaling mechanism for regulation was provided by the steroid hormone, 1,25(OH)$_2$D$_3$, combining with its receptor and translocating to the nucleus to influence transcription through a vitamin D responsive element in target genes [134]. Finally, a membrane-bound receptor complex involving a 130 kDa glycoprotein (gp130) [128] provided for osteoclast formation under the influence of the group of cytokines that use this signaling mechanism. In mouse co-cultures, simultaneous treatment with IL-6 and its soluble receptor (sIL-6R) induced osteoclast formation, but when added separately they were ineffective. The other cytokines in this group, IL-11, leukemia inhibitory factor (LIF), and oncostatin M (OSM), all of which use gp130 as a common transducer, also stimulated osteoclast formation. In later experiments using cells from IL-6R-overexpressing transgenic mice in crossover co-cultures with cells from wild-type mice, expression of IL-6R by osteoblast lineage cells was shown to be indispensable for the induction of osteoclasts [135]. This clear demonstration that IL-6 stimulation of osteoclast formation required the cytokine to act upon the osteoblast, despite the fact that osteoclasts possessed its receptor [136], illustrated the power of *ex vivo* experimentation with cells from genetically modified animals to study osteoclast formation, an approach which has proved itself repeatedly since that time.

Despite the three main classes of initial signaling mechanisms, it seemed that a common downstream pathway was a membrane-bound stromal factor [130]. It was assumed that these agents must converge at some stage before finally generating this crucial membrane factor [137]. Of the many multifunctional cytokines that had some role in osteoclast formation, none fulfilled the requirements for such a factor. This included M-CSF which, despite its essential role in stimulating both proliferation and differentiation of osteoclast progenitors, inhibited the bone resorbing activity of isolated osteoclasts.

The discovery of osteoprotegerin (OPG), a soluble member of the TNF receptor superfamily, revealed it as a powerful inhibitor of osteoclast formation [138,139]. This provided the means of identifying and cloning the elusive osteoclastogenic factor, which proved to be a TNF ligand family member that came to be called receptor activator of nuclear factor κB ligand (RANKL), the common factor mediating osteoclast formation in response to all known stimuli [140,141]. Osteoblasts/stromal cells are also the source of M-CSF, which plays a crucial role in osteoclast formation by promoting precursor proliferation. As a membrane protein, RANKL fulfilled earlier predictions that osteoclast differentiation required contact-dependent activation of hemopoietic precursors. This communication with the hemopoietic lineage results from RANKL

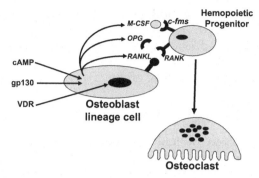

FIGURE 2.2 **Regulation of osteoclast formation by cells of the osteoblast lineage.** RANKL and M-CSF are required as products of the osteoblast lineage to promote osteoclast formation from hemopoietic precursors. OPG is the decoy receptor for RANKL in its interaction with receptor, RANK (see text).

binding to its receptor, RANK, on osteoclast precursors, thereby initiating signaling essential for osteoclast differentiation. Figure 2.2 summarizes these control mechanisms, illustrating the regulated production of RANKL required for osteoclast formation and maintenance of activity. The bone-resorbing cytokines and hormones, with disparate signaling mechanisms, converge in promoting RANKL production, with the decoy receptor OPG having an essential physiological role as a paracrine inhibitor of osteoclast formation that is produced by the osteoblast lineage and binds RANKL to limit its activation of osteoclast formation through its receptor, RANK.

All of these discoveries have been validated by studies in genetically altered mice, establishing clearly the essential physiological role of these TNF ligand and receptor family members in controlling osteoclast formation and activity. First, transgenic overexpression of OPG in mice results in osteopetrosis because of failure to form osteoclasts [138]. Genetic ablation of OPG, on the other hand, leads to severe high turnover osteoporosis [142]. Results of *ex vivo* studies of bone organ cultures and cells from the latter animals were consistent with the concept of OPG being constantly produced, and acting physiologically as a paracrine "brake" on RANKL action, with its production varied under the influence of local and hormonal factors [143]. Removal of the stimulatory pathway by genetic ablation of RANKL also resulted in osteopetrosis since RANKL is necessary for normal osteoclast formation [144]. Finally, genetic ablation of RANK also leads to osteopetrosis [145]. Because this signaling pathway also functions in immune cells, RANK null mice have severe abnormalities in that system, reflecting an intriguing link with the immune system, which was evident very early in the discovery process [146,147]. Furthermore, production of soluble RANKL by activated T cells *in vitro* directly stimulated osteoclast formation [148].

Physiological control of bone resorption is thus dependent on the functions of RANKL to promote osteoclast formation, survival, and activity [149]. The concepts resulting from these discoveries are summarized in Fig. 2.2. By treating with RANKL and M-CSF it became possible to generate osteoclasts in relatively large numbers without the need for stromal/osteoblastic precursors, including the generation of human osteoclasts from peripheral blood [150,151]. As predicted, osteotropic hormones and cytokines, including $1,25(OH)_2D_3$, IL-11, PTH, and PGE_2, stimulated RANKL production by the osteoblast lineage, thereby triggering osteoclast development, and the same treatments reduced production of the RANKL decoy receptor, OPG [152,153]. The functions of RANKL extend to pathological states of increased bone resorption, where increased local RANKL production contributes to osteoclast-mediated bone destruction in disease states such as breast cancer metastases to bone [154], rheumatoid arthritis [148,152], multiple myeloma [155], and osteoporosis [156]. The firm view took hold that RANKL–RANK signaling required a contact-dependent process in exerting its physiological function as the essential regulator of osteoclast formation [157–159].

While the prevailing concept is that physiological generation of osteoclasts requires direct contact between the participating cells, there is in vitro evidence that extracellular RANKL can be cleaved to a soluble form by certain enzymes [160]. These include the metalloproteinase TNF-alpha convertase (TACE) [161], MMP14 [162], and a disintegrin and metalloproteinase (ADAM) 10 [163]. It would be important to know whether there are circumstances in physiological osteoclastogenesis in which free RANKL becomes available. This will be discussed further below, with respect to the formation of osteoclasts in bone remodeling, and especially in light of the finding that isolated osteocytes produce copious amounts of RANKL [105,106]. It seems likely therefore that free RANKL would be generated in certain pathological states where proteases are abundant, for example in the inflammatory states of rheumatoid arthritis and periodontal bone disease where activated T cells produce abundant RANKL[146,148] while abundant MMP14 is produced in the rheumatoid synovium [164]. In addition free RANKL may be generated in metastatic bone disease. Prostate cancer cells were found to process RANKL to a soluble form that promoted osteoclast formation [162], and RANKL was shed by the action of tumor-derived MT1-MMP on LNCaP prostate cancer cells implanted intratibially in immune-deficient mice [165]. In a model of breast cancer metastasis to bone, osteoclast-derived cathepsin G at the tumor–bone interface appeared to initiate

shedding of free RANKL [166]. Further in vivo evidence was obtained in orchiectomized rats, in which free RANKL was increased several-fold in marrow and MMP-14 was involved as the responsible sheddase enzyme [167]. The role of shedding in RANKL action needs close attention, particularly to address the question of shedding in normal physiology, and how this process may make RANKL available to osteoclast precursors not immediately apposed to the RANKL-producing cells.

BONE REMODELING

The changes taking place in bone shape during skeletal growth are determined by bone modeling, which takes place from the beginning of skeletogenesis during fetal life until the end of the second decade when the longitudinal growth of the skeleton is completed. In the bone remodeling that occurs throughout life, small packets of bone are resorbed by osteoclasts, followed by the recruitment of osteoblast precursors that differentiate to replace the amount of removed bone. Modeling differs from remodeling in that bone is formed at sites that have not undergone prior resorption, thus resulting in a change in the shape or macroarchitecture of the bone. Modeling determines the size and shape of bone, such as the simultaneous widening of long bones and development of medullary cavity by bone formation at the periosteal surface and resorption at the endosteal surface, respectively.

The remodeling process takes place asynchronously throughout the skeleton at anatomically distinct sites termed basic multicellular units (BMUs). The resorption activity in a BMU in adult human bone takes approximately 3 weeks and the formation response 3 to 4 months. The process is such that remodeling replaces about 5–10% of the skeleton each year, with the entire adult human skeleton replaced in 10 years. This process is an integral part of the calcium homeostatic system and provides a crucial mechanism for adaptation to physical stress, the removal of old bone, and the repair of damaged bone. It is thus central to the maintenance of the mechanical integrity of the skeleton and the repair of damaged bone [168–171].

In order to maintain the mass of bone, remodeling must achieve a balance in which the resorbed bone at each BMU is fully replaced. This requirement that resorption is followed by an equal amount of formation has come to be known as "coupling." However, the effects of growth and ageing during life, including changes in mechanical stress, mean that this theory of equal bone replacement often does not hold true. During growth there is a positive balance, with the amount of bone replaced at individual BMUs exceeding that lost

[169] and with ageing a negative balance at individual BMUs results in gradual bone loss [172], accelerating over the years of the menopause that are associated with a net bone loss.

It was considered for many years that bone remodeling is controlled primarily by the actions upon bone of circulating hormones, such as PTH, 1,25(OH)$_2$ vitamin D$_3$, and sex steroids. Discoveries of the last two decades have revealed that locally generated cytokines are the key influences, influencing bone cell communication and subsequent function in complex ways, and often are themselves regulated by the hormones. Next we aim to discuss remodeling briefly in a way that might best be related to the many influences on remodeling that will be described in other chapters that introduce even more recently discovered influences external to bone, such as leptin, the sympathetic and central nervous systems, neuropeptide Y, and serotonin, which in their actions extend the repertoires of communicating roles of locally generated cytokines.

Activation of Remodeling in the BMU

The first essential step in the remodeling cycle is the generation of active osteoclasts from hemopoietic precursors. Regardless of the source of the initiation signal, osteoclasts are likely derived from early and late precursors available in marrow adjacent to activation sites, or could be recruited from blood at the bone interface through a sinus structure of bone remodeling compartments (BRCs) [173]. This concept has been extended to provide a mechanism by which mesenchymal and hemopoietic stem cells that can become either osteoblasts or osteoclasts circulate and so may arrive at the BRC via capillaries penetrating the canopy that overlies the BRC [174–176]. As mentioned above, osteoblast progenitors may reside as pericytes associated with vascular structures in the marrow, with several studies suggesting that common progenitors may give rise to cells forming the blood vessel and multipotent perivascular cells [21,23,177,178]. Osteoclast formation can take place rapidly *in vivo*, and it is appealing to consider that this might be made possible by niches of partially differentiated cells available in the BRC [179]. Only recently evidence was obtained for this possibility, with the discovery of the "osteoclast niche"—cell cycle-arrested quiescent osteoclast precursors (QuOPs) that are RANK and c-fms positive that can be detected along bone surfaces near to osteoblasts [180]. QuOPs are capable of rapid differentiation into osteoclasts. In addition to providing a potential source of osteoclasts for the rapid initiation of the remodeling sequence, their existence might explain why injection of PTH *in vivo* can induce active osteoclasts in less

than 30 minutes [101]. Figure 2.3 illustrates events taking place in the BMU, with resorption of a certain amount of bone taking place, and followed by recruitment of osteoblast precursors to differentiate and replace the lost bone.

Cancellous bone remodeling starts on the bone surface, initiated by any of several possible stimuli. Among these are pressure changes sensed by osteocytes resulting in signals delivered to surface cells, damage in the form of microcracks in bone that lead to osteocyte stimulation or even apoptosis, and the release of signals from other nearby bone cells which may include known cytokines and prostanoids. Chemoattractants for osteoclast precursors may include factors from the bone matrix itself [181], factors produced by cells of the osteoblast lineage [182], or signals from apoptotic osteocytes. Osteoclasts are formed by the attraction of hematopoietic myelomonocytic precursors to the resorption site, followed by their fusion, and attachment of the subsequent multinucleated cell to the bone surface. Earlier in this chapter the role of osteocyte-derived sclerostin in bone formation was discussed. There is increasing evidence that osteocyte-derived signals can contribute to the recruitment and formation of osteoclasts [183–185]. When the dentin matrix protein-1 (DMP-1) promoter was used to generate mice expressing diphtheria toxin (DT) receptor specifically in osteocytes, and DT was used to kill the osteocytes [88], increased RANKL mRNA was detected in bones shortly after osteocyte killing. This was associated with increased osteoclast formation and bone resorption, supporting the idea that viable osteocytes prevent osteoclast recruitment and activation, whereas the reverse accompanies osteocyte death. The idea of osteocyte regulation of resorption is strengthened further by the evidence that osteocytes are an abundant and necessary source of RANKL production [105,106] (see above), a discovery which needs to be extended to help us understand how osteocyte-derived RANKL is regulated and presented to osteoclast precursors.

Cessation of Resorption in the BMU

Once a BMU is activated, resorption within that site must be limited. If it were to continue unchecked, resorption would be excessive. A novel aspect of signaling in osteoclast development that could be relevant to the control of osteoclasts in the BMU is the ability of RANKL to limit its own osteoclastogenic effect by promoting interferon-β (IFN-β) production by monocytic osteoclast precursors [186]. This inhibits osteoclast formation by preventing RANKL-induced expression of c-fos, an essential transcription factor in osteoclast differentiation, identified by the

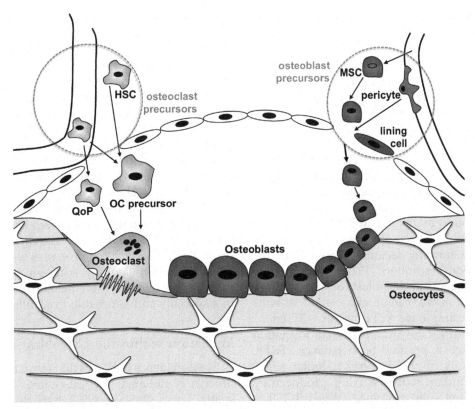

FIGURE 2.3   Cellular events in the BMU. Under the canopy generated by bone lining cells, osteoclasts are formed from hemopoietic precursors supplied from marrow and the bloodstream, and from partially differentiated osteoclasts termed quiescent osteoclast precursors (QoP). On the right side of the diagram, precursors of osteoblasts come from mesenchymal stem cells in the marrow, from blood, and from pericytes, and differentiate within the BMU through the osteoblast precursor stage to fully functional synthesizing osteoblasts; lining cells may also differentiate into active osteoblasts. Osteocytes communicate with the surface cells, particularly osteoblasts, through their canaliculae.

osteopetrosis of c-*fos*-null mice due to failed osteoclast formation [187]. RANKL-induced IFN-β provides an appealing mechanism to control osteoclast differentiation, since it would be contained within the osteoclast itself and would regulate osteoclast formation within the BMU. A further possible mechanism of osteoclast restraint within the BMU might come from reverse signaling through osteoblast-derived EphB4 acting on ephrinB2 in the osteoclast to restrict osteoclast formation [188].

How do the osteoclasts know when to stop resorbing within the BMU? Cell death is a likely determinant, but its regulation *in vivo* remains obscure. There are some candidate regulators of the process, including matrix-derived TGFβ [189], and estrogen enhancing osteoclast apoptosis through the mediation of Fas ligand [190]. Some insights into control of apoptosis arise from genetic and pharmacological studies showing that inhibition of acidification of the resorption space by blockade of either ClC-7 or the V-type H+ATPase of the osteoclast results in prolonged osteoclast survival [191,192]. This might suggest a role for acidification in determining

osteoclast lifespan, perhaps even through TGFβ activation. In determining how resorption ends in the BMU, focus on regulation of osteoclast apoptosis in that microenvironment could be helpful.

The Reversal Phase

In the "reversal" phase of remodeling, when resorption pits are prepared for the engagement of osteoblast precursors in bone formation, mesenchymal cells may be responsible for the enzymatic activity, most likely metalloproteinases, that degrades accumulated collagen fragments on the bone surface [193,194]. They then go on to lay down a thin layer of collagen along the Howship's lacuna, closely associated with a cement line, an RGD-containing extracellular matrix protein containing abundant osteopontin [195] which interacts with integrin receptors $\alpha_v\beta_3$ in osteoclasts and primarily $\alpha_v\beta_5$ in osteoblasts. These integrin receptors were shown not only to mediate cell attachment of both cell types to the bone matrix, but also to act as signal transducing receptors [196]. It is not yet fully established what influence osteopontin has on osteoclast or osteoblast activity but it appears to be required for a normal response of bone to mechanical unloading.

COUPLING OF BONE FORMATION TO RESORPTION IN THE BMU

Growth Factor Mediation

The coupling of osteoblast-mediated bone formation to bone resorption depends on understanding how osteoblast lineage cells, forming bone within the BMU during balanced bone remodeling, replace almost precisely the amount of bone that was resorbed. A favored hypothesis has been that this "coupling" is regulated by bone forming factors released from the matrix during bone resorption [197]. Indeed, many growth factors mitogenic to osteoblasts or which stimulate bone formation *in vivo* can be extracted from bone matrix [198]. The example we will consider is TGFβ.

BMPs injected into bone stimulate bone formation locally and produce a positive bone balance. TGFβ, from the same family of proteins, has a similar effect, and bone is an abundant source of TGFβ, produced by all osteoblast lineage cells examined. When TGFβ is injected next to the periosteum or endosteum, local bone formation is substantially augmented in rats and other species [199,200]. At the same time, endocortical resorption is increased; thus TGFβ seems to stimulate both resorption and formation; however, the local balance is clearly positive. It was proposed that TGFβ, which is produced as an inactive precursor in bone and is present in the matrix, can be activated by acidification or proteolytic cleavage by resorbing osteoclasts [201]. TGFβ may also be released from latent complexes at appropriate sites in the matrix by plasmin generated locally by plasminogen activators, in a manner controlled temporally and spatially by hormones and cytokines [202]. It remains to be established to what extent growth factors can survive the proteolytic cleavage of the acidic hydrolases present in resorption lacunae. Evidence from mouse genetics suggests that active TGFβ1 released during bone resorption might couple bone formation to resorption by inducing the migration of bone mesenchymal stem cells to sites that have been resorbed, thus making them available for differentiation and bone formation in remodeling [203]. This would provide an attractive explanation for the concept that in remodeling, osteoblasts are recruited from a pool of stem cells, and need to be attracted to remodeling sites to be differentiated and replenish the osteoblast population. Consistent with this idea, when bone resorption was inhibited with a bisphosphonate, so too was the release of active TGFβ, and the recruitment of Sca-1+ve stem cells to remodeling sites [204];

this was associated with decreased bone formation. It remains difficult to see how tight quantitative control of the amount of active TGFβ can be exercised if it depends solely on the acid pH at resorption sites. It may be that the necessary quantitative control is left to the next stage—influences upon the stem cells when they reach the remodeling site. Furthermore, while an action of TGFβ to promote stem cell migration to appropriate sites is plausible, such an effect might contribute to the overall process by which bone formation follows upon bone resorption. It fits less easily as a mechanism applied to rapid changes in bone remodeling.

This model of coupling in the BMU by growth factor release from the matrix raises a number of questions that relate to the time course and the distance between the resorption and formation processes and whether activation can be controlled with sufficient precision to ensure that they are released from the matrix in active form and in a spatially and temporally controlled manner.

Mediation within the Osteoblast Lineage

Some evidence indicates that once the bone formation process is initiated, the osteoblasts themselves sense spatial limits [205], perhaps through paracrine mediators or gap junction communication among the osteoblasts themselves [206]. The ability of cells to respond to topography would not be unique to osteoblasts. Osteoblast precursors have been shown to respond to changes in surface topography, whether the change is larger or smaller than the cell itself [207]. Altered nanotopography induces formation of osteoblast filipodia, important for topographical sensing, followed by cytoskeletal changes involving cell adhesion and differentiation as well as altered expression of osteocalcin and osteopontin. Regulation could also be provided by osteocytes, most notably by the production of sclerostin. Physiologically, rapid changes in osteocyte production of sclerostin could signal to surface cells to limit the filling of remodeling spaces by osteoblasts, in addition to keeping lining cells in a quiescent state on nonremodeling bone surfaces [78], as discussed above.

Another possible local control mechanism within the osteoblast lineage comes with the finding that PTH and PTHrP promote production by osteoblast lineage cells of ephrinB2 which acts through its receptor, EphB4, to promote osteoblast differentiation and bone formation within the BMU [208]. Ephrin/Eph family members are recognized as local mediators of cell function and tissue remodeling in a diverse range of cells through contact-dependent processes in development and in maturity [209,210]. Some evidence suggests that osteoclast-derived ephrinB2 acts through a contact-dependent mechanism on EphB4 in osteoblasts, to promote osteoblast differentiation and bone formation, and that through reverse signaling, osteoblast-derived EphB4 acts upon ephrinB2 in osteoclasts to suppress osteoclast formation [188]. The latter mechanism would require osteoblast—osteoclast contact, with evidence for the proximity of EphB4-positive osteoblast precursors to osteoclasts being provided by De Freitas et al. [211]. In the same work ephrinB2-positive osteoblasts were close to bone formation sites, with the overall conclusion that the ephrin/Eph signaling pathway could function both within the osteoblast lineage to favor formation of bone [208], and between osteoblast and osteoclast to limit resorption [188]. These mechanisms warrant further study since pharmacological manipulation of ephrinB2/EphB4 signaling might be an attractive means of regulating the volumes of bone formed in the BMU.

Can Osteoclasts Generate Bone-forming Activities?

Observations made in genetically manipulated mice and human genetics suggest that the osteoclast itself could also be the source of an activity that contributes to the fine control of osteoblast function in bone remodeling. In individuals with the osteopetrotic syndrome, ADOII, due to inactivating mutations in the chloride-7 channel (ClC-7), bone resorption is deficient because of failure of osteoclast acidification. Bone formation in these patients is nevertheless normal, rather than diminished as might be expected because of the greatly impaired resorption [212]. Furthermore, in mice deficient in c-src [213,214], cathepsin K [215], or tyrosine phosphatase epsilon [216], bone resorption is inhibited without inhibition of formation, and v-ATPase V0 subunit D2-deficient mice exhibit failure of fusion of osteoclast precursors accompanied by increased bone formation [217]. In these knockout mice while resorption is greatly reduced osteoclast numbers are not; in some, osteoclast numbers are increased because of reduced osteoclast apoptosis. A possible explanation for the normal level of bone formation in these mice is that these osteoclasts, although unable to resorb bone, are nevertheless capable of generating a factor (or factors) contributing to bone formation. On the other hand, mice lacking c-fos, which are unable to generate osteoclasts, have reduced bone formation as well as resorption [187]. Studies with other mutant mice, with specific inactivation of each of the two alternative signaling pathways through gp130, led to the conclusion that that resorption alone was insufficient to promote the coupled bone formation, but active osteoclasts are the likely source [218,219].

Several osteoclast-derived factors are candidate "coupling factors," one possibility being cardiotropin-1 (CT-1), a member of the family of cytokines that signal through the gp130 transducer that is expressed in differentiated osteoclasts but not in the osteoblast lineage [51]. As well as indirectly stimulating osteoclast differentiation through stimulation of RANKL production, CT-1, like LIF and IL-11[220,221], powerfully stimulates bone formation using a mechanism that begins with rapidly increased expression of the C/EBPδ transcription factor [51]. Intriguingly, CT-1, like oncostatin M, LIF, and PTH, also profoundly decreases sclerostin mRNA expression by osteocytes [52], thus introducing the concept that osteoclasts might communicate with the osteoblast lineage by signaling directly to osteocytes. CT-1 may be a coupling factor that signals from the osteoclast to the osteoblast in more than one way to promote bone formation and contribute to the regulated process of remodeling in the BMU. Some further possibilities arise from in vitro studies suggesting that osteoclast-derived Wnt 10b, BMP6, and sphingosine-1-phosphate produced by osteoclasts can also enhance osteoblast differentiation [222]. The possibility of osteoclast-derived ephrinB2 acting through a contact-dependent mechanism on EphB4 in the osteoblast to promote osteoblast differentiation and bone formation has been discussed above.

BONE AS AN ENDOCRINE ORGAN

The cells of bone communicate among themselves, both within and between lineages, with the matrix they have synthesized, and the vasculature and the immune cells in the marrow. These processes are governed by many locally produced cytokines and growth factors, whose functions in skeletal biology have been revealed in the last few decades by a variety of approaches, beginning with careful structural analyses as a base, and progressing to application of cell biology, pharmacology and genetics, both mouse and human. A remarkable number of bone phenotypes have emerged with genetic manipulation of cytokines and their receptors. These discoveries tell us that skeletal physiology is regulated through the brain and peripheral sympathetic nervous system and, most recently, that the skeleton behaves as an endocrine organ. A number of chapters in this book will review those discoveries and their implications.

Two major osteoblast lineage-derived hormones have been discovered. These are fibroblast growth factor 23 (FGF23) [223], which controls inorganic phosphate metabolism and mineralization, and osteocalcin. Osteocalcin has multiple endocrine targets, affecting energy metabolism by acting upon the pancreatic β-cell to promote insulin release and enhancing insulin responsiveness [224] and promoting testosterone production by actions on the Leydig cell of the testis [225] (see Chapter 11, From Gonads to Bone, and Back). The idea that the skeleton is simply a support for the musculature and a protective casing for marrow immune cells and hemopoietic functions is no longer tenable. Discoveries of the last few years establish the evolutionary importance of the skeleton for survival. Its interactions with muscle and its own internal functions have substantial energy requirements, e.g. the constant, multi-site skeletal remodeling events that take place throughout life. Hence, the development of a bone-based endocrine control system to link bone to energy metabolism is logical. The evolutionary role of the skeleton is further illustrated by the discovery of an osteocalcin contribution to male fertility.

The concept is therefore developed of the skeleton as a ductless gland, producing a hormone, on the one hand in response to environmental influences upon energy requirements, and on the other, to the maintenance of male fertility. Given that the skeleton functions as an endocrine organ, it is important to specify the origin of such hormones: which bone cell, at what stage of differentiation, and in response to what signals? Evidence so far points to the osteoblast lineage, perhaps not surprisingly because these are the only locally residing bone cells. All others are wandering cells (i.e. osteoclasts and bone marrow cells derived from hemopoietic precursors). By the use of the term osteoblast lineage, we do not necessarily mean the bone matrix-producing osteoblast. In the case of FGF23, the osteocyte, the terminally differentiated osteoblast, is the hormone-producing cell. The osteocyte contributes to both bone formation and resorption, and is considered to provide a singularly important system of communication to respond to requirements such as loading. Which cells within the osteoblast lineage produce osteocalcin as a hormone is less clear. The stage of differentiation must be late because that is when osteocalcin is expressed. These all present important questions to be answered, and many will be addressed in accompanying chapters.

Acknowledgments

Work from the authors' laboratories was supported by Project Grants from the National Health and Medical Research Council of Australia, and by the Victorian Government OIS Program.

References

[1] Civitelli R. Cell—cell communication in the osteoblast/osteocyte lineage. Arch Biochem Biophys 2008 May 15;473(2):188—92.

[2] Peck WA, Birge Jr SJ, Fedak SA. Bone cells: biochemical and biological studies after enzymatic isolation. Science 1964 Dec 11;146:1476—7.

[3] Luben RA, Wong GL, Cohn DV. Biochemical characterization with parathormone and calcitonin of isolated bone cells: provisional identification of osteoclasts and osteoblasts. Endocrinology 1976 Aug;99(2):526—34.

[4] Partridge NC, Alcorn D, Michelangeli VP, Ryan G, Martin TJ. Morphological and biochemical characterization of four clonal osteogenic sarcoma cell lines of rat origin. Cancer Res 1983 Sep;43(9):4308—14.

[5] Majeska RJ, Rodan SB, Rodan GA. Parathyroid hormone-responsive clonal cell lines from rat osteosarcoma. Endocrinology 1980 Nov;107(5):1494—503.

[6] Crawford A, Atkins D, Martin TJ. Rat osteogenic sarcoma cells: comparison of the effects of prostaglandins E1, E2, I2 (prostacyclin), 6-keto F1alpha and thromboxane B2 on cyclic AMP production and adenylate cyclase activity. Biochem Biophys Res Commun 1978 Jun 29;82(4):1195—201.

[7] Partridge NC, Alcorn D, Michelangeli VP, Kemp BE, Ryan GB, Martin TJ. Functional properties of hormonally responsive cultured normal and malignant rat osteoblastic cells. Endocrinology 1981 Jan;108(1):213—9.

[8] Partridge NC, Kemp BE, Livesey SA, Martin TJ. Activity ratio measurements reflect intracellular activation of adenosine 3′,5′-monophosphate-dependent protein kinase in osteoblasts. Endocrinology 1982 Jul;111(1):178—83.

[9] Sudo H, Kodama HA, Amagai Y, Yamamoto S, Kasai S. In vitro differentiation and calcification in a new clonal osteogenic cell line derived from newborn mouse calvaria. J Cell Biol 1983 Jan;96(1):191—8.

[10] Allan EH, Ho PW, Umezawa A, Hata J, Makishima F, Gillespie MT, et al. Differentiation potential of a mouse bone marrow stromal cell line. J Cell Biochem 2003 Sep 1;90(1):158—69.

[11] Stein GS, Lian JB, Gerstenfeld LG, Shalhoub V, Aronow M, Owen T, et al. The onset and progression of osteoblast differentiation is functionally related to cellular proliferation. Connect Tissue Res 1989;20(1—4):3—13.

[12] Bianco P, Robey PG, Simmons PJ. Mesenchymal stem cells: revisiting history, concepts, and assays. Cell Stem Cell 2008 Apr 10;2(4):313—9.

[13] Bianco P, Robey PG, Saggio I, Riminucci M. "Mesenchymal" stem cells in human bone marrow (skeletal stem cells): a critical discussion of their nature, identity, and significance in incurable skeletal disease. Hum Gene Ther 2010 Sep;21(9):1057—66.

[14] Friedenstein AJ. Precursor cells of mechanocytes. Int Rev Cytol 1976;47:327—59.

[15] Bab I, Ashton BA, Syftestad GT, Owen ME. Assessment of an in vivo diffusion chamber method as a quantitative assay for osteogenesis. Calcif Tissue Int 1984 Jan;36(1):77—82.

[16] Friedenstein AJ, Latzinik NV, Gorskaya UF, Sidorovich SY. Radiosensitivity and postirradiation changes of bone marrow clonogenic stromal mechanocytes. Int J Radiat Biol Relat Stud Phys Chem Med 1981 May;39(5):537—46.

[17] Friedenstein AJ. Osteogenic stem cells. In: Heerschje JNM, Kanis JA, editors. Bone and Mineral Research. Amsterdam: Elsevier; 1990. p. 243—72.

[18] Lundberg P, Allison SJ, Lee NJ, Baldock PA, Brouard N, Rost S, et al. Greater bone formation of Y2 knockout mice is associated with increased osteoprogenitor numbers and altered Y1 receptor expression. J Biol Chem 2007 Jun 29;282(26):19082—91.

[19] Kalajzic I, Staal A, Yang WP, Wu Y, Johnson SE, Feyen JH, et al. Expression profile of osteoblast lineage at defined stages of differentiation. J Biol Chem 2005 Jul 1;280(26):24618—26.

[20] Paic F, Igwe JC, Nori R, Kronenberg MS, Franceschetti T, Harrington P, et al. Identification of differentially expressed genes between osteoblasts and osteocytes. Bone 2009 Oct;45(4):682—92.

[21] Modder UI, Khosla S. Skeletal stem/osteoprogenitor cells: current concepts, alternate hypotheses, and relationship to the bone remodeling compartment. J Cell Biochem 2008 Feb 1; 103(2):393–400.

[22] Otsuru S, Tamai K, Yamazaki T, Yoshikawa H, Kaneda Y. Circulating bone marrow-derived osteoblast progenitor cells are recruited to the bone-forming site by the CXCR4/stromal cell-derived factor-1 pathway. Stem Cells 2008 Jan;26(1): 223–34.

[23] Doherty MJ, Ashton BA, Walsh S, Beresford JN, Grant ME, Canfield AE. Vascular pericytes express osteogenic potential in vitro and in vivo. J Bone Miner Res 1998 May;13(5):828–38.

[24] Kalajzic Z, Li H, Wang LP, Jiang X, Lamothe K, Adams DJ, et al. Use of an alpha-smooth muscle actin GFP reporter to identify an osteoprogenitor population. Bone 2008 Sep;43(3):501–10.

[25] Dellavalle A, Sampaolesi M, Tonlorenzi R, Tagliafico E, Sacchetti B, Perani L, et al. Pericytes of human skeletal muscle are myogenic precursors distinct from satellite cells. Nat Cell Biol 2007 Mar;9(3):255–67.

[26] Fujisaki J, Wu J, Carlson AL, Silberstein L, Putheti P, Larocca R, et al. In vivo imaging of Treg cells providing immune privilege to the haematopoietic stem-cell niche. Nature 2011 Jun 9; 474(7350):216–9.

[27] Simmons PJ, Torok-Storb B. Identification of stromal cell precursors in human bone marrow by a novel monoclonal antibody, STRO-1. Blood 1991 Jul 1;78(1):55–62.

[28] Gronthos S, Zannettino AC, Graves SE, Ohta S, Hay SJ, Simmons PJ. Differential cell surface expression of the STRO-1 and alkaline phosphatase antigens on discrete developmental stages in primary cultures of human bone cells. J Bone Miner Res 1999 Jan;14(1):47–56.

[29] Stewart K, Walsh S, Screen J, Jefferiss CM, Chainey J, Jordan GR, et al. Further characterization of cells expressing STRO-1 in cultures of adult human bone marrow stromal cells. J Bone Miner Res 1999 Aug;14(8):1345–56.

[30] Aubin JE. Regulation of osteoblast formation and function. Rev Endocr Metab Disord 2001 Jan;2(1):81–94.

[31] Aubin JE. Advances in the osteoblast lineage. Biochem Cell Biol 1998;76(6):899–910.

[32] Stein GS, Lian JB. Molecular mechanisms mediating proliferation/differentiation interrelationships during progressive development of the osteoblast phenotype. Endocr Rev 1993 Aug;14(4):424–42.

[33] Karsenty G. Minireview: transcriptional control of osteoblast differentiation. Endocrinology 2001 Jul;142(7):2731–3.

[34] Karsenty G, Kronenberg HM, Settembre C. Genetic control of bone formation. Annu Rev Cell Dev Biol 2009;25:629–48.

[35] Ducy P, Starbuck M, Priemel M, Shen J, Pinero G, Geoffroy V, et al. A Cbfa1-dependent genetic pathway controls bone formation beyond embryonic development. Genes Dev 1999 Apr 15;13(8):1025–36.

[36] Thirunavukkarasu K, Miles RR, Halladay DL, Yang X, Galvin RJ, Chandrasekhar S, et al. Stimulation of osteoprotegerin (OPG) gene expression by transforming growth factor-beta (TGF-beta). Mapping of the OPG promoter region that mediates TGF-beta effects. J Biol Chem 2001 Sep 28;276(39): 36241–50.

[37] Nakashima K, Zhou X, Kunkel G, Zhang Z, Deng JM, Behringer RR, et al. The novel zinc finger-containing transcription factor osterix is required for osteoblast differentiation and bone formation. Cell 2002 Jan 11;108(1):17–29.

[38] Yang X, Matsuda K, Bialek P, Jacquot S, Masuoka HC, Schinke T, et al. ATF4 is a substrate of RSK2 and an essential regulator of osteoblast biology; implication for Coffin–Lowry syndrome. Cell 2004 Apr 30;117(3):387–98.

[39] Sabatakos G, Sims NA, Chen J, Aoki K, Kelz MB, Amling M, et al. Overexpression of DeltaFosB transcription factor(s) increases bone formation and inhibits adipogenesis. Nat Med 2000 Sep;6(9):985–90.

[40] Shirakabe K, Terasawa K, Miyama K, Shibuya H, Nishida E. Regulation of the activity of the transcription factor Runx2 by two homeobox proteins, Msx2 and Dlx5. Genes Cells 2001 Oct;6(10):851–6.

[41] el Ghouzzi V, Le Merrer M, Perrin-Schmitt F, Lajeunie E, Benit P, Renier D, et al. Mutations of the TWIST gene in the Saethre–Chotzen syndrome. Nat Genet 1997 Jan;15(1):42–6.

[42] Howard TD, Paznekas WA, Green ED, Chiang LC, Ma N, Ortiz de Luna RI, et al. Mutations in TWIST, a basic helix–loop–helix transcription factor, in Saethre–Chotzen syndrome. Nat Genet 1997 Jan;15(1):36–41.

[43] Gutierrez S, Javed A, Tennant DK, van Rees M, Montecino M, Stein GS, et al. CCAAT/enhancer-binding proteins (C/EBP) beta and delta activate osteocalcin gene transcription and synergize with Runx2 at the C/EBP element to regulate bone-specific expression. J Biol Chem 2002 Jan 11;277(2):1316–23.

[44] Wu M, Hesse E, Morvan F, Zhang JP, Correa D, Rowe GC, et al. Zfp521 antagonizes Runx2, delays osteoblast differentiation in vitro, and promotes bone formation in vivo. Bone 2009 Apr;44(4):528–36.

[45] Barak Y, Nelson MC, Ong ES, Jones YZ, Ruiz-Lozano P, Chien KR, et al. PPAR gamma is required for placental, cardiac, and adipose tissue development. Mol Cell 1999 Oct;4(4):585–95.

[46] Tanaka T, Yoshida N, Kishimoto T, Akira S. Defective adipocyte differentiation in mice lacking the C/EBPbeta and/or C/EBP-delta gene. EMBO J 1997 Dec 15;16(24):7432–43.

[47] Quach JM, Walker EC, Allan E, Solano M, Yokoyama A, Kato S, et al. Zinc finger protein 467 is a novel regulator of osteoblast and adipocyte commitment. J Biol Chem 2011 Feb 11;286(6): 4186–98.

[48] Justesen J, Stenderup K, Ebbesen EN, Mosekilde L, Steiniche T, Kassem M. Adipocyte tissue volume in bone marrow is increased with aging and in patients with osteoporosis. Biogerontology 2001;2(3):165–71.

[49] Martin RB, Chow BD, Lucas PA. Bone marrow fat content in relation to bone remodeling and serum chemistry in intact and ovariectomized dogs. Calcif Tissue Int 1990 Mar;46(3):189–94.

[50] Ahdjoudj S, Lasmoles F, Holy X, Zerath E, Marie PJ. Transforming growth factor beta2 inhibits adipocyte differentiation induced by skeletal unloading in rat bone marrow stroma. J Bone Miner Res 2002 Apr;17(4):668–77.

[51] Walker E, McGregor N, Poulton I, Pompolo S, Allan E, Quinn J, et al. Cardiotrophin-1 is an osteoclast-derived stimulus of bone formation required for normal bone remodeling. J Bone Miner Res 2008 Dec;23:2025–32.

[52] Walker EC, McGregor NE, Poulton IJ, Solano M, Pompolo S, Fernandes TJ, et al. Oncostatin M promotes bone formation independently of resorption through the leukemia inhibitory factor receptor. J Clin Invest 2010; in press.

[53] Boyden LM, Mao J, Belsky J, Mitzner L, Farhi A, Mitnick MA, et al. High bone density due to a mutation in LDL-receptor-related protein 5. N Engl J Med 2002 May 16;346(20):1513–21.

[54] Gong Y, Slee RB, Fukai N, Rawadi G, Roman-Roman S, Reginato AM, et al. LDL receptor-related protein 5 (LRP5) affects bone accrual and eye development. Cell 2001 Nov 16;107(4):513–23.

[55] Rawadi G, Vayssiere B, Dunn F, Baron R, Roman-Roman S. BMP-2 controls alkaline phosphatase expression and osteoblast mineralization by a Wnt autocrine loop. J Bone Miner Res 2003 Oct;18(10):1842–53.

[56] Kato M, Patel MS, Levasseur R, Lobov I, Chang BH, Glass 2nd DA, et al. Cbfa1-independent decrease in osteoblast proliferation, osteopenia, and persistent embryonic eye vascularization in mice deficient in Lrp5, a Wnt coreceptor. J Cell Biol 2002 Apr 15;157(2):303–14.

[57] Babij P, Zhao W, Small C, Kharode Y, Yaworsky PJ, Bouxsein ML, et al. High bone mass in mice expressing a mutant LRP5 gene. J Bone Miner Res 2003 Jun;18(6):960–74.

[58] Glass 2nd DA, Karsenty G. In vivo analysis of Wnt signaling in bone. Endocrinology 2007 Jun;148(6):2630–4.

[59] Morvan F, Boulukos K, Clement-Lacroix P, Roman Roman S, Suc-Royer I, Vayssiere B, et al. Deletion of a single allele of the Dkk1 gene leads to an increase in bone formation and bone mass. J Bone Miner Res 2006 Jun;21(6):934–45.

[60] Kulkarni NH, Onyia JE, Zeng Q, Tian X, Liu M, Halladay DL, et al. Orally bioavailable GSK-3alpha/beta dual inhibitor increases markers of cellular differentiation in vitro and bone mass in vivo. J Bone Miner Res 2006 Jun;21(6):910–20.

[61] Glass 2nd DA, Bialek P, Ahn JD, Starbuck M, Patel MS, Clevers H, et al. Canonical Wnt signaling in differentiated osteoblasts controls osteoclast differentiation. Dev Cell 2005 May;8(5):751–64.

[62] Kramer I, Halleux C, Keller H, Pegurri M, Gooi JH, Weber PB, et al. Osteocyte Wnt/beta-catenin signaling is required for normal bone homeostasis. Mol Cell Biol 2010 Jun;30(12):3071–85.

[63] Kubota T, Michigami T, Sakaguchi N, Kokubu C, Suzuki A, Namba N, et al. Lrp6 hypomorphic mutation affects bone mass through bone resorption in mice and impairs interaction with Mesd. J Bone Miner Res 2008 Oct;23(10):1661–71.

[64] Holmen SL, Zylstra CR, Mukherjee A, Sigler RE, Faugere MC, Bouxsein ML, et al. Essential role of beta-catenin in postnatal bone acquisition. J Biol Chem 2005 Jun 3;280(22):21162–8.

[65] Yadav VK, Ryu JH, Suda N, Tanaka KF, Gingrich JA, Schutz G, et al. Lrp5 controls bone formation by inhibiting serotonin synthesis in the duodenum. Cell 2008 Nov 28;135(5):825–37.

[66] Yadav VK, Balaji S, Suresh PS, Liu XS, Lu X, Li Z, et al. Pharmacological inhibition of gut-derived serotonin synthesis is a potential bone anabolic treatment for osteoporosis. Nat Med 2010 Mar;16(3):308–12.

[67] Inose H, Zhou B, Yadav VK, Guo XE, Karsenty G, Ducy P. Efficacy of serotonin inhibition in mouse models of bone loss. J Bone Miner Res 2011 Sep;26(9):2002–11.

[68] Cui Y, Niziolek PJ, MacDonald BT, Zylstra CR, Alenina N, Robinson DR, et al. Lrp5 functions in bone to regulate bone mass. Nat Med 2011 Jun;17(6):684–91.

[69] Bonewald LF. The amazing osteocyte. J Bone Miner Res 2011 Feb;26(2):229–38.

[70] Holmbeck K, Bianco P, Pidoux I, Inoue S, Billinghurst RC, Wu W, et al. The metalloproteinase MT1-MMP is required for normal development and maintenance of osteocyte processes in bone. J Cell Sci 2005 Jan 1;118(Pt 1):147–56.

[71] Wetterwald A, Hoffstetter W, Cecchini MG, Lanske B, Wagner C, Fleisch H, et al. Characterization and cloning of the E11 antigen, a marker expressed by rat osteoblasts and osteocytes. Bone 1996 Feb;18(2):125–32.

[72] Loots GG, Kneissel M, Keller H, Baptist M, Chang J, Collette NM, et al. Genomic deletion of a long-range bone enhancer misregulates sclerostin in Van Buchem disease. Genome Res 2005 Jul;15(7):928–35.

[73] Balemans W, Patel N, Ebeling M, Van Hul E, Wuyts W, Lacza C, et al. Identification of a 52 kb deletion downstream of the SOST gene in patients with van Buchem disease. J Med Genet 2002 Feb;39(2):91–7.

[74] Balemans W, Ebeling M, Patel N, Van Hul E, Olson P, Dioszegi M, et al. Increased bone density in sclerosteosis is due to the deficiency of a novel secreted protein (SOST). Hum Mol Genet 2001 Mar 1;10(5):537–43.

[75] Li X, Ominsky MS, Warmington KS, Morony S, Gong J, Cao J, et al. Sclerostin antibody treatment increases bone formation, bone mass, and bone strength in a rat model of postmenopausal osteoporosis. J Bone Miner Res 2009 Apr;24(4):578–88.

[76] Eddleston A, Marenzana M, Moore AR, Stephens P, Muzylak M, Marshall D, et al. A short treatment with an antibody to sclerostin can inhibit bone loss in an ongoing model of colitis. J Bone Miner Res 2009 Oct;24(10):1662–71.

[77] Padhi D, Jang G, Stouch B, Fang L, Posvar E. Single-dose, placebo-controlled, randomized study of AMG 785, a sclerostin monoclonal antibody. J Bone Miner Res 2011 Jan;26(1):19–26.

[78] van Bezooijen RL, ten Dijke P, Papapoulos SE, Lowik CW. SOST/sclerostin, an osteocyte-derived negative regulator of bone formation. Cytokine Growth Factor Rev 2005 Jun;16(3):319–27.

[79] Keller H, Kneissel M. SOST is a target gene for PTH in bone. Bone 2005 Aug;37(2):148–58.

[80] Genetos DC, Yellowley CE, Loots GG. Prostaglandin E2 signals through PTGER2 to regulate sclerostin expression. PLoS ONE 2011;6(3):e17772.

[81] Genetos DC, Toupadakis CA, Raheja LF, Wong A, Papanicolaou SE, Fyhrie DP, et al. Hypoxia decreases sclerostin expression and increases Wnt signaling in osteoblasts. J Cell Biochem 2010 May 15;110(2):457–67.

[82] Powell Jr WF, Barry KJ, Tulum I, Kobayashi T, Harris SE, Bringhurst FR, et al. Targeted ablation of the PTH/PTHrP receptor in osteocytes impairs bone structure and homeostatic calcemic responses. J Endocrinol 2011 Apr;209(1):21–32.

[83] Schipani E, Lanske B, Hunzelman J, Luz A, Kovacs CS, Lee K, et al. Targeted expression of constitutively active receptors for parathyroid hormone and parathyroid hormone-related peptide delays endochondral bone formation and rescues mice that lack parathyroid hormone-related peptide. Proc Natl Acad Sci USA 1997 Dec 9;94(25):13689–94.

[84] de Souza RL, Pitsillides AA, Lanyon LE, Skerry TM, Chenu C. Sympathetic nervous system does not mediate the load-induced cortical new bone formation. J Bone Miner Res 2005 Dec;20(12):2159–68.

[85] Sawakami K, Robling AG, Ai M, Pitner ND, Liu D, Warden SJ, et al. The Wnt co-receptor LRP5 is essential for skeletal mechanotransduction but not for the anabolic bone response to parathyroid hormone treatment. J Biol Chem 2006 Aug 18;281(33):23698–711.

[86] Robling AG, Bellido T, Turner CH. Mechanical stimulation in vivo reduces osteocyte expression of sclerostin. J Musculoskelet Neuronal Interact 2006 Oct–Dec;6(4):354.

[87] Moustafa A, Sugiyama T, Prasad J, Zaman G, Gross TS, Lanyon LE, et al. Mechanical loading-related changes in osteocyte sclerostin expression in mice are more closely associated with the subsequent osteogenic response than the peak strains engendered. Osteoporos Int 2011 May 15.

[88] Tatsumi S, Ishii K, Amizuka N, Li M, Kobayashi T, Kohno K, et al. Targeted ablation of osteocytes induces osteoporosis with defective mechanotransduction. Cell Metab 2007 Jun;5(6):464–75.

[89] Gaudio A, Pennisi P, Bratengeier C, Torrisi V, Lindner B, Mangiafico RA, et al. Increased sclerostin serum levels associated with bone formation and resorption markers in patients

with immobilization-induced bone loss. J Clin Endocrinol Metab 2010 May;95(5):2248—53.

[90] Lin C, Jiang X, Dai Z, Guo X, Weng T, Wang J, et al. Sclerostin mediates bone response to mechanical unloading through antagonizing Wnt/beta-catenin signaling. J Bone Miner Res 2009 Oct;24(10):1651—61.

[91] Tian X, Jee WS, Li X, Paszty C, Ke HZ. Sclerostin antibody increases bone mass by stimulating bone formation and inhibiting bone resorption in a hindlimb-immobilization rat model. Bone 2011 Feb;48(2):197—201.

[92] Papanicolaou SE, Phipps RJ, Fyhrie DP, Genetos DC. Modulation of sclerostin expression by mechanical loading and bone morphogenetic proteins in osteogenic cells. Biorheology 2009;46(5):389—99.

[93] Niikura T, Hak DJ, Reddi AH. Global gene profiling reveals a downregulation of BMP gene expression in experimental atrophic nonunions compared to standard healing fractures. J Orthop Res 2006 Jul;24(7):1463—71.

[94] Hak DJ, Makino T, Niikura T, Hazelwood SJ, Curtiss S, Reddi AH. Recombinant human BMP-7 effectively prevents non-union in both young and old rats. J Orthop Res 2006 Jan;24(1):11—20.

[95] Mantila Roosa SM, Liu Y, Turner CH. Gene expression patterns in bone following mechanical loading. J Bone Miner Res 2011 Jan;26(1):100—12.

[96] Heller-Steinberg M. Ground substance, bone salts, and cellular activity in bone formation and destruction. Am J Anat 1951 Nov;89(3):347—79.

[97] Belanger LF, Robichon J. Parathormone-induced osteolysis in dogs. a microradiographic and alpharadiographic survey. J Bone Joint Surg Am 1964 Jul;46:1008—12.

[98] Belanger LF. Osteocytic osteolysis. Calcif Tissue Res 1969 Aug 11;4(1):1—12.

[99] Teti A, Zallone A. Do osteocytes contribute to bone mineral homeostasis? Osteocytic osteolysis revisited. Bone 2009 Jan;44(1):11—6.

[100] Boyde A. Evidence against osteocytic osteolysis. In: Jee WSS, Parfitt AM, editors. Bone Histomorphometry Third International Workshop. Paris: Societe Nouvelle de Publications Medicales et Dentaires; 1980.

[101] Holtrop ME, King GJ, Cox KA, Reit B. Time-related changes in the ultrastructure of osteoclasts after injection of parathyroid hormone in young rats. Calcif Tissue Int 1979 Apr 17;27(2):129—35.

[102] Parfitt AM. The cellular basis of bone turnover and bone loss: a rebuttal of the osteocytic resorption—bone flow theory. Clin Orthop Relat Res 1977;(127)::236—47.

[103] Qing H, Ardeshirpor L, Dusevich V, Wysolmerski J, Bonewald LF. Osteocyte perilacunar remodeling is regulated hormonally, but not by mechanical unloading. J Bone Min Res 2009;29(Suppl 1):S440.

[104] Bonewald L. The holy grail of high bone mass. Nat Med 2011 Jun;17(6):657—8.

[105] Nakashima T, Hayashi M, Fukunaga T, Kurata K, Oh-Hora M, Feng JQ, et al. Evidence for osteocyte regulation of bone homeostasis through RANKL expression. Nat Med 2011;17(10):1231—4.

[106] Xiong J, Onal M, Jilka RL, Weinstein RS, Manolagas SC, O'Brien CA. Matrix-embedded cells control osteoclast formation. Nat Med 2011;17(10):1235—41.

[107] Kogianni G, Mann V, Noble BS. Apoptotic bodies convey activity capable of initiating osteoclastogenesis and localized bone destruction. J Bone Miner Res 2008 Jun;23(6):915—27.

[108] Kolliker A. Die Normal Resorption des Knochengewebes und ihre Bedeutung die Entstehung der Typischen Knochenformen. Liepzig: Vogel FCW 1873.

[109] Holtrop ME, King GJ. The ultrastructure of the osteoclast and its functional implications. Clin Orthop Relat Res 1977 Mar—Apr;(123)::177—96.

[110] Vaes G. Cellular biology and biochemical mechanism of bone resorption. A review of recent developments on the formation, activation, and mode of action of osteoclasts. Clin Orthop Relat Res 1988 Jun;(231)::239—71.

[111] Baron R. Molecular mechanisms of bone resorption: therapeutic implications. Rev Rhum Engl Ed 1996 Nov;63(10): 633—8.

[112] Arnett TR, Dempster DW. Protons and osteoclasts. J Bone Miner Res 1990 Nov;5(11):1099—103.

[113] Burger EH, van der Meer JW, Nijweide PJ. Osteoclast formation from mononuclear phagocytes: role of bone-forming cells. J Cell Biol 1984 Dec;99(6):1901—6.

[114] Scheven BA, Visser JW, Nijweide PJ. In vitro osteoclast generation from different bone marrow fractions, including a highly enriched haematopoietic stem cell population. Nature 1986 May 1—7;321(6065):79—81.

[115] Nicholson GC, Moseley JM, Sexton PM, Mendelsohn FA, Martin TJ. Abundant calcitonin receptors in isolated rat osteoclasts. Biochemical and autoradiographic characterization. J Clin Invest 1986 Aug;78(2):355—60.

[116] Tonna EA. Osteoclasts and the aging skeleton: a cytological, cytochemical and autoradiographic study. Anat Rec 1960 Jul;137:251—69.

[117] Young RW. Cell proliferation and specialization during endochondral osteogenesis in young rats. J Cell Biol 1962 Sep;14: 357—70.

[118] Rasmussen H, Bordier P. The Physiological Basis of Metabolic Bone Disease. Baltimore: Williams and Wilkins, Waverley Press; 1974.

[119] Kahn AJ, Simmons DJ. Investigation of cell lineage in bone using a chimaera of chick and quial embryonic tissue. Nature 1975 Nov 27;258(5533):325—7.

[120] Nijweide PJ, Burger EH, Feyen JH. Cells of bone: proliferation, differentiation, and hormonal regulation. Physiol Rev 1986 Oct;66(4):855—86.

[121] Loutit JF, Townsend KM. Longevity of osteoclasts in radiation chimaeras of osteopetrotic beige and normal mice. Br J Exp Pathol 1982 Apr;63(2):221—3.

[122] Martin TJ, Partridge NC, Greaves M, Atkins D, Ibbotson KJ. Prostaglandin effects on bone and role in cancer hypercalcaemia. In: MacIntyre I, Szelke M, editors. Molecular Endocrinology. Amsterdam: Elsevier; 1979. p. 251—64.

[123] Rodan GA, Martin TJ. Role of osteoblasts in hormonal control of bone resorption—a hypothesis. Calcif Tissue Int 1981;33(4): 349—51.

[124] Chambers TJ. cof bone resorption. Clin Orthop Relat Res 1980 Sep;(151):283—93.

[125] Chambers TJ. The pathobiology of the osteoclast. J Clin Pathol 1985 Mar;38(3):241—52.

[126] Akatsu T, Takahashi N, Udagawa N, Sato K, Nagata N, Moseley JM, et al. Parathyroid hormone (PTH)-related protein is a potent stimulator of osteoclast-like multinucleated cell formation to the same extent as PTH in mouse marrow cultures. Endocrinology 1989 Jul;125(1):20—7.

[127] Akatsu T, Takahashi N, Udagawa N, Imamura K, Yamaguchi A, Sato K, et al. Role of prostaglandins in interleukin-1-induced bone resorption in mice in vitro. J Bone Miner Res 1991 Feb;6(2):183—9.

[128] Tamura T, Udagawa N, Takahashi N, Miyaura C, Tanaka S, Yamada Y, et al. Soluble interleukin-6 receptor triggers osteoclast formation by interleukin 6. Proc Natl Acad Sci USA 1993 Dec 15;90(24):11924—8.

[129] Takahashi N, Yamana H, Yoshiki S, Roodman GD, Mundy GR, Jones SJ, et al. Osteoclast-like cell formation and its regulation by osteotropic hormones in mouse bone marrow cultures. Endocrinology 1988 Apr;122(4):1373–82.

[130] Suda T, Takahashi N, Martin TJ. Modulation of osteoclast differentiation. Endocr Rev 1992 Feb;13(1):66–80.

[131] Takahashi N, Akatsu T, Udagawa N, Sasaki T, Yamaguchi A, Moseley JM, et al. Osteoblastic cells are involved in osteoclast formation. Endocrinology 1988 Nov;123(5):2600–2.

[132] Yamashita T, Asano K, Takahashi N, Akatsu T, Udagawa N, Sasaki T, et al. Cloning of an osteoblastic cell line involved in the formation of osteoclast-like cells. J Cell Physiol 1990 Dec;145(3): 587–95.

[133] Udagawa N, Takahashi N, Akatsu T, Sasaki T, Yamaguchi A, Kodama H, et al. The bone marrow-derived stromal cell lines MC3T3-G2/PA6 and ST2 support osteoclast-like cell differentiation in cocultures with mouse spleen cells. Endocrinology 1989 Oct;125(4):1805–13.

[134] Kitazawa R, Kitazawa S. Vitamin D(3) augments osteoclastogenesis via vitamin D-responsive element of mouse RANKL gene promoter. Biochem Biophys Res Commun 2002 Jan 18;290(2):650–5.

[135] Udagawa N, Takahashi N, Katagiri T, Tamura T, Wada S, Findlay DM, et al. Interleukin (IL)-6 induction of osteoclast differentiation depends on IL-6 receptors expressed on osteoblastic cells but not on osteoclast progenitors. J Exp Med 1995 Nov 1;182(5):1461–8.

[136] Gao Y, Morita I, Maruo N, Kubota T, Murota S, Aso T. Expression of IL-6 receptor and GP130 in mouse bone marrow cells during osteoclast differentiation. Bone 1998 May;22(5):487–93.

[137] Martin TJ, Ng KW. Mechanisms by which cells of the osteoblast lineage control osteoclast formation and activity. J Cell Biochem 1994 Nov;56(3):357–66.

[138] Simonet WS, Lacey DL, Dunstan CR, Kelley M, Chang MS, Luthy R, et al. Osteoprotegerin: a novel secreted protein involved in the regulation of bone density. Cell 1997 Apr 18;89(2):309–19.

[139] Tsuda E, Goto M, Mochizuki S, Yano K, Kobayashi F, Morinaga T, et al. Isolation of a novel cytokine from human fibroblasts that specifically inhibits osteoclastogenesis. Biochem Biophys Res Commun 1997 May 8;234(1):137–42.

[140] Lacey DL, Timms E, Tan HL, Kelley MJ, Dunstan CR, Burgess T, et al. Osteoprotegerin ligand is a cytokine that regulates osteoclast differentiation and activation. Cell 1998 Apr 17;93(2): 165–76.

[141] Yasuda H, Shima N, Nakagawa N, Yamaguchi K, Kinosaki M, Mochizuki S, et al. Osteoclast differentiation factor is a ligand for osteoprotegerin/osteoclastogenesis-inhibitory factor and is identical to TRANCE/RANKL. Proc Natl Acad Sci USA 1998 Mar 31;95(7):3597–602.

[142] Bucay N, Sarosi I, Dunstan CR, Morony S, Tarpley J, Capparelli C, et al. osteoprotegerin-deficient mice develop early onset osteoporosis and arterial calcification. Genes Dev 1998 May 1;12(9):1260–8.

[143] Udagawa N, Takahashi N, Yasuda H, Mizuno A, Itoh K, Ueno Y, et al. Osteoprotegerin produced by osteoblasts is an important regulator in osteoclast development and function. Endocrinology 2000 Sep;141(9):3478–84.

[144] Kong YY, Feige U, Sarosi I, Bolon B, Tafuri A, Morony S, et al. Activated T cells regulate bone loss and joint destruction in adjuvant arthritis through osteoprotegerin ligand. Nature 1999 Nov 18;402(6759):304–9.

[145] Dougall WC, Glaccum M, Charrier K, Rohrbach K, Brasel K, De Smedt T, et al. RANK is essential for osteoclast and lymph node development. Genes Dev 1999 Sep 15;13(18):2412–24.

[146] Wong BR, Josien R, Lee SY, Sauter B, Li HL, Steinman RM, et al. TRANCE (tumor necrosis factor [TNF]-related activation-induced cytokine), a new TNF family member predominantly expressed in T cells, is a dendritic cell-specific survival factor. J Exp Med 1997 Dec 15;186(12):2075–80.

[147] Anderson DM, Maraskovsky E, Billingsley WL, Dougall WC, Tometsko ME, Roux ER, et al. A homologue of the TNF receptor and its ligand enhance T-cell growth and dendritic-cell function. Nature 1997 Nov 13;390(6656):175–9.

[148] Horwood NJ, Kartsogiannis V, Quinn JM, Romas E, Martin TJ, Gillespie MT. Activated T lymphocytes support osteoclast formation in vitro. Biochem Biophys Res Commun 1999 Nov;265(1):144–50.

[149] Jimi E, Akiyama S, Tsurukai T, Okahashi N, Kobayashi K, Udagawa N, et al. Osteoclast differentiation factor acts as a multifunctional regulator in murine osteoclast differentiation and function. J Immunol 1999 Jul 1;163(1):434–42.

[150] Quinn JM, Neale S, Fujikawa Y, McGee JO, Athanasou NA. Human osteoclast formation from blood monocytes, peritoneal macrophages, and bone marrow cells. Calcif Tissue Int 1998 Jun;62(6):527–31.

[151] Matsuzaki K, Udagawa N, Takahashi N, Yamaguchi K, Yasuda H, Shima N, et al. Osteoclast differentiation factor (ODF) induces osteoclast-like cell formation in human peripheral blood mononuclear cell cultures. Biochem Biophys Res Commun 1998 May 8;246(1):199–204.

[152] Horwood NJ, Elliott J, Martin TJ, Gillespie MT. Osteotropic agents regulate the expression of osteoclast differentiation factor and osteoprotegerin in osteoblastic stromal cells. Endocrinology 1998 Nov;139(11):4743–6.

[153] Lee SK, Lorenzo JA. Parathyroid hormone stimulates TRANCE and inhibits osteoprotegerin messenger ribonucleic acid expression in murine bone marrow cultures: correlation with osteoclast-like cell formation. Endocrinology 1999 Aug;140(8): 3552–61.

[154] Thomas RJ, Guise TA, Yin JJ, Elliott J, Horwood NJ, Martin TJ, et al. Breast cancer cells interact with osteoblasts to support osteoclast formation. Endocrinology 1999 Oct;140(10):4451–8.

[155] Lai FP, Cole-Sinclair M, Cheng WJ, Quinn JM, Gillespie MT, Sentry JW, et al. Myeloma cells can directly contribute to the pool of RANKL in bone bypassing the classic stromal and osteoblast pathway of osteoclast stimulation. Br J Haematol 2004 Jul;126(2):192–201.

[156] Eghbali-Fatourechi G, Khosla S, Sanyal A, Boyle WJ, Lacey DL, Riggs BL. Role of RANK ligand in mediating increased bone resorption in early postmenopausal women. J Clin Invest 2003 Apr;111(8):1221–30.

[157] Suda T, Takahashi N, Udagawa N, Jimi E, Gillespie MT, Martin TJ. Modulation of osteoclast differentiation and function by the new members of the tumor necrosis factor receptor and ligand families. Endocr Rev 1999 Jun;20(3):345–57.

[158] Boyle WJ, Simonet WS, Lacey DL. Osteoclast differentiation and activation. Nature 2003 May 15;423(6937):337–42.

[159] Teitelbaum SL, Ross FP. Genetic regulation of osteoclast development and function. Nat Rev Genet 2003 Aug;4(8):638–49.

[160] Hikita A, Tanaka S. Ectodomain shedding of receptor activator of NF-kappaB ligand. Adv Exp Med Biol 2007;602:15–21.

[161] Lum L, Wong BR, Josien R, Becherer JD, Erdjument-Bromage H, Schlondorff J, et al. Evidence for a role of a tumor necrosis factor-alpha (TNF-alpha)-converting enzyme-like protease in shedding of TRANCE, a TNF family member involved in osteoclastogenesis and dendritic cell survival. J Biol Chem 1999 May 7;274(19):13613–8.

[162] Lynch CC, Hikosaka A, Acuff HB, Martin MD, Kawai N, Singh RK, et al. MMP-7 promotes prostate cancer-induced

osteolysis via the solubilization of RANKL. Cancer Cell 2005 May;7(5):485−96.

[163] Hikita A, Yana I, Wakeyama H, Nakamura M, Kadono Y, Oshima Y, et al. Negative regulation of osteoclastogenesis by ectodomain shedding of receptor activator of NF-kappaB ligand. J Biol Chem 2006 Dec 1;281(48):36846−55.

[164] Yamanaka H, Makino K, Takizawa M, Nakamura H, Fujimoto N, Moriya H, et al. Expression and tissue localization of membrane-types 1, 2, and 3 matrix metalloproteinases in rheumatoid synovium. Lab Invest 2000 May;80(5):677−87.

[165] Sabbota AL, Kim HR, Zhe X, Fridman R, Bonfil RD, Cher ML. Shedding of RANKL by tumor-associated MT1-MMP activates Src-dependent prostate cancer cell migration. Cancer Res 2010 Jul 1;70(13):5558−66.

[166] Wilson TJ, Nannuru KC, Futakuchi M, Sadanandam A, Singh RK. Cathepsin G enhances mammary tumor-induced osteolysis by generating soluble receptor activator of nuclear factor-kappaB ligand. Cancer Res 2008 Jul 15;68(14):5803−11.

[167] Proell V, Xu H, Schuler C, Weber K, Hofbauer LC, Erben RG. Orchiectomy upregulates free soluble RANKL in bone marrow of aged rats. Bone 2009 Oct;45(4):677−81.

[168] Frost. Dynamics of bone remodeling. Bone Biodyn 1964;1964: 315−33.

[169] Parfitt AM. The coupling of bone formation to bone resorption: a critical analysis of the concept and of its relevance to the pathogenesis of osteoporosis. Metab Bone Dis Relat Res 1982;4(1):1−6.

[170] Eriksen EF. Normal and pathological remodeling of human trabecular bone: three dimensional reconstruction of the remodeling sequence in normals and in metabolic bone disease. Endocr Rev 1986 Nov;7(4):379−408.

[171] Martin TJ, Gooi JH, Sims NA. Molecular mechanisms in coupling of bone formation to resorption. Crit Rev Eukaryot Gene Expr 2009;19:73−88.

[172] Lips P, Courpron P, Meunier PJ. Mean wall thickness of trabecular bone packets in the human iliac crest: changes with age. Calcif Tissue Res 1978 Nov 10;26(1):13−7.

[173] Hauge EM, Qvesel D, Eriksen EF, Mosekilde L, Melsen F. Cancellous bone remodeling occurs in specialized compartments lined by cells expressing osteoblastic markers. J Bone Miner Res 2001 Sep;16(9):1575−82.

[174] Fujikawa Y, Quinn JM, Sabokbar A, McGee JO, Athanasou NA. The human osteoclast precursor circulates in the monocyte fraction. Endocrinology 1996 Sep;137(9):4058−60.

[175] Eghbali-Fatourechi GZ, Modder UI, Charatcharoenwitthaya N, Sanyal A, Undale AH, Clowes JA, et al. Characterization of circulating osteoblast lineage cells in humans. Bone 2007 May;40(5):1370−7.

[176] Eriksen EF, Eghbali-Fatourechi GZ, Khosla S. Remodeling and vascular spaces in bone. J Bone Miner Res 2007 Jan;22(1):1−6.

[177] Howson KM, Aplin AC, Gelati M, Alessandri G, Parati EA, Nicosia RF. The postnatal rat aorta contains pericyte progenitor cells that form spheroidal colonies in suspension culture. Am J Physiol Cell Physiol 2005 Dec;289(6):C1396−407.

[178] Matsumoto T, Kawamoto A, Kuroda R, Ishikawa M, Mifune Y, Iwasaki H, et al. Therapeutic potential of vasculogenesis and osteogenesis promoted by peripheral blood CD34-positive cells for functional bone healing. Am J Pathol 2006 Oct;169(4): 1440−57.

[179] Yamamoto Y, Udagawa N, Matsuura S, Nakamichi Y, Horiuchi H, Hosoya A, et al. Osteoblasts provide a suitable microenvironment for the action of receptor activator of nuclear factor-kappaB ligand. Endocrinology 2006 Jul;147(7):3366−74.

[180] Mizoguchi T, Muto A, Udagawa N, Arai A, Yamashita T, Hosoya A, et al. Identification of cell cycle-arrested quiescent osteoclast precursors in vivo. J Cell Biol 2009 Feb 23;184(4): 541−54.

[181] Malone JD, Kahn AJ, Teitelbaum SL. Dissociation of organic acid secretion from macrophage mediated bone resorption. Biochem Biophys Res Commun 1982 Sep 30;108(2):468−73.

[182] Yu X, Huang Y, Collin-Osdoby P, Osdoby P. Stromal cell-derived factor-1 (SDF-1) recruits osteoclast precursors by inducing chemotaxis, matrix metalloproteinase-9 (MMP-9) activity, and collagen transmigration. J Bone Miner Res 2003 Aug;18(8):1404−18.

[183] Verborgt O, Gibson GJ, Schaffler MB. Loss of osteocyte integrity in association with microdamage and bone remodeling after fatigue in vivo. J Bone Miner Res 2000 Jan;15(1):60−7.

[184] Verborgt O, Tatton NA, Majeska RJ, Schaffler MB. Spatial distribution of Bax and Bcl-2 in osteocytes after bone fatigue: complementary roles in bone remodeling regulation? J Bone Miner Res 2002 May;17(5):907−14.

[185] Noble BS, Peet N, Stevens HY, Brabbs A, Mosley JR, Reilly GC, et al. Mechanical loading: biphasic osteocyte survival and targeting of osteoclasts for bone destruction in rat cortical bone. Am J Physiol Cell Physiol 2003 Apr;284(4):C934−43.

[186] Takayanagi H, Kim S, Matsuo K, Suzuki H, Suzuki T, Sato K, et al. RANKL maintains bone homeostasis through c-Fos-dependent induction of interferon-beta. Nature 2002 Apr 18;416(6882):744−9.

[187] Grigoriadis AE, Wang ZQ, Cecchini MG, Hofstetter W, Felix R, Fleisch HA, et al. c-Fos: a key regulator of osteoclast-macrophage lineage determination and bone remodeling. Science 1994 Oct 21;266(5184):443−8.

[188] Zhao C, Irie N, Takada Y, Shimoda K, Miyamoto T, Nishiwaki T, et al. Bidirectional ephrinB2-EphB4 signaling controls bone homeostasis. Cell Metab 2006 Aug;4(2):111−21.

[189] Hughes DE, Boyce BF. Apoptosis in bone physiology and disease. Mol Pathol 1997 Jun;50(3):132−7.

[190] Nakamura T, Imai Y, Matsumoto T, Sato S, Takeuchi K, Igarashi K, et al. Estrogen prevents bone loss via estrogen receptor alpha and induction of Fas ligand in osteoclasts. Cell 2007 Sep 7;130(5):811−23.

[191] Henriksen K, Gram J, Schaller S, Dahl BH, Dziegiel MH, Bollerslev J, et al. Characterization of osteoclasts from patients harboring a G215R mutation in ClC-7 causing autosomal dominant osteopetrosis type II. Am J Pathol 2004 May;164(5): 1537−45.

[192] Karsdal MA, Henriksen K, Sorensen MG, Gram J, Schaller S, Dziegiel MH, et al. Acidification of the osteoclastic resorption compartment provides insight into the coupling of bone formation to bone resorption. Am J Pathol 2005 Feb;166(2): 467−76.

[193] Everts V, Delaisse JM, Korper W, Jansen DC, Tigchelaar-Gutter W, Saftig P, et al. The bone lining cell: its role in cleaning Howship's lacunae and initiating bone formation. J Bone Miner Res 2002 Jan;17(1):77−90.

[194] Perez-Amodio S, Beertsen W, Everts V. (Pre-)osteoclasts induce retraction of osteoblasts before their fusion to osteoclasts. J Bone Miner Res 2004 Oct;19(10):1722−31.

[195] Chen D, Zhao M, Mundy GR. Bone morphogenetic proteins. Growth Factors 2004 Dec;22(4):233−41.

[196] Hynes RO. Integrins: versatility, modulation, and signaling in cell adhesion. Cell 1992 Apr 3;69(1):11−25.

[197] Mohan S, Baylink DJ. Bone growth factors. Clin Orthop Relat Res 1991 Feb;(263):30−48.

[198] Hauschka PV, Mavrakos AE, Iafrati MD, Doleman SE, Klagsbrun M. Growth factors in bone matrix. Isolation of multiple types by affinity chromatography on heparin-Sepharose. J Biol Chem 1986 Sep 25;261(27):12665−74.

[199] Critchlow MA, Bland YS, Ashhurst DE. The effects of age on the response of rabbit periosteal osteoprogenitor cells to exogenous transforming growth factor-beta 2. J Cell Sci 1994 Feb;107(Pt 2):499–516.

[200] Joyce ME, Roberts AB, Sporn MB, Bolander ME. Transforming growth factor-beta and the initiation of chondrogenesis and osteogenesis in the rat femur. J Cell Biol 1990 Jun;110(6): 2195–207.

[201] Bonewald LF, Wakefield L, Oreffo RO, Escobedo A, Twardzik DR, Mundy GR. Latent forms of transforming growth factor-beta (TGF beta) derived from bone cultures: identification of a naturally occurring 100-kDa complex with similarity to recombinant latent TGF beta. Mol Endocrinol 1991 Jun;5(6):741–51.

[202] Martin TJ, Allan EH, Fukumoto S. The plasminogen activator and inhibitor system in bone remodelling. Growth Regul 1993 Dec;3(4):209–14.

[203] Tang Y, Wu X, Lei W, Pang L, Wan C, Shi Z, et al. TGF-beta1-induced migration of bone mesenchymal stem cells couples bone resorption with formation. Nat Med 2009 Jul;15(7):757–65.

[204] Wu X, Pang L, Lei W, Lu W, Li J, Li Z, et al. Inhibition of Sca-1-positive skeletal stem cell recruitment by alendronate blunts the anabolic effects of parathyroid hormone on bone remodeling. Cell Stem Cell 2010 Nov 5;7(5):571–80.

[205] Gray C, Boyde A, Jones SJ. Topographically induced bone formation in vitro: implications for bone implants and bone grafts. Bone 1996 Feb;18(2):115–23.

[206] Stains JP, Civitelli R. Gap junctions in skeletal development and function. Biochim Biophys Acta 2005 Dec 20;1719(1–2):69–81.

[207] Dalby MJ, McCloy D, Robertson M, Agheli H, Sutherland D, Affrossman S, et al. Osteoprogenitor response to semi-ordered and random nanotopographies. Biomaterials 2006 May;27(15):2980–7.

[208] Allan EH, Hausler KD, Wei T, Gooi JH, Quinn JM, Crimeen-Irwin B, et al. EphrinB2 regulation by PTH and PTHrP revealed by molecular profiling in differentiating osteoblasts. J Bone Miner Res 2008 Aug;23(8):1170–81.

[209] Gale NW, Holland SJ, Valenzuela DM, Flenniken A, Pan L, Ryan TE, et al. Eph receptors and ligands comprise two major specificity subclasses and are reciprocally compartmentalized during embryogenesis. Neuron 1996 Jul;17(1):9–19.

[210] Pasquale EB. Eph receptor signalling casts a wide net on cell behaviour. Nat Rev Mol Cell Biol 2005 Jun;6(6):462–75.

[211] Luiz de Freitas PH, Li M, Ninomiya T, Nakamura M, Ubaidus S, Oda K, et al. Intermittent PTH administration stimulates pre-osteoblastic proliferation without leading to enhanced bone formation in osteoclast-less c-fos(−/−) mice. J Bone Miner Res 2009 Sep;24(9):1586–97.

[212] Del Fattore A, Peruzzi B, Rucci N, Recchia I, Cappariello A, Longo M, et al. Clinical, genetic, and cellular analysis of 49 osteopetrotic patients: implications for diagnosis and treatment. J Med Genet 2006 Apr;43(4):315–25.

[213] Soriano P, Montgomery C, Geske R, Bradley A. Targeted disruption of the c-src proto-oncogene leads to osteopetrosis in mice. Cell 1991 Feb 22;64(4):693–702.

[214] Kornak U, Kasper D, Bosl MR, Kaiser E, Schweizer M, Schulz A, et al. Loss of the ClC-7 chloride channel leads to osteopetrosis in mice and man. Cell 2001 Jan 26;104(2):205–15.

[215] Pennypacker B, Shea M, Liu Q, Masarachia P, Saftig P, Rodan S, et al. Bone density, strength, and formation in adult cathepsin K (−/−) mice. Bone 2009 Feb;44(2):199–207.

[216] Chiusaroli R, Knobler H, Luxenburg C, Sanjay A, Granot-Attas S, Tiran Z, et al. Tyrosine phosphatase epsilon is a positive regulator of osteoclast function in vitro and in vivo. Mol Biol Cell 2004 Jan;15(1):234–44.

[217] Lee SH, Rho J, Jeong D, Sul JY, Kim T, Kim N, et al. v-ATPase V0 subunit d2-deficient mice exhibit impaired osteoclast fusion and increased bone formation. Nat Med 2006 Dec;12(12): 1403–9.

[218] Sims NA, Jenkins BJ, Quinn JM, Nakamura A, Glatt M, Gillespie MT, et al. Glycoprotein 130 regulates bone turnover and bone size by distinct downstream signaling pathways. J Clin Invest 2004 Feb;113(3):379–89.

[219] Martin TJ, Sims NA. Osteoclast-derived activity in the coupling of bone formation to resorption. Trends Mol Med 2005 Feb;11(2):76–81.

[220] Takeuchi Y, Watanabe S, Ishii G, Takeda S, Nakayama K, Fukumoto S, et al. Interleukin-11 as a stimulatory factor for bone formation prevents bone loss with advancing age in mice. J Biol Chem 2002 Dec 13;277(50):49011–8.

[221] Cornish J, Callon K, King A, Edgar S, Reid IR. The effect of leukemia inhibitory factor on bone in vivo. Endocrinology 1993 Mar;132(3):1359–66.

[222] Pederson L, Ruan M, Westendorf JJ, Khosla S, Oursler MJ. Regulation of bone formation by osteoclasts involves Wnt/BMP signaling and the chemokine sphingosine-1-phosphate. Proc Natl Acad Sci USA 2008 Dec 30;105(52):20764–9.

[223] Shimada T, Mizutani S, Muto T, Yoneya T, Hino R, Takeda S, et al. Cloning and characterization of FGF23 as a causative factor of tumor-induced osteomalacia. Proc Natl Acad Sci USA 2001 May 22;98(11):6500–5.

[224] Ferron M, Wei J, Yoshizawa T, Del Fattore A, DePinho RA, Teti A, et al. Insulin signaling in osteoblasts integrates bone remodeling and energy metabolism. Cell 2010 Jul 23;142(2): 296–308.

[225] Oury F, Sumara G, Sumara O, Ferron M, Chang H, Smith CE, et al. Endocrine regulation of male fertility by the skeleton. Cell 2011 Mar 4;144(5):796–809.

3

The Central Control of Bone Mass

Shu Takeda

Keio University, Tokyo, Japan

INTRODUCTION

All homeostatic functions including bone remodeling are regulated by the central nervous system, specifically by the hypothalamus. Indeed, the existence of a neuronal regulatory system for bone remodeling has long been mentioned in the clinical literature. Osteoporosis is a well-known complication of stroke, spinal cord injury, and peripheral neuropathy [1]. In addition, various neuropeptides and neurotransmitters are expressed in bone [2,3]. However, until recently, the physiological role of these molecules was unknown. The first molecular demonstration of the central control of bone remodeling, i.e. control of bone remodeling by leptin, was performed a decade ago [4]. Since then, cell-type specific genetic manipulation in mice has allowed studies to uncover the unappreciated role of neuropeptides and neurotransmitters in bone remodeling.

LEPTIN

Leptin is a 16-kDa peptide hormone secreted by adipocytes that was identified through the positional cloning of the mutation in morbidly obese (*ob/ob*) mice [5]. Subsequently, it was shown that leptin functions in various physiological processes beyond its role in energy metabolism; those are reproduction, immune regulation, and hematopoietic cell differentiation [6]. Therefore, mice lacking either functional leptin or the leptin receptor (*ob/ob* or *db/db* mice, respectively) develop obesity, hypogonadotropic hypogonadism, among other abnormalities [6]. Most of the actions of leptin are mediated through the functional form of its receptor, OBRb, which is located in the central nervous system [7]. Indeed, the intracerebroventricular infusion of leptin rescues most, if not all, of the phenotypes observed in *ob/ob* mice [6].

In 2000 it was shown that, despite their hypogonadism *ob/ob* and *db/db* mice have increased bone mass (Fig. 3.1). A histomorphometric analysis revealed that this increase in bone mass results from a nearly two-fold increase in bone formation overcoming the increase in bone resorption that hypogonadism creates. Although this phenotype is observed in both male and female mice, the strongest effect is observed in the vertebrae of females [4]. Interestingly, leptin only affects trabecular bone, as cortical bone is not affected in *ob/ob* mice [4,8]. Conversely, overexpression of *leptin* in the liver of mice using the serum amyloid P promoter or the apolipoprotein E promoter resulted in low bone mass due to a decrease in bone formation [9]. Moreover, several mouse models of lipodystrophy caused by the overexpression of the dominant negative form of b-ZIP or the hypomorphic allele of *PPARγ*, which are both transcription factors essential for adipocyte differentiation, have increased bone mass despite decreased serum leptin levels and body weight [9,10]. Thus, leptin signaling regulates bone mass accrual regardless of its influence on body weight, the analysis of the bone phenotype of the *ob/ob* mice was the first indication that the high bone mass, reported in obese patients, may not be a mere consequence of their obesity.

That intracerebroventricular (ICV) infusions of leptin in *ob/ob* or wild-type mice decrease bone mass, whereas leptin treatment has no detectable effects on osteoblasts, provided the first indication that this hormone uses a central neuronal relay to regulate bone mass (Fig. 3.1) [4]. In contrast, other studies have reported the putative effects of leptin on osteoblasts [11–13]; however, most of these studies used pharmacological doses of leptin, calling into question their relevance to physiology. The best evidence that leptin acts centrally to regulate bone mass accrual came from *in vivo* experiments. Mice lacking the leptin receptor in neurons have

Translational Endocrinology of Bone
DOI: http://dx.doi.org/10.1016/B978-0-12-415784-2.00003-8

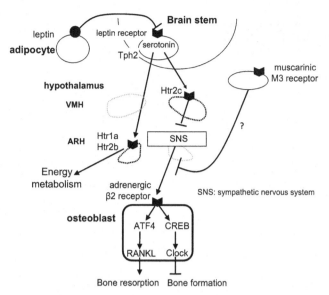

FIGURE 3.1 **Control of bone remodeling by leptin, sympathetic nervous system and serotonin.** Leptin secreted by adipocytes binds its receptor in the brain stem and inhibits serotonin synthesis. Subsequently, serotonin inhibits sympathetic nervous system activity, which, in turn, decreases bone mass.

The leptin-mediated decrease in bone mass has been observed in other species. The decrease in bone mass due to ICV infusion of leptin has been verified in both rats and sheep [19,20]. More importantly, patients harboring a mutation in the leptin gene have increased bone mass [9]. Lipodystrophic patients, whose serum leptin levels are extremely low due to the absence of adipocytes, develop advanced bone age and osteosclerotic lesions [9]. In most large-scale human epidemiological studies, the serum concentration of leptin is negatively associated with bone mineral density after adjusting fat mass and other covariates [21–25], which is consistent with data obtained from mouse studies; however, this association is not observed in smaller studies [26]. The serum concentration of leptin is correlated with body mass index; thus, in obesity, serum leptin levels increase but do not reduce body weight (leptin resistance). Therefore, caution should be taken when evaluating the "net" effect of serum leptin on bone. In addition, the differences in the skeletal sites, gender, and ages affected by leptin require further clarification.

a bone phenotype similar as the one seen *db/db* mice, whereas mice overexpressing leptin or mice lacking the leptin receptor in osteoblasts have no overt bone abnormalities [14]. Interestingly, the amount of leptin required to normalize bone mass is significantly less than the one needed to normalize food intake [9]. In addition, *ob/+* mice have increased bone mass with normal appetite and body weight and 4-week-old *ob/ob* mice have normal body weight but increased bone mass [4]. These results imply that the function of leptin in bone is as important as its function in energy metabolism.

The regulation of food intake and energy expenditure is primarily controlled by the hypothalamus, which receives adipostatic signals, including leptin, from the peripheral adipose tissue [15]. Neurons of the hypothalamic arcuate nucleus (ARH) and ventromedial nucleus (VMH) express *OBRb* at high level and play an important role in leptin regulation [16]. In the ARH, leptin affects the proopiomelanocortin (POMC) and AgRP/NPY pathways, which lead to an increase and decrease in food intake, respectively [17]. Ablating the ARH by lesioning causes body weight gain, which is not ameliorated by the ICV infusion of leptin, indicating that leptin requires an intact ARH to affect body weight [18]. In contrast, the ablation of the VMH by lesioning leads to an increase in bone mass accompanied by body weight gain [18]. Importantly, ICV infusion of leptin does not affect the bone mass in the VMH-lesioned mice. These results demonstrated the importance of the integrity of VMH for leptin to decrease bone mass.

SYMPATHETIC NERVOUS SYSTEM (SNS)

The nature of the signaling machinery downstream of leptin that mediates its influence on bone mass accrual was characterized using parabiotic mice [18]. Two *ob/ob* mice were surgically united to allow exchange of blood. This was followed by ICV infusion of leptin to only one mouse of each pair. The mouse that was directly infused with leptin lost bone, whereas the contralateral mouse did not, indicating the neuronal nature of the molecule involved in the leptin-dependent signaling pathway for bone remodeling. *Ob/ob* mice display low SNS activity [27], and ICV infusion or injection of leptin into the VMH, which is needed for leptin regulation of bone mass, into *ob/ob* or wild-type mice increases SNS activity [28], indicating that the SNS might be involved in the leptin-dependent bone remodeling signaling pathway. Clinically, complex regional pain syndrome type I, or reflex sympathetic dystrophy, which develops after trauma, is characterized by the local activation of the SNS accompanied with osteoporosis [29].

The SNS ligands norepinephrine and epinephrine are synthesized from dopamine by the action of dopamine β-hydroxylase (DBH). *Dbh−/−* mice are unable to produce norepinephrine and epinephrine and display an increased bone mass due to an increase in bone formation, similar what is observed in *ob/ob* mice [18]. Among the many adrenergic receptors (ARs), the adrenergic β2 (adrb2) receptor is the most abundantly expressed in bone. *Adrb2−/−* mice have increased bone mass [30] and wild-type mice treated with propranolol, a non-selective β blocker, gain bone mass, whereas wild-type mice treated with isopropanol, a non-selective β agonist, or clenbuterol or salbutamol, adrb2-selective agonists, see their bone mass decrease [31]. Moreover, the b2AR agonist decreases the BMD and bone mechanical strength in rats [32]. Thus, these results indicate that the SNS regulates bone remodeling (Fig. 3.1). Notably, adrb2−/− mice have no endocrine abnormalities that would affect bone mass, such as an increase in corticosterone concentration or decrease in sex steroid concentration, which indicates that the bone abnormalities in adrb2−/− mice are not secondary to any endocrine abnormalities.

Mice with reduced SNS activity (Dbh−/−, adrb2−/− mice and propranolol-treated wild-type mice) do not lose bone mass even upon ICV infusion of leptin, indicating that the SNS is the primary downstream pathway of leptin (Fig. 3.1) [18,30]. Moreover, osteoblast-specific adrb2−/− mice recapitulate the bone abnormalities of adrb2−/− mice [33], indicating that it is the adrb2 expressed in osteoblasts and not in other cell types that is responsible for the bone-altering effect of the sympathetic nervous system.

The increase in the bone formation in adb2−/− mice is accompanied by an increase in osteoblast number. The molecular machinery involved in the SNS, altering osteoblast proliferation and hence bone remodeling, involves two different pathways: molecular clocks and AP-1 family transcription factors [34].

The molecular clock is conserved from bacteria to humans, and exists in all cell types of the body. The mammalian molecular clock is composed of the positive regulators Bmal1 and clock, which work as heterodimeric partners, and the negative regulators period (per) 1 and 2 and cryptochrome (cry) 1 and 2, which regulate the 24-h circadian rhythm [35]. The diurnal variation in the markers of bone mineral metabolism has been documented in pre- and early postmenopausal women [36].

Mice lacking both Per genes or both Cry genes have increased bone mass in vertebrae and long bones due to an increase in osteoblast proliferation, similar to that seen in ob/ob and Adrb2−/− mice [34]. Mice deficient in the clock genes are not leptin- or sympathetic-tone deficient but, instead, are resistant to the leptin-mediated decrease in bone mass. These results suggested that the molecular clock is located downstream of the leptin−SNS pathway. That osteoblast-specific per1/2-deficient mice have increased bone mass due to an increase in osteoblast proliferation established that the increase in osteoblast proliferation in the clock gene-mutated mice is cell autonomous [34]. Molecular experiments revealed that in osteoblasts, Per1 and Per2 negatively regulate the expression of c-myc and the G1 cyclins and thereby osteoblast proliferation and that

the absence of Per1 and Per2 or Cry1 and Cry2 leads to an increase in bone mass accrual (Fig. 3.1) [34]. In contrast, AP-1 stimulates the expression of c-myc and the G1 cyclins [34]. Upon stimulation of the SNS through the Adrb2, phosphorylation of cAMP response element binding protein (CREB) is inhibited by an unknown mechanism [33] that results in the downregulation of further downstream effectors, such as the molecular clock and AP-1 transcription factors. Accordingly, osteoblast-specific CREB-deficient mice have low bone mass due to a decrease in bone formation. Thus, in general, the SNS decreases bone formation [34].

The characterization of the neuronal regulation of bone formation implies that bone resorption is also neuronally regulated. This suspicion was reinforced by the fact that Adrb2−/− mice not only have increased bone formation, but they also have decreased bone resorption [30]. In addition, leptin ICV infusion increases bone resorption in wild-type mice [30]. Although Adrb2 is expressed in osteoclasts, the effect of sympathetic signaling on bone resorption occurs through the osteoblasts. Upon stimulation of Adrb2, ATF4 is activated through phosphorylation by protein kinase A in osteoblasts. Activated ATF4 induces the expression of receptor activator of nuclear factor kappa-B ligand (Rankl) eventually causing an increase in bone resorption [30]. Indeed, RANKL expression is decreased in Adrb2−/− mice and osteoblast-specific inactivation of ATF4 results in the inhibition of bone resorption. Therefore, leptin−SNS activity stimulates bone resorption through the osteoblasts (Fig. 3.1).

The various mouse models of osteoporosis, such as ovariectomy- [18], unloading- [37], or depression-induced bone loss [38], are all ameliorated by treatment with β-blockers. These results imply that, at least in mice, the pathogenesis of osteoporosis includes a neural component. However, there are some conflicting reports, and these discrepancies might be related to the amount of β-blockers used in each study: low doses of propranolol, which does not affect cardiovascular functions, increase bone formation parameters, and increasing the doses of propranolol progressively decreases its beneficial effects on bone [39]. In addition, mice lacking Adrb2 and Adrb1 have reduced bone mass. Because mouse osteoblasts do not express Adrb1, and because Adrb1/2−/− mice have lower serum IGF-1 concentrations, it is likely that Adrb1 exerts its action on bone indirectly [40]. In addition, mice lacking all three b-receptors have increased bone mass, indicating that adrb3 is also involved in bone remodeling [41].

Many epidemiological studies have confirmed the effect of β-blockers on bone mass or fracture [42,43]. Although there are some conflicting results showing either the beneficial or neutral effects of β-blockers on the prevention of osteoporotic fractures, a meta-analysis of eight studies demonstrated that the use of β-blockers is associated with the reduction of hip or general fracture [43]. The absence of a protective effect of β-blockers on fracture also supports the specificity of the beta-adrenergic pathway. One trial, which did not include the use of β1-blocker, failed to demonstrate a protective effect [44]. This result indicates that in humans, β1 receptor signaling is also related to the protective effect of β-blockers on bone, or alternatively, that this study did not have enough statistical power to detect an effect.

Because β-blockers are already widely used in clinical medicine, they could also be easily applied to the treatment of osteoporosis. However, because most of the studies addressing the relationship between β-blockers and osteoporotic fracture are observational studies, long-term prospective randomized clinical trials are needed.

Other adrenergic and muscarinic receptors are also involved in bone remodeling. *M3 muscarinic receptor−/−* and neuron-specific *M3 muscarinic receptor*-deficient mice, which both have increased SNS activity, have reduced bone mass due to a decrease in bone formation and an increase in bone resorption [45], whereas the osteoblast-specific *M3 muscarinic receptor−/−* mice do not have bone abnormalities (Fig. 3.1) [45]. These results demonstrate that the parasympathetic nervous system affects bone mass by targeting neurons, and the balance between the parasympathetic and autonomic nervous systems defines bone mass. Moreover, *α2Aα2C adrenergic receptor−/−* mice have increased bone mass despite an increase in the activity of the sympathetic nervous system, and selective α2 adrenergic receptor agonists increase osteoclast formation [46], indicating that α2-adrenergic receptors are also involved in bone remodeling. Whether these observations might be applied to humans remains unknown.

SEROTONIN

The technological advances allowing for neuron-specific deletion of a gene of interest have greatly contributed to our understanding of how bone remodeling is controlled by the central nervous system. Steroidogenic factor-1 (SF-1) is a nuclear receptor that regulates adrenal and reproductive development and function, and it is expressed in the adrenal glands, gonads, and in the VMH in the hypothalamus [47]. Thus, SF-1 promoter-driven *Cre* mice crossed with leptin receptor floxed mice only lack leptin receptor in SF-1 positive neurons within the VMH; these mice are obese but

only on a high-fat diet, indicating that the fundamental role of leptin, namely the control of appetite in animals fed a normal diet, was not reproduced [48]. In addition, these mice do not have any bone abnormalities. These results contrasted with the chemical ablation of the VMH that resulted in increased bone mass [48], thus suggesting that leptin targets other neuronal populations and that signal emanating from these neurons may signal to the VMH neurons to regulate SNS activity and bone metabolism. This hypothesis was recently verified.

Serotonin is a monoamine neurotransmitter that is primarily found in the gastrointestinal (GI) tract and central nervous system (CNS) [49]. It is synthesized in two steps: first, L-tryptophan is hydroxylated into L-5-hydroxytryptophan by a specific tryptophan hydroxylase (Tph) in a rate-limiting manner; second, Tph is decarboxylated by an L-amino acid decarboxylase. Clinically, tryptophan has antidepressant activities, and the expression of 5-HIAA, a primary serotonin metabolite, is reduced in the cerebrospinal fluid of depressed patients, indicating that the serotonin concentration in the central nervous system is a determinant of mood and behavior. Indeed, selective serotonin reuptake inhibitors, which increase the extracellular levels of serotonin by inhibiting its reuptake into presynaptic cells and thereby raising the levels of serotonin in the synaptic cleft available to bind to the postsynaptic receptor, are often prescribed for the treatment of depression and anxiety disorders. Interestingly, patients with carcinoid syndrome, which is characterized by a marked elevation of serotonin in the serum produced by carcinoid tumors in the gastrointestinal tract, do not demonstrate a change in mental status or autonomic nervous system activity [50]; these symptoms are associated with increased serotonin levels in the brain. In a contrast, the deletion of the Tph1 gene, which is expressed in the gastrointestinal tract and not in the brain, does not affect the serotonin concentrations in the brain or the mental status of mice [51]. These results suggest that serotonin does not cross the blood−brain barrier and, more importantly, that there must be another enzyme in the brain that compensates for the loss of Tph1. *Tph2* was later cloned and identified as a tryptophan hydroxylase (Tph) in the brain. In *Tph2−/−* mice, serotonin is undetectable in the brain whereas the serum serotonin levels are normal [52]. Epidemiological studies have revealed that the use of selective serotonin reuptake inhibitor (SSRI) antidepressants is associated with hip fractures or reduced bone mineral densities [53−55], indicating a role for serotonin in bone remodeling in humans. Consistent with this observation, serotonin transporter, i.e. 5-hydroxy-tryptamine transporter (5-HTT), knockout mice, which are unable to reuptake serotonin, also have reduced bone mass [56].

In contrast to the increase in bone mass observed in *Tph1−/−* mice (see chapter 5), *Tph2−/−* mice harbor a low bone mass secondary to a decrease in bone formation and an increase in bone resorption. Moreover, they also show a decrease in appetite and body weight and an increase in energy expenditure [52]. The bone phenotype of *Tph2−/−* mice mirrors the one observed in *Adrb2−/−* mice. In fact, the serum concentration of catecholamine, and hence the sympathetic nervous system activity, is increased in *Tph2−/−* mice [52]. Because leptin also uses the sympathetic nervous system to regulate bone remodeling, the interaction of the leptin- and serotonin-signaling pathways was investigated. First, it was shown that *ObRb* is expressed in the serotonin-producing neurons in the raphe nuclei of the brainstem. Second, leptin localizes to the leptin receptors in the serotonin-producing neurons when infused ICV. Third, the serotonin concentration in the brain of *ob/ob* mice increases, and leptin ICV infusions alter serotonin turnover, synthesis, and distribution, resulting in a decrease in serotonin concentrations in the brain. These results revealed a functional interaction between serotonin and leptin. The most rigorous proof was obtained by the selective inactivation of *ObRb* in serotonin-producing neurons using serotonin transporter promoter-driven cre mice [52]. These (serotonergic neuron-specific, *ObRb*-deficient) mice have hyperphagia, reduced energy expenditure and increased bone mass due to an increase in bone formation and decreased bone resorption. Hence, they are a phenocopy of *ob/ob* mice. Most importantly, the absence of one allele of *Tph2* reduces serotonin concentrations in the brain of *ob/ob* mice and results in the normalization of food intake, energy expenditure, and bone mass, thereby formally establishing the link between leptin signaling in the brain and serotonin in the regulation of energy and bone metabolism. Furthermore, only serotonergic neuron-specific, *ObRb*-deficient mice, not ARH-specific *ObRb*-deficient mice developed obesity, reduced energy expenditure, and increased bone mass, indicating that serotonergic neurons in the brainstem are the primary, if not the sole, pathway by which leptin regulates energy and bone metabolism (Fig. 3.1) [52].

Serotonin binds 14 different receptors, which are arranged in seven different groups (Htr1-7) [49]. Among these receptors, Htr2c is most abundantly expressed in the hypothalamus, especially in the SF1-expressing VMH. In addition, serotonergic neurons in the brainstem project to the VMH. Both *Htr2c−/−* mice and, more importantly, *Htr2c+/−/Tph2+/−* mice have the same low bone mass phenotype as *Tph2−/−* mice, demonstrating a genetic link between Tph2 and Htr2c in the regulation of bone metabolism (Fig. 3.1). Furthermore, the restoration of Htr2c expression only in the SF-1 positive neurons is sufficient to rescue the bone abnormalities in Htr2c mice, i.e. the reduced bone mass, decreased bone formation, and increased bone resorption, which are all induced by SNS activity, establishing that Htr2c in the *Sf-1*-positive VMH neurons is responsible for the serotonin modulation of SNS activity and bone remodeling. Molecular analysis revealed that serotonin activates CaMKK-β, CaMK-IV, and the downstream target Creb via phosphorylation in the VMH neurons, and the activation of Creb downregulates SNS activity [57].

Serotonergic neurons in the brainstem also project into the ARH. Among the many 5-HT receptors, increased levels of Htr1a and modest levels of Htr2b and Htr2c are expressed in the ARH. In the ARH, α-MSH, produced by proteolytic processing of POMC, and its receptor MC4R play a major role in the regulation of food intake and energy metabolism [58]. *Htr1a−/−*, *Pomc*-specific *Htr1a*-deficient, or *Pomc*-specific *Htr2b*-deficient mice, but not *Htr2c−/−* mice, exhibit a decrease in food intake and an increase in MC4R and POMC expression. Thus, Htr1a and Htr2b exert some physiological function in the regulation of food intake (Fig. 3.1). However, it remains unclear if there is any genetic link between *Tph2* and *Htr1a* or *Htr2b*, i.e. if serotonin acts via Htr1a and Htr2b to regulate food intake. In addition, energy expenditure is not altered in either the *Htr1a−/−* or *Pomc*-specific *Htr2b*-deficient mice, which indicates that other receptors and pathways are responsible for the increase in energy expenditure observed in *Tph2−/−* mice. In the ARH, serotonin binding to Htr1a, which is a Gs protein-coupled receptor, activates CREB by inducing its phosphorylation; CREB then decreases expression of *Mc4R* and *Pomc*, thereby stimulating appetite. Indeed, compound heterozygous *Htr1a+/−*, POMC-specific Creb-deficient heterozygote mice are lean and have decreased appetites [59]. Further analyses have revealed that leptin, serotonin, and Htr1a-dependent signaling are also involved in neuropeptide VF, a satiety factor, and aspartoacylase 3, both of which are mutated in patients with increased appetites [59]. Moreover, the Htr1a antagonist LY426965 decreases food intake and body weight in *ob/ob* mice; however, energy expenditure is not affected.

Thus, leptin first binds to ObRb in serotonin-producing neurons, and decreases the synthesis of serotonin in these neurons that project into the VMH and ARH. Subsequently, the decreased serotonin content in the VMH upregulates SNS activity via Htr2c to regulate bone metabolism; the decreased serotonin content in the ARH, presumably via Htr1a and Htr2b, activates the POMC–MC4R pathway to regulate energy metabolism.

In contrast, a recent report suggests that leptin regulates serotonin synthesis not by acting in serotonergic neurons but through an interneuron yet to be identified

[60]. The reason for this negative data is unknown and requires further investigation.

NEUROMEDIN U

Neuromedin U (NMU) was first isolated in 1985 from the porcine spinal cord and named for its ability to contract smooth uterine muscles. It was later identified in many species from goldfish to humans [61]. NMU exists in two major forms: a longer 23- to 25-amino acid peptide and a truncated 8- to 9-amino acid C-terminal fragment [61]. Both the long and truncated forms share two characteristics that are necessary for the function of NMU: the amidation of the C-terminus and a conserved C-terminal pentapeptide. In humans, NMU is produced as a pre-peptide that comprises 174 amino acids, which include 34 signal peptides; NMU is secreted and subsequently cleaved to become the mature peptide NMU-25.

NMU is expressed in various tissues, but is most abundant in the gastrointestinal tract. Interestingly, in the intestine, NMU is primarily expressed in the enteric nervous system and not in the smooth muscle layers or the mucosal endocrine cells. Although it is potentially secreted into the circulatory system as a hormone, based on the absence of its expression in endocrine cells and its low concentration in the plasma, NMU likely acts locally as a neuropeptide [61]. In the brain, NMU is present in the striatum and hypothalamus [61].

Two NMU receptors, NMUR1 and NMUR2, have been identified [62]. Both of these receptors belong to the GPCR family, and they share 51% protein sequence identity in humans. In fact, after these receptors were cloned, NMU was characterized as their ligand [61]. NMU has a similar binding affinity and comparable activity with NMUR1 and NMUR2. Therefore, the differences between the physiological functions of NMUR1 and NMUR2 originate from differences in their expression patterns. NMU1R is broadly expressed in regions of peripheral tissue, such as the gastrointestinal tract and the adrenal cortex, but is not expressed in the central nervous system [61]. NMU2R is also expressed, to a lesser extent, in the peripheral tissues, but is primarily expressed in the central nervous system.

Nmu−/− mice [63] have increased bone mass due to an increase in bone formation that is accompanied by an increase in osteoblast proliferation, without alteration of osteoblast differentiation. Cultured Nmu−/− osteoblasts proliferate normally, which indicates that the abnormalities in Nmu−/− osteoblast proliferation are not cell autonomous. In contrast, one report suggested that NMU affects osteoblast proliferation by acting on the osteoblast, although the observed effect was modest [64]. Nevertheless, ICV infusion of NMU decreases bone mass in Nmu−/− mice, which indicates that NMU regulates bone metabolism through the central nervous system (Fig. 3.2) [63]. Because NMU acts as a local factor and not as a hormone, there must be a source of NMU that is responsible for its action on bone; however, this source remains unknown.

The functional relationship between NMU and leptin on bone metabolism was examined in two experiments involving leptin ICV infusions into Nmu−/− mice and NMU into ob/ob mice [63]. After the ICV infusion of leptin, Nmu−/− mice decrease bone mass, which indicates that, similar to its regulation of energy metabolism, NMU does not require leptin to regulate bone mass. Leptin ICV infusion does not decrease bone mass in Nmu−/− mice but rather increases bone mass, which indicates that leptin requires intact NMU signaling to affect bone but does not solely rely on NMU signaling to affect bone. Interestingly, Nmu−/− mice lack a diurnal rhythm of food intake. Moreover, expression of the clock genes was downregulated in Nmu−/− bones, this may explain why Nmu−/− mice develop a high bone mass phenotype and leptin ICV infusion causes a paradoxical increase in their bone mass similar to mice lacking the clock genes (Fig. 3.2).

NMU ICV infusions stimulate the HPA axis and lead to an increase in the secretion of glucocorticoids [65]. Because glucocorticoids are detrimental to bone, it is conceivable that the catabolic action of NMU in bone involves the HPA pathway. However, given that a small decrease in the serum glucocorticoid level does not necessarily lead to an increase in bone mass [66], the increased bone mass observed in Nmu−/− mice, which is accompanied by a small decline in serum glucocorticoid levels [67], is not solely related to reduced

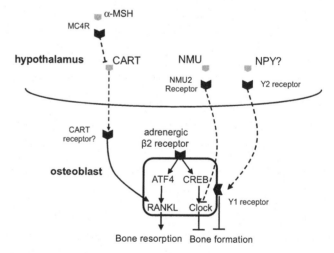

FIGURE 3.2 **Control of bone remodeling by orexigenic/anorexigenic neuropeptides.** Various neuropeptides expressed in the hypothalamic area are involved in bone remodeling. However, the precise molecular action for bone remodeling is unknown.

glucocorticoid secretion; therefore, another mechanism should be involved. Moreover, although acute ICV infusion of NMU induces glucocorticoid secretion and decreases bone mass, it does not elevate serum glucocorticoid levels [68]. These results suggest that the HPA pathway is not the major pathway for the NMU-dependent regulation of bone metabolism.

In humans, the Ala19Glu polymorphism of the NMU gene is associated with obesity [69], which suggests that NMU is also involved in energy metabolism in humans. It would be interesting to study the bone abnormalities in these polymorphic patients.

Because recent reports have shown that leptin acts on the brainstem to regulate energy and bone metabolism [52], it would be interesting to determine if NMU also acts through the brainstem where NMU receptors are expressed.

NEUROPEPTIDE Y (NPY) AND NPY RECEPTORS

NPY is expressed in the central and peripheral nervous system and has various physiological actions, including the regulation of food intake. Currently, five NPY receptors (Y1, 2, 4, 5, and 6) have been identified [70]. In addition, the Y signaling system is composed of multiple endogenous ligands, including neuropeptide Y (NPY), peptide YY (PYY), and pancreatic polypeptide (PP) [70]. The functions of NPY include the regulation of anxiety-related behavior, cardiovascular and memory function, and energy metabolism. Notably, increased NPY expression in the hypothalamus leads to increased food intake and obesity in mice on a high-sucrose diet [71]. In addition, body weight and food intake is reduced when *ob/ob* mice are crossed with *NPY−/−* mice. Consistent with this observation, NPY-ergic neurons project into the ARH in the hypothalamus, which is a critical nucleus for energy metabolism. The analysis of knockout mice has revealed that Y1 and Y5 are important for appetite regulation [70].

Y2−/− or hypothalamic-specific *Y2−/−* mice develop an increased bone mass phenotype in long bones but not in the vertebrae, which is accompanied by an increase in bone formation due to increased osteoblast activity without a change in osteoblast proliferation. In contrast, bone resorption is unchanged in *Y2−/−* mice. Thus, Y2 signaling affects bone formation through the central nervous system (Fig. 3.2) [72]. Interestingly, NPY-ergic neuron-specific Y2 receptor-deficient mice develop mild phenotypes in trabecular bone and no abnormalities in cortical bone, indicating that the main pathway downstream of Y2 receptor

signaling in the hypothalamus does not involve the NPY neurons [73].

Y1−/− mice also have increased bone mass due to an increase in bone formation, despite increased osteoclast surfaces [74]. However, hypothalamus-specific *Y1−/−* mice have normal bone mass, suggesting that Y1 receptor signaling affects bone remodeling peripherally. Accordingly, treatment of wild-type calvarial osteoblasts with NPY reduces cell numbers and inhibits the cAMP response to PTH in mice, and these effects are abolished in *Y1−/−* osteoblasts cultures, all data suggesting that Y1 regulates bone mass by acting directly on bone cells (Fig. 3.2).

Y1−/−/Y2−/− mice do not have more severe phenotypes than *Y1−/−* mice, indicating that Y1 and Y2 are located in the same signaling pathway. Indeed, the germline deletion of Y2 significantly reduces the expression of Y1 in osteoblasts, which potentially explains the increased bone mass observed in Y2-deficient mice (Fig. 3.2) [75].

Though *Y4−/−* mice have normal bone, *Y2/Y4* double mutant mice have a higher bone mass than *Y2−/−* mice due to an increase in the rate of bone formation. Notably, serum leptin levels in *Y2/Y4* double mutant mice are lower than in *Y2* single mutant mice, suggesting an indirect effect on bone remodeling through leptin signaling by Y4 [76]. To date, there is no evidence of an interaction between Y receptor signaling and the SNS in bone remodeling.

The ligand responsible for the Y receptor-dependent bone remodeling has been investigated. ICV infusions or viral delivery of NPY into the ARH causes bone loss in wild-type mice. Because *NPY−/−* mice have normal bone mass, a ligand other than NPY is responsible for the Y2 receptor-dependent bone regulation. However, in contrast, an increased bone mass in *NPY−/−* mice has also been reported. This discrepancy could be attributed to the difference in background. In the periphery, NPY is expressed in osteocytes at higher level than in osteoblasts, and its expression is reduced through mechanical loading. Given that osteocytes are considered as a mechanosensor, NPY might play a role in the stimulation of bone formation upon loading [77].

COCAINE- AND AMPHETAMINE-REGULATED TRANSCRIPTS

The increased bone mass phenotype in *ob/ob* mice is due to a decrease in SNS activity. Increased bone resorption was initially considered to be due to hypogonadism. However, gonadectomized *Adrb2−/−* mice, which should recapitulate the bone phenotype of *ob/ob* mice, have decreased bone resorption, which suggests that SNS is not the sole mediator of the action of leptin in bone resorption. One characteristic change in *ob/ob* mice is a reduction of CART expression [30]. CART is a neuropeptide expressed broadly in the central nervous system, including the ARH where it is co-expressed with *Pomc*, and in peripheral organs, such as the pancreas and adrenal gland [78], but it is not expressed in bone. ICV infusions of CART decrease food intake, whereas antisera against CART increase food intake [78]. CART expression is almost undetectable in *ob/ob* mice, and leptin ICV infusions into *ob/ob* mice restore its expression. Thus, CART is a neuropeptide which is located downstream of leptin signaling although *Cart−/−* mice have normal appetite [78].

Cart−/− mice demonstrate a reduced bone mass phenotype due to an increase in bone resorption and osteoclast number, while bone formation is unchanged [30], indicating that CART regulates bone resorption *in vivo*. The decreased *Cart* expression in *ob/ob* mice explains their increase in bone resorption. In addition, *Cart−/−* mice lose bone mass to a greater extent than wild-type mice in response to leptin ICV infusion, further indicating that CART is involved in the leptin-dependent bone resorption *in vivo*.

CART is not expressed in bone, *Cart−/−* pre-osteoclasts normally differentiate into osteoclasts upon stimulation with RANKL and M-CSF and CART treatment of osteoclasts does not affect their differentiation; thus, CART does not directly act on osteoclasts to regulate bone resorption. Instead, in *Cart−/−* bones, expression of *Rankl* is increased, which indicates that CART regulates bone resorption through osteoblasts (Fig. 3.2).

Interestingly, ICV infusions or viral delivery of CART in the hypothalamus do not rescue the bone resorption phenotype of *Cart−/−* mice; instead, *Cart* overexpression in bone, which leads to an increase in serum CART concentrations, increases bone mass in wild-type mice and *Cart−/−* mice, indicating that CART regulates bone remodeling as a hormone (Fig. 3.2) [79]. Considering that CART does not affect osteoclastogenesis when added in culture, CART must regulate bone remodeling indirectly via organs other than bone by an unidentified mechanism. In addition, the observation that CART polymorphisms affect bone mass in postmenopausal women suggests that CART regulates bone remodeling in other species [80]. However, the identification of CART receptor has not been achieved yet.

MELANOCORTIN AND MC4R

Melanocortins, namely α-MSH, β-MSH, γ-MSH, and adrenocorticotropic hormone, are biologically active neuropeptides processed from the single precursor protein proopiomelanocortin (POMC) [58]. The cell bodies of the POMC neurons are located in the ARH and the nucleus tractus solitarius of the brainstem. Both of these areas have well-defined functions related to appetite and food intake. Five melanocortin receptors (MC1R-5R) belonging to the G-protein coupled receptor family have been characterized to date. Of these, MC3R and MC4R are expressed in the hypothalamus and demonstrate high binding affinity to α-MSH. α-MSH, MC3R, and MC4R are critically involved in the regulation of energy metabolism. Specifically, *POMC−/−*, *Mc4r−/−*, and *Mc3r−/−* mice all develop obesity due to an increase in food intake and reduced locomotor activity [58].

Mc4r−/− mice have high bone mass due to a decrease in bone resorption. CART expression is upregulated in the hypothalamus of *Mc4r−/−* mice and the serum CART levels are increased in these mice. Importantly, the increased bone mass phenotype of *Mc4r−/−* and *Mc4r+/−* mice is either ameliorated or normalized upon deletion of one allele of *Cart*, which decreases CART expression without altering the metabolic characteristics of the *Mc4r* mutant mice [81]. Thus, the melanocortin-Mc4R pathway regulates bone mass indirectly by altering CART expression (Fig. 3.2). Accordingly, patients with an *MC4R* mutation also have increased bone mass due to a decrease in bone resorption, which is accompanied by an increase in CART serum concentration as observed in *Mc4r* mutant mice. Importantly, this increased bone mass is not ameliorated by decreasing body weight, further suggesting that the regulation of bone remodeling by MC4R is independent from its action in energy metabolism.

THE CANNABINOID SYSTEM

Cannabinoids are a class of compounds that include plant, synthetic, and endogenous cannabinoids, such as 2-arachidonolglycerol (2-AG) [82]. Cannabinoids display analgesic, psychotropic, and orexigenic effects by binding and modulating the cannabinoid type 1 and 2 receptors (CB1 and CB2, respectively). CB1 is expressed in the central and peripheral neurons, including the SNS, and peripheral tissues, including the gastrointestinal tract, immune cells, and osteoclasts [82]. CB2 is primarily expressed in peripheral tissues, including osteoblasts and osteoclasts.

CB1−/− mice have increased bone mass at a young age and reduced bone mass at an older age in a CD1 background and when backcrossed on a C57BL/6 background [83,84]. This reduced bone mass phenotype is accompanied by an increase in bone resorption. The molecular basis for the phenotypic differences between the backgrounds is not known.

CB1 signaling inhibits the release of norepinephrine by the SNS, which indicates that the reduced bone mass in *CB1−/−* mice might be partly due to an increase in SNS activity [85]. Traumatic brain injury (TBI) accelerates fracture healing in the appendicular skeleton. It was shown that TBI decreases the norepinephrine content in bone via 2-AG and cannabinoid receptor 1 signaling, and a beta agonist rescues the TBI-induced stimulation of osteogenesis [85]. This effect was reduced in *CB1−/−* mice, and the administration of 2-AG to wild-type mice recapitulates the accelerated fracture healing. Thus, these results suggest that the activation of CB1 inhibits SNS activity by regulating the release of NE release.

CB1 also regulates osteoblast and adipocyte differentiation in mesenchymal stromal cells [86]. Osteoblast differentiation is reduced, whereas adipocyte differentiation is increased in bone marrow stromal cells from *CB1−/−* mice or in wild-type cells treated with a CB1 antagonist. The CB1 signaling pathway activates CREB and PPARγ phosphorylation, which accelerates adipocyte differentiation [86]. It has also been shown that the CB1 antagonist/inverse agonist directly regulates osteoclast differentiation and protects against osteoporosis [87].

CB2 is also involved in bone remodeling. *CB2−/−* mice have reduced bone mass with an increase in bone formation and a further increase in bone resorption [88]. A CB2 agonist prevents osteoporosis by increasing bone formation and inhibiting bone resorption [89]. In human studies, single nucleotide polymorphisms and haplotypes encompassing the CNR2 gene encoding CB2 are significantly associated with the susceptibility locus on the human 1p36 chromosome for reduced bone mineral density. No association was found with CNR1, which encodes the CB1 gene in humans [90]. Recently, other receptors and channels related to the endocannabinoid system, including TRPV1 and GPR55, have emerged as molecules involved in bone remodeling [91−93]. Thus, cannabinoids and their receptors regulate bone remodeling by directly affecting bone cells and thorough neuronal pathways.

OTHER CENTRAL HORMONES AND NEUROPEPTIDES REGULATING BONE REMODELING

Melanin concentrating hormone (MCH) is highly expressed in the hypothalamus and has been implicated in the regulation of energy homeostasis. *Mchr1−/−* mice develop osteoporosis in the cortical bone, whereas the amount of trabecular bone is unaffected. This osteoporosis is caused by an increase in bone resorption by an unidentified mechanism [94].

IL-1 is a proinflammatory cytokine produced by many cell types. It binds to two known receptors, IL-1RI and IL-1RII, to exert its action. In addition, the IL-1 receptor antagonist (IL-1ra), a highly selective endogenous competitive IL-1 inhibitor that binds to but does not activate IL-1RI and IL-1RII, inhibits IL-1 signaling. IL-1 receptor I-deficient mice are protected from ovariectomy-induced osteoporosis, and the administration of IL-1ra inhibits bone resorption in ovariectomized mice, indicating a peripheral role for IL-1 in postmenopausal osteoporosis [95,96]. In addition, a central role of IL-1 in regulating bone remodeling has been uncovered [97]. The overexpression of IL-1ra in the central nervous system using the glial fibrillary acidic protein (GFAP) promoter causes bone loss by causing a two-fold increase in bone resorption [97], indicating that IL-1 signaling in the central nervous system is required for the maintenance of normal bone mass.

Oxytocin is a small neuropeptide produced in the hypothalamus, which travels to the posterior lobe of the pituitary where it is released into general circulation. Classically, oxytocin is known to regulate lactation and social behaviors. Surprisingly, oxytocin−/− and oxytocin receptor−/− mice develop osteoporosis via impaired bone formation. Oxytocin stimulates osteoblast differentiation by inducing BMP-2 expression [98]. Thus, oxytocin possesses dual roles in osteoclasts by stimulating osteoclast differentiation through activating NF-kB signaling and by inhibiting bone resorption. The ICV infusion of oxytocin does not affect bone mass and supports the notion that oxytocin regulates bone remodeling by directly acting on bone cells. However, the physiological relevance of MCH, IL-1ra, and oxytocin on bone remodeling in humans remains unknown.

References

[1] Jiang SD, Dai LY, Jiang LS. Osteoporosis after spinal cord injury. Osteoporos Int 2006 Feb;17(2):180−92.

[2] Chenu C. Glutamatergic regulation of bone resorption. J Musculoskelet Neuronal Interact 2002 Sep;2(5):423−31.

[3] Hukkanen M, Konttinen YT, Santavirta S, Paavolainen P, Gu XH, Terenghi G, et al. Rapid proliferation of calcitonin gene-related peptide-immunoreactive nerves during healing of rat tibial fracture suggests neural involvement in bone growth and remodelling. Neuroscience 1993 Jun;54(4):969−79.

[4] Ducy P, Amling M, Takeda S, Priemel M, Schilling AF, Beil FT, et al. Leptin inhibits bone formation through a hypothalamic relay: a central control of bone mass. Cell 2000 Jan 21;100(2):197−207.

[5] Ahima RS, Flier JS. Leptin. Annu Rev Physiol 2000;62:413−37.

[6] Friedman JM, Halaas JL. Leptin and the regulation of body weight in mammals. Nature 1998;395(6704):763−70.

[7] Tartaglia LA. The leptin receptor. J Biol Chem 1997 March 7, 1997;272(10):6093−6.

[8] Hamrick MW, Pennington C, Newton D, Xie D, Isales C. Leptin deficiency produces contrasting phenotypes in bones of the limb and spine. Bone 2004 Mar;34(3):376—83.

[9] Elefteriou F, Takeda S, Ebihara K, Magre J, Patano N, Kim CA, et al. Serum leptin level is a regulator of bone mass. Proc Natl Acad Sci USA 2004 Mar 2;101(9):3258—63.

[10] Cock TA, Back J, Elefteriou F, Karsenty G, Kastner P, Chan S, et al. Enhanced bone formation in lipodystrophic PPARgamma(hyp/hyp) mice relocates haematopoiesis to the spleen. EMBO Rep 2004 Oct;5(10):1007—12.

[11] Steppan C, Crawford D, Chidsey-Frink K, Ke H, Swick A. Leptin is a potent stimulator of bone growth in ob/ob mice. Regul Pept 2000 Aug;92(1—3):73—8.

[12] Thomas T, Gori F, Khosla S, Jensen MD, Burguera B, Riggs BL. Leptin acts on human marrow stromal cells to enhance differentiation to osteoblasts and to inhibit differentiation to adipocytes. Endocrinology 1999 Apr;140(4):1630—8.

[13] Reseland JE, Syversen U, Bakke I, Qvigstad G, Eide LG, Hjertner O, et al. Leptin is expressed in and secreted from primary cultures of human osteoblasts and promotes bone mineralization. J Bone Miner Res 2001 Aug;16(8):1426—33.

[14] Shi Y, Yadav VK, Suda N, Liu XS, Guo XE, Myers Jr MG, et al. Dissociation of the neuronal regulation of bone mass and energy metabolism by leptin in vivo. Proc Natl Acad Sci USA 2008 Dec 23;105(51):20529—33.

[15] Ahima RS, Osei SY. Leptin signaling. Physiol Behav 2004 Apr;81(2):223—41.

[16] Gautron L, Elmquist JK. Sixteen years and counting: an update on leptin in energy balance. J Clin Invest 2011 Jun 1;121(6):2087—93.

[17] Ahima RS, Saper CB, Flier JS, Elmquist JK. Leptin regulation of neuroendocrine systems. Front Neuroendocrinol 2000 Jul;21(3):263—307.

[18] Takeda S, Elefteriou F, Levasseur R, Liu X, Zhao L, Parker KL, et al. Leptin regulates bone formation via the sympathetic nervous system. Cell 2002 Nov 1;111(3):305—17.

[19] Pogoda P, Egermann M, Schnell JC, Priemel M, Schilling AF, Alini M, et al. Leptin inhibits bone formation not only in rodents, but also in sheep. J Bone Miner Res 2006 Oct;21(10):1591—9.

[20] Guidobono F, Pagani F, Sibilia V, Netti C, Lattuada N, Rapetti D, et al. Different skeletal regional response to continuous brain infusion of leptin in the rat. Peptides 2006 Jun;27(6):1426—33.

[21] Weiss LA, Barrett-Connor E, von Muhlen D, Clark P. Leptin predicts BMD and bone resorption in older women but not older men: the Rancho Bernardo study. J Bone Miner Res 2006 May;21(5):758—64.

[22] Blum M, Harris SS, Must A, Naumova EN, Phillips SM, Rand WM, et al. Leptin, body composition and bone mineral density in premenopausal women. Calcif Tissue Int 2003 Jul;73(1):27—32.

[23] Ruhl CE, Everhart JE. Relationship of serum leptin concentration with bone mineral density in the United States population. J Bone Min Res 2002 Oct;17(10):1896—903.

[24] Sato M, Takeda N, Sarui H, Takami R, Takami K, Hayashi M, et al. Association between serum leptin concentrations and bone mineral density, and biochemical markers of bone turnover in adult men. J Clin Endocrinol Metab 2001 Nov 1;86(11):5273—6.

[25] Garnett SP, Hogler W, Blades B, Baur LA, Peat J, Lee J, et al. Relation between hormones and body composition, including bone, in prepubertal children. Am J Clin Nutr 2004 Oct;80(4):966—72.

[26] Roemmich JN, Clark PA, Mantzoros CS, Gurgol CM, Weltman A, Rogol AD. Relationship of leptin to bone mineralization in children and adolescents. J Clin Endocrinol Metab 2003 Feb 1;88(2):599—604.

[27] Bray GA, York DA. The MONA LISA hypothesis in the time of leptin. Recent Prog Horm Res 1998;53:95—117.

[28] Satoh N, Ogawa Y, Katsuura G, Numata Y, Tsuji T, Hayase M, et al. Sympathetic activation of leptin via the ventromedial hypothalamus: leptin-induced increase in catecholamine secretion. Diabetes 1999;48(9):1787—93.

[29] Kurvers HA. Reflex sympathetic dystrophy: facts and hypotheses. Vasc Med 1998;3(3):207—14.

[30] Elefteriou F, Ahn JD, Takeda S, Starbuck M, Yang X, Liu X, et al. Leptin regulation of bone resorption by the sympathetic nervous system and CART. Nature 2005 Mar 24;434(7032):514—20.

[31] Bonnet N, Brunet-Imbault B, Arlettaz A, Horcajada MN, Collomp K, Benhamou CL, et al. Alteration of trabecular bone under chronic beta2 agonists treatment. Med Sci Sports Exerc 2005 Sep;37(9):1493—501.

[32] Bonnet N, Beaupied H, Vico L, Dolleans E, Laroche N, Courteix D, et al. Combined effects of exercise and propranolol on bone tissue in ovariectomized rats. J Bone Miner Res 2007 Apr;22(4):578—88.

[33] Kajimura D, Hinoi E, Ferron M, Kode A, Riley KJ, Zhou B, et al. Genetic determination of the cellular basis of the sympathetic regulation of bone mass accrual. J Exp Med 2011 Apr 11;208(4):841—51.

[34] Fu L, Patel MS, Bradley A, Wagner EF, Karsenty G. The molecular clock mediates leptin-regulated bone formation. Cell 2005 Sep 9;122(5):803—15.

[35] Green CB, Takahashi JS, Bass J. The meter of metabolism. Cell 2008 Sep 5;134(5):728—42.

[36] Schlemmer A, Hassager C, Jensen SB, Christiansen C. Marked diurnal variation in urinary excretion of pyridinium cross-links in premenopausal women. J Clin Endocrinol Metab 1992 Mar;74(3):476—80.

[37] Kondo H, Nifuji A, Takeda S, Ezura Y, Rittling SR, Denhardt DT, et al. Unloading induces osteoblastic cell suppression and osteoclastic cell activation to lead to bone loss via sympathetic nervous system. J Biol Chem 2005 Aug 26;280(34):30192—200.

[38] Yirmiya R, Goshen I, Bajayo A, Kreisel T, Feldman S, Tam J, et al. Depression induces bone loss through stimulation of the sympathetic nervous system. Proc Natl Acad Sci USA 2006 Nov 7;103(45):16876—81.

[39] Bonnet N, Laroche N, Vico L, Dolleans E, Benhamou CL, Courteix D. Dose effects of propranolol on cancellous and cortical bone in ovariectomized adult rats. J Pharmacol Exp Ther 2006 Sep;318(3):1118—27.

[40] Pierroz DD, Muzzin P, Glatt V, Bouxsein ML, Rizzoli R, Ferrari SL. Bone loss following ovariectomy is maintained in absence of adrenergic receptor β1 and β2 signaling. J Bone Miner Res 2005;20:S277.

[41] Bouxsein ML, Devlin MJ, Glatt V, Dhillon H, Pierroz DD, Ferrari SL. Mice lacking beta-adrenergic receptors have increased bone mass but are not protected from deleterious skeletal effects of ovariectomy. Endocrinology 2009 Jan;150(1):144—52.

[42] Pasco JA, Henry MJ, Sanders KM, Kotowicz MA, Seeman E, Nicholson GC. Beta-adrenergic blockers reduce the risk of fracture partly by increasing bone mineral density: Geelong Osteoporosis Study. J Bone Miner Res 2004 Jan;19(1):19—24.

[43] Wiens M, Etminan M, Gill SS, Takkouche B. Effects of antihypertensive drug treatments on fracture outcomes: a meta-analysis of observational studies. J Intern Med 2006 Oct;260(4):350—62.

[44] Levasseur R, Dargent-Molina P, Sabatier JP, Marcelli C, Breart G. Beta-blocker use, bone mineral density, and fracture risk in older women: results from the Epidemiologie de l'Osteoporose prospective study. J Am Geriatr Soc 2005 Mar; 53(3):550−2.

[45] Shi Y, Oury F, Yadav VK, Wess J, Liu XS, Guo XE, et al. Signaling through the M(3) muscarinic receptor favors bone mass accrual by decreasing sympathetic activity. Cell Metab 2010 Mar 3; 11(3):231−8.

[46] Fonseca TL, Jorgetti V, Costa CC, Capelo LP, Covarrubias AE, Moulatlet AC, et al. Double disruption of alpha2A- and alpha2C-adrenoceptors results in sympathetic hyperactivity and high-bone-mass phenotype. J Bone Miner Res 2011 Mar;26(3):591−603.

[47] Schimmer BP, White PC. Minireview: steroidogenic factor 1: its roles in differentiation, development, and disease. Mol Endocrinol 2010 Jul;24(7):1322−37.

[48] Dhillon H, Zigman JM, Ye C, Lee CE, McGovern RA, Tang V, et al. Leptin directly activates SF1 neurons in the VMH, and this action by leptin is required for normal body-weight homeostasis. Neuron 2006 Jan 19;49(2): 191−203.

[49] Ducy P, Karsenty G. The two faces of serotonin in bone biology. J Cell Biol 2010 Oct 4;191(1):7−13.

[50] Serotonin Sjoerdsma A. N Engl J Med 1959 Jul 30;261(5):231−7. concl.

[51] Yadav VK, Ryu JH, Suda N, Tanaka KF, Gingrich JA, Schutz G, et al. Lrp5 controls bone formation by inhibiting serotonin synthesis in the duodenum. Cell 2008 Nov 28;135(5):825−37.

[52] Yadav VK, Oury F, Suda N, Liu ZW, Gao XB, Confavreux C, et al. A serotonin-dependent mechanism explains the leptin regulation of bone mass, appetite, and energy expenditure. Cell 2009 Sep 4;138(5):976−89.

[53] Richards JB, Papaioannou A, Adachi JD, Joseph L, Whitson HE, Prior JC, et al. Effect of selective serotonin reuptake inhibitors on the risk of fracture. Arch Intern Med 2007 January 22, 2007;167(2):188−94.

[54] Diem SJ, Blackwell TL, Stone KL, Yaffe K, Haney EM, Bliziotes MM, et al. Use of antidepressants and rates of hip bone loss in older women: the study of osteoporotic fractures. Arch Intern Med 2007 Jun 25;167(12):1240−5.

[55] Haney EM, Chan BK, Diem SJ, Ensrud KE, Cauley JA, Barrett-Connor E, et al. Association of low bone mineral density with selective serotonin reuptake inhibitor use by older men. Arch Intern Med 2007 Jun 25;167(12):1246−51.

[56] Warden SJ, Robling AG, Sanders MS, Bliziotes MM, Turner CH. Inhibition of the serotonin (5-hydroxytryptamine) transporter reduces bone accrual during growth. Endocrinology 2005 Feb;146(2):685−93.

[57] Oury F, Yadav VK, Wang Y, Zhou B, Liu XS, Guo XE, et al. CREB mediates brain serotonin regulation of bone mass through its expression in ventromedial hypothalamic neurons. Genes Dev 2010 Oct 15;24(20):2330−42.

[58] Cone RD. Studies on the physiological functions of the melanocortin system. Endocr Rev 2006 Dec;27(7):736−49.

[59] Yadav VK, Oury F, Tanaka KF, Thomas T, Wang Y, Cremers S, et al. Leptin-dependent serotonin control of appetite: temporal specificity, transcriptional regulation, and therapeutic implications. J Exp Med 2011 Jan 17;208(1): 41−52.

[60] Lam DD, Leinninger GM, Louis GW, Garfield AS, Marston OJ, Leshan RL, et al. Leptin does not directly affect CNS serotonin neurons to influence appetite. Cell Metab 2011 May 4;13(5):584−91.

[61] Brighton PJ, Szekeres PG, Willars GB. Neuromedin U and its receptors: structure, function, and physiological roles. Pharmacol Rev 2004 Jun;56(2):231−48.

[62] Howard AD, Wang R, Pong SS, Mellin TN, Strack A, Guan XM, et al. Identification of receptors for neuromedin U and its role in feeding. Nature 2000 Jul 6;406(6791):70−4.

[63] Sato S, Hanada R, Kimura A, Abe T, Matsumoto T, Iwasaki M, et al. Central control of bone remodeling by neuromedin U. Nat Med 2007 Oct;13(10):1234−40.

[64] Rucinski M, Ziolkowska A, Tyczewska M, Szyszka M, Malendowicz LK. Neuromedin U directly stimulates growth of cultured rat calvarial osteoblast-like cells acting via the NMU receptor 2 isoform. Int J Mol Med 2008 Sep;22(3):363−8.

[65] Hanada T, Date Y, Shimbara T, Sakihara S, Murakami N, Hayashi Y, et al. Central actions of neuromedin U via corticotropin-releasing hormone. Biochem Biophys Res Commun 2003 Nov 28;311(4):954−8.

[66] Braatvedt GD, Joyce M, Evans M, Clearwater J, Reid IR. Bone mineral density in patients with treated Addison's disease. Osteoporos Int 1999;10(6):435−40.

[67] Hanada R, Teranishi H, Pearson JT, Kurokawa M, Hosoda H, Fukushima N, et al. Neuromedin U has a novel anorexigenic effect independent of the leptin signaling pathway. Nat Med 2004 Oct;10(10):1067−73.

[68] Peier A, Kosinski J, Cox-York K, Qian Y, Desai K, Feng Y, et al. The antiobesity effects of centrally administered neuromedin U and neuromedin S are mediated predominantly by the neuromedin U receptor 2 (NMUR2). Endocrinology 2009 Jul;150(7):3101−9.

[69] Hainerova I, Torekov SS, Ek J, Finkova M, Borch-Johnsen K, Jorgensen T, et al. Association between neuromedin U gene variants and overweight and obesity. J Clin Endocrinol Metab 2006 Dec;91(12):5057−63.

[70] Lin S, Boey D, Herzog H. NPY and Y receptors: lessons from transgenic and knockout models. Neuropeptides 2004 Aug;38(4):189−200.

[71] Kaga T, Inui A, Okita M, Asakawa A, Ueno N, Kasuga M, et al. Modest overexpression of neuropeptide Y in the brain leads to obesity after high-sucrose feeding. Diabetes 2001 May;50(5): 1206−10.

[72] Baldock PA, Sainsbury A, Couzens M, Enriquez RF, Thomas GP, Gardiner EM, et al. Hypothalamic Y2 receptors regulate bone formation. J Clin Invest 2002;109(7):915−21.

[73] Shi YC, Lin S, Wong IP, Baldock PA, Aljanova A, Enriquez RF, et al. NPY neuron-specific Y2 receptors regulate adipose tissue and trabecular bone but not cortical bone homeostasis in mice. PLoS One 2010;5(6):e11361.

[74] Baldock PA, Allison SJ, Lundberg P, Lee NJ, Slack K, Lin EJ, et al. Novel role of Y1 receptors in the coordinated regulation of bone and energy homeostasis. J Biol Chem 2007 Jun 29;282(26): 19092−102.

[75] Lundberg P, Allison SJ, Lee NJ, Baldock PA, Brouard N, Rost S, et al. Greater bone formation of Y2 knockout mice is associated with increased osteoprogenitor numbers and altered Y1 receptor expression. J Biol Chem 2007 Jun 29;282(26):19082−91.

[76] Sainsbury A, Baldock PA, Schwarzer C, Ueno N, Enriquez RF, Couzens M, et al. Synergistic effects of Y2 and Y4 receptors on adiposity and bone mass revealed in double knockout mice. Mol Cell Biol 2003 Aug;23(15):5225−33.

[77] Igwe JC, Jiang X, Paic F, Ma L, Adams DJ, Baldock PA, et al. Neuropeptide Y is expressed by osteocytes and can inhibit osteoblastic activity. J Cell Biochem 2009 Oct 15;108(3): 621−30.

[78] Rogge G, Jones D, Hubert GW, Lin Y, Kuhar MJ. CART peptides: regulators of body weight, reward and other functions. Nat Rev Neurosci 2008 Oct;9(10):747−58.

[79] Singh MK, Elefteriou F, Karsenty G. Cocaine and amphetamine-regulated transcript may regulate bone remodeling as a circulating molecule. Endocrinology 2008 Aug;149(8):3933–41.

[80] Guerardel A, Tanko LB, Boutin P, Christiansen C, Froguel P. Obesity susceptibility CART gene polymorphism contributes to bone remodeling in postmenopausal women. Osteoporos Int 2006 Jan;17(1):156–7.

[81] Ahn JD, Dubern B, Lubrano-Berthelier C, Clement K, Karsenty G. Cart overexpression is the only identifiable cause of high bone mass in melanocortin 4 receptor deficiency. Endocrinology 2006 Jul;147(7):3196–202.

[82] Miller LK, Devi LA. The highs and lows of cannabinoid receptor expression in disease: mechanisms and their therapeutic implications. Pharmacol Rev 2011 Sep;63(3):461–70.

[83] Idris AI, van 't Hof RJ, Greig IR, Ridge SA, Baker D, Ross RA, et al. Regulation of bone mass, bone loss and osteoclast activity by cannabinoid receptors. Nat Med 2005 Jul;11(7):774–9.

[84] Tam J, Ofek O, Fride E, Ledent C, Gabet Y, Muller R, et al. Involvement of neuronal cannabinoid receptor CB1 in regulation of bone mass and bone remodeling. Mol Pharmacol 2006 Sep;70(3):786–92.

[85] Tam J, Trembovler V, Di Marzo V, Petrosino S, Leo G, Alexandrovich A, et al. The cannabinoid CB1 receptor regulates bone formation by modulating adrenergic signaling. Faseb J 2008 Jan;22(1):285–94.

[86] Idris AI, Sophocleous A, Landao-Bassonga E, Canals M, Milligan G, Baker D, et al. Cannabinoid receptor type 1 protects against age-related osteoporosis by regulating osteoblast and adipocyte differentiation in marrow stromal cells. Cell Metabolism 2009;10(2):139–47.

[87] Idris AI. Cannabinoid receptors as target for treatment of osteoporosis: a tale of two therapies. Current Neuropharmacol 2010;8(3):243–53.

[88] Ofek O, Karsak M, Leclerc N, Fogel M, Frenkel B, Wright K, et al. Peripheral cannabinoid receptor, CB2, regulates bone mass. Proc Natl Acad Sci USA 2006 Jan 17;103(3):696–701.

[89] Sophocleous A, Landao-Bassonga E. van 't Hof RJ, Idris AI, Ralston SH. The type 2 cannabinoid receptor regulates bone mass and ovariectomy-induced bone loss by affecting osteoblast differentiation and bone formation. Endocrinology 2011 June 1, 2011;152(6):2141–9.

[90] Karsak M, Cohen-Solal M, Freudenberg J, Ostertag A, Morieux C, Kornak U, et al. Cannabinoid receptor type 2 gene is associated with human osteoporosis. Hum Mol Genet 2005 Nov 15;14(22):3389–96.

[91] Idris AI, Landao-Bassonga E, Ralston SH. The TRPV1 ion channel antagonist capsazepine inhibits osteoclast and osteoblast differentiation in vitro and ovariectomy induced bone loss in vivo. Bone 2010 Apr;46(4):1089–99.

[92] Rossi F, Siniscalco D, Luongo L, De Petrocellis L, Bellini G, Petrosino S, et al. The endovanilloid/endocannabinoid system in human osteoclasts: possible involvement in bone formation and resorption. Bone 2009 Mar;44(3):476–84.

[93] Whyte LS, Ryberg E, Sims NA, Ridge SA, Mackie K, Greasley PJ, et al. The putative cannabinoid receptor GPR55 affects osteoclast function in vitro and bone mass in vivo. Proc Natl Acad Sci USA 2009 Sep 22;106(38):16511–6.

[94] Bohlooly YM, Mahlapuu M, Andersen H, Astrand A, Hjorth S, Svensson L, et al. Osteoporosis in MCHR1-deficient mice. Biochem Biophys Res Commun 2004 Jun 11;318(4):964–9.

[95] Kitazawa R, Kimble RB, Vannice JL, Kung VT, Pacifici R. Interleukin-1 receptor antagonist and tumor necrosis factor binding protein decrease osteoclast formation and bone resorption in ovariectomized mice. J Clin Invest 1994 Dec; 94(6):2397–406.

[96] Lorenzo JA, Naprta A, Rao Y, Alander C, Glaccum M, Widmer M, et al. Mice lacking the type I interleukin-1 receptor do not lose bone mass after ovariectomy. Endocrinology 1998 Jun;139(6):3022–5.

[97] Bajayo A, Goshen I, Feldman S, Csernus V, Iverfeldt K, Shohami E, et al. Central IL-1 receptor signaling regulates bone growth and mass. Proc Natl Acad Sci USA 2005 Sep 6; 102(36):12956–61.

[98] Tamma R, Colaianni G, Zhu LL, DiBenedetto A, Greco G, Montemurro G, et al. Oxytocin is an anabolic bone hormone. Proc Natl Acad Sci USA 2009 Apr 28;106(17):7149–54.

4

Neuropeptide Y and Bone Formation

Dr. Paul A. Baldock

University of New South Wales, Sydney, Australia

THE NEUROPEPTIDE Y SYSTEM

NPY is one of the most widely expressed neuropeptides in neural tissues, being expressed in both central and peripheral nervous systems. In the brain, NPY has a complex distribution, with marked expression in a number of regions, with the highest expression levels occurring within the hypothalamus. More specifically, the hypothalamic NPY-ergic neurons are distributed most prominently in the arcuate nucleus [1]. In peripheral nervous tissue, NPY is found in the sympathetic nervous system, co-stored and co-released with noradrenaline during nerve stimulation [2]. While NPY expression was initially discovered in neural tissue, it is increasingly being characterized in peripheral tissues. Importantly, NPY is known to be expressed in osteoblastic cells [3,4]. In addition to NPY, two other ligands of the NPY family exist; peptide YY (PYY) and pancreatic polypeptide (PP). In contrast to NPY, these are both gut-derived peptides with PYY being mainly produced by the endocrine L cells of the colon, rectum, small intestine, stomach, and pancreas [5], and PP being primarily produced in F type cells of the pancreas [6].

All three of these ligands bind a family of G-protein coupled receptors termed the Y receptors. To date, five receptors have been cloned and classified as the Y1, Y2, Y4, Y5, and y6 [7–9], although evidence exists suggesting the possibility of further receptors in this family [10,11]. All Y receptors are expressed in higher organisms including man, although the y6 receptor is absent in the rat and present in a truncated form in the primate and human genome [8]. In the brain, all Y receptors have been demonstrated in high concentration in regions involved in energy intake and energy expenditure, such as the hypothalamus [12]. Due to the initial lack of pharmacological tools, functions of the different Y receptors in vivo have been studied in knockout and transgenic mouse models. However, over recent times various Y receptor selective agonists and antagonists

have also been developed and tested. NPY and PYY have similar receptor binding profiles, with greatest affinity for the Y2 receptors, followed by Y1, Y5, and the least affinity for Y4 receptors [9,10]. Both NPY and PYY can be further processed by a specific protease, dipeptididyl peptidase-IV (DPPIV), which removes the first two amino acids from the N-terminus, producing the truncated forms NPY3-36 or PYY3-36 [13,14]. This post-translational modification specifically attenuates the affinity of the ligands for the Y1 receptor. Thus NPY3-36 and PYY3-36 have affinity for Y2 but not Y1 receptors. In contrast, PP prefers the Y4 receptor with much lower affinity to the other Y receptors.

The Y receptor family displays a high degree of sequence divergence; however, they all use similar signal transduction pathways, acting through G_i or G_o proteins. Functionally, Y receptors have all been shown to mediate their response through inhibiting the accumulation of cyclic adenosine monophosphate (cAMP) [8] (Fig. 4.1). Y receptor signaling has also been shown to induce extracellularly regulated kinase (ERK) phosphorylation, thus indicating the involvement of mitogen-activated protein kinase (MAPK) pathways [21]. This effect has been shown to involve intermediary protein kinase C (PKC) [15] and phosphatidylinositol (PI)-3-kinase [16]. Most Y receptors display post-synaptic/post-junctional expression; however, Y2 receptors are more often pre-synaptic/pre-junctional, with their activation suppressing neurotransmitter release [17,18].

Through their actions on Y these receptors, the NPY family of peptides regulates numerous and diverse physiological processes, perhaps most notably stimulation of food intake and conservation of energy homeostasis [19]. Recently, however, a number of studies have demonstrated their requirement for normal bone homoeostasis. As detailed below, our understanding of the NPY family and its role in the regulation of bone mass is rapidly increasing, and is revealing the marked influence upon the maintenance of bone mass.

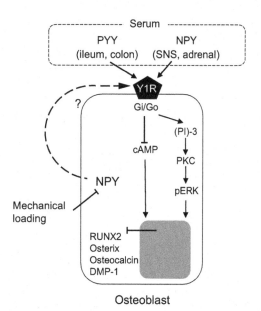

FIGURE 4.1 Local actions of NPY ligands on osteoblast activity. Osteoblasts express the Y1 receptor, which signals NPY and PYY. These ligands originate from the GI tract and adrenals, but NPY is also released from sympathetic neurons (SNS). These act upon the Y1 receptor to inhibit cyclic AMP accumulation and to stimulate ERK phosphorylation. These pathways result in an inhibition of osteoblast gene expression and ultimately and reduction in cell activity. In addition, osteoblast produce NPY, which is regulated by mechanical load; this NPY may be available to signal local Y1 receptors in an autocrine/paracrine manner.

In addition it is revealing an interconnection of skeletal biology with other organ systems, in particular, energy homeostasis, one of NPY's primary regulatory actions.

NEUROPEPTIDE Y AND BONE HOMEOSTASIS

NPY-immunoreactive fibers were identified in bone tissue some time ago, associated with blood vessels. This anatomical localization led to a presumed role of NPY in vasoregulation within the marrow [20–23]. However, NPY-immunoreactive fibers have also been shown located close to opposing osteoblasts and bone lining cells [23,24], suggesting the possibility of direct actions on bone cells. Moreover, in its role as a critical mediator of energy homoeostasis, NPY responds within the hypothalamus to changes in serum leptin [25]. In this manner, the identification of centrally mediated skeletal effects in response to altered leptin signaling indicated the possibility of central actions of NPY, and was the first to be investigated.

Central Actions of NPY on Bone Homoeostasis

The closely integrated biology of leptin and NPY within the hypothalamus rendered NPY as an early candidate for the downstream affecter of the central

leptin pathway to bone. Indeed, an experiment in the initial central leptin manuscript demonstrated that intra-cerebroventricular infusion of NPY into wild-type mice produced a significant reduction in cancellous bone volume [26]. In subsequent studies, the site of NPY action elucidated by demonstrating a similarly anti-osteogenic response following viral vector-mediated overexpression of NPY confined specifically to the hypothalamus [19,27]. The skeletal response to elevated hypothalamic NPY was rapid and cell specific. Tibial bone mineral content was significantly reduced (20%) 3 weeks after viral injection. This bone loss was associated with reductions in mineral apposition rate (up to seven-fold), indicating an inhibition of osteoblast activity, on cortical and cancellous surfaces, with no change in osteoblast number or indices of bone resorption. Interestingly, in the hypothalamus, NPY acts to trigger starvation responses; among these are increased food intake and reduced energy expenditure [19]. Thus the continuous NPY production by the viral construct is perceived within the hypothalamus as a marker of significant calorie deprivation, triggering the starvation responses. As a result, the NPY overexpressing mice increased their body weight by 60% over the 3-week period, while load bearing bone mass (such as the tibiae) was markedly reduced. This result highlights the powerful interactions between the central perceptions of nutritional status, such as elevated NPY expression, and the maintenance of bone mass, and is discussed in more detail in later sections and elsewhere in this volume.

Consistent with a role of central NPY to tonically inhibit osteoblast activity, NPY-null mice display skeleton-wide increases in bone mass. This high bone mass results from an increase in mineral apposition rate in cortical and cancellous surfaces, in axial and appendicular regions [28]. Thus it represents an opposing change to those evident following central NPY overexpression. This increase in osteoblastic activity is supported by increased expression of bone osteogenic transcription factors, RUNX2, and Osterix in bone of NPY-null mice [4]. Despite the consistency of the skeletal response between elevated and reduced NPY, these findings are in contrast to the initial examination of vertebral cancellous bone in NPY knockout mice, which did not detect a difference [29]. Nevertheless, in recent years the NPY-ergic neurons of the hypothalamus have emerged as inhibitors of bone formation.

Local Actions of NPY on Osteoblast Activity

In addition to skeletal changes following alterations in hypothalamic NPY expression, there are non-central actions of the NPY system that alter skeletal homeostasis. NPY knockout mice display elevated osteoblast activity; however, reintroduction of NPY into the hypothalamus of these mice is not sufficient to completely normalize osteoblast function, suggesting the existence of non-central actions in NPY to regulate bone mass [36]. Indeed, NPY has direct effects upon osteoblast activity. NPY treatment of *in vitro* osteoblastic cell lines inhibited the cAMP response to a number of factors including PTH, noradrenaline, and forskolin [3,30,31]. Thus bone cells express functional Y receptors and identify a possible regulatory role for NPY in the periphery. NPY has been shown to inhibit the isoprenaline-induced differentiation of osteoblasts from bone marrow stromal cells [32]. Moreover, NPY administration decreases cell numbers in osteoblast cultures, in a Y1 receptor-dependent manner [33,34]. In differentiated cultures, NPY reduced the expression of late stage genes (osteocalcin and DMP-1) and reduced mineral deposition, consistent with an increase in Y1 receptor expression with maturation in these cells [3]. Interestingly, osteoblasts also produce NPY, but reduce this expression in response to mechanical load [3]; thereby releasing the tonic inhibition of osteoblast activity and contributing to the increase in bone formation. As such, osteoblastic NPY production may be integrated into this fundamental skeletal response, highlighting the importance of neuropeptide signaling to bone biology.

In addition to effects on bone formation, evidence suggests that NPY may also be involved in the control of bone resorption. Loss of NPY Y1 receptor in mice (discussed below) produced an increase in osteoclast surface, without an increase in mineralizing surface [33]. *In vitro*, NPY treatment of osteoblastic cells inhibited RANKL expression and a transient increase in osteoprotegerin (OPG) [35]. NPY has also been shown to selectively inhibit osteoclastogenesis in mouse bone marrow cells induced by isoproterenol and parathyroid hormone (PTH), respectively. This occurred through inhibition of cAMP and RANKL production in a pathway dependent upon intact Y1 receptor signaling [32]. The stimulation of RANKL production by both isoproterenol and PTH is mediated via the cAMP/protein kinase A (PKA) pathway [32]. However, NPY alone did not alter osteoclast formation or osteoclastogenesis induced by $1,25(OH)_2$ vitamin D which utilizes a different signal transduction pathway, or soluble RANKL [33], leading to the suggestion that NPY inhibited osteoclastogenesis by interfering with β-adrenergic-induced cAMP production by stromal cells. Therefore, NPY's effect upon osteoclasts is likely mediated through alterations in osteoblast behavior.

OTHER NPY LIGANDS

Peptide YY

Peptide YY is a member of the NPY family, released in response to feeding by L cells in the ileum and colon;

however, low levels have been detected in the brain stem [6]. Two forms of PYY exist in the circulation, the full length PYY1-36 and the more abundant PYY3-36, produced through action of DPPIV [13,14]. The full length peptide binds both Y1 and Y2 receptors with high affinity, while the short form binds only NPY Y2 receptor [8].

While the link between PYY and food intake is well established, the link between PYY and bone requires further investigation. However, several clinical disorders show alterations in PYY levels as well as altered bone metabolism, which together suggest a negative skeletal effect of PYY. The dramatic reduction in bone mass in anorexia nervosa patients has been significantly associated with the greater PYY levels evident in these individuals [36], particularly at the spine [37]. In anorexia nervosa patients, baseline PYY levels were inversely associated with changes in whole body bone mass [38], consistent with the anti-osteogenic actions of NPY [36]. PYY is also elevated in amenorrheic athletes, and was found to be negatively associated with lumbar BMD Z-scores and the bone formation marker, procollagen type I N-terminal propeptide (PINP), compared to eumenorrheic athletes [39]. This negative association between serum PYY and BMD among premenopausal, exercising women with amenorrhea was confirmed in a subsequent study [40].

Importantly, PYY may play a broader role in the maintenance of bone mass. Obesity is associated with lower levels of PYY [41] and greater BMD [42]. While, in addition, a recent cross-sectional study in healthy premenopausal women reported that circulating PYY has a significant, negative association with total body and hip bone mass [43]. Of interest, variation in PYY explained nearly 9% of the variance in hip bone mineral density in these women, suggesting that PYY may provide a marked determinant of bone mass in the general population. A more detailed understanding of the relationship between PYY and bone is clearly required, particularly with regard to the skeletal effect of increased PYY levels. Together, these disorders suggest a negative correlation between PYY levels and BMD; however, whether these represent a direct effect of PYY on bone or an indirect result of the response to altered energy metabolism remains to be determined.

In contrast to these human studies, a report of the first PYY-null mouse model indicated that knockout of the PYY gene, and with it loss of both forms of PYY, is associated with a reduction in total BMD, BMC, and bone strength [44]. Cancellous bone mass and volume were reduced in the lumbar vertebrae. This is an interesting finding, standing in contrast to the increased bone mass following deletion of NPY and the similar increases in bone mass following deletion of the PYY receptors, Y1R and Y2R, as detailed below. These contradictory findings warrant further investigation into the skeletal effects of PYY. Indeed, ongoing murine studies in an independent PYY KO and PYY overexpressing model (manuscript in preparation), indicate a negative relationship between PYY and bone mass, consistent with emerging human data.

Pancreatic Polypeptide

Pancreatic polypeptide (PP), the third member of the neuropeptide Y family, is released in response to feeding primarily by F type cells in the pancreas [6]. Of all the NPY receptors, PP binds most predominantly to the Y4 receptor. Data do exist suggesting PP may play a role in bone. Both PP and Y4 receptor are found in the transformed murine osteoblastic cell line MC3T3-E1, with PP treatment stimulating differentiation of these cells, suggesting a role for PP in osteoblast differentiation [45]. This is supported by findings from Y4 receptor knockout mice, in which osteoblast number is decreased [46]. However, this role in osteoblast differentiation did not result in altered bone mass in mouse models. Investigation of three related models, Y4 receptor knockout mice, PP knockout mice, and PP transgenic mice [44,46], all have unaltered bone mass. In addition, PP overexpression does not alter bone turnover, including osteoblast surface or number [46]. Interestingly, in male mice, Y2RY4R double knockout produces a greater increase in cancellous bone volume than in mice with deficiency of either the Y2R or Y4 receptor alone. However, this is likely an indirect action through altered leptin production [46] as discussed below. Thus the existence and nature of pancreatic polypeptides' action in bone is uncertain.

THE NPY RECEPTORS

Y1 Receptor

The Y1 receptor, so named because it was the first to be successfully cloned [47], consists of 384 amino acids and binds the NPY family of ligands with the following order of potency: NPY = PYY >> PP [47,48]. Y1 receptor expression, ascribed using mRNA and/or protein detection, was detected in the hypothalamus and hippocampus, several thalamic and amygdaloid nuclei of the rat and mouse [49,50]. In the hypothalamus of humans, as in rodents, Y1 receptor mRNA was detected in the arcuate and paraventricular nuclei [51]. In the periphery, initial rodent studies identified Y1 receptor expression in colon [52], pancreatic β cells [53], and visceral adipose tissues [54]. In subsequent human studies, the Y1 receptor is expressed in the epithelium and mucosal nerves of the colon, in the kidney, adrenal gland, heart, and placenta [55]. Y1 receptor expression

has been detected in bone tissue [3,4], in mesenchymal stem cells and osteoprogenitor cells [56] as well as the osteoblastic lineage, increasing with differentiation [3]. Y1 is also widely expressed in the myeloid lineage, including osteoclasts [57].

Y1 Receptor Control of Bone Homeostasis

Germline deletion of Y1 receptors results a generalized increase in bone mass both cancellous and cortical envelopes, with consistent changes in femoral, tibial, and vertebral bones [33]. Similar to results from NPY-null mice, these anabolic changes were the result of elevation in osteoblast activity. However, this effect was mediated by hypothalamic Y1 receptors. Specific deletion of Y1 receptors from the hypothalamus had no effects on bone homeostasis. This suggested a direct action of Y1 receptor on bone, consistent with the known Y1 receptor expression in osteoblastic and bone marrow stromal cells [4,33]. Indeed, osteoblast-specific Y1 receptor deletion resulted in a similar bone phenotype as those seen in germline Y1 deletion [58]. These bone changes occurred in the absence of obesity, hyperinsulinemia or other metabolic changes reported in germline Y1R knockout mice [33]. Moreover, the greater bone resorption and RANKL:OPG of germline Y1R KO mice was absent in the osteoblastic Y1 knockout mice, indicating maturation-dependent effects of Y1 to regulate osteoclastogenesis. These findings highlight that antagonizing Y1 receptors may have beneficial effects on bone mass.

The Y2 Receptor

The Y2 receptor is a highly conserved 381 amino acid protein that has maintained over 90% identity between orders of mammals [59]. The Y2 receptor binds to NPY and PYY with equally high affinity, but with low affinity for PP [8,9]. In addition, the Y2 receptor, but not Y1R, exhibits high affinity to NPY3-36 and PYY3-36 [9], produced endogenously by a specific protease, dipeptididyl peptidase-IV (DPPIV) [14], itself a pharmacological target [60]. Thus DPPIV treatment would block Y1 receptor (osteoblastic) signaling but not alter Y2 receptor (hypothalamic) signaling. Currently, no assay available is able to consistently distinguish between these truncated variants of NPY or PYY. This may contribute to variation in response reported studies examining these peptides under varying physiological conditions.

The Y2 receptor is expressed predominantly in a presynaptic location, acting to suppress the release of neurotransmitters into the synaptic cleft [63]. It is the most prominent Y-receptor in the central nervous system, representing approximately two thirds of the total binding capacity for NPY [11]. In the brain, Y2 receptor mRNA can be found within the hypothalamus, hippocampus, and amygdala, as well as in specific nuclei of the brain stem [61]. Y2 receptors regulate a wide variety of physiological functions, including circadian rhythm [62,63], vasoconstriction [22,64], angiogenesis [65], gastric emptying [66], and stress-coping behaviors [67]. Activation of Y2 receptors promotes the induction of satiety, generating great interest in Y2R as a potential anti-obesity treatment using compounds such as PYY3-36. Importantly, central Y2 receptors expression in the arcuate nucleus of the hypothalamus and the area postreama in the brain stem [61] are exposed with circulating factors, such as PYY, and are areas known to have a semi-permeable blood–brain barrier [68]. These regions are also important for NPY's response to changes in other circuiting factors such as leptin [69], as discussed below.

Y2 Receptor Control of Bone Homeostasis

A significant role for Y2 receptors in the regulation of bone metabolism has been revealed following study of Y2 receptor knockout mice. Germline deletion of Y2 receptors resulted in a skeleton-wide increase in bone mass, with a two-fold greater cancellous bone volume and significantly greater cortical bone mass, compared with control mice [34,70,71]. This increase was associated with an increase in osteoblast activity, specifically an increase in mineral apposition rate, with no differences in mineralizing surface or osteoblast number. Moreover, bone turnover was unaltered, as osteoclast surface was not different from control. Thus Y2R signaling regulates the activity of osteoblastic cells but does not alter cell number.

The alterations in bone mass were accompanied by changes in body composition, with increased lean mass and reduced fat mass. This promotion of lean mass at the expense of fat mass is consistent with alterations in the hypothalamo–pituitary–somatotropic axis [72]. Indeed, within the hypothalamus, Y2 receptors co-localize with GHRH neurons [73]. This Y2 receptor-mediated regulation of the somatotropic axis highlights the central actions of these receptors, and moreover the potential for the skeletal phenotype to be the result of signaling within the brain. Indeed, hypothalamus-specific deletion of Y2 receptors recapitulated the bone phenotype observed in germline Y2 knockout mice [71]. This finding demonstrates the key role of hypothalamic Y2 receptors in regulating bone metabolism. Moreover, these studies identify multiple advantages of antagonizing Y2 receptor as a therapy in osteoporotic populations; stimulating bone formation, while also stimulating lean mass: an action important in those

with lower body weight who represent a high fracture-risk population [74].

Despite the isolation of the skeletal effects of Y2 receptors to the hypothalamus, the specific neuronal species responsible remain to be defined. A recent study, however, investigated the role of NPY signals in the Y2 receptor pathway to bone. Ablation of hypothalamic Y2 receptors specifically from NPY-ergic neurons resulted in moderate increases in cancellous bone volume, and no effect on cortical bone mass [75]. Thus within the hypothalamus, the Y2 receptor pathway to bone is mediated through neuronal populations other than NPY neurons, and, in addition, the NPY pathway to bone is not signaled through Y2 receptors. A number of potential signaling pathways for hypothalamic NPY remain to be investigated. Y5 receptors, which are expressed in the paraventricular nucleus, a critical nucleus for NPY-ergic neurons, represent one such unexplored pathway by which arcuate NPY-ergic neurons may affect bone. Y5 receptors are co-expressed on NPY target neurons along with Y1 receptors. Previous studies indicate that deletion of Y1 receptors from the paraventricular nucleus does not alter bone mass [33]. Deletion of Y1R may not be sufficient to block the NPY pathway to bone. Conversely, Y5R may be the sole receptor to transduce the signal resulting from altered NPY expression in the arcuate, a known site of NPY signaling to bone [19]. Also, sympathetic neurons emanating from the paraventricular nucleus may be responsible for the efferent pathway (unpublished observation) (Fig. 4.2). These possibilities indicate that there may be multiple neural species capable of mediating hypothalamic NPY-ergic signals to bone, and, moreover, that NPY and Y2 receptor pathways to bone are distinct, highlighting the complexity of neural control of bone mass.

The Y4 Receptor

The Y4 receptor shows a unique ligand binding profile, preferentially binding the NPY family ligand pancreatic polypeptide (PP) [76]. Y4 receptor mRNA has been identified in the brain stem, with a dense population of high-affinity Y4 receptors in the dorsal vagal complex of the brain stem [76]. This site is critical to reception of neuronal signals from organs in the periphery, with an incomplete blood–brain barrier, permitting the entry of small peptide hormones. The presence of Y4 receptors has also been reported in the lateral hypothalamic area, specifically in orexin-containing neurons [76]. In peripheral tissues, Y4 receptors are predominantly expressed in the heart, gastrointestinal tract, skeletal muscle, pancreas, testis, and uterus [76].

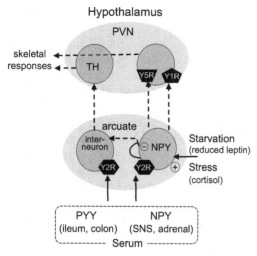

FIGURE 4.2 Proposed hypothalamic NPY pathways to bone. Circulating starvation signals, such as reduced leptin, or stress indices, such as elevated cortisol, act upon NPY-ergic neurons in the arcuate nucleus to increase NPY production. Experimental overexpression of NPY in this region produces marked bone anabolic suppression; however, the pathway mediating this action is unknown. Several possibilities exist for the NPY pathway to bone. [1] NPY-ergic neurons of the arcuate synapse in the paraventricular nucleus (PVN) with neurons expressing Y1 and Y5 receptors. Loss of Y1R in these neurons does not alter bone, thus Y5R alone or both Y1R and Y5R may be required for signal transduction. [2] NPY-ergic neurons in the arcuate also alter TH-positive neurons in the PVN, by an indirect pathway involving non-NPY-ergic inter-neurons. These TH-positive neurons may alter bone homeostasis. In addition, circulating NPY and PYY signal directly upon Y2 receptors in the arcuate to suppress NPY through Y2 signaling, but also stimulate TH-positive neurons in the PVN. Deletion of Y2 receptors increases bone mass by non-NPY neurons, thus activity of this TH-dependent pathway may be important to hypothalamic control of bone mass.

Y4 Receptor Control of Bone Homeostasis

A potential for Y4 receptors to regulate bone mass was hypothesized following the finding that serum levels of PP, the Y4 ligand, were markedly elevated in Y2 receptor knockout mice [71]. However, there was no alteration in bone mass in PP transgenic mice or following germline deletion of Y4 receptors [46]. Interestingly, coincident deletion of Y2 and Y4 receptors increased cancellous bone volume in male mice to a significantly greater extent than that observed in Y2R KO mice [46,77], associated with a general increase in bone turnover. Importantly, they showed significant reductions in cortical bone mass that were not evident in either single receptor knockout model [46]. The synergistic interaction between Y2 and Y4 receptors also had implications for obesity as the male Y2RY4R KO mice displayed a lean phenotype and reduced body weight despite hyperphagia, with reduced white adipose tissue mass and hypoleptinemia [46]. The reduced leptin levels suggested a mechanism for the additive increase in bone

mass observed in the male Y2RY4R KO mice. Indeed, female Y2RY4R KO mice did not have a reduction in leptin levels, nor did they display the additional increase in cancellous bone volume [19]. This indicates a potential interaction between the NPY and leptin pathways to bone (discussed below).

NPY INTERACTION WITH LEPTIN IN THE CONTROL OF BONE HOMEOSTASIS

Leptin biology led to the discovery of a central control of bone mass [26]. Interestingly, both leptin and NPY affect, albeit to different extents, energy homeostasis. In particular, both are fundamental to the response to calorie depravation. Leptin circulates as a marker of peripheral adipose mass, with NPY a critical downstream mediator of the central response to leptin deficiency [26]. In the arcuate nucleus, expression of NPY is inversely related to the decrease in leptin due to starvation [78–80] and in leptin-deficient *ob/ob* mice [81], as a result of direct leptin receptor signaling in NPY-ergic neurons in that region [25]. Administration of leptin to *ob/ob* mice reduces the elevated levels of NPY [82], while central injection of NPY mimics many of the characteristics of leptin deficiency, including hyperphagia, decreased thermogenesis, hyperinsulinemia, and the development of obesity [19]. Deletion of NPY does not affect appetite but partially corrects the obesity phenotype of *ob/ob* mice [82]. Thus their shared biology in the control of energy homeostasis suggests the possibility of a shared control of bone homeostasis.

Consistent with this shared biology, several lines of evidence suggest commonalities between the leptin- and NPY-mediated pathways to bone. The dual Y receptor and leptin-deficient mice, Y1R*ob/ob* and Y2R*ob/ob*, did not show an additive effect on cancellous bone volume or formation [34]. However, as mentioned above, hypoleptinaemic male Y2RY4R double knockout mice revealed a synergistic increase in cancellous bone volume, compared with normoleptinaemic Y2R and female Y2RY4R mice [46]. Moreover, these male Y2RY4R double knockout mice displayed the increase in cancellous and decrease in cortical bone mass characteristic of the leptin-deficient skeletal phenotype evident in *ob/ob* mice [34] and following chronic calorie restriction [83]. The involvement of central NPY signaling in the Y2RY4R model was confirmed by a later study [84]. Thus it appears that leptin-induced, NPY-mediated signals may combine to control bone mass.

However, in addition, evidence from numerous studies indicates the existence of distinct pathways for NPY and leptin to bone. Administration of NPY into the CSF of wild-type mice, mimicking the increase in *ob/ob*, induced a reduction in cancellous bone volume, the opposite of that evident in *ob/ob* mice, suggesting that NPY and leptin may use different pathways to control bone mass [26]. Chemical ablation techniques, used to destroy entire hypothalamic regions, suggest that the leptin pathway to cancellous bone originates from a region without NPY expression [85,86]. Gain-of-function experiments, however, showed that leptin can signal in the hypothalamus when introduced in wild-type mice through viral-mediated methods [87].

However, the most definitive evidence for separate pathways was provided by the examination of cortical bone in Y2R KO and *ob/ob* mice. In contrast to its effect on cancellous bone, leptin deficiency has been reported to reduce cortical mass by some [19,34,88–91], but not all, studies [26]. This is in contrast to the increase in cortical bone mass resulting from loss of NPY or Y-receptor signaling, as outlined above. This opposing relationship is further enhanced following correction for the greater body weight of *ob/ob* [34]. In addition, exogenous elevation of central NPY levels, as evident in *ob/ob* did not block the Y2R KO mediated anabolic response, even in the presence of elevated serum leptin [19]. Thus it appears that although related in their expression in some regions of the hypothalamus, the afferent pathways mediating the skeletal effects of NPY and Y2R and that of leptin appear distinct.

NPY'S COORDINATION OF BODY WEIGHT AND BONE MASS

NPY has proven an important regulator of skeletal and adipose homeostasis, through actions within the hypothalamus and the periphery (Fig. 4.3). In the hypothalamus, the skeletal and adipose responses mediated by NPY expression originate from within the arcuate nucleus. This anatomical consistency suggested the possibility of integration of these two processes within the brain. While the degree to which these processes are interrelated remains to be elucidated, existing evidence indicates a degree of connection between the NPY-mediated control in energy and skeletal homeostasis. Elevation of hypothalamic NPY expression, as evident following negative energy balance, triggers energy conservation and with it an inhibition in bone formation [26,92]. Consistently, when NPY is exogenously elevated in the same hypothalamic nuclei, mimicking the central response to starvation, the inhibition of bone formation persists. Intriguingly, this NPY-induced reduction in bone mass occurs despite being accompanied by marked increase in weight, white adipose tissue mass, and circulating leptin levels. In this manner, the perception by the brain of the body's starvation state appears to play an important role in

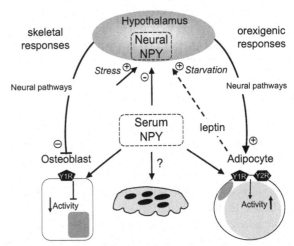

FIGURE 4.3 **Central and peripheral regulation of bone and fat mass by NPY and its receptors.** Central pathways originate with increased NPY expression in NPY-ergic neurons in the hypothalamus. These neurons are also known to induce skeletal and orexigenic responses. NPY is also produced by peripheral sources, most notably during stress (sympathetic neurons/adrenals) and can signal directly to Y1 receptors on osteoblasts and Y1 and Y2 receptors on adipocytes. NPY stimulates adipose accrual, increasing serum leptin, a major regulator of central NPY. NPY may also act upon osteoclasts.

determining the tonic levels of bone formation occurring in the periphery. Thus when the brain perceives the body is starving, then bone formation is altered accordingly. The exogenous NPY experiment illustrates that this regulatory pathway is active independently of local mechanical loading, as bone mass decreases in line with greater central NPY, despite greater loading induced by the increase in body weight [19]. Thus although there is a strong and positive link between body weight and bone mass due to mechanical loading, the central perception of energy status, and with it body weight, may have an important impact on peripheral activity of osteoblasts and osteocytes, through NPY-mediated processes.

Conversely, hypothalamic NPY level is decreased during times of energy excess or after short-term overfeeding with increased serum leptin levels [26,93]. As evident in the mice model lacking NPY, the reduction of NPY is associated with an increase in bone mass and greater osteoblast activity [28]. Such a calorie intake-induced inhibition of central NPY would act to ensure mechanical competence of the skeleton during times of increased weight bearing. Therefore, central NPY, acting in response to indicators of energy status, could act to coordinate bone mass to body weight [28,94] as a pathway operating in addition to the well-defined actions of mechanical loading. NPY is expressed in both osteoblast and adipocytes, thus NPY may also play a role in direct signaling between bone and fat. However, this remains to be determined.

INTERACTIONS BETWEEN NPY AND SEX HORMONES IN THE CONTROL OF BONE HOMEOSTASIS

Sex hormone levels play a fundamental role in the maintenance of bone mass and the etiology of osteoporosis. The expression of estrogen and androgen receptors on bone cells and the response of bone cells to sex steroid treatment *in vitro* highlight the importance of direct actions of these hormones on bone homeostasis. However, far less appreciated is the evidence of indirect actions, suggesting that estrogen signaling in the brain contributes to the regulation of the skeleton. Indeed, central estrogen signaling, examined by intracerebroventricular estrogen replacement in ovariectomized mice, provides at least one third of the total cancellous bone response to estrogen supplementation [95]. Part of this regulation could involve NPY signaling, as estrogen is known to inversely regulate hypothalamic NPY expression [96]. Estrogen deficiency therefore may contribute to bone loss by increasing hypothalamic NPY expression, which in turn would suppress osteoblast activity while also promoting fat gain, both of which are characteristic responses to ovariectomy [97] and experimental central NPY overexpression [19,28]. Consistent with such a mechanism, mean wall thickness, a direct measure of osteoblast activity, is reduced following ovariectomy [98]. Further insight into the role of NPY in mediating bone loss and fat gain in response to sex steroid deficiency is required in order to properly assess the potential therapeutic utility of NPY modulation in postmenopausal populations.

In addition to interactions with estrogen signaling, NPY has also been shown to interact with androgen signaling. Despite similarities in the skeletal responses to Y1 and Y2 receptor deletion, important differences in the effect of androgen deficiency are apparent in these models. In male Y1R KO mice, the characteristic increase in osteoblast activity evident in these animals was abolished by orchidectomy, while no such effect was evident in ovariectomized female Y1R KO [27] or orchidectomized male Y1R KO mice [70]. This finding suggests that intact androgen signaling may be required for the bone anabolic responses mediated by Y1 deletion. As the Y1 receptor effect occurs locally within the osteoblast [58], this study identifies the osteoblast as a novel site of interaction between classic endocrine and neural pathways in the regulation of bone homeostasis. Reduced androgen levels are a known risk factor for fracture in men [99] and are associated with reduced bone mass in women [100], and it may be that these relationships are in part the result of loss of Y1-mediated effects in bone. Studies such as these are revealing a significant level of integration between neural and endocrine signaling in the regulation of tissue homeostasis. They offer the exciting potential to modify existing endocrine-based models of disease and, moreover, may identify novel therapeutic strategies.

CONCLUSION

The NPY family of peptides and receptors influences numerous homeostatic processes and represents a complex and wide-reaching regulatory apparatus. Its actions in bone, to modulate osteoblast activity, and potentially osteoclast activity, appear as a consistent and powerful response to alterations in both central and peripheral aspects of this regulatory network. The studies outlined above have provided interesting information regarding osteoblast and osteoclast biology. However, it is through system-wide analysis of NPY biology that we are gaining entirely novel insights into the interaction of skeletal processes with other organ systems. Most noticeably at present, these interactions have been defined between skeletal and energy homeostasis, thereby providing a weight-independent system for matching of body weight to bone mass. However, ongoing studies suggest further interactions, involving endocrine pathways, glucose homeostasis, as well as local actions in bone such as mechanical loading. This potential for neural pathways to expand our knowledge of human biology has yet to be fully realized. Excitingly, the constant development of murine models, pharmacological agents, and analytical tools indicates a continued analysis of NPY biology, and with it novel opportunities for biological and therapeutic insight.

References

[1] Bai FL, Yamano M, Shiotani Y, Emson PC, Smith AD, Powell JF, et al. An arcuato-paraventricular and -dorsomedial hypothalamic neuropeptide Y-containing system which lacks noradrenaline in the rat. Brain Res 1985 Apr 1;331(1):172–5.

[2] Ekblad E, Edvinsson L, Wahlestedt C, Uddman R, Hakanson R, Sundler F. Neuropeptide Y co-exists and co-operates with noradrenaline in perivascular nerve fibers. Regul Pept 1984 Apr;8(3):225–35.

[3] Igwe JC, Jiang X, Paic F, Ma L, Adams DJ, Baldock PA, et al. Neuropeptide Y is expressed by osteocytes and can inhibit osteoblastic activity. J Cell Biochem 2009 Oct 15;108(3):621–30.

[4] Lee NJ, Doyle KL, Sainsbury A, Enriquez RF, Hort YJ, Riepler SJ, et al. Critical role for Y1 receptors in mesenchymal progenitor cell differentiation and osteoblast activity. J Bone Miner Res 2010 Aug;25(8):1736–47.

[5] Ekblad E, Sundler F. Distribution of pancreatic polypeptide and peptide YY. Peptides 2002 Feb;23(2):251–61.

[6] Hazelwood RL. The pancreatic polypeptide (PP-fold) family: gastrointestinal, vascular, and feeding behavioral implications. Proc Soc Exp Biol Med 1993 Jan;202(1):44–63.

[7] Berglund MM, Hipskind PA, Gehlert DR. Recent developments in our understanding of the physiological role of PP-fold peptide receptor subtypes. Exp Biol Med (Maywood) 2003 Mar;228(3):217—44.

[8] Blomqvist AG, Herzog H. Y-receptor subtypes—how many more? Trends Neurosci 1997 Jul;20(7):294—8.

[9] Michel MC, Beck-Sickinger A, Cox H, Doods HN, Herzog H, Larhammar D, et al. XVI. International Union of Pharmacology recommendations for the nomenclature of neuropeptide Y, peptide YY, and pancreatic polypeptide receptors. Pharmacol Rev 1998 Mar;50(1):143—50.

[10] Dumont Y, Moyse E, Fournier A, Quirion R. Evidence for the existence of an additional class of neuropeptide Y receptor sites in rat brain. J Pharmacol Exp Ther 2005 Oct;315(1):99—108.

[11] Lin S, Boey D, Couzens M, Lee N, Sainsbury A, Herzog H. Compensatory changes in [125I]-PYY binding in Y receptor knockout mice suggest the potential existence of further Y receptor(s). Neuropeptides 2005 Feb;39(1):21—8.

[12] Fetissov S, Kopp J, Hokfelt T. Distribution of NPY receptors in the hypothalamus. Neuropeptides 2004 Aug;38(4):175—88.

[13] Mentlein R. Dipeptidyl-peptidase IV (CD26)—role in the inactivation of regulatory peptides. Regul Pept 1999 Nov 30;85(1): 9—24.

[14] Unniappan S, McIntosh CH, Demuth HU, Heiser U, Wolf R, Kieffer TJ. Effects of dipeptidyl peptidase IV on the satiety actions of peptide YY. Diabetologia 2006 Aug;49(8):1915—23.

[15] Cho YR, Kim CW. Neuropeptide Y promotes beta-cell replication via extracellular signal-regulated kinase activation. Biochem Biophys Res Commun 2004 Feb 13;314(3):773—80.

[16] Keffel S, Schmidt M, Bischoff A, Michel MC. Neuropeptide-Y stimulation of extracellular signal-regulated kinases in human erythroleukemia cells. J Pharmacol Exp Ther 1999 Dec; 291(3):1172—8.

[17] King PJ, Williams G, Doods H, Widdowson PS. Effect of a selective neuropeptide Y Y(2) receptor antagonist, BIIE0246 on neuropeptide Y release. Eur J Pharmacol 2000 May 12;396(1): R1—3.

[18] Wahlestedt C, Yanaihara N, Hakanson R. Evidence for different pre- and post-junctional receptors for neuropeptide Y and related peptides. Regul Pept 1986 Feb;13(3—4):307—18.

[19] Baldock PA, Sainsbury A, Allison S, Lin EJ, Couzens M, Boey D, et al. Hypothalamic control of bone formation: distinct actions of leptin and Y2 receptor pathways. J Bone Miner Res 2005;20(10):1851—7.

[20] Ahmed M, Bjurholm A, Kreicbergs A, Schultzberg M. Neuropeptide Y. tyrosine hydroxylase and vasoactive intestinal polypeptide-immunoreactive nerve fibers in the vertebral bodies, discs, dura mater, and spinal ligaments of the rat lumbar spine. Spine (Phila Pa 1976). 1993 Feb;18(2):268—73.

[21] Bjurholm A, Kreicbergs A, Terenius L, Goldstein M, Schultzberg M. Neuropeptide Y-, tyrosine hydroxylase- and vasoactive intestinal polypeptide-immunoreactive nerves in bone and surrounding tissues. J Auton Nerv Syst 1988 Dec; 25(2—3):119—25.

[22] Malmstrom RE. Vascular pharmacology of BIIE0246, the first selective non-peptide neuropeptide YY(2) receptor antagonist, in vivo. Br J Pharmacol 2001 Aug;133(7):1073—80.

[23] Sisask G, Bjurholm A, Ahmed M, Kreicbergs A. The development of autonomic innervation in bone and joints of the rat. J Auton Nerv Syst 1996 Jun 10;59(1—2):27—33.

[24] Hill EL, Elde R. Distribution of CGRP-, VIP-, D beta H-, SP-, and NPY-immunoreactive nerves in the periosteum of the rat. Cell Tissue Res 1991 Jun;264(3):469—80.

[25] Mercer JG, Hoggard N, Williams LM, Lawrence CB, Hannah LT, Morgan PJ, et al. Coexpression of leptin receptor and preproneuropeptide Y mRNA in arcuate nucleus of mouse hypothalamus. J Neuroendocrinol 1996;8(10):733—5.

[26] Ducy P, Amling M, Takeda S, Priemel M, Schilling AF, Beil FT, et al. Leptin inhibits bone formation through a hypothalamic relay: a central control of bone mass. Cell 2000 Jan 21;100(2): 197—207.

[27] Allison SJ, Baldock PA, Enriquez RF, Lin E, During M, Gardiner EM, et al. Critical interplay between neuropeptide Y and sex steroid pathways in bone and adipose tissue homeostasis. J Bone Miner Res 2009 Feb;24(2):294—304.

[28] Baldock PA, Lee NJ, Driessler F, Lin S, Allison S, Stehrer B, et al. Neuropeptide Y knockout mice reveal a central role of NPY in the coordination of bone mass to body weight. PLoS One 2009;4(12):e8415.

[29] Elefteriou F, Takeda S, Liu X, Armstrong D, Karsenty G. Monosodium glutamate-sensitive hypothalamic neurons contribute to the control of bone mass. Endocrinology 2003 Sep;144(9): 3842—7.

[30] Bjurholm A. Neuroendocrine peptides in bone. Int Orthop 1991;15(4):325—9.

[31] Bjurholm A, Kreicbergs A, Schultzberg M, Lerner UH. Neuroendocrine regulation of cyclic AMP formation in osteoblastic cell lines (UMR-106-01, ROS 17/2.8, MC3T3-E1, and Saos-2) and primary bone cells. J Bone Miner Res 1992;7(9):1011—9.

[32] Amano S, Arai M, Goto S, Togari A. Inhibitory effect of NPY on isoprenaline-induced osteoclastogenesis in mouse bone marrow cells. Biochim Biophys Acta 2007 Jun;1770(6):966—73.

[33] Baldock PA, Allison SJ, Lundberg P, Lee NJ, Slack K, Lin EJ, et al. Novel role of Y1 receptors in the coordinated regulation of bone and energy homeostasis. J Biol Chem 2007 May 9;282(26):19092—102.

[34] Baldock PA, Allison SJ, McDonald MM, Sainsbury A, Enriquez R, Little DG, et al. Hypothalamic regulation of cortical bone mass: opposing activity of Y2 receptor and leptin pathways. J Bone Miner Res 2006;21:1600—7.

[35] Teixeira L, Sousa DM, Nunes AF, Sousa MM, Herzog H, Lamghari M. NPY revealed as a critical modulator of osteoblast function in vitro: new insights into the role of Y1 and Y2 receptors. J Cell Biochem 2009 Aug 1;107(5):908—16.

[36] Misra M, Miller KK, Tsai P, Gallagher K, Lin A, Lee N, et al. Elevated peptide YY levels in adolescent girls with anorexia nervosa. J Clin Endocrinol Metab 2006 Mar;91(3):1027—33.

[37] Utz AL, Lawson EA, Misra M, Mickley D, Gleysteen S, Herzog DB, et al. Peptide YY (PYY) levels and bone mineral density (BMD) in women with anorexia nervosa. Bone 2008 Jul;43(1):135—9.

[38] Misra M, Prabhakaran R, Miller KK, Goldstein MA, Mickley D, Clauss L, et al. Prognostic indicators of changes in bone density measures in adolescent girls with anorexia nervosa-II. J Clin Endocrinol Metab 2008 Apr;93(4):1292—7.

[39] Russell M, Stark J, Nayak S, Miller KK, Herzog DB, Klibanski A, et al. Peptide YY in adolescent athletes with amenorrhea, eumenorrheic athletes and non-athletic controls. Bone 2009 Jul;45(1):104—9.

[40] Toombs RJ, Scheid JL, Williams NI, De Souza MJ. PYY is negatively associated with bone mineral density in exercising women with amenorrhea. Medicine & Science in Sports & Exercise 2010;42(5):701. doi: 10.1249/01.MSS.0000386039.50422.f7.

[41] Batterham RL, Cohen MA, Ellis SM, Le Roux CW, Withers DJ, Frost GS, et al. Inhibition of food intake in obese subjects by peptide YY3-36. N Engl J Med 2003 Sep 4;349(10):941—8.

[42] Reid IR. Relationships among body mass, its components, and bone. Bone 2002 Nov;31(5):547—55.

[43] Scheid JL, Toombs RJ, Ducher G, Gibbs JC, Williams NI, De Souza MJ. Estrogen and peptide YY are associated with bone

mineral density in premenopausal exercising women. Bone 2011 Aug;49(2):194−201.

[44] Wortley KE, Garcia K, Okamoto H, Thabet K, Anderson KD, Shen V, et al. Peptide YY regulates bone turnover in rodents. Gastroenterology 2007 Nov;133(5):1534−43.

[45] Hosaka H, Nagata A, Yoshida T, Shibata T, Nagao T, Tanaka T, et al. Pancreatic polypeptide is secreted from and controls differentiation through its specific receptors in osteoblastic MC3T3-E1 cells. Peptides 2008 Aug;29(8):1390−5.

[46] Sainsbury A, Baldock PA, Schwarzer C, Ueno N, Enriquez RF, Couzens M, et al. Synergistic effects of Y2 and Y4 receptors on adiposity and bone mass revealed in double knockout mice. Mol Cell Biol 2003 Aug;23(15):5225−33.

[47] Herzog H, Hort YJ, Ball HJ, Hayes G, Shine J, Selbie LA. Cloned human neuropeptide Y receptor couples to two different second messenger systems. Proc Natl Acad Sci USA 1992 Jul 1;89(13): 5794−8.

[48] Larhammar D, Blomqvist AG, Yee F, Jazin E, Yoo H, Wahlested C. Cloning and functional expression of a human neuropeptide Y/peptide YY receptor of the Y1 type. J Biol Chem 1992 Jun 5;267(16):10935−8.

[49] Eva C, Keinanen K, Monyer H, Seeburg P, Sprengel R. Molecular cloning of a novel G protein-coupled receptor that may belong to the neuropeptide receptor family. FEBS Lett 1990 Oct 1;271(1−2):81−4.

[50] Kopp J, Xu ZQ, Zhang X, Pedrazzini T, Herzog H, Kresse A, et al. Expression of the neuropeptide Y Y1 receptor in the CNS of rat and of wild-type and Y1 receptor knock-out mice. Focus on immunohistochemical localization. Neuroscience 2002; 111(3):443−532.

[51] Jacques D, Tong Y, Dumont Y, Shen SH, Quirion R. Expression of the neuropeptide Y Y1 receptor mRNA in the human brain: an in situ hybridization study. Neuroreport 1996 Apr 10;7(5): 1053−6.

[52] Goumain M, Voisin T, Lorinet AM, Laburthe M. Identification and distribution of mRNA encoding the Y1, Y2, Y4, and Y5 receptors for peptides of the PP-fold family in the rat intestine and colon. Biochem Biophys Res Commun 1998 Jun 9;247(1):52−6.

[53] Morgan DG, Kulkarni RN, Hurley JD, Wang ZL, Wang RM, Ghatei MA, et al. Inhibition of glucose stimulated insulin secretion by neuropeptide Y is mediated via the Y1 receptor and inhibition of adenylyl cyclase in RIN 5AH rat insulinoma cells. Diabetologia 1998 Dec;41(12):1482−91.

[54] Yang K, Guan H, Arany E, Hill DJ, Cao X. Neuropeptide Y is produced in visceral adipose tissue and promotes proliferation of adipocyte precursor cells via the Y1 receptor. FASEB J 2008 Jul;22(7):2452−64.

[55] Wharton J, Gordon L, Byrne J, Herzog H, Selbie LA, Moore K, et al. Expression of the human neuropeptide tyrosine Y1 receptor. Proc Natl Acad Sci USA 1993 Jan 15;90(2):687−91.

[56] Lundberg P, Allison SJ, Lee NJ, Baldock PA, Brouard N, Rost S, et al. Greater bone formation of Y2 knockout mice is associated with increased osteoprogenitor numbers and altered Y1 receptor expression. J Biol Chem 2007 Jun 29;282(26):19082−91.

[57] Wheway J, Mackay CR, Newton RA, Sainsbury A, Boey D, Herzog H, et al. A fundamental bimodal role for neuropeptide Y1 receptor in the immune system. J Exp Med 2005 Dec 5;202(11):1527−38.

[58] Lee NJ, Nguyen AD, Enriquez RF, Doyle KL, Sainsbury A, Baldock PA, et al. Osteoblast specific Y1 receptor deletion enhances bone mass. Bone 2010 Oct 30;30:30.

[59] Gerald C, Walker MW, Vaysse PJ, He C, Branchek TA, Weinshank RL. Expression cloning and pharmacological characterization of a human hippocampal neuropeptide Y/peptide

[60] Maes MB, Scharpe S, De Meester I. Dipeptidyl peptidase II (DPPII), a review. Clin Chim Acta 2007 May 1;380(1−2):31−49.

[61] Parker RM, Herzog H. Regional distribution of Y-receptor subtype mRNAs in rat brain. Eur J Neurosci 1999 Apr;11(4): 1431−48.

[62] Golombek DA, Biello SM, Rendon RA, Harrington ME. Neuropeptide Y phase shifts the circadian clock in vitro via a Y2 receptor. Neuroreport 1996 May 17;7(7):1315−9.

[63] Huhman KL, Gillespie CF, Marvel CL, Albers HE. Neuropeptide Y phase shifts circadian rhythms in vivo via a Y2 receptor. Neuroreport 1996 May 17;7(7):1249−52.

[64] Pheng LH, Perron A, Quirion R, Cadieux A, Fauchere JL, Dumont Y, et al. Neuropeptide Y-induced contraction is mediated by neuropeptide Y Y2 and Y4 receptors in the rat colon. Eur J Pharmacol 1999 Jun 11;374(1):85−91.

[65] Zukowska-Grojec Z, Karwatowska-Prokopczuk E, Rose W, Rone J, Movafagh S, Ji H, et al. Neuropeptide Y: a novel angiogenic factor from the sympathetic nerves and endothelium. Circ Res 1998 Jul 27;83(2):187−95.

[66] Chen CH, Stephens Jr RL, Rogers RC. PYY and NPY: control of gastric motility via action on Y1 and Y2 receptors in the DVC. Neurogastroenterol Motil 1997 Jun;9(2):109−16.

[67] Heilig M. The NPY system in stress, anxiety and depression. Neuropeptides 2004 Aug;38(4):213−24.

[68] Broadwell RD, Brightman MW. Entry of peroxidase into neurons of the central and peripheral nervous systems from extracerebral and cerebral blood. J Comp Neurol 1976 Apr 1;166(3):257−83.

[69] Schwartz MW, Baskin DG, Bukowski TR, Kuijper JL, Foster D, Lasser G, et al. Specificity of leptin action on elevated blood glucose levels and hypothalamic neuropeptide Y gene expression in ob/ob mice. Diabetes 1996 Apr;45(4):531−5.

[70] Allison SJ, Baldock P, Sainsbury A, Enriquez R, Lee NJ, Lin EJ, et al. Conditional deletion of hypothalamic Y2 receptors reverts gonadectomy-induced bone loss in adult mice. J Biol Chem 2006 Jun 19;281(33):23436−44.

[71] Baldock PA, Sainsbury A, Couzens M, Enriquez RF, Thomas GP, Gardiner EM, et al. Hypothalamic Y2 receptors regulate bone formation. J Clin Invest 2002 Apr;109(7):915−21.

[72] Ho KK, O'Sullivan AJ, Hoffman DM. Metabolic actions of growth hormone in man. Endocr J 1996 Oct;43(63):S57−63.

[73] Lin S, Lin EJ, Boey D, Lee NJ, Slack K, During MJ, et al. Fasting inhibits the growth and reproductive axes via distinct Y2 and Y4 receptor-mediated pathways. Endocrinology 2007 May; 148(5):2056−65.

[74] Nguyen ND, Center JR, Eisman JA, Nguyen TV. Bone loss, weight loss, and weight fluctuation predict mortality risk in elderly men and women. J Bone Miner Res 2007 Aug;22(8):1147−54.

[75] Shi YC, Lin S, Wong IP, Baldock PA, Aljanova A, Enriquez RF, et al. NPY neuron-specific Y2 receptors regulate adipose tissue and trabecular bone but not cortical bone homeostasis in mice. PLoS One 2010;5(6):e11361.

[76] Darby K, Eyre HJ, Lapsys N, Copeland NG, Gilbert DJ, Couzens M, et al. Assignment of the Y4 receptor gene (PPYR1) to human chromosome 10q11.2 and mouse chromosome 14. Genomics 1997 Dec 15;46(3):513−5.

[77] Lee NJ, Allison S, Enriquez RF, Sainsbury A, Herzog H, Baldock PA. Y2 and Y4 receptor signalling attenuates the skeletal response of central NPY. J Mol Neurosci Feb;43(2)123−31.

[78] Schwartz MW, Dallman MF, Woods SC. Hypothalamic response to starvation: implications for the study of wasting disorders. Am J Physiol 1995;269(5 Pt 2):R949−57.

YY Y2 receptor subtype. J Biol Chem 1995 Nov 10;270(45): 26758−61.

[79] Spanswick D, Smith MA, Groppi VE, Logan SD, Ashford ML. Leptin inhibits hypothalamic neurons by activation of ATP-sensitive potassium channels. Nature 1997; 390(6659):521−5.

[80] Spiegelman BM, Flier JS. Adipogenesis and obesity: rounding out the big picture. Cell 1996;87(3):377−89.

[81] Wilding JP, Gilbey SG, Bailey CJ, Batt RA, Williams G, Ghatei MA, et al. Increased neuropeptide-Y messenger ribonucleic acid (mRNA) and decreased neurotensin mRNA in the hypothalamus of the obese (ob/ob) mouse. Endocrinology 1993;132(5):1939−44.

[82] Stephens TW, Basinski M, Bristow PK, Bue-Valleskey JM, Burgett SG, Craft L, et al. The role of neuropeptide Y in the antiobesity action of the obese gene product. Nature 1995;377(6549):530−2.

[83] Hamrick MW, Ding KH, Ponnala S, Ferrari SL, Isales CM. Caloric restriction decreases cortical bone mass but spares trabecular bone in the mouse skeleton: implications for the regulation of bone mass by body weight. J Bone Miner Res 2008 Jun;23(6):870−8.

[84] Lee NJ, Allison S, Enriquez RF, Sainsbury A, Herzog H, Baldock PA. Y2 and Y4 receptor signalling attenuates the skeletal response of central NPY. J Mol Neurosci 2011 Feb;43(2): 123−31.

[85] Takeda S, Elefteriou F, Levasseur R, Liu X, Zhao L, Parker KL, et al. Leptin regulates bone formation via the sympathetic nervous system. Cell 2002 Nov 1;111(3):305−17.

[86] Yadav VK, Oury F, Suda N, Liu ZW, Gao XB, Confavreux C, et al. A serotonin-dependent mechanism explains the leptin regulation of bone mass, appetite, and energy expenditure. Cell 2009 Sep 4;138(5):976−89.

[87] Iwaniec UT, Boghossian S, Lapke PD, Turner RT, Kalra SP. Central leptin gene therapy corrects skeletal abnormalities in leptin-deficient ob/ob mice. Peptides 2007 May;28(5):1012−9.

[88] Hamrick MW, Pennington C, Newton D, Xie D, Isales C. Leptin deficiency produces contrasting phenotypes in bones of the limb and spine. Bone 2004 Mar;34(3):376−83.

[89] Lorentzon M, Landin K, Mellstrom D, Ohlsson C. Leptin is a negative independent predictor of areal BMD and cortical bone size in young adult Swedish men. J Bone Miner Res 2006 Dec;21(12):1871−8.

[90] Steppan CM, Crawford DT, Chidsey-Frink KL, Ke H, Swick AG. Leptin is a potent stimulator of bone growth in ob/ob mice. Regulatory peptides 2000 Aug 25;92(1−3): 73−8.

[91] Takeshita N, Mutoh S, Yamaguchi I. Osteopenia in genetically diabetic DB/DB mice and effects of 1alpha-hydroxyvitamin D3 on the osteopenia. Basic Research Group. Life sciences 1995 Feb 17;56(13):1095−101.

[92] Baldock PA, Sainsbury A, Allison S, Lin EJ, Couzens M, Boey D, et al. Hypothalamic control of bone formation: distinct actions of leptin and y2 receptor pathways. J Bone Miner Res 2005 Oct;20(10):1851−7.

[93] Sipols AJ, Baskin DG, Schwartz MW. Effect of intracerebroventricular insulin infusion on diabetic hyperphagia and hypothalamic neuropeptide gene expression. Diabetes 1995 Feb;44(2):147−51.

[94] Zengin A, Zhang L, Herzog H, Baldock PA, Sainsbury A. Neuropeptide Y and sex hormone interactions in humoral and neuronal regulation of bone and fat. Trends Endocrinol Metab 2010 Jul;21(7):411−8.

[95] Andersson N, Islander U, Egecioglu E, Lof E, Swanson C, Moverare-Skrtic S, et al. Investigation of central versus peripheral effects of estradiol in ovariectomized mice. J Endocrinol 2005 Nov;187(2):303−9.

[96] Clegg DJ, Brown LM, Zigman JM, Kemp CJ, Strader AD, Benoit SC, et al. Estradiol-dependent decrease in the orexigenic potency of ghrelin in female rats. Diabetes 2007 Apr;56(4): 1051−8.

[97] Baldock PA, Morris HA, Need AG, Moore RJ, Durbridge TC. Variation in the short-term changes in bone cell activity in three regions of the distal femur immediately following ovariectomy. J Bone Miner Res 1998 Sep;13(9):1451−7.

[98] Malluche HH, Faugere MC, Rush M, Friedler R. Osteoblastic insufficiency is responsible for maintenance of osteopenia after loss of ovarian function in experimental beagle dogs. Endocrinology 1986 Dec;119(6):2649−54.

[99] Meier C, Nguyen TV, Handelsman DJ, Schindler C, Kushnir MM, Rockwood AL, et al. Endogenous sex hormones and incident fracture risk in older men: the Dubbo Osteoporosis Epidemiology Study. Arch Intern Med 2008 Jan 14;168(1): 47−54.

[100] Hofbauer LC, Khosla S, Dunstan CR, Lacey DL, Spelsberg TC, Riggs BL. Estrogen stimulates gene expression and protein production of osteoprotegerin in human osteoblastic cells. Endocrinology 1999 Sep;140(9):4367−70.

Serotonin: The Central Link between Bone Mass and Energy Metabolism

Vijay K. Yadav

Wellcome Trust Sanger Institute, Cambridge, UK

The skeleton is among the largest organ systems in vertebrates, and functions to support organs, shelter hematopoiesis, and regulate metabolism [1,2]. In order to perform these functions properly bones are continuously remodeled through a homeostatic process known as bone remodeling [3]. Bone remodeling is carried out by bone remodeling units (BRUs) that are composed of osteoblasts—the cells that make new bone—and osteoclasts—the cells that resorb the old bone matrix. These BRUs function tirelessly in the skeleton throughout adulthood giving humans a new skeleton every 8–10 years [4,5]. To function, these BRUs need a proper inflow of energy, mostly in the form of glucose, to the skeleton. Therefore perturbations in any aspect of energy inflow or utilization in the body have a strong impact on the processes of bone remodeling. For example, obesity or high body mass index often leads to an increase in bone mass while chronic low appetite disorders such as anorexia often result in a decrease in bone mass [6–9]. In order to understand how perturbations in energy metabolism affect bone remodeling, one needs to look at this process, on which organismal function depends, in greater detail.

ENERGY METABOLISM AND ITS REGULATION

Energy metabolism can be defined as the processes that underlie food intake, burning the food to release energy, and storing the excess for the time of energy shortage [10–12]. These processes typically take the form of complex metabolic pathways within the cell, generally categorized as being either catabolic or anabolic. These events then provide a source of energy at the cellular level. As the organisms evolved from simpler metabolisms in invertebrates to the more complex ones in vertebrates, the organisms faced three challenges. First, they needed a mechanism to regulate how much excess energy can be stored and in which form; second, there arose a need for specialized cell types to store excess energy typically in the form of fat so that its deposition can be better regulated; and third, they needed a mechanism to coordinately adjust energy flux through various organs in response to changing nutritional status. Organisms coped with these three challenges by storing fat, predominantly, in the specialized cell types called adipocytes, and regulated the energy metabolism status of different tissues/organs through hormonal signals that acted on multiple organs to coordinate their energy flux [13,14]. Regulation of whole body energy metabolism and bone mass through an adipocyte-secreted hormone called leptin provides a beautiful illustration of how multiple functions are coordinated by the energy stores of the body—the adipose tissue, and how organs in turn regulate this store.

PERTURBATIONS IN ENERGY METABOLISM AND BONE MASS

The fact that high body mass index protects from osteoporosis raised questions about the physiological pathways that are involved in this effect [15]. Just 12 years ago, many possibilities existed to explain this protective effect of obesity on bone. Let us look at them in the context of what we know today. First, increased body mass index and mechanical loading on the bone result in increased bone mass. Although mechano-sensing has many fundamental roles to play in the regulation of localized changes in bone, the protective effects of weight have also been observed in non-weight-bearing bones suggesting the involvement of other factors [15–18]. The second possibility was that higher insulin levels in obese people result in an increase in bone cell functions and bone mass. We now know that obesity is a state of insulin resistance or less insulin signaling in the target cell types; therefore, in the light of recent demonstrations that insulin signaling in osteoblasts increases bone mass we would expect that obesity would result in a low bone mass phenotype, but this, in general, is not the case [19–21]. Third, the higher fat amount during obesity results in increased aromatization of androgens to estrogens through fat [22]. Studies in model organisms have provided experimental evidence that high bone mass in obese mice is observed in the presence of hypogonadism or low steroid milieu and therefore increased aromatization alone cannot explain higher bone mass during obesity [23]. The fourth possibility was that adipocytes secrete some factors that regulate bone mass. The discovery of leptin, an adipocyte-derived hormone regulating several homeostatic functions, raised the possibility that this might be one of the hormones that regulate bone mass. I will describe the series of studies through which leptin regulation of bone mass was identified; this will illustrate beautifully how advances in mouse molecular genetics have not only helped identify how leptin regulates bone mass, but have transformed the approaches we use today to address questions of physiology, i.e. interactions between organ systems.

DISCOVERY OF LEPTIN REGULATION OF BONE MASS

Leptin is a circulatory hormone that is predominantly expressed in the adipose tissue [24]. It was first identified by classical positional cloning experiments while trying to identify the genes responsible for obesity in the obese mouse model [25]. Once identified, the gene was therefore named Ob gene, and its product leptin (Greek, *leptos*; thin). Since its discovery in 1994 it has taken scientists through voyages of discovery from regulation of appetite to reproduction to bone mass. Long before leptin was discovered it was well recognized that obesity was a protective factor for osteoporosis and reduces fracture risk. However, it was not clear where this protective effect originated. Identification of leptin as a hormone that acted through the brain to regulate appetite provided a means to test whether leptin is among the factors involved in the protective effect of obesity on bone loss.

Leptin is released in the circulation in response to changes in nutritional status, travels to the brain, and acts through its cognate receptor (Obrb) to achieve its function [26–29]. To test whether leptin regulates bone mass, genetic and pharmacological approaches have been used in the past in different species. Analysis of loss of function mouse models for leptin (*ob/ob* mice) demonstrated that the absence of leptin results in a high bone mass phenotype at both the axial and appendicular skeleton [23]. This high bone mass phenotype was due to an increase in bone formation rate without much effect on osteoblast numbers or surface indicating that leptin deficiency affects the function of osteoblasts, and not their differentiation or proliferation [23]. In addition this high bone mass phenotype existed in the presence of higher bone resorption that is observed in leptin-deficient mice [23]. The high bone mass phenotype in leptin-deficient mice persisted even when obesity was abrogated in the *ob/ob* mice by feeding them a low fat diet, reiterating that the bone phenotype is not secondary to the high body mass index that is observed in the absence of leptin [23]. Intracerebroventricular (ICV) infusion of leptin provided one of the most convincing pieces of evidence for the central action of leptin as an inhibitor of bone mass accrual [23,30]. Administration of small quantities of leptin (in nanograms) through osmotic pumps, which importantly did not leak into the periphery, resulted in a decrease in bone mass that mirrored histological, cellular, and molecular bone phenotype observed in the leptin-deficient mice [23,30,31].

Like the *ob/ob* mice, the *db/db* mice that have a loss of function mutation in the leptin receptor (Obrb), are obese [24,32,33]. Analysis of the bone phenotype in these mice revealed a three-fold increase in bone volume compared to wild-type mice [23]. Histological and histomorphometric analysis of aged *db/db* mice revealed that this high bone mass phenotype, which was observed in the trabecular compartment, was due to their increased bone formation rate, and was identical to what had been observed in *ob/ob* mice [23]. These genetic studies using mice that lacked leptin or its signaling in all the cells of the body demonstrated that the adipocyte-secreted hormone leptin signals through the brain to affect bone mass, and provided the first ever experimental evidence of the central control of bone mass [23].

Studies carried out in multiple bony vertebrates have confirmed the central nature of leptin regulation of bone mass, and have elucidated the conserved function this hormone has across vertebrates [34,35]. Parallel to the elucidation of this central mode of leptin action on bone, it has been proposed that leptin could also regulate bone mass through local means [36]. This hypothesis is based on studies injecting pharmacological amounts (μg/day) of leptin in wild-type mice or by infusing leptin in the *ob/ob* mice [37]. The fact that the peripheral signaling through leptin needs higher doses (μg to mg/day) to see small effects on bone mass while a strong effect on bone is seen when ng quantities of leptin are infused in the brain demonstrates that central regulation of bone mass accrual through leptin is more sensitive, like its regulation of appetite and other functions.

GAIN OF FUNCTION OF LEPTIN SIGNALING AND BONE MASS

High bone mass observed in the loss of function mouse models of leptin synthesis or action raises the question of effect of a gain of function of leptin signaling on bone mass. To mediate its functions leptin binds to its receptor, Obrb, linked to the JAK—STAT signaling pathway [38]. Leptin binding activates Jak resulting in phosphorylation of several key residues on the intracellular region of the receptor. Some of these phosphorylated residues then activate downstream effectors by recruiting them to the plasma membrane while others act to limit the signaling through Obrb to bring the receptor back to unstimulated condition. Tyr985 phosphorylation results in recruitment of Socs3 to the leptin receptor that inhibits signaling through Obrb. Accordingly, mutation of this residue in Obrb (Y985L) results in gain of function of leptin signaling *in vitro* and *in vivo* (*l/l* mice) [39]. *l/l* mice only display phenotypes that are very sensitive to leptin signaling as the Y985L mutation results in only a partial gain of function. Therefore, *l/l* mice reveal function(s) of leptin requiring a lower threshold of signaling. These *l/l* mice have normal appetite when fed a normal chow, breed normally but are osteoporotic [39,40]. This suggests that the threshold of leptin signaling required to affect bone mass in rodents is much lower than the one needed to affect appetite and other functions under normal conditions.

FACTORS DOWNSTREAM OF LEPTIN REGULATION OF BONE MASS

Leptin regulates a multitude of factors in the brain and most, if not all, are located in the hypothalamus. Therefore, the initial search for leptin's anti-osteogenic mediator(s) zeroed in on the hypothalamus as it was the best characterized downstream target of leptin action [41]. The hypothalamus harbors a constellation of subtypes of neurons that are downstream of leptin signaling, ventromedial (VMH) and arcuate (ARC) being the most prominent among these nuclei [41,42]. In a hope to identify the site of leptin's antiosteogenic action Takeda et al. destroyed, through chemical lesioning, either VMH or arcuate nuclei [30]. The ablation of VMH neurons by gold thioglucose (GTG) led to a high bone mass phenotype similar to what is observed in leptin receptor-deficient mice. However, ablation of ARC neurons by monosodium glutamate (MSG) resulted in no alterations in bone mass despite the expected effects on appetite [30,43]. Mice that had the VMH lesion no longer responded to ICV infusion of leptin in the regulation of bone mass, demonstrating that a distinct subset of hypothalamic neurons lies downstream of leptin regulation of bone mass (VMH) and appetite (ARC) [30,43]. The next obvious problem was to identify the neuromediator in these hypothalamic neurons that regulated bone mass. The candidate(s) for such a neuromediator in the hypothalamus included Pomc, Cart, Npy, Agrp, and more recently neuromedin U (NMU). Let us look at these molecules briefly as they increase the molecular repertoire through which the brain regulates bone, before we move on to the site where leptin action initiates the regulation of bone mass.

Cocaine- and amphetamine-regulated transcript (Cart) is a neuropeptide expressed in the hypothalamus that is upregulated by leptin [44]. Consistent with this, leptin-deficient mice have a lower expression of Cart [30]. In the hunt to identify other neuromediators that can explain leptin regulation of bone mass Elefteriou et al. inactivated Cart in mice [45]. *Cart−/−* mice have a low bone mass phenotype that is due to an increase in bone resorption without much effect on bone formation demonstrating that it is a positive regulator of bone mass [45]. Surprisingly, however, leptin was still able to decrease bone mass, and in fact leptin decreases bone mass more severely in *Cart−/−* mice than the wild-type mice [45]. This fact underscored that Cart is a powerful inhibitor of bone resorption. Later studies have revealed that this function of Cart is mediated through a local action in the bone [46]. Cart overexpression in osteoblasts but not the hypothalamus results in an increase in bone mass by affecting *Rankl* expression that is a mirror image of what is observed in the *Cart−/−* mice [46]. These studies have identified Cart as an important regulator of bone resorption and bone mass.

Neuropeptide Y (Npy) is one of the most abundant peptides in the nervous system, and leptin inhibits its expression [43,47]. Npy acts through at least five receptors (Y1, Y2, Y4, Y5, and Y6). All of these receptors are expressed in the hypothalamus and several respond to other ligands, including peptide YY and pancreatic polypeptide (PP), which makes the mechanistic dissection of Npy-ergic signaling difficult. A high percentage of arcuate Npy-positive neurons, however, co-express the Y2 receptor, and mice that lack it in all the cells have increased osteoblast activity and a high bone mass phenotype, suggesting that central Y2 receptor inhibits bone formation [48,49]. Conditional hypothalamic Y2 receptor deletion recapitulated the bone phenotype of complete null mice confirming the cellular origin of the effect to the hypothalamus [50]. The fact that leptin infusion has the same effect on bone and Npy is increased in the hypothalamus of *ob/ob* mice suggests that Npy may not be a modulator of leptin regulation of bone mass directly, but it may act parallel to this neural circuit. In addition it is also possible that dose and frequency used for the Npy infusions do not mimic the physiological rhythm through which Npy functions.

Neuromedin U (NMU) is a neuromediator that has been very recently described as a downstream mediator of leptin in the hypothalamus. NMU regulates appetite and activates sympathetic tone, as demonstrated by the development of obesity in NMU-deficient mice [51–53]. While trying to identify the downstream target of leptin action in the hypothalamus Sato et al. tested the importance of NMU in leptin-dependent regulation of bone formation [54]. Analysis of NMU-deficient mice revealed a high bone mass phenotype caused by an increase in bone formation. Experimental evidence points towards NMU playing an important role in leptin regulation of bone mass through the brain. First, NMU receptors NMU1R and NMU2R are expressed in the brain and not detectable in bone [54]. Second, NMU does not directly affect osteoblast proliferation or function *in vitro*. Third, NMU acts centrally and not peripherally as the high bone mass of NMU-deficient mice can be rescued by NMU ICV infusion [54]. The fact that NMU ICV infusion could decrease the high bone mass of leptin-deficient mice indicated that NMU acts downstream of leptin to regulate bone formation. Interestingly, NMU-deficient mice were resistant to the anti-osteogenic effect of leptin and beta-adrenergic receptor agonists [54]. However, osteoblast number surprisingly increased in NMU-deficient mice treated with leptin ICV, suggesting that other mediators are involved in leptin action on osteoblasts.

These findings, all based on mutant animal models and *in vivo* studies, thus identified NMU, Cart, and Npy as three molecules, regulated by leptin, that regulate bone cell functions. In contrast to these three mediators, analysis of Pomc or Agrp knockout mice did not reveal any changes in bone mass. Despite the discovery of these three neuromediators, we still did not know whether these molecules were directly or indirectly regulated by leptin to regulate bone mass. Investigation of these questions had to wait for the generation of tools for the conditional mutagenesis in mouse that allowed investigators to ask this question genetically using the leptin receptor floxed mice and cell type-specific Cre drivers.

LEPTIN ACTS IN THE BRAIN TO REGULATE BONE MASS

Leptin receptor deletion in all the neurons using *Nestin-Cre* mice led to the expected obesity and a high bone mass phenotype [40,55]. The high bone mass phenotype in these mice was due to a high bone formation rate and existed in the presence of high bone resorption parameters, and recapitulated the high bone mass phenotype observed in the *db/db* mice that have deficiency in the leptin receptor signaling throughout the body [40]. This phenotype was present in both trabecular and cortical compartments of the axial and appendicular skeleton. These studies demonstrated that leptin regulates bone mass through leptin receptor and this site is present in the brain. Is this site the hypothalamus? The leptin receptor has been deleted in two distinct populations of the hypothalamus, VMH and ARC, using Cre drivers specific for these locations, *Sf1-Cre* and *Pomc-Cre*, respectively. Surprisingly, however, these mutant mice lacking leptin receptor in VMH or ARC neurons or both have normal bone mass parameters at both the axial and appendicular skeleton [56]. Taken as it is these studies suggested that leptin does not regulate bone mass through the hypothalamus, so where does leptin signal in the brain to regulate bone mass?

NEUROTRANSMITTER PROFILING IN LEPTIN-DEFICIENT MICE BRAIN POINTS TO SEROTONIN AS A TARGET OF LEPTIN

A simple way to address the leptin site of action is to carry out a profiling of different neurotransmitters in the brain, and that is exactly what was done. HPLC profiling of the neurotransmitter levels in the leptin-deficient *ob/ob* mice in comparison with wild-type mice revealed that 1-month-old leptin-deficient animals that had obesity and a high bone mass phenotype have significantly higher content of serotonin in their brain stem, and these levels became more severe as the animals aged [57]. This was consistent with earlier studies that reported increased turnover of serotonin upon leptin infusion [58]. These results suggested that serotonin, directly or indirectly, is inhibited by leptin signaling in the brain. We decided to follow this lead further to understand the importance of high serotonin levels in leptin-deficient mice in the regulation of bone mass. The first questions that come to mind are what is serotonin, and does it regulate bone mass?

Serotonin

Serotonin (5-hydroxytryptamine) is a small molecule that functions both as a neurotransmitter in the central nervous system and as a hormone in the periphery. Serotonin is synthesized through a multistep pathway in which L-tryptophan is converted into L-5OH-tryptophan by an enzyme called tryptophan hydroxylase (Tph). L-5OH-tryptophan is then converted to serotonin by an aromatic L-amino acid decarboxylase [59,60]. There are two Tph genes: *Tph1* and *Tph2*. *Tph1* is expressed mostly in enterochromaffin cells of the gut and is responsible for most of the serotonin present in the blood [61]. On the other hand, the gene *Tph2* is expressed exclusively in serotonergic neurons of the brainstem and is responsible for the production of serotonin in the brain [59]. These two pools of serotonin, one in the blood and the other in the brain, never cross over; therefore these should be viewed from a functional point of view as two distinct molecules [60]. Brain-derived serotonin (BDS) acts as a neurotransmitter, while gut-derived serotonin (GDS) acts as a hormone and regulates a wide variety of processes [62]. The importance of serotonin in the regulation of bone mass is underscored by two clinical observations. First, depressed patients, who allegedly have low serotonergic tone, also have low bone mass [63]; and second, serotonin reuptake inhibitors (SSRIs) when taken for a long time often decrease bone mass [64].

Brain-derived Serotonin Regulates Bone

To determine whether BDS affects bone mass *Tph2*, the gene that encodes for serotonin synthesis in the brain was inactivated by replacing it with a LacZ reporter [57]. This genetic manipulation resulted in barely detectable serotonin levels in *Tph2−/−* mice while it did not have any effect on peripheral serotonin production [57]. This fact is consistent with the serotonin not being able to cross the blood−brain barrier. Histological, histomorphometric, and microcomputed tomography (uCT) analyses of bones performed in 4-, 6-, and 12-week-old wild-type and *Tph2−/−* mice revealed that the absence of serotonin in the brain resulted, at all time points, in a severe low bone mass phenotype affecting axial (vertebrae) and appendicular (long bones) skeleton [57]. This phenotype was secondary to a decrease in bone formation parameters (osteoblast numbers and bone formation rate) and to an increase in bone resorption parameters (osteoclast surface and circulating levels of deoxypridinoline). These results demonstrated that BDS is a positive and powerful regulator of bone mass accrual acting on both arms of bone remodeling [57].

High Sympathetic Tone in BDS-deficient Mice

The cellular phenotype in the bone seen in *Tph2−/−* mice, i.e. a decrease in bone formation and an increase in bone resorption, is the mirror image of what is observed in mice lacking the b2 adrenergic receptor (*Adrb2−/−* mice) [45]. Adrb2 is the receptor that mediates the effect of sympathetic tone on bone mass that is in turn under the regulation of leptin [30]. In addition, there is indirect evidence in patients for the existence of sympathetic

regulation of bone mass. First, patients with reflex sympathetic dystrophy or complex regional pain syndrome suffer from local osteoporosis caused by decreased bone formation in face of elevated sympathetic tone [65]. Second, patients on β-adrenergic blockers seem to have decreased risk of fracture that is associated with an increase in BMD [66].

Analysis of markers of the sympathetic tone, norepinephrine content in the brain, epinephrine elimination in the urine, and *Ucp1* expression in brown fat in the *Tph2−/−* mice revealed a marked increase in all these markers [57]. Two correlative observations indicated that BDS regulation of sympathetic tone and bone mass occurs through the hypothalamic VMH neurons. First, chemical destruction of the VMH neurons results in a decreased sympathetic tone and increase in bone mass, while the opposite is the case for the BDS regulation of bone mass, i.e. increased sympathetic tone and a decreased bone mass. Second, leptin-induced changes in catecholamine secretion occur through the VMH neurons [67,68]. This suggested that VMH neurons are somehow linked with the serotonergic neurons.

Neuroanatomical tracing using fluorescent dextran, a sugar that is pumped through the axonal structures from the site of its application to the end site, revealed that serotonergic and VMH neurons are anatomically connected to each other [57]. If serotonin synthesized in the brainstem is acting on the VMH neurons, serotonin receptors must be expressed on the VMH neurons. Among the 14 serotonin receptors Htr2c is one of the highly expressed receptors in the hypothalamus and is localized to the VMH neurons. Analysis of mice that lack *Htr2c* in all the cells revealed that these mice had a low bone mass phenotype like the BDS-deficient mice [57]. This low bone mass phenotype was due to an increase in bone resorption and a decrease in bone formation and existed in the presence of a high sympathetic tone. These neuroanatomical and genetic studies revealed that serotonin acts on the VMH neurons through Htr2c to inhibit sympathetic tone and positively regulate bone mass [57].

Existence of Low Fat Mass in *Tph2−/−* Mice Reveals a New Function of an Old Neurotransmitter

Tph2-deficient animals, in addition to being severely osteoporotic, have a dramatic decrease in their adipose mass [57]. This observation was not entirely surprising since serotonin is known to play important roles in many other physiological processes. This prompted us to analyze in great detail their energy metabolism phenotype. Detailed studies revealed that the decrease in their fat mass was due, in part, to the fact that these mice ate less and spent much more energy compared to their wild-type littermates [57]. This regulation of appetite through serotonin occurs as early as 1 month of age when *Htr2c*-deficient mice have a normal appetite, fat pad weight, and body weight suggesting involvement of additional serotonin receptors in the regulation of appetite and energy expenditure through serotonin at this age [57].

One of the neuroanatomical sites through which appetite is regulated in the brain is the arcuate neurons in the hypothalamus [11,69]. Two experimental evidences indicated that serotonin synthesized in the brainstem regulates appetite through the arcuate neurons in the hypothalamus. First, neuroanatomical tracing experiments revealed that serotonin neurons are connected with the arcuate neurons. Second, co-*in situ* hybridization analysis showed that arcuate neurons express two of the serotonin receptors, namely *Htr1a* and *2b* [57]. Analysis of mice that lack *Htr1a* and *Htr2b* in the *Pomc*-expressing neurons of the arcuate revealed that these two receptors regulate appetite, and mice that lack both of these receptors on the arcuate neurons have more severe appetite phenotype than their individual counterparts [57,70]. These studies established that serotonin acts through Htr1a and 2b on the ARC neurons to regulate appetite and Htr2c on VMH neurons to regulate bone [57].

SEROTONIN USES CREB IN ARC AND VMH NEURONS TO REGULATE TWO DIFFERENT FUNCTIONS

To understand the downstream effector of serotonin signaling in the arcuate and VMH neurons, *ex vivo* and *in vivo* approaches were used. Analysis of serotonin signaling using hypothalamic slices revealed that serotonin treatment increased the phosphorylation and nuclear localization of Creb in both the VMH and ARC neurons [70,71]. This signaling event could be abrogated, or dramatically reduced, on the VMH or ARC nuclei specifically when *Htr2c* or *Htr1a* knockout explants were used for this analysis demonstrating that it is a specific effect through these receptors [70,71]. This revealed that Creb signaling is active downstream of Htr2c and Htr1a receptors in the VMH and ARC neurons, respectively. Consistent with this model, inactivation of *Creb* in the VMH nuclei resulted in a low bone mass phenotype due to similar dysregulation of sympathetic tone as observed in the *Htr2c−/−* mice [57,71]. This signaling event was confirmed through genetic epistasis experiments since the *Htr2c+/−; Creb+/−* mice had a more severe decrease in bone mass than the individual mice alone [71]. On the other hand, when *Creb* was genetically inactivated in the ARC nuclei these mice had a decrease in appetite

without any effect on their bone mass [70]. Generation of double heterozygous mice revealed that Creb is downstream of the Htr1a receptor in the ARC neurons.

This body of work illustrating a link between the brainstem and hypothalamus does not contradict or exclude a more recent proposal that serotonin uses an interneuron to signal in the hypothalamus [72]. In addition the lower severity of bone phenotype in the *Htr2c−/−* mice compared to *Tph2−/−* mice suggests that there are other receptors of serotonin, perhaps expressed in the hypothalamus or other locations in the brain that mediate leptin-dependent serotonin regulation of bone mass. These studies have illustrated the importance of the serotonin–hypothalamus axis and future studies shall be directed towards understanding the importance of direct and indirect relay of serotonin to the hypothalamic neurons to regulate bone and appetite.

Increase in Brain Serotonin Signaling and Bone Mass

Serotonin once released outside the cells is inactivated by either metabolizing it through the enzymes or is taken back in the cells through a transporter (HTT) to curtail its effect on the receptors. This metabolism of serotonin has long been utilized to cure patients with depression by elevating their extracellular concentration of serotonin in the brain and thereby increasing serotonin signaling. This raises the question of what effect an increase in serotonin signaling has on the bone mass. Selective serotonin reuptake inhibitors (SSRIs) are a class of drugs that blocks the transporter HTT and increase serotonin signaling [73]. Based on these effects, this class of drugs is prescribed to cure many psychiatric disorders associated with diminished serotonin signaling and their therapeutic actions are diverse, ranging from efficacy in the treatment of depression to panic disorders. The plethora of receptors and metabolic pathways for serotonin are candidates to mediate not only the therapeutic actions of SSRIs, but also their side effects [62,64]. Richards et al. [64], while studying a cohort of community-dwelling adults, revealed that patients that were taking SSRIs had an increased risk of hip fractures. Because SSRIs have the ability to cross the blood–brain barrier it raised the question as to the site of action of these drugs to produce their deleterious actions on bone.

Multiple studies using different approaches have tried to understand the deleterious consequences of SSRIs on bone. Battaglino et al. gave animals SSRIs and looked at the alterations in bone mass in these animals; they observed an increase in trabecular bone mass in the animals that received SSRI treatment [74]. These results, given the effects of SSRIs in humans, were surprising at the time they were reported, but we should view them in the context that SSRIs cross the blood–brain barrier and affect both the central and peripheral serotonin compartments. Likely, the observed effects were due to the fact that under the conditions tested in their study SSRIs were having more profound influences on the BDS, a positive regulator of bone mass. Gustafsson et al., on the other hand, used naïve rats and injected them daily with serotonin as a model of serotonin effect on bone mass. Their analysis revealed site-specific alterations in the long bones [75]. Trabecular bone mass decreased while cortical thickness increased in the long bones. The negative influence of serotonin injections on the trabecular bone mass in their study conforms to the SSRIs increasing peripheral serotonin and earlier mouse genetic studies. Warden et al., taking a genetic approach for a model of chronic use of SSRIs, reported that mice that lack serotonin transporter ($Htt-/-$ mice) have decreased bone mass at both cortical and trabecular sites [76]. This is consistent with the clinical reports that show that patients taking SSRIs often have a decrease in bone mass. Surprisingly, however, $Htt-/-$ mice have barely detectable levels of serotonin in their blood and a two-fold reduction in brain serotonin content (VKY, unpublished observations). This raised the question, if both pools of serotonin are decreased in an animal model what phenotype would be apparent? The only way one can decrease serotonin pools consistently in the body is by removing the enzymes that synthesize serotonin. When both of these genes were inactivated in mice, mutant animals were not able to synthesize any serotonin, and most scientists would have predicted that mice will die *in utero* due to the versatile nature of serotonin in biology of different organs. Surprisingly, however, these serotonin-free ($Tph1-/-$; $Tph2-/-$) mice were alive, and until 6 months of age there was no physical abnormality detectable. This generation of mice allowed us to ask which pool of serotonin dominates over regulation of bone mass. Analysis of serotonin-free mice revealed that these mice had a low bone mass phenotype demonstrating that despite accounting for >5% of total serotonin pool in the body, BDS dominates in the overall regulation of bone mass [57]. Since SSRIs cross blood–brain barrier, and osteoporosis and fracture risk are increased only when they are used chronically, development of SSRIs with selective central actions would be worth exploring in the future for curing depression while maximizing the positive influence of serotonin on bone.

Leptin Inhibits Serotonin

Brain-derived serotonin and its signaling-deficient mice collectively have three known functional defects, i.e. a decrease in bone mass and appetite, and an increase in energy expenditure [57]. Serotonin uses distinct receptors expressed on ARC or VMH nuclei to regulate bone mass and appetite [57]; at present we do not know what site or receptor serotonin utilizes to regulate energy expenditure. Although originally we sought to address leptin regulation of bone mass it did not take us long to realize that these three functions of serotonin are a mirror image of the leptin functions. Serotonin regulates these functions in the opposite manner to leptin. So does leptin signal in the serotonergic neurons to inhibit serotonin production that in turn signals in the hypothalamic neurons?

Several experimental evidences pointed towards the validity of this hypothesis. First, ObRb, the signaling form of the leptin receptor, was expressed in $Tph2$-expressing neurons [57]. Several previous studies corroborate the expression of leptin receptors and function on the serotonergic neurons [77–82]. Second, analysis of ob/ob mice revealed an increase in $Tph2$ expression and, conversely, serotonin content was higher in the brainstem of ob/ob mice [57]. Third, leptin ICV infusion decreased $Tph2$ expression in a time- and dose-dependent manner in wild-type mice [57]. Electrophysiological studies with the brain slices prepared from wild-type mice demonstrated experimentally that leptin receptors on the serotonin neurons are functional as the action potential (AP) frequency of these neurons decreased in the presence of leptin. This decrease in the AP frequency was absent in the mice that lacked the leptin receptors on serotonin neurons only revealing that these are serotonin neurons and not the neighboring neurons on which leptin acts. These data pointed towards a model whereby leptin regulates bone mass accrual through a double inhibitory loop. Leptin inhibits synthesis of BDS, which in turn reduces the sympathetic tone; as a result leptin prevents bone mass accrual.

LEPTIN RECEPTOR DELETION ON SEROTONIN NUCLEI RESULTS IN INCREASED APPETITE

The ultimate proof of a physiological pathway that connects two cell types can come from the conditional gene mutagenesis. To understand whether leptin receptor expression on the serotonergic nuclei results in alterations in synthesis and secretion of the serotonin machinery, leptin receptor floxed mice were crossed with a battery of *Sert-Cre* driver [57]. *Sert-Cre* is driven by the *Sert* promoter elements and is expressed highly in the serotonergic nuclei in the brain starting from the early embryonic stages. Generation of *Obrb floxed*; *Sert-Cre* ($Obrb_{Sert}-/-$) animals revealed that these animals had very low levels of the *Obrb* mRNA and protein, and when challenged with leptin they were quiescent electrophysiologically. Ablation of *Obrb* on these neurons resulted in an increase in *Tph2* expression and serotonin content in the brainstem [57]. The first phenotype that was noticeable upon looking in these cages where litters containing wild-type and *Obrb*~Sert~−/− animals were present was that some mice were obese. Genotype analysis confirmed that the animals that were looking obese were *Sert-Cre*+ animals. As these mutant animals aged their obesity became more severe. This alteration in the leptin receptor population in the serotonin neurons resulted in similar cellular and molecular changes in the hypothalamus as observed in the leptin-deficient mice. On the other hand, leptin receptor deletion in ARC neurons or VMH neurons did not result in any significant changes in appetite. These studies demonstrated that leptin uses serotonin as one of its downstream mediators to affect hypothalamic regulation of appetite [57].

Two immediate questions were raised by the discovery that leptin inhibits serotonin to regulate appetite. First, is this phenotype serotonin neuron specific, as the *Cre* driver that was used to demonstrate the leptin action on serotonin neurons is also expressed on many peripheral cell types? Second, is this a developmental effect of leptin receptor deletion or does leptin regulate appetite through serotonin postnatally? These questions were next addressed using an *ERT2-Cre* line that was driven by the *Tph2* promoter elements. This *Cre* driver was silent in the absence of tamoxifen, but Cre was exclusively expressed in the serotonin neurons of the brain once these animals were injected with tamoxifen, and was not detectable in any other region of the brain or peripheral tissues [70]. When this *Tph2ERT2-Cre* driver was used to delete *Obrb* postnatally it resulted in an increase in the serotonin content in the brain stem, and an increase in appetite. This phenotype was, however, less severe than the phenotype observed in the *db/db* mice suggesting that other molecular players are also involved in the leptin regulation of appetite [23,70]. The use of this *Tph2ERT2-Cre* driver cleared many of the questions that were surrounding leptin action on serotonin neurons, and confirmed the importance of this brainstem—hypothalamus axis in adult mice.

Let us rewind from the regulation of appetite to regulation of bone through leptin. Mice that lacked *Obrb* on serotonin neurons (*Obrb*~Sert~−/− mice) are obese and have a low sympathetic tone. Histological and histomorphometric analysis of 3-month-old animals confirmed that, as expected, these mice had a high bone mass phenotype that was due to an increase in osteoblast and osteoclast functions. This phenotype was similar at cellular and molecular levels to the leptin or its receptor-deficient animals and was associated with a decreased sympathetic tone in these animals [23,57]. Similar to what was observed in the regulation of appetite, leptin receptor deletion in ARC neurons or VMH

neurons did not result in any significant changes in bone mass [57].

Together these studies unraveled an unanticipated molecular link between leptin and serotonin and revealed how leptin orchestrates two of its main functions, i.e. energy and bone metabolism through a common mediator, serotonin, and by utilizing different receptors on distinct neurons in the hypothalamus (Fig. 5.1). It makes sense from an organismal point of view to have a single molecule regulating multiple functions to reduce the energetic costs of this regulation, and at the same time making the system more efficient.

Are Other Functions of Leptin Going through the Brain—Osteoblast Axis?

Leptin regulates insulin secretion besides its well-established role in regulating appetite, bone mass, and reproduction. This regulation occurs through the direct effect of leptin on the pancreas and through its indirect effects occurring via the brain [83]. Consistent with leptin being an inhibitor of insulin secretion, *ob/ob* mice have higher insulin levels since birth [84]. Hinoi et al., while elucidating this regulation, identified that one mechanism through which leptin decreases insulin secretion is via bone [84]. Leptin upregulates the sympathetic tone that impinges on bone to regulate Esp expression. Esp is a phosphatase that decreases osteocalcin bioavailability that, in turn, regulates insulin secretion [85]. In the context of the recent demonstration that insulin signaling in osteoblasts is a positive regulator of bone mass, this study identifies a feedback loop through which leptin coordinates energy metabolism and bone mass [19].

Potential for Pharmacological Inhibition of Serotonin Pathways in the Treatment of Energy and Bone Metabolism

These studies have revealed that leptin affects bone and energy metabolism by regulating serotonin synthesis in the brain. Serotonin, in turn, acts on the hypothalamus and uses distinct receptors to regulate appetite and bone mass. These studies thus provide a new means through which these functions can be therapeutically targeted. Involvement of specific serotonin receptors on hypothalamic neurons that regulate appetite and bone mass provides an opportunity to pharmacologically target these specific receptors for the treatment of osteoporosis and appetite. However, the fact that each of these serotonin receptors participates in multiple physiologic processes presents a challenge, since even a drug targeting a single serotonin receptor is likely to affect multiple body systems.

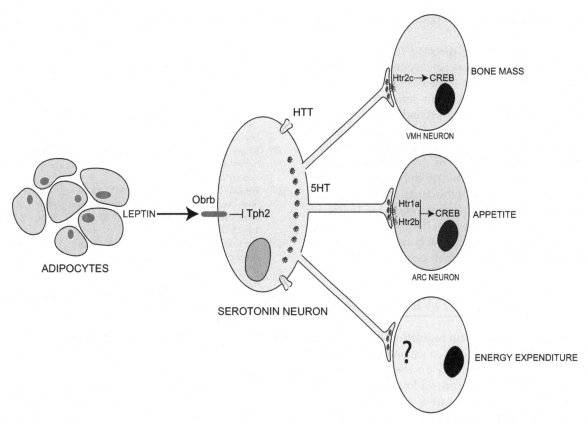

FIGURE 5.1 **Serotonin-dependent neuronal relay in the leptin regulation of bone mass, appetite, and energy expenditure.** Leptin inhibits synthesis and release of brain-derived serotonin, among other neuronal relays, which favors bone mass accrual and appetite through its action on ventromedial and arcuate hypothalamic neurons. VMH, ventromedial hypothalamus; ARC, arcuate; HTT, 5-hydroxytryptamine transporter. Structures not to scale. Please see color plate section.

Leptin-dependent serotonin control of bone mass seems to be more complex yet amenable to therapeutic interventions if we can selectively target the downstream events. Small molecules that target *Tph2* expression or activity can be used for increasing bone mass. However, it will also result in an increase in appetite, as BDS is a positive regulator of food intake. The same would be the case if we can find ways to increase signaling specifically in the brain through brain-selective SSRIs. Htr2c agonists may be more selective as they would only regulate bone as demonstrated by mouse and human genetic studies, but their clinical use would be limited by their effects on other organ systems, such as on the sympathetic tone [57,86]. Despite these complexities in the regulation of bone mass through serotonin relay in the brain, future studies might be able to dissociate the downstream events, and the serotonergic system in the brain may very well become a way to increase bone mass in future.

In contrast, the regulation of bone serotonergic pathways downstream of leptin in the regulation of appetite seems simpler and could be targeted to regulate appetite disorders. Serotonin favors appetite through Htr1a receptors expressed on the hypothalamus, therefore use of antagonists that target Htr1a receptor should decrease appetite. In a proof of principle study it was shown that LY426965, a small molecule potent inhibitor of Htr1a receptor, when fed to mice daily led to a significant decrease in their appetite and caused them to gain less weight compared to vehicle-treated control mice [70]. Most importantly, a single dose of LY426965 could decrease appetite when administered to 4-week-old *ob/ob* mice. Food intake in LY426965-treated *ob/ob* animals was ~24% lower than in vehicle-treated mice, demonstrating that inhibition of signaling through Htr1a in leptin deficiency or resistance can reduce appetite. The fact that this compound did not fully rescue the appetite phenotype caused by the absence of leptin is consistent with the notion that serotonin also decreases appetite by signaling through Htr2b receptor, and possibly through other systems in the brain. LY426965 could rescue, partially, the hyperphagia of *ob/ob* mice when it was administered chronically in 4-week-old *ob/ob* mice, and lead to a significant decrease in the obesity phenotype of *ob/ob* mice (~27%), without affecting the energy expenditure. This result is consistent with the notion that one mechanism whereby leptin inhibits appetite is by decreasing serotonin synthesis and release from serotonergic neurons and signaling through the Htr1a receptor [57].

Future studies should be directed towards a better understanding of the serotonergic system in the brain and address several specific issues: first, the threshold levels at which activation in brain serotonin signaling increases bone and appetite; second, to analyze in more detail downstream targets of serotonin in this regulation, and how bone and appetite are coordinated under specific physiological or pathological stimuli such as stress or physical activity; third, to thoroughly characterize the side effects of the drugs that have potential to target this pathway on other systems in the body; and fourth, and most importantly, if these types of drugs can be used to treat obesity or low bone mass disorders in other genetic models of human diseases.

PERSPECTIVE

Since the discovery of leptin regulation of bone in the year 2000 to the realization of a common central control of bone and energy metabolism downstream of leptin through serotonin, we have come a long way in understanding the way appetite centers are regulated and coordinated to provide sufficient energy to the energy-driven processes such as bone metabolism [87]. Bones, in turn, feed back to the energy metabolic centers, though indirectly under the regulation of leptin, by secreting osteocalcin—a hormone that regulates glucose homeostasis and thereby provides energy for the bone remodeling units. These studies have been made possible through the use of modern mouse molecular genetics that has given us new tools to identify leptin's site and mechanism of action. Understanding the biology of leptin in these processes has led to the identification of novel therapeutic targets for regulation of appetite—Htr1a antagonists, and bone mass—Tph2/Htr2c agonists. These and many such studies have raised the hope that, perhaps one day, we will find cure for osteoporosis and obesity—two of mankind's most common metabolic diseases of 21st century.

Acknowledgment

This work was supported by the Wellcome Trust (Grant Number: 098051). My sincere apologies to researchers whose work has not been discussed due to the space constraints.

References

[1] Rodan GA, Martin TJ. Therapeutic approaches to bone diseases. Science 2000;289:1508–14.

[2] Karsenty G. Bone endocrine regulation of energy metabolism and male reproduction. C R Biol Oct 2012;334(10):720–4.

[3] Crockett JC, Rogers MJ, Coxon FP, Hocking LJ, Helfrich MH. Bone remodelling at a glance. J Cell Sci Apr 1 2011;124(Pt 7):991–8.

[4] Teitelbaum SL. Bone resorption by osteoclasts. Science 2000;289:1504–8.

[5] Ducy P, Schinke T, Karsenty G. The osteoblast: a sophisticated fibroblast under central surveillance. Science 2000;289:1501–4.

[6] Legroux-Gerot I, Vignau J, D'Herbomez M, Collier F, Marchandise X, Duquesnoy B, et al. Evaluation of bone loss and its mechanisms in anorexia nervosa. Calcif Tissue Int 2007 Sep;81(3):174–82.

[7] Misra M, Klibanski A. The neuroendocrine basis of anorexia nervosa and its impact on bone metabolism. Neuroendocrinology 2011;93(2):65–73.

[8] Felson DT, Zhang Y, Hannan MT, Anderson JJ. Effects of weight and body mass index on bone mineral density in men and women: the Framingham study. J Bone Miner Res 1993;8(5):567–73.

[9] Tremollieres FA, Pouilles JM, Ribot C. Vertebral postmenopausal bone loss is reduced in overweight women: a longitudinal study in 155 early postmenopausal women. J Clin Endocrinol Metab 1993;77:683–6.

[10] Saper CB, Chou TC, Elmquist JK. The need to feed: homeostatic and hedonic control of eating. Neuron 2002 Oct 10;36(2):199–211.

[11] Elmquist J, Zigman J, Lutter M. Molecular determinants of energy homeostasis. Am J Psychiatry 2006 Jul;163(7):1137.

[12] Spiegelman BM, Flier JS. Obesity and the regulation of energy balance. Cell 2001 Feb 23;104(4):531–43.

[13] Lindsley JE, Rutter J. Nutrient sensing and metabolic decisions. Comp Biochem Physiol B Biochem Mol Biol 2004 Dec;139(4):543–59.

[14] Salway JG. Metabolism at a Glance.. Third Edition. Oxford: Blackwell Publishing Ltd; 2004.

[15] Glauber HS, Vollmer WM, Nevitt MC, Ensrud KE, Orwoll ES. Body weight versus body fat distribution, adiposity, and frame size as predictors of bone density. J Clin Endocrinol Metab 1995 Apr;80(4):1118–23.

[16] Reid IR, Plank LD, Evans MC. Fat mass is an important determinant of whole body bone density in premenopausal women but not in men. J Clin Endocrinol Metab 1992 Sep;75(3):779–82.

[17] Reid IR, Ames R, Evans MC, Sharpe S, Gamble G, France JT, et al. Determinants of total body and regional bone mineral density in normal postmenopausal women—a key role for fat mass. J Clin Endocrinol Metab 1992 Jul;75(1):45–51.

[18] Revilla M, Villa LF, Hernandez ER, Sanchez-Atrio A, Cortes J, Rico H. Influence of weight and gonadal status on total and regional bone mineral content and on weight-bearing and non-weight-bearing bones, measured by dual-energy X-ray absorptiometry. Maturitas 1997 Sep;28(1):69–74.

[19] Clemens TL, Karsenty G. The osteoblast: an insulin target cell controlling glucose homeostasis. J Bone Miner Res Apr 2011;26(4):677–80.

[20] Fulzele K, Clemens TL. Novel functions for insulin in bone. Bone 2012 Feb;50(2):452–6.

[21] Ferron M, Wei J, Yoshizawa T, Del Fattore A, DePinho RA, Teti A, et al. Insulin signaling in osteoblasts integrates bone remodeling and energy metabolism. Cell. 2010 Jul 23; 142(2):296–308.

[22] Schindler AE, Ebert A, Friedrich E. Conversion of androstenedione to estrone by human tissue. J Clin Endocrinol Metab 1972 Oct;35(4):627–30.

[23] Ducy P, Amling M, Takeda S, Priemel M, Schilling AF, Beil FT, et al. Leptin inhibits bone formation through a hypothalamic relay: a central control of bone mass. Cell 2000 Jan 21;100(2):197–207.

[24] Friedman JM, Halaas JL. Leptin and the regulation of body weight in mammals. Nature 1998;395(6704):763−70.

[25] Zhang Y, Proenca R, Maffei M, Barone M, Leopold L, Friedman JM. Positional cloning of the mouse obese gene and its human homologue. Nature 1994;372:425−32.

[26] Chehab FF, Qiu J, Ogus S. The use of animal models to dissect the biology of leptin. Recent Prog Horm Res. 2004;59:245−66.

[27] Unger RH, Elmquist JK. Movin' on up: adipocytes become regulators of nutrient homeostasis. Cell Metab 2006 Mar;3(3):147−8.

[28] Grill HJ. Leptin and the systems neuroscience of meal size control. Front Neuroendocrinol 2010;Jan;31(1):61−78.

[29] Ahima RS, Flier JS. Leptin. Annu Rev Physiol 2000;62:413−37.

[30] Takeda S, Elefteriou F, Levasseur R, Liu X, Zhao L, Parker KL, et al. Leptin regulates bone formation via the sympathetic nervous system. Cell 2002 Nov 1;111(3):305−17.

[31] Elefteriou F, Takeda S, Ebihara K, Magre J, Patano N, Kim CA, et al. Serum leptin level is a regulator of bone mass. Proc Natl Acad Sci USA 2004 Mar 2;101(9):3258−63.

[32] Tartaglia LA, Dembski M, Weng X, Deng N, Culpepper J, Devos R, et al. Identification and expression cloning of a leptin receptor, OB-R. Cell 1995;83(7):1263−71.

[33] Flier JS, Elmquist JK. Energetic pursuit of leptin function. Nat Biotechnol 1997 Jan;15(1):20−1.

[34] Pogoda P, Egermann M, Schnell JC, Priemel M, Schilling AF, Alini M, et al. Leptin inhibits bone formation not only in rodents, but also in sheep. J Bone Miner Res 2006 Oct;21(10):1591−9.

[35] Guidobono F, Pagani F, Sibilia V, Netti C, Lattuada N, Rapetti D, et al. Different skeletal regional response to continuous brain infusion of leptin in the rat. Peptides 2006 Jun;27(6):1426−33.

[36] Cornish J, Callon KE, Bava U, Lin C, Naot D, Hill BL, et al. Leptin directly regulates bone cell function in vitro and reduces bone fragility in vivo. J Endocrinol 2002 Nov;175(2):405−15.

[37] Bartell SM, Rayalam S, Ambati S, Gaddam DR, Hartzell DL, Hamrick M, et al. Central (ICV) leptin injection increases bone formation, bone mineral density, muscle mass, serum IGF-1, and the expression of osteogenic genes in leptin-deficient ob/ob mice. J Bone Miner Res Aug;2010;26(8):1710−20.

[38] Bjorbaek C, Kahn BB. Leptin signaling in the central nervous system and the periphery. Recent Prog Horm Res 2004;59:305−31.

[39] Bjornholm M, Munzberg H, Leshan RL, Villanueva EC, Bates SH, Louis GW, et al. Mice lacking inhibitory leptin receptor signals are lean with normal endocrine function. J Clin Invest 2007 May;117(5):1354−60.

[40] Shi Y, Yadav VK, Suda N, Liu XS, Guo XE, Myers Jr MG, et al. Dissociation of the neuronal regulation of bone mass and energy metabolism by leptin in vivo. Proc Natl Acad Sci USA 2008 Dec 23;105(51):20529−33.

[41] Elmquist JK. Hypothalamic pathways underlying the endocrine, autonomic, and behavioral effects of leptin. Physiol Behav 2001 Nov−Dec;74(4−5):703−8.

[42] Elmquist JK, Ahima RS, Elias CF, Flier JS, Saper CB. Leptin activates distinct projections from the dorsomedial and ventromedial hypothalamic nuclei. Proc Natl Acad Sci USA 1998 Jan 20;95(2):741−6.

[43] Elefteriou F, Takeda S, Liu X, Armstrong D, Karsenty G. Monosodium glutamate-sensitive hypothalamic neurons contribute to the control of bone mass. Endocrinology 2003 Sep;144(9):3842−7.

[44] Elias CF, Lee C, Kelly J, Aschkenasi C, Ahima RS, Couceyro PR, et al. Leptin activates hypothalamic CART neurons projecting to the spinal cord. Neuron 1998 Dec;21(6):1375−85.

[45] Elefteriou F, Ahn JD, Takeda S, Starbuck M, Yang X, Liu X, et al. Leptin regulation of bone resorption by the sympathetic nervous system and CART. Nature 2005 Mar 24;434(7032):514−20.

[46] Singh MK, Elefteriou F, Karsenty G. Cocaine and amphetamine-regulated transcript may regulate bone remodeling as a circulating molecule. Endocrinology 2008 Aug;149(8):3933−41.

[47] Baldock PA, Sainsbury A, Allison S, Lin EJ, Couzens M, Boey D, et al. Hypothalamic control of bone formation: distinct actions of leptin and y2 receptor pathways. J Bone Miner Res 2005 Oct;20(10):1851−7.

[48] Lundberg P, Allison SJ, Lee NJ, Baldock PA, Brouard N, Rost S, et al. Greater bone formation of Y2 knockout mice is associated with increased osteoprogenitor numbers and altered Y1 receptor expression. J Biol Chem 2007 Jun 29;282(26):19082−91.

[49] Baldock PA, Sainsbury A, Couzens M, Enriquez RF, Thomas GP, Gardiner EM, et al. Hypothalamic Y2 receptors regulate bone formation. J Clin Invest 2002;109(7):915−21.

[50] Baldock PA, Allison S, McDonald MM, Sainsbury A, Enriquez RF, Little DG, et al. Hypothalamic regulation of cortical bone mass: opposing activity of Y2 receptor and leptin pathways. J Bone Miner Res 2006 Oct;21(10):1600−7.

[51] Peier A, Kosinski J, Cox-York K, Qian Y, Desai K, Feng Y, et al. The antiobesity effects of centrally administered neuromedin U and neuromedin S are mediated predominantly by the neuromedin U receptor 2 (NMUR2). Endocrinology 2009 Jul;150(7):3101−9.

[52] Doggrell SA. Neuromedin U—a new target in obesity. Expert Opin Ther Targets 2005 Aug;9(4):875−7.

[53] Howard AD, Wang R, Pong SS, Mellin TN, Strack A, Guan XM, et al. Identification of receptors for neuromedin U and its role in feeding. Nature 2000 Jul 6;406(6791):70−4.

[54] Sato S, Hanada R, Kimura A, Abe T, Matsumoto T, Iwasaki M, et al. Central control of bone remodeling by neuromedin U. Nat Med 2007 Sep 16. in press.

[55] Cohen P, Zhao C, Cai X, Montez JM, Rohani SC, Feinstein P, et al. Selective deletion of leptin receptor in neurons leads to obesity. J Clin Invest 2001;108(8):1113−21.

[56] Dhillon H, Zigman JM, Ye C, Lee CE, McGovern RA, Tang V, et al. Leptin directly activates SF1 neurons in the VMH, and this action by leptin is required for normal body-weight homeostasis. Neuron 2006 Jan 19;49(2):191−203.

[57] Yadav VK, Oury F, Suda N, Liu ZW, Gao XB, Confavreux C, et al. A serotonin-dependent mechanism explains the leptin regulation of bone mass, appetite, and energy expenditure. Cell 2009 Sep 4;138(5):976−89.

[58] Calapai G, Corica F, Corsonello A, Sautebin L, Di Rosa M, Campo GM, et al. Leptin increases serotonin turnover by inhibition of brain nitric oxide synthesis. J Clin Invest 1999 Oct;104(7):975−82.

[59] Walther DJ, Peter JU, Bashammakh S, Hortnagl H, Voits M, Fink H, et al. Synthesis of serotonin by a second tryptophan hydroxylase isoform. Science 2003 Jan 3;299(5603):76.

[60] Mann JJ, McBride PA, Brown RP, Linnoila M, Leon AC, DeMeo M, et al. Relationship between central and peripheral serotonin indexes in depressed and suicidal psychiatric inpatients. Arch Gen Psychiatry 1992 Jun;49(6):442−6.

[61] Gershon MD, Tack J. The serotonin signaling system: from basic understanding to drug development for functional GI disorders. Gastroenterology 2007 Jan;132(1):397−414.

[62] Heath MJ, Hen R. Serotonin receptors. Genetic insights into serotonin function. Curr Biol 1995 Sep 1;5(9):997−9.

[63] Eskandari F, Martinez PE, Torvik S, Phillips TM, Sternberg EM, Mistry S, et al. Low bone mass in premenopausal women with depression. Arch Intern Med 2007 Nov 26;167(21):2329−36.

[64] Richards JB, Papaioannou A, Adachi JD, Joseph L, Whitson HE, Prior JC, et al. Effect of selective serotonin reuptake inhibitors on the risk of fracture. Arch Intern Med 2007 Jan 22;167(2): 188–94.

[65] Schwartzman RJ. New treatments for reflex sympathetic dystrophy. N Engl J Med 2000 Aug 31;343(9):654–6.

[66] Pasco JA, Henry MJ, Sanders KM, Kotowicz MA, Seeman E, Nicholson GC. Beta-adrenergic blockers reduce the risk of fracture partly by increasing bone mineral density: Geelong Osteoporosis Study. J Bone Miner Res 2004 Jan;19(1):19–24.

[67] Ruffin M, Nicolaidis S. Electrical stimulation of the ventromedial hypothalamus enhances both fat utilization and metabolic rate that precede and parallel the inhibition of feeding behavior. Brain Res 1999;846(1):23–9.

[68] Satoh N, Ogawa Y, Katsuura G, Numata Y, Tsuji T, Hayase M, et al. Sympathetic activation of leptin via the ventromedial hypothalamus: leptin-induced increase in catecholamine secretion. Diabetes 1999;48(9):1787–93.

[69] Hill J, Elmquist JK, Elias CF. Hypothalamic pathways linking energy balance and reproduction. Am J Physiol Endocrinol Metab 2008 Feb 19.

[70] Yadav VK, Oury F, Tanaka KF, Thomas T, Wang Y, Cremers S, et al. Leptin-dependent serotonin control of appetite: temporal specificity, transcriptional regulation, and therapeutic implications. J Exp Med 2011 Jan 17;208(1):41–52.

[71] Oury F, Yadav VK, Wang Y, Zhou B, Liu XS, Guo XE, et al. CREB mediates brain serotonin regulation of bone mass through its expression in ventromedial hypothalamic neurons. Genes Dev 2010 Oct 15;24(20):2330–42.

[72] Lam DD, Leinninger GM, Louis GW, Garfield AS, Marston OJ, Leshan RL, et al. Leptin does not directly affect CNS serotonin neurons to influence appetite. Cell Metab 2011; 13(5):584–91.

[73] Mann JJ. The medical management of depression. N Engl J Med 2005 Oct 27;353(17):1819–34.

[74] Battaglino R, Vokes M, Schulze-Spate U, Sharma A, Graves D, Kohler T, et al. Fluoxetine treatment increases trabecular bone formation in mice. J Cell Biochem 2007 Apr 15;100(6):1387–94.

[75] Gustafsson BI, Westbroek I, Waarsing JH, Waldum H, Solligard E, Brunsvik A, et al. Long-term serotonin administration leads to higher bone mineral density, affects bone

architecture, and leads to higher femoral bone stiffness in rats. J Cell Biochem 2006 Apr 15;97(6):1283–91.

[76] Warden SJ, Robling AG, Sanders MS, Bliziotes MM, Turner CH. Inhibition of the serotonin (5-hydroxytryptamine) transporter reduces bone accrual during growth. Endocrinology 2005 Feb;146(2):685–93.

[77] Scott MM, Lachey JL, Sternson SM, Lee CE, Elias CF, Friedman JM, et al. Leptin targets in the mouse brain. J Comp Neurol 2009 Jun 10;514(5):518–32.

[78] Hay-Schmidt A, Helboe L, Larsen PJ. Leptin receptor immunoreactivity is present in ascending serotonergic and catecholaminergic neurons of the rat. Neuroendocrinology 2001 Apr;73(4):215–26.

[79] Fernandez-Galaz MC, Diano S, Horvath TL, Garcia-Segura LM. Leptin uptake by serotonergic neurones of the dorsal raphe. J Neuroendocrinol 2002 Jun;14(6):429–34.

[80] Fei H, Okano HJ, Li C, Lee GH, Zhao C, Darnell R, et al. Anatomic localization of alternatively spliced leptin receptors (Ob-R) in mouse brain and other tissues. Proc Natl Acad Sci USA 1997;94(13):7001–5.

[81] Elmquist JK, Bjorbaek C, Ahima RS, Flier JS, Saper CB. Distributions of leptin receptor mRNA isoforms in the rat brain. J Comp Neurol 1998;395(4):535–47.

[82] Elmquist JK, Ahima RS, Maratos-Flier E, Flier JS, Saper CB. Leptin activates neurons in ventrobasal hypothalamus and brainstem. Endocrinology 1997 Feb;138(2):839–42.

[83] Kieffer TJ, Habener JF. The adipoinsular axis: effects of leptin on pancreatic beta-cells. Am J Physiol Endocrinol Metab 2000 Jan;278(1):E1–E14.

[84] Hinoi E, Gao N, Jung DY, Yadav V, Yoshizawa T, Myers Jr MG, et al. The sympathetic tone mediates leptin's inhibition of insulin secretion by modulating osteocalcin bioactivity. J Cell Biol 2008 Dec 29;183(7):1235–42.

[85] Lee NK, Sowa H, Hinoi E, Ferron M, Ahn JD, Confavreux C, et al. Endocrine regulation of energy metabolism by the skeleton. Cell 2007 Aug 10;130(3):456–69.

[86] Heisler LK, Cowley MA, Kishi T, Tecott LH, Fan W, Low MJ, et al. Central serotonin and melanocortin pathways regulating energy homeostasis. Ann N Y Acad Sci 2003 Jun;994:169–74.

[87] Karsenty G, Oury F. Biology without Walls: The Novel Endocrinology of Bone. Annu Rev Physiol 2012;74:87–105.

6

Gastrointestinal Tract and the Control of Bone Mass

Thorsten Schinke, Michael Amling

University Medical Center Hamburg-Eppendorf, Hamburg, Germany

It is obvious that the skeleton does not exist by itself, but that it is under the influence of several other organs, which are in turn regulated by bone-derived hormones. Likewise, osteoporosis, the most common bone remodeling disorder, is not only caused by intrinsic defects of bone cell differentiation or function, but also by defects of other sites in the organism that indirectly influence bone-forming osteoblasts or bone-resorbing osteoclasts. Based on these arguments it is important not only to identify, but also to understand all relevant interactions between the skeleton and other tissues to ensure an appropriate treatment of the respective patients. This chapter will focus on novel findings obtained from clinical studies and mouse models that demonstrate the importance of intact gastric acidification for calcium homeostasis and skeletal integrity. Given the high prevalence of hypochlorhydria in the aged population, it is indeed important to address the question of whether an increased gastric pH is a relevant risk factor for osteoporosis, and, if so, if these individuals would profit from specific calcium supplementation. Moreover, the following discussion of the current knowledge regarding these questions provides another example for the critical importance of a complete osteologic patient assessment and for the requirement of *in vivo* models to understand bone as an integral part of the organism.

THE RELEVANCE OF THE GASTROINTESTINAL TRACT FOR THE SKELETON

The gastrointestinal tract, which can be grossly divided into the stomach and the intestine, is surely not part of the skeleton, yet there are some aspects of gastroenterology that are highly relevant for osteology.

First, one of the most important hormones of bone biology, namely vitamin D, primarily acts in the intestine, where it induces the expression of specific genes required for calcium absorption [1]. Second, inflammatory diseases affecting the gastrointestinal tract, such as Morbus Crohn or ulcerative colitis, are often associated with decreased bone mineral density, and it is still under debate whether this is a consequence of malabsorption or rather of inflammatory processes [2]. Third, one of the most relevant negative regulators of bone formation, namely peripheral serotonin, is primarily expressed by enterochromaffin cells in the duodenum, and it is remarkable that an inhibitor of the rate-limiting enzyme for peripheral serotonin synthesis causes an osteoanabolic effect in preclinical models, although it specifically acts in the gut [3]. Fourth, the recent identification of proton pump inhibitors as potential risk factors for osteoporosis has paved the way to reevaluate the previously suggested importance of gastric acidification for calcium homeostasis and skeletal integrity [4]. While the relevance of duodenal serotonin synthesis for bone biology is discussed in another chapter of this book, this chapter will particularly focus on the impact of gastric acidification on the skeleton. In our opinion, this aspect of bone biology is particularly important, since many osteoporotic patients are also characterized by hypochlorhydria; in other words, if we understand how an increased gastric pH affects bone remodeling, we might be able to treat these patients in the most efficient way.

HYPOCHLORHYDRIA, A MAJOR PUBLIC HEALTH PROBLEM

Hypochlorhydria (HCH) is defined as a pathological condition characterized by reduced or even absent (achlorhydria) acid secretion through parietal cells of the stomach [5]. The most common cause of spontaneous HCH is chronic atrophic gastritis, which can either be the result of *H. pylori* infection or of an autoimmune reaction [6]. Since both conditions are frequently asymptomatic and therefore remain undiagnosed in many cases, there is yet no consensus regarding the actual prevalence of HCH [7]. However, based on epidemiologic studies, it has been estimated that more than 30% of individuals older than 60 years are affected by chronic gastritis, which includes the so-called developed countries [5,7−9]. While this already implies that HCH is one of the most common pathologies in the aged population, the theoretical problem becomes even more obvious when the cases of iatrogenic HCH are included.

Although the intake of antacids or antihistamines can cause a transient increase of the gastric pH, the major class of drugs causing persistent HCH is the so-called proton pump inhibitors (PPIs) [10]. These compounds have been developed as specific antagonists of the H^+/K^+-ATPase, which represents an enzyme complex expressed by parietal cells that is required for gastric acidification [11]. PPIs are widely used, not only to prevent gastric ulcers, but even more to treat individuals with gastroesophageal reflux disease. Underscoring the fact that gastric pathologies are extremely common, PPIs are some of the best-selling drugs worldwide, and some lower-dosage variants are even available without prescription [10]. Only in the US are there more than 100 million prescriptions filled per year, and there are more than 20 million people using PPIs, mostly to prevent the uncomfortable symptoms of gastroesophageal reflux. Based on these arguments, it is obvious that the continuous usage of PPIs is a relevant factor that substantially increases the prevalence of HCH, especially in the elderly. In conclusion, while osteoporosis has already been recognized as one of the most common disorders in the aged population, the same is surely true for HCH. Moreover, even if there would be no association between the two pathologies, it is evident that a large subgroup of osteoporotic individuals is also characterized by impaired gastric acidification.

PROTON PUMP INHIBITORS AND OSTEOPOROSIS

One of the major reasons for the large number of individuals using PPIs is surely that these drugs are generally well tolerated and relieve the irritating symptoms of gastroesophageal reflux without causing other ones. There is, however, increasing evidence for specific adverse effects of chronic PPI usage, which are likely explained by the fact that the gastric pH in the respective individuals is pathologically increased [12,13]. These side effects include enhanced susceptibility to infections, increased risk of heart failure (when PPIs are used in combination with drugs suppressing blood coagulation) and a higher rate of skeletal fractures. For obvious reasons this chapter will solely focus on the adverse effect of chronic PPI therapy on the skeleton, a matter that has arisen based on the outcome of a clinical study published in 2006 [14]. Given their hypothesis that PPIs could have a dual effect on the skeleton, namely impaired bone mineralization due to calcium malabsorption and/or decreased bone resorption due to inhibition of osteoclast-mediated extracellular acidification, the authors aimed at analyzing a possible association between PPI therapy and fracture risk. They therefore conducted a case−control study using the General Practice Research Database in the UK and specifically included individuals older than 50 years. They observed a significant association of hip fractures with PPI therapy for more than 1 year, most importantly the strength of this association was correlated with increased PPI dose and duration of usage [14]. A similar study performed in Denmark at the same time confirmed these observations, although these authors did not identify a dose−response relationship in their population, which did, however, include individuals of all ages [15].

Given the important clinical impact of these findings, it is not surprising that subsequent studies have been performed by various investigators (summarized in Table 6.1), and while some of them confirmed an association of PPI therapy with hip fracture incidence, others did not [16−21]. For obvious reasons the conflicting outcome of these studies has initiated a debate into whether PPI therapy should be considered as an additional risk factor for osteoporosis [22]. Although there is as yet no consensus regarding this question, there are a few conclusions that can be drawn from the combined efforts of many investigators. First, there is ample evidence for an increased fracture risk in individuals receiving PPI therapy for more than 5 years [17,23]. Second, the reported association between PPI therapy and osteoporotic fractures is rather moderate, since the adjusted odds ratios were all below 2.0 [24]. And third, it appears that PPI therapy is specifically associated with increased fracture risk, when it is combined with other risk factors for osteoporosis [19,22]. Taken together and regardless of the open questions, these arguments have led to the consensus that PPI therapy should be restricted to appropriate indications and not be applied at higher doses or longer durations than necessary [23,25].

TABLE 6.1 Summary of Published Clinical Studies Analyzing the Association of PPI Therapy and Fracture Risk

Study	Country	Type of study	# individuals	PPI fracture association Hip	Other sites
Yang et al., 2006 [15]	UK	Case–control	13,556 cases 153,386 controls	Yes	Not reported
Vestergaard et al., 2006 [16]	Denmark	Case–control	124,655 cases 373,962 controls	Yes	Yes
Targownik et al., 2008 [17]	Canada	Case–control	15,792 cases 47 289 controls	Yes[1]	Yes[1]
Yu et al., 2008 [18]	USA	Cohort	721 PPI users 10,373 controls	No	Yes
Kaye et al., 2008 [19]	UK	Case–control	1098 cases 10,923 controls	No[2]	Not reported
Roux et al., 2009 [20]	Germany UK	Cohort	61 PPI users 1150 controls	Not reported	Yes
Gray et al., 2010 [21]	USA	Cohort	3396 PPI users 127,756 controls	No	Yes
Corley et al., 2010 [22]	USA	Case–control	33,752 cases 130,471 controls	Yes[3]	Not reported

[1]Only after 7 years of PPI therapy.
[2]In individuals without additional risk factors for hip fractures.
[3]Only in individuals with at least one additional risk factor for hip fractures.

HOW ARE PROTON PUMP INHIBITORS AFFECTING THE SKELETON?

Since intact gastric acidification is physiologically relevant in several regards, it is obvious that raising the gastric pH by PPI therapy can potentially affect the organism in multiple ways [5]. Therefore, it is virtually impossible to rule out that impaired absorption of certain vitamins and trace elements, bacterial overgrowth in the intestine, or even disturbed functions of enterochromaffin cells can partially explain the adverse effects of long-term PPI usage on the skeleton. There are, however, two major hypotheses being discussed in the field to explain the association of PPI therapy and fracture risk. First, since osteoclasts are acid-producing cells and since a PPI-mediated inhibition of their resorptive capacity has been demonstrated *in vitro*, PPIs could potentially interfere with physiological bone remodeling [26]. Second, since skeletal integrity relies on sufficient calcium supply, it is that PPI-induced calcium malabsorption may trigger secondary hyperparathyroidism and thereby increased fracture risk. In this regard it is important to state that none of the clinical studies summarized in Table 6.1 has addressed these two possibilities, for instance by analyzing serum markers of bone remodeling and/or calcium homeostasis. However, while there is one publication reporting decreased urinary levels of bone resorption markers in individuals receiving the PPI omeprazole [27],

there are several studies addressing the impact of omeprazole on intestinal calcium absorption, and again there were conflicting results [28].

For instance, there are three published studies showing that the postprandial increment in serum calcium is significantly reduced by omeprazole, either in healthy individuals or in hemodialysis patients [29–31]. In contrast, two studies, both determining calcium absorption by different means, failed to detect an influence of omeprazole in healthy individuals [32,33]. Another study specifically analyzed the absorption of calcium carbonate, representing the most common calcium supplement, which is widely used to prevent or to treat osteoporosis. Using a ^{45}Ca tracing technology the authors were able to demonstrate that omeprazole decreased the fractional absorption of calcium carbonate by more than 40% in a group of healthy women aged between 65 and 89 years [34]. They thereby confirmed previous data demonstrating that calcium carbonate, in contrast to calcium citrate, is poorly absorbed in patients with achlorhydria [35]. Interestingly, however, the malabsorption of calcium carbonate in these individuals was only seen when they were fasted; this underscores the difficulties to draw definite conclusions in this regard, since the effects of HCH on calcium absorption apparently depend on the size and type of meal being applied to the study subjects [28]. Moreover, since none of the above-mentioned studies involved more than 30 individuals, it is essentially still unknown whether PPIs act on the skeleton through a negative effect on calcium homeostasis.

GASTRECTOMY AND OSTEOMALACIA, AN ASSOCIATION NOT TO BE FORGOTTEN

This heading represents the title of a case report published 1999 [36]. Although the authors did not confirm their diagnosis by non-decalcified histology of a bone biopsy, they reported on a patient who had undergone partial gastrectomy and pancreatectomy 5 years earlier, where they observed secondary hyperparathyroidism and osteomalacia (based on X-ray and serum analysis). Importantly, all of these pathologies were markedly improved by supplementing calcium and vitamin D, thereby underscoring the authors' conclusion that gastrectomy primarily affects calcium homeostasis and skeletal mineralization [36]. They hereby refer to a previously published histomorphometric analysis of transiliac bone biopsy specimens from 68 individuals who had undergone partial or total gastrectomy [37]. In addition to a significant reduction of the trabecular bone volume, when compared to biopsies from healthy volunteers, these authors observed increased osteoid thickness (one of the histological features of osteomalacia) in 56% of gastrectomized patients, which is indeed an association that should

not be forgotten. In fact, most of the clinical studies addressing the impact of gastrectomy on the skeleton have focused on the assessment of bone mineral density using dual-energy X-ray absorptiometry [38–47]. Thus, although these studies have clearly demonstrated a high prevalence of osteoporosis in gastrectomized patients, they usually did not address the question of whether the decreased bone mineral density in these individuals is primarily caused by impaired matrix mineralization, rather than by impaired bone remodeling. This paucity of knowledge is best explained by the fact that the definite diagnosis of osteomalacia requires the application of non-decalcified histology of bone biopsy specimens, which can only be performed by specialized departments.

In this regard we would like to report on our own unpublished findings, where we took advantage of the Hamburg Bone Register, a collection of non-decalcified iliac crest bone biopsies from individuals with various disorders [48]. Here we retrospectively analyzed patient files and non-decalcified bone sections from 12 individuals who had undergone total gastrectomy at least 4 years prior to biopsy. Using van Kossa/van Gieson staining followed by quantitative histomorphometry we observed a pathological increase of non-mineralized osteoid in all cases, which was accompanied by reduced serum calcium levels (Fig. 6.1A). In addition, all of the patient biopsies were characterized by an accumulation of fibrous tissue and increased osteoclastogenesis, two typical features of secondary hyperparathyroidism

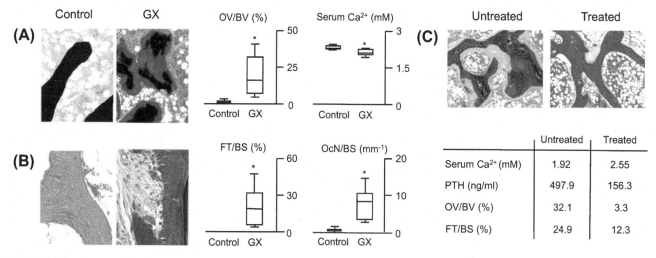

FIGURE 6.1 Osteomalacia in gastrectomized patients. (A) von Kossa/van Gieson staining of sections from non-decalcified bone biopsies derived from gastrectomized (GX) patients revealed a pathological enrichment of osteoid. Quantification of the osteoid volume per bone volume (OV/BV) and serum calcium is given on the right. Boxes include data from the 25th to 75th percentile. $n = 12$ individuals per group. *$p < 0.05$ compared to the control group. (B) Goldner staining revealed fibroosteoclasia in the GX patients. Quantification of fibrous tissue per bone surface (FT/BS) and osteoclast number per bone surface (OcN/BS) is given on the right. $n = 12$ individuals per group. *$p < 0.005$ compared to the control group. (C) Goldner staining of sections from non-decalcified bone biopsies derived from one patient before supplementation with calcium and vitamin D3 (untreated) and 1 year thereafter (treated). Quantification of serum calcium, PTH, OV/BV, and FT/BS is given below. Please see color plate section.

(Fig. 6.1B). Since a second biopsy was taken from one of the patients after supplementation with calcium and vitamin D3 for 1 year, we were able to demonstrate that even a partial normalization of calcium homeostasis can almost fully rescue the defects of skeletal mineralization (Fig. 6.1C). These findings are an important contribution to our attempts of understanding the influence of the gastrointestinal tract on the skeleton. What they show is that the stomach is required for intact calcium homeostasis and proper mineralization of the bone matrix. What they imply is that any impairment of gastric acidification could result in the same pathologies, although the consequences might be less severe and can potentially be counteracted by actions in the kidney or in bone.

OSTEOPETRORICKETS, A RARE DISORDER CAUSED BY A COMBINED ACIDIFICATION DEFECT OF OSTEOCLASTS AND PARIETAL CELLS

Osteopetrorickets (OPR) is a term introduced to describe a condition, where osteopetrosis is accompanied by hypocalcemia and defects of skeletal mineralization [49,50]. While the clinical literature on OPR is mostly based on case reports, a spontaneously arising osteopetrotic mouse strain termed oc/oc has been described to display OPR in 1985, and only in the latter case the diagnosis was supported by non-decalcified histology [50]. Fifteen years after this fairly important observation the phenotype of the oc/oc mice could be attributed to a 1.6 kb deletion of the Tcirg1 gene, whose targeted deletion in mice had previously been shown to cause osteopetrosis [51,52]. Tcirg1 is now known to encode a subunit of the vacuolar proton pump, which is of critical importance in osteoclasts to facilitate extracellular acidification of the resorption lacunae [53–56]. Homozygous inactivating mutations of the TCIRG1 gene in humans have been identified in about 50% of individuals with infantile malignant osteopetrosis, an inherited disorder of osteoclast dysfunction, which is accompanied by bone marrow displacement and severe immunological defects, unless it is treated by hematopoietic stem cell transplantation [57–60]. Given the importance of these findings it is somehow surprising that the initial description of an OPR phenotype in oc/oc mice has essentially been neglected, which is again best explained by the fact that the subsequent analysis of bone biopsies from Tcirg1-deficient mice and patients has only been performed following decalcification of the samples, thus excluding the possibility to diagnose skeletal mineralization defects.

In this regard it was again important that we had access to the Hamburg Bone Register, which allowed us to retrospectively analyze non-decalcified sections of iliac crest biopsies from 21 individuals with diagnosed osteopetrosis. Despite the unfortunate fact that we were not able to retrieve genotype data from the respective individuals we made an important observation. While all 21 biopsies were characterized by the expected increase of the trabecular bone volume, there were striking differences in terms of osteoid accumulation. In fact, while there was no increase in the osteoid volume in 11 cases, the other 10 cases displayed severe osteomalacia [61]. Since this finding demonstrated that osteopetrosis and osteopetrorickets are distinct diseases with comparable prevalence, we utilized mouse models of both conditions to find a cellular and molecular explanation for the observed differences. In a comparative analysis of Src−/− and oc/oc mice we were able to demonstrate that the Src−/− mice only displayed osteopetrosis, while the oc/oc mice displayed OPR [61]. After ruling out a cell-autonomous defect of skeletal mineralization caused by Tcirg1 deficiency, we reasoned that the disturbance of skeletal mineralization in oc/oc mice is the consequence of impaired calcium homeostasis, which was further underscored by the postnatal onset of the OPR phenotype. Likewise, while the serum levels of calcium and PTH were not significantly different between wild-type (WT) and Src−/− mice, the oc/oc mice displayed severe hypocalcemia and a more than 10-fold increase of the serum PTH levels [61]. Since we did not observe increased renal calcium loss in oc/oc mice, we asked the question whether Tcirg1 would be required for proper calcium absorption and monitored its expression in the gastrointestinal tract. Here we found that Tcirg1, a gene previously thought to be specifically expressed by osteoclasts, was also expressed in the stomach. This was further confirmed by immunohistochemistry on human stomach sections, where the TCIRG1 protein was detected in parietal cells [61].

Since this suggested a functional relevance of the vacuolar proton pump in gastric acidification, we next measured the gastric pH in oc/oc mice and observed a significant increase compared to WT littermates. That this previously identified role of TCIRG1 is also relevant in humans was further supported by the diagnosis of HCH in an individual with TCIRG1-dependent OPR [61]. These results led us to hypothesize that HCH-dependent calcium malabsorption is normally counteracted by osteoclast-dependent calcium mobilization from the bone matrix, and that the severe hypocalcemia in oc/oc mice is explained by the coexistence of HCH and osteoclast dysfunction. To test this hypothesis we took advantage of the Src−/− mice and crossed them with mice lacking the gastrin receptor Cckbr, which are known to display HCH [62]. Here we observed that osteoid enrichment was only present in mice lacking both genes, and that the additional deletion of the *Cckbr* gene from the *Src−/−* mice converted their osteopetrotic phenotype into OPR [61]. Taken together, these results demonstrated that OPR is the consequence of a combined acidification defect of osteoclasts and parietal cells. In addition, they suggested that in the absence of an osteoclast defect, HCH could negatively affect the skeleton by a PTH-dependent increase of bone resorption.

ANIMAL MODELS OF IMPAIRED GASTRIC ACIDIFICATION

Since these findings underscore the value of loss-of-function mouse models to understand human pathologies, it is important to discuss some of the published animal studies regarding a possible connection between gastric acidification, calcium homeostasis, and skeletal integrity. In fact, there are many data on the analysis of gastrectomized animals, mostly using rats. However, although all of them essentially confirmed that gastrectomy results in a reduction of bone mineral density, the underlying mechanisms have been discussed controversially [63–71]. For instance, while some investigators detected secondary hyperparathyroidism in their models, others did not, and similar inconsistencies were reported in terms of bone matrix mineralization. In this regard it is particularly important that some studies have been performed in pigs, and here the gastrectomy-induced decrease in bone mineral density was accompanied by calcium malabsorption and secondary hyperparathyroidism [65]. Another highly relevant observation came from a primarily surgical study in rats [63]. Here the authors observed that serum calcium levels were significantly reduced following either gastrectomy or parathyroidectomy, but only to a moderate extent. In contrast, when both surgical procedures were sequentially performed in either way serum calcium immediately dropped to a lethal concentration [63]. Taken together, these data provide evidence for the requirement of PTH to counteract calcium malabsorption caused by impaired gastric acidification. The most relevant question, however, is if the same applies for states of moderate HCH, for instance following PPI administration.

In this regard it is somehow surprising that only a few animal studies have been published so far that address the impact of PPIs on the skeleton. Nevertheless, while one study using omeprazole in rats has essentially confirmed the negative impact of PPIs on bone mineral density, one study has focused on the analysis of a mouse model lacking the PPI target protein [72,73]. These mice carry a targeted deletion of the *Atp4b* gene, which encodes the β-subunit of the H^+/K^+-ATPase, and

they are not able to facilitate gastric acidification [74]. *Atp4b*-deficient mice display a low bone mass phenotype associated with reduced biomechanical strength, and their PTH serum levels were found significantly increased compared to WT controls [73]. Taken together, these findings support the ones that we obtained through the analysis of mice lacking the gastrin receptor Cckbr [61]. These mice display HCH, and when we analyzed their skeletal phenotype by non-decalcified histology we observed progressive osteoporosis accompanied by cortical porosity, but no enrichment of non-mineralized osteoid. Although the skeletal changes in these mice were readily explained by a hyperparathyroidism-related increase in osteoclastogenesis, we performed one additional experiment to confirm this hypothesis. We fed *Cckbr*-deficient mice for 1 year with four different diets being different in two regards, calcium content (0.8% vs. 2%) and type of calcium (calcium carbonate vs. calcium gluconate). When we subsequently analyzed the four groups of mice we observed that the severe disturbances of bone remodeling and calcium homeostasis were fully prevented by the diet containing 2% calcium gluconate, and that calcium gluconate, even at the lower dose, was more effective than calcium carbonate in terms of improving the phenotype [61]. These results are potentially important for two reasons. First, they demonstrate that the osteoporotic phenotype in a mouse model of HCH is normalized by calcium supplementation. Second, they underscore the relevance of applying specific calcium supplements, since they are readily explained by the fact that calcium gluconate is known to have a greater solubility at neutral pH compared to calcium carbonate [75].

CALCIUM SUPPLEMENTATION IN CLINICAL PRACTICE

Although it is generally difficult to translate findings from mouse models into human pathology, one possibility should at least be considered. Indeed, if HCH primarily affects the skeleton through calcium malabsorption and secondary hyperparathyroidism, the problems discussed above might easily be solved by supplementing with the right form of calcium. This could be particularly relevant for individuals diagnosed with osteoporosis, for which supplementation with calcium and vitamin D is generally recommended in addition to anti-resorptive medication [75–77]. If we assume that many of them additionally display spontaneous or iatrogenic HCH, it is important to discuss the currently available calcium supplements and their potential impact for this subgroup of patients. In the US the two most commonly applied forms of calcium are calcium carbonate and calcium citrate. For reasons of cost-effectiveness calcium carbonate is principally preferred, although its absorption at neutral pH is much lower compared to calcium citrate. Likewise, calcium carbonate is contraindicated in patients with achlorhydria, for whom supplementation with calcium citrate is recommended [75]. In the light of this knowledge, it is remarkable that calcium citrate supplements are not available in pharmacy stores throughout Germany, which underscores that the fundamental differences between the two supplements are not yet fully appreciated. Nevertheless, there is another type of calcium supplement available in Germany, which contains calcium gluconate and is thus applicable for patients with achlorhydria.

Coming from the data obtained with *Cckbr*-deficient mice, in whom osteoporosis is fully prevented by calcium gluconate but not by calcium carbonate supplementation, there is one important question that needs to be addressed: Should osteoporotic individuals with HCH receive calcium citrate or gluconate, instead of calcium carbonate? This question is not easy to answer, since the absorption of calcium carbonate does not solely depend on gastric pH, but also on the way of administration [35]. Moreover, there are no clinical studies so far, where the benefits of the different calcium forms on skeletal integrity have been directly compared in a cohort of individuals suffering from HCH and osteoporosis. There are, however, some clinical studies comparing the effects of calcium carbonate and calcium citrate on calcium homeostasis and bone turnover in postmenopausal women with unknown gastric status [78–83]. While Heller et al. reported that calcium citrate was better absorbed than calcium carbonate in their cohort of 25 postmenopausal women [80], Heaney et al. did not observe differential effects of the two calcium supplements on serum calcium and PTH in their cohort of 24 postmenopausal women [81]. In this regard it is interesting to mention a third study involving 40 postmenopausal women by Kenny et al. These authors did not detect differences in serum calcium and PTH either, but they observed that supplementation with calcium citrate resulted in a significant decrease of four different bone resorption markers, which were all unaffected by supplementation with calcium carbonate [82]. In conclusion, although there are good reasons to think about the choice of calcium supplements to treat osteoporotic individuals with HCH in the most efficient way, there is as yet no consensus, as there is only indirect evidence.

CONCLUDING REMARKS

As is probably true for the majority of scientific questions, there are many more experiments required to fully uncover the role of the gastrointestinal tract in the control of bone mass. Nevertheless, some current conclusions are certainly validated by the studies described above. First, given the high prevalence of HCH and osteoporosis in the aged population, it is evident that a large subgroup of osteoporotic patients displays impaired gastric acidification. Second, while long-term and high-dose administration of PPIs increases the risk of skeletal fractures, gastrectomy has a profound negative effect on bone mass and matrix mineralization. Third, several animal studies have demonstrated that impaired gastric acidification negatively affects calcium homeostasis, which is counteracted by secondary hyperparathyroidism. And fourth, at neutral pH and in fasted patients with achlorhydria, calcium citrate and calcium gluconate are much better absorbed than calcium carbonate. What are the implications of this surely important information? In our opinion, it is most important to create an awareness of a potential problem that might be solved easily, as discussed above. In fact, it is certainly possible to include questions about gastric status in the anamnesis or to determine serum gastrin levels as a readout for HCH. In addition, it might be useful to monitor parameters of calcium homeostasis and bone turnover in individuals with osteoporosis and HCH, and this should be done at baseline and after several weeks of calcium supplementation. And finally, one has to ask the simple question again: Should osteoporotic individuals with HCH be supplemented with calcium citrate or gluconate? In the absence of randomized, double-blind, placebo-controlled clinical studies addressing exactly this question the answer might be simple as well: Why not?

References

[1] Bouillon R, Van Cromphaut S, Carmeliet G. Intestinal calcium absorption: molecular vitamin D mediated mechanisms. J Cell Biochem 2008;88:332–9.
[2] Ghishan FK, Kiela PR. Advances in the understanding of mineral and bone metabolism in inflammatory bowel diseases. Am J Physiol Gastrointest Liver Physiol 2011;300:G191–201.
[3] Karsenty G, Gershon MD. The importance of the gastrointestinal tract in the control of bone mass accrual. Gastroenterology 2011;141:439–42.
[4] Ngamruengphong S, Leontiadis GI, Radhi S, Dentino A, Nugent K. Proton pump inhibitors and risk of fracture: a systematic review and meta-analysis of observational studies. Am J Gastroenterol 2011;106:1209–18.
[5] Kassarjian Z, Russell RM. Hypochlorhydria: a factor in nutrition. Annu Rev Nutr 1989;9:271–85.
[6] Kuipers EJ, Grool TA. The dynamics of gastritis. Curr Gastroenterol Rep 2001;3:509–15.
[7] Sipponen P, Härkönen M. Hypochlorhydric stomach: a risk condition for calcium malabsorption and osteoporosis? Scand J Gastroenterol 2010;45:133–8.
[8] Aoki K, Kihaile PE, Wenyuan Z, Xianghang Z, Castro M, Disla M, et al. Comparison of prevalence of chronic atrophic gastritis in Japan, China, Tanzania, and the Dominican Republic. Ann Epidemiol 2005;15:598–606.

[9] Valle J, Kekki M, Sipponen P, Ihamäki T, Siurala M. Long-term course and consequences of Helicobacter pylori gastritis. Results of a 32-year follow-up study. Scand J Gastroenterol 1996;31:546–50.

[10] Mullin JM, Gabello M, Murray LJ, Farrell CP, Bellows J, Wolov KR, et al. Proton pump inhibitors: actions and reactions. Drug Discov Today 2009;14:647–60.

[11] Yao X, Forte JG. Cell biology of acid secretion by the parietal cell. Annu Rev Physiol 2003;65:103–31.

[12] Madanick RD. Proton pump inhibitor side effects and drug interactions: much ado about nothing? Cleve Clin J Med 2011;78:39–49.

[13] Sheen E, Triadafilopoulos G. Adverse effects of long-term proton pump inhibitor therapy. Dig Dis Sci 2011;56:931–50.

[14] Yang YX, Lewis JD, Epstein S, Metz DC. Long-term proton pump inhibitor therapy and risk of hip fracture. JAMA 2006;296:2947–53.

[15] Vestergaard P, Rejnmark L, Mosekilde L. Proton pump inhibitors, histamine H2 receptor antagonists, and other antacid medications and the risk of fracture. Calcif Tissue Int 2006;79:76–83.

[16] Targownik LE, Lix LM, Metge CJ, Prior HJ, Leung S, Leslie WD. Use of proton pump inhibitors and risk of osteoporosis-related fractures. CMAJ 2008;179:319–26.

[17] Yu EW, Blackwell T, Ensrud KE, Hillier TA, Lane NE, Orwoll E, et al. Acid-suppressive medications and risk of bone loss and fracture in older adults. Calcif Tissue Int 2008;83:251–9.

[18] Kaye JA, Jick H. Proton pump inhibitor use and risk of hip fractures in patients without major risk factors. Pharmacotherapy 2008;28:951–9.

[19] Roux C, Briot K, Gossec L, Kolta S, Blenk T, Felsenberg D, et al. Increase in vertebral fracture risk in postmenopausal women using omeprazole. Calcif Tissue Int 2009;84:13–9.

[20] Gray SL, LaCroix AZ, Larson J, Robbins J, Cauley JA, Manson JE, et al. Proton pump inhibitor use, hip fracture, and change in bone mineral density in postmenopausal women: results from the Women's Health Initiative. Arch Intern Med 2010;170:765–71.

[21] Corley DA, Kubo A, Zhao W, Quesenberry C. Proton pump inhibitors and histamine-2 receptor antagonists are associated with hip fractures among at-risk patients. Gastroenterology 2010;139:93–101.

[22] Pitts CJ, Kearns AE. Update on medications with adverse skeletal effects. Mayo Clin Proc 2011;86:338–43.

[23] Fournier MR, Targownik LE, Leslie WD. Proton pump inhibitors, osteoporosis, and osteoporosis-related fractures. Maturitas 2009;64:9–13.

[24] Laine L. Proton pump inhibitors and bone fractures? Am J Gastroenterol 2009;104:S21–6.

[25] Heidelbaugh JJ, Goldberg KL, Inadomi JM. Overutilization of proton pump inhibitors: a review of cost-effectiveness and risk. Am J Gastroenterol 2009;104:S27–32.

[26] Mattsson JP, Väänänen K, Wallmark B, Lorentzon P. Omeprazole and bafilomycin, two proton pump inhibitors: differentiation of their effects on gastric, kidney and bone H(+)-translocating ATPases. Biochim Biophys Acta 1991;1065:261–8.

[27] Mizunashi K, Furukawa Y, Katano K, Abe K. Effect of omeprazole, an inhibitor of H+, K(+)-ATPase, on bone resorption in humans. Calcif Tissue Int 1993;53:21–5.

[28] Insogna KL. The effect of proton pump-inhibiting drugs on mineral metabolism. Am J Gastroenterol 2009;104:S2–4.

[29] Graziani G, Como G, Badalamenti S, Finazzi S, Malesci A, Gallieni M, et al. Effect of gastric acid secretion on intestinal phosphate and calcium absorption in normal subjects. Nephrol Dial Transplant 1995;10:1376–80.

[30] Hardy P, Sechet A, Hottelart C, Oprisiu R, Abighanem O, Said S, et al. Inhibition of gastric secretion by omeprazole and efficiency of calcium carbonate on the control of hyperphosphatemia in patients on chronic hemodialysis. Artif Organs 1998;22:569–73.

[31] Graziani G, Badalamenti S, Como G, Gallieni M, Finazzi S, Angelini C, et al. Calcium and phosphate plasma levels in dialysis patients after dietary Ca-P overload. Role of gastric acid secretion. Nephron 2002;91:474–9.

[32] Serfaty-Lacrosniere C, Wood RJ, Voytko D, Saltzman JR, Pedrosa M, Sepe TE, et al. Hypochlorhydria from short-term omeprazole treatment does not inhibit intestinal absorption of calcium, phosphorus, magnesium or zinc from food in humans. J Am Coll Nutr 1995;14:364–8.

[33] Hansen KE, Jones AN, Lindstrom MJ, Davis LA, Ziegler TE, Penniston KL, et al. Do proton pump inhibitors decrease calcium absorption? J Bone Miner Res 2010;25:2786–95.

[34] O'Connell MB, Madden DM, Murray AM, Heaney RP, Kerzner LJ. Effects of proton pump inhibitors on calcium carbonate absorption in women: a randomized crossover trial. Am J Med 2005;118:778–81.

[35] Recker RR. Calcium absorption and achlorhydria. N Engl J Med 1985;313:70–3.

[36] Efstathiadou Z, Bitsis S, Tsatsoulis A. Gastrectomy and osteomalacia: an association not to be forgotten. Horm Res 1999;52:295–7.

[37] Bisballe S, Eriksen EF, Melsen F, Mosekilde L, Sørensen OH, Hessov I. Osteopenia and osteomalacia after gastrectomy: interrelations between biochemical markers of bone remodelling, vitamin D metabolites, and bone histomorphometry. Gut. 32:1303–7.

[38] Nishimura O, Furumoto T, Nosaka K, Kouno K, Sumikawa M, Hisaki T, et al. Bone disorder following partial and total gastrectomy with reference to bone mineral content. Jpn J Surg 1986;16:98–105.

[39] Imamura M, Yamauchi H, Fukushima K, Sasaki I, Ouchi A. Bone metabolism following gastric surgery: microdensitometry and single-photon absorptiometry. Tohoku J Exp Med 1988;156:237–49.

[40] Resch H, Pietschmann P, Pernecker B, Krexner E, Willvonseder R. The influence of partial gastrectomy on biochemical parameters of bone metabolism and bone density. Clin Investig 1992;70:426–9.

[41] Inoue K, Shiomi K, Higashide S, Kan N, Nio Y, Tobe T, et al. Metabolic bone disease following gastrectomy: assessment by dual energy X-ray absorptiometry. Br J Surg 1992;79:321–4.

[42] Mellström D, Johansson C, Johnell O, Lindstedt G, Lundberg PA, Obrant K, et al. Osteoporosis, metabolic aberrations, and increased risk for vertebral fractures after partial gastrectomy. Calcif Tissue Int 1993;53:370–7.

[43] Zittel TT, Zeeb B, Maier GW, Kaiser GW, Zwirner M, Liebich H, et al. High prevalence of bone disorders after gastrectomy. Am J Surg 1997;174:431–8.

[44] Schmiedl A, Schwille PO, Stühler C, Göhl J, Rümenapf G. Low bone mineral density after total gastrectomy in males: a preliminary report emphasizing the possible significance of urinary net acid excretion, serum gastrin and phosphorus. Clin Chem Lab Med 1999;37:739–44.

[45] Adachi Y, Shiota E, Matsumata T, Iso Y, Yoh R, Kitano S. Osteoporosis after gastrectomy: bone mineral density of lumbar spine assessed by dual-energy X-ray absorptiometry. Calcif Tissue Int 2000;66:119–22.

[46] Heiskanen JT, Kröger H, Pääkkönen M, Parviainen MT, Lamberg-Allardt C, Alhava E. Bone mineral metabolism after total gastrectomy. Bone 2001;28:123–7.

[47] Lim JS, Kim SB, Bang HY, Cheon GJ, Lee JI. High prevalence of osteoporosis in patients with gastric adenocarcinoma following gastrectomy. World J Gastroenterol 2007;13:6492–7.

[48] Seitz S, Priemel M, Zustin J, Beil FT, Semler J, Minne H, et al. Paget's disease of bone: histologic analysis of 754 patients. J Bone Miner Res 2009;24:62–9.

[49] Kaplan FS, August CS, Fallon MD, Gannon F, Haddad JG. Osteopetrorickets. The paradox of plenty. Pathophysiology and treatment. Clin Orthop Relat Res 1993;294:64–78.

[50] Banco R, Seifert MF, Marks Jr SC, McGuire JL. Rickets and osteopetrosis: the osteosclerotic (oc) mouse. Clin Orthop Relat Res 1985;201:238–46.

[51] Scimeca JC, Franchi A, Trojani C, Parrinello H, Grosgeorge J, Robert C, et al. The gene encoding the mouse homologue of the human osteoclast-specific 116-kDa V-ATPase subunit bears a deletion in osteosclerotic (oc/oc) mutants. Bone 2000;26:207–13.

[52] Li YP, Chen W, Liang Y, Li E, Stashenko P. Atp6i-deficient mice exhibit severe osteopetrosis due to loss of osteoclast-mediated extracellular acidification. Nat Genet 1999;23:447–51.

[53] Kornak U, Schulz A, Friedrich W, Uhlhaas S, Kremens B, Voit T, et al. Mutations in the a3 subunit of the vacuolar H(+)-ATPase cause infantile malignant osteopetrosis. Hum Mol Genet 2000;9:2059–63.

[54] Sobacchi C, Frattini A, Orchard P, Porras O, Tezcan I, Andolina M, et al. The mutational spectrum of human malignant autosomal recessive osteopetrosis. Hum Mol Genet 2001;10:1767–73.

[55] Taranta A, Migliaccio S, Recchia I, Caniglia M, Luciani M, De Rossi G, et al. Genotype-phenotype relationship in human ATP6i-dependent autosomal recessive osteopetrosis. Am J Pathol 2003;162:57–68.

[56] Del Fattore A, Peruzzi B, Rucci N, Recchia I, Cappariello A, Longo M, et al. Clinical, genetic, and cellular analysis of 49 osteopetrotic patients: implications for diagnosis and treatment. J Med Genet 2006;43:315–25.

[57] Tolar J, Teitelbaum SL, Orchard PJ. Osteopetrosis. N Engl J Med 2004;351:2839–49.

[58] Del Fattore A, Cappariello A, Teti A. Genetics, pathogenesis and complications of osteopetrosis. Bone 2008;42:19–29.

[59] Villa A, Guerrini MM, Cassani B, Pangrazio A, Sobacchi C. Infantile malignant, autosomal recessive osteopetrosis: the rich and the poor. Calcif Tissue Int 2009;84:1–12.

[60] Steward CG. Hematopoietic stem cell transplantation for osteopetrosis. Pediatr Clin North Am 2010;57:171–80.

[61] Schinke T, Schilling AF, Baranowsky A, Seitz S, Marshall RP, Linn T, et al. Impaired gastric acidification negatively affects calcium homeostasis and bone mass. Nat Med 2009;15:674–81.

[62] Langhans N, Rindi G, Chiu M, Rehfeld JF, Ardman B, Beinborn M, Kopin AS. Abnormal gastric histology and decreased acid production in cholecystokinin-B/gastrin receptor-deficient mice. Gastroenterology 1997;112:280–6.

[63] Axelson J, Persson P, Gagnemo-Persson R, Håkanson R. Importance of the stomach in maintaining calcium homoeostasis in the rat. Gut 1991;32:1298–302.

[64] Rümenapf G, Schwille PO, Erben RG, Schreiber M, Fries W, Schmiedl A, Hohenberger W. Osteopenia following total gastrectomy in the rat—state of mineral metabolism and bone histomorphometry. Eur Surg Res 1997;29:209–21.

[65] Maier GW, Kreis ME, Zittel TT, Becker HD. Calcium regulation and bone mass loss after total gastrectomy in pigs. Ann Surg 1997;225:181–92.

[66] Rümenapf G, Schwille PO, Erben RG, Schreiber M, Bergé B, Fries W, et al. Gastric fundectomy in the rat: effects on mineral and bone metabolism, with emphasis on the gastrin-calcitonin-parathyroid hormone-vitamin D axis. Calcif Tissue Int 1998;63:433–41.

[67] Lehto-Axtelius D, Stenström M, Johnell O. Osteopenia after gastrectomy, fundectomy or antrectomy: an experimental study in the rat. Regul Pept 1998;78:41–50.

[68] Mühlbauer RC, Schenk RK, Chen D, Lehto-Axtelius D, Håkanson R. Morphometric analysis of gastrectomy-evoked osteopenia. Calcif Tissue Int 1998;62:323–6.

[69] Suzuki Y, Fukushima S, Iwai T, Ishibashi Y, Omura N, Hanyu N, et al. Bisphosphonate incadronate prevents total gastrectomy-induced osteopenia in rats. Bone 2004;35:1346–52.

[70] Dobrowolski PJ, Piersiak T, Surve VV, Kruszewska D, Gawron A, Pacuska P, et al. Dietary alpha-ketoglutarate reduces gastrectomy-evoked loss of calvaria and trabecular bone in female rats. Scand J Gastroenterol 2008;43:551–8.

[71] Königsrainer I, Königsrainer A, Maier GW. Preserving duodenal passage for bone mineralization: Billroth I versus Billroth II reconstruction after partial gastrectomy in growing minipigs. J Surg Res 2009;155:321–9.

[72] Cui GL, Syversen U, Zhao CM, Chen D, Waldum HL. Long-term omeprazole treatment suppresses body weight gain and bone mineralization in young male rats. Scand J Gastroenterol 2001;36:1011–5.

[73] Fossmark R, Stunes AK, Petzold C, Waldum HL, Rubert M, Lian AM, et al. Decreased bone mineral density and reduced bone quality in H+/K+ATPase beta-subunit deficient mice. J Cell Biochem 2011 [Epub ahead of print].

[74] Scarff KL, Judd LM, Toh BH, Gleeson PA, Van Driel IR. Gastric H(+), K(+)-adenosine triphosphatase beta subunit is required for normal function, development, and membrane structure of mouse parietal cells. Gastroenterology 1999;117:605–18.

[75] Straub DA. Calcium supplementation in clinical practice: a review of forms, doses, and indications. Nutr Clin Pract 2007;22:286–96.

[76] Shea B, Wells G, Cranney A, Zytaruk N, Robinson V, Griffith L, et al. Meta-analyses of therapies for postmenopausal osteoporosis. VII. Meta-analysis of calcium supplementation for the prevention of postmenopausal osteoporosis. Endocr Rev 2002;23:552–9.

[77] Jackson RD, LaCroix AZ, Gass M, Wallace RB, Robbins J, et al. Calcium plus vitamin D supplementation and the risk of fractures. N Engl J Med 2006;354:669–83.

[78] Sakhaee K, Bhuket T, Adams-Huet B, Rao DS. Meta-analysis of calcium bioavailability: a comparison of calcium citrate with calcium carbonate. Am J Ther 1999;6:313–21.

[79] Heller HJ, Stewart A, Haynes S, Pak CY. Pharmacokinetics of calcium absorption from two commercial calcium supplements. J Clin Pharmacol 1999;39:1151–4.

[80] Heller HJ, Greer LG, Haynes SD, Poindexter JR, Pak CY. Pharmacokinetic and pharmacodynamic comparison of two calcium supplements in postmenopausal women. J Clin Pharmacol 2000;40:1237–44.

[81] Heaney RP, Dowell MS, Bierman J, Hale CA, Bendich A. Absorbability and cost effectiveness in calcium supplementation. J Am Coll Nutr 2001;20:239–46.

[82] Kenny AM, Prestwood KM, Biskup B, Robbins B, Zayas E, Kleppinger A, et al. Comparison of the effects of calcium loading with calcium citrate or calcium carbonate on bone turnover in postmenopausal women. Osteoporos Int 2004;15:290–4.

[83] Thomas SD, Need AG, Tucker G, Slobodian P, O'Loughlin PD, Nordin BE. Suppression of parathyroid hormone and bone resorption by calcium carbonate and calcium citrate in postmenopausal women. Calcif Tissue Int 2008;83:81–4.

7

Gut-derived Serotonin and Bone Formation

Patricia Ducy

Columbia University Medical Center, New York, NY, USA

The bone resorption side of bone remodeling has been known for decades to be regulated by hormones, namely parathyroid hormone (PTH) and sex steroid hormones. Over the last 15 years, and for a large part owing to the development of mouse genetics, this type of regulation has been broadened to include the bone formation process as well. These regulation hormones previously known to regulate energy metabolism such as insulin and leptin have also been shown to control either bone resorption or both resorption and formation [1,2]. More recently, an unexpected player has been added to this growing list of hormones influencing bone remodeling: serotonin. More specifically, gut-derived serotonin has been shown to act negatively on bone formation by inhibiting osteoblast proliferation [3]. Not only has this regulation revealed a novel interaction between gut and bone cells, further adding weight to the emerging notion of a link between food intake and bone mass, it has also opened new avenues to search for an anabolic treatment of bone loss disorders. This chapter proposes to review the current knowledge on the biology of gut-derived serotonin and its influence on bone mass accrual. It will also discuss the therapeutic potential of specifically targeting serotonin synthesis in gut to treat osteoporosis.

SEROTONIN: A TALE OF GUTS AND BRAIN

Serotonin (or 5-hydroxytryptophan, 5-HT) was first identified in the 1940s as a factor released from platelets during blood clotting and promoting vasoconstriction [4,5]. It became quickly evident that serotonin was the same factor that had been previously identified as "enteramine," a smooth muscle cell-contracting substance stored in large amounts in the enterochromaffin cells of the gastrointestinal tract [6]. Shortly after these discoveries serotonin was isolated from brain extracts and the three major pools of serotonin, i.e. gut, platelets and brain, were therefore identified [7]. It then became apparent that there was a functional dissociation between the central and peripheral pools of serotonin. This early observation was later reinforced when it was shown that while serotonin is synthesized both in gut and in brain it cannot cross the blood–brain barrier and therefore its central and peripheral pools remain separated [8,9]. In this chapter serotonin synthesized in the brain will be referred to as central serotonin while serotonin produced in the periphery will be referred to as gut-derived serotonin.

Serotonin is synthesized in a two-step process [10,11]. L-tryptophan is first hydroxylated into L-5-hydroxytryptophan by a specific tryptophan hydroxylase (Tph) and this product is then decarboxylated by an aromatic L-amino acid decarboxylase (Fig. 7.1). To be active Tph requires the presence of a cofactor, (6R)-L-erythro-5,6,7,8-tetrahydrobiopterin (BH4), and of molecular oxygen as an additional substrate (Fig. 7.1A). The first step of this biosynthesis cascade is rate limiting, and the availability of tryptophan as well as Tph levels and function are therefore key regulators of the production of serotonin. Once synthesized serotonin is actively transported by the vesicular monoamine transporter (VMAT) and stored in secretory granules [12–14]. Serotonin exerts its effects via 14 specific receptors (Htrs) organized in seven subtypes, which except for one (Htr3, a member of the ligand-gated ion channel receptor superfamily) are all G-protein coupled receptors (GPCRs) [15,16]. Importantly, depending on the receptor subtype serotonin signaling can elicit either a decrease or an increase in cellular levels of cAMP; hence serotonin can either have a positive or a negative effect on cAMP-dependent mechanisms.

Most (95%) of the serotonin present in the body is produced by enterochromaffin cells of the gut [17,18] (Fig. 7.2). These cells are part of the enteroendocrine

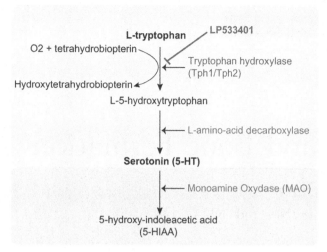

FIGURE 7.1   Mechanism of serotonin biosynthesis (yellow box) and degradation (gray box). Enzymes are in blue. LP533401 (in red) inhibits Tph activity, and thereby serotonin production, by preventing binding of its tetrahydrobiopterin cofactor. Please see color plate section.

system, which regroup more than 10 different types of secretory cells responsible for the production of gastrin, somatostatin, ghrelin, and glucagon-like peptide 1 (GLP-1) among other factors [19–21]. Unlike

most endocrine cells that are usually located within a specific endocrine organ, enteroendocrine cells are scattered within the epithelial cells lining the stomach, small intestine, and colon [17]. Although it was long thought that enterochromaffin cells originate from neural crest cells, recent studies using lineage tracing have clearly established that they are derived from the endoderm, not the neuroectoderm [22,23]. Their differentiation is under the control of a cascade of b-HLH transcription factors in which initial determination by Math1 is a key step [22,24]. During mouse embryogenesis the first serotonin immuno-positive enterochromaffin cells appear relatively late, i.e. around embryonic day 15 (E15) [25]. Beyond development, enterochromaffin cells are renewed from a large pool of stem cells located at the basis of some crypt-villus unit of the gut [17,18,26]. Mature enterochromaffin cells are located on the basal lamina of the gut epithelium, projecting into the gut lumen with their apical portion. While they are widely expressed within the stomach, small intestine, and large intestine in human, in mice they are more restricted to the small intestine, and in particular to the duodenum [17]. Serotonin is released from these cells by translocation of the secretory granules to the cell membrane and exocytosis upon

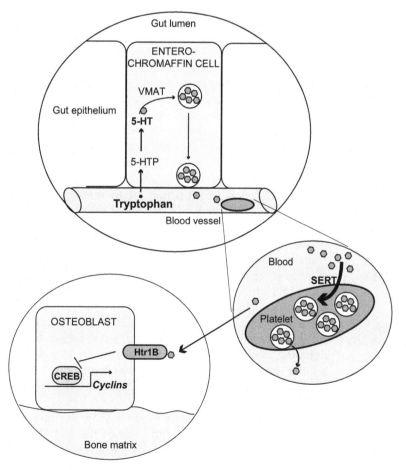

FIGURE 7.2   Schematic representation of the functional link between gut-derived serotonin and bone formation. Serotonin is synthesized in enterochromaffin cells located within the gut epithelium via the enzymatic transformation of tryptophan (see Fig. 7.1 for details). Following its association with the VMAT transporter it is stored in secretory granules before being released into the general circulation where most (95%) of it is absorbed by platelets through the SERT transporter. The remaining amount of circulating serotonin can reach bone and bind to osteoblasts that express the Htr1b receptor. This binding triggers a signaling cascade that results in the decreased expression and activity of the transcription factor CREB. As a result expression of *Cyclins* is lowered and osteoblast proliferation is decreased. Please see color plate section.

stimulation by a wide variety of signals including acid pH, hypertonic glucose, caffeine, amino acid presence and β-adrenergic stimulation [17,27−29]. Somatostatin signaling, in contrast, inhibits the secretion of serotonin [30,31].

Approximately 95% of the amount of serotonin released in blood by enterochromaffin cells is absorbed and stored in platelets, which have the ability to uptake serotonin through a specific transporter termed 5-HT transporter (5HTT) or serotonin transporter (SERT) [32,33] (Fig. 7.2). SERT belongs to a large superfamily of sodium/chloride-dependent transporters harboring 12 transmembrane domains, which also include transporters for norepinephrine and dopamine [34]. It is encoded by the Solute carrier family 6 member 4 (*Slc6a4*) gene, which is expressed in the central and peripheral nervous systems as well as in enterochromaffin cells, platelets, pulmonary endothelium and placental syncytiotrophoblasts, all cells where serotonin signaling has been shown to have a direct impact [32,33,35−40]. SERT expression has also been observed in osteoblasts and osteoclasts but its function in these cells has not been fully elucidated yet since only mice globally deficient in SERT have been analyzed for skeletal abnormalities [41−44]. SERT biology has been most extensively studied at the neuronal synapse where it is key to regulate the flux of serotonin. A minor fraction (5%) of the body's serotonin is synthesized in the brain, where it functions as a neuromediator [15,45]. Upon its release by neurons of the brainstem serotonin signals to receptors expressed by the post-synaptic neuron [15,16]. To regulate this process and also, presumably, to prevent the serotonin receptors from desensitization, a common feature of GPCR signaling, SERT expressed by the pre-synaptic neuron binds and transports serotonin across the cell membrane for its internalization [46,47]. This is the process targeted by serotonin reuptake inhibitors (SSRIs), a class of drugs widely used to treat mood disorders, which enhances serotonin signaling by increasing its persistence at the synaptic junction [46,48,49]. SERT is therefore critical to terminate serotonergic signaling. It is also required for serotonin elimination, a process that occurs mostly in lung and liver in the periphery. Indeed, the enzymes that catabolize serotonin, i.e. monoamine oxidases are localized intracellularly and thus require its transport across the cell membrane [39]. The main metabolite resulting from the enzymatic degradation of serotonin, 5-hydroxy-indoleacetic acid (5-HIAA), is then excreted in the urine (Fig. 7.1).

As mentioned above serotonin is produced both peripherally and centrally. However, because serotonin cannot cross the blood−brain barrier, altering its levels peripherally does not influence its central concentration, or vice versa [8,9]. This is exemplified by the fact that patients with carcinoid syndrome do not develop associated mental disorders or migraines despite having a massive elevation of circulating serotonin [45,50]. This dissociation also exists at the genetic level. For a long time the only known Tph-encoding gene was *Tph1*, the gene responsible for serotonin production in the gut. However, when *Tph1*-deficient mice were generated they had normal levels of brain serotonin and did not show signs of neurological disorders or behavioral abnormalities indicating that another gene, brain specific, was responsible for the synthesis of serotonin in the central nervous system [51,52]. This pivotal observation led to the identification of a second Tph-encoding gene, *Tph2*, which is specifically expressed in neurons [52,53].

That serotonin biosynthesis is synthesized by two distinct genes and that it does not cross the blood−brain barrier created the opportunity to study separately the role of each pool of serotonin using mouse genetic experiments. This approach was instrumental in showing that both central and gut serotonin regulate bone mass accrual but do it in opposite manners and through different pathways [54−57]. The role and mechanism of action of central serotonin is the topic of Chapter 5 and will not be reviewed here.

REGULATION OF BONE FORMATION BY GUT-DERIVED SEROTONIN

As powerful as mouse genetics is in demonstrating the consequences of missing a gene, some phenotypes are harder to detect than others and might therefore be overlooked until a specific interest in the organ or function they affect develops and specific techniques are applied. For instance, because they do not cause pain or visible distress and in most cases cannot be revealed by a mere physical examination, abnormalities of bone remodeling often remain undetected. Hence, when *Tph1*-deficient mice were initially analyzed no bone phenotype was detected and their study focused mainly on the many expected functions of gut-derived serotonin. Not surprisingly, these analyses revealed abnormalities in cardiovascular function and platelet function [51,58,59]. They also identified a mild defect in hematopoiesis and a requirement for expression of maternal *Tph1* in the placenta during early development [36,60−62]. In contrast, despite the logical assumption that a paracrine activity of gut-derived serotonin could be key to bowel movement gastrointestinal tract motility is not affected in a clearly detrimental manner in the absence of Tph1. Accordingly, recent studies have shown that such function is regulated by the Tph2-dependent serotonin originating from enteric neurons [53].

The potent function of gut-derived serotonin on bone mass accrual was revealed when mice deficient in Tph1 in gut cells only were generated [3]. This conditional approach has the advantage of bypassing any potential embryonic abnormality that could derive from either a decrease in maternal circulating levels of serotonin or the decrease expression of maternal *Tph1* in placenta when heterozygous mutant mice are intercrossed. Furthermore, since this conditional deletion does not result in a total absence of circulating serotonin these mice do not show the defect in hemostasis observed in the globally *Tph1*-deficient mice [3,59]. Surprisingly, given the low bone mass phenotype of the *Tph2*-null mice [54], *Tph1* gut-specific deficient mice show high bone mass [3]. This phenotype is dominant, i.e. it is also present in heterozygous mutant mice. This phenotype is sufficiently strong that in both homozygous and heterozygous mice, it counterbalances the deleterious effect of ovariectomy on bone mass [3,63]. In agreement with the late expression of serotonin by enterochromaffin cells during embryogenesis, this phenotype only appears postnatally. At the cellular level it is characterized by a sole increase in bone formation; all parameters of bone resorption are unaffected. Once more, this differs from serotonin central effect on bone mass that involves both bone formation and bone resorption [3,54,57]. The high bone mass phenotype of the *Tph1* gut-specific-deficient mice is caused by an increase in osteoblast number and the bone formation rate that is secondary to enhanced osteoblast proliferation. Accordingly, expression of *CycD1*, *D2*, and *E1* in bone is increased in absence of gut-derived serotonin and serotonin decreases the expression of these genes in primary cultures of mouse osteoblasts without affecting *Runx2*, *Osx*, or *Atf4* expression [3].

Expression of only three of the 14 known serotonin receptors, Htr1b, Htr2a, and Htr2b, can be detected to a significant level in cultured mouse primary osteoblasts, with Htr1b being the most highly expressed [3]. Mutant mice harboring either a global deletion of *Htr2a* or an osteoblast-specific deletion of *Htr2b* do not display a skeletal phenotype comparable to the one displayed by *Tph1*-deficient mice thus ruling out that these receptors are necessary and sufficient for serotonin's inhibitory activity on osteoblasts [3]. In contrast, mice with an osteoblast-specific deletion of *Htr1b* show a bone phenotype of the same anabolic nature and with the same onset than the one observed in *Tph1* gut-specific-deficient mice [3]. In addition, as it is the case for *Tph1* inactivation, *Htr1b* haploinsufficiency also leads to a significant bone phenotype, further illustrating both the similarities between these pathways and their importance for bone formation [3].

From a molecular point of view *Htr1b* inactivation also has the same molecular signature as deletion of *Tph1* in gut cells; expression of *Cyclin D1, D2,* and *E1* is affected whereas expression of *Runx2, Osx,* or *Atf4* is not [3]. Htr1b belongs to a subfamily of serotonin receptors that are coupled to G_i/G_o and mediate inhibitory signals via decreased cAMP production and PKA- dependent phosphorylation [64]. Accordingly, treatment of primary osteoblasts with serotonin decreases phosphorylation of CREB on its Serine 133, which is a known target of PKA [3]. This, in turn, prevents binding of CREB to the promoter of *Cyclin D1,* a known target gene of CREB transcriptional activity in osteoblasts [65,66] (Fig. 7.2). Both of these effects of serotonin are blocked when *Htr1b*-deficient osteoblasts are used indicating that this receptor is necessary to mediate serotonin signaling in these cells. Further evidence that gut-derived serotonin, Htr1b, and CREB belong to the same signaling cascade *in vivo* comes from genetic epistasis experiments [3]. This approach, which is commonly used by geneticists to define genetic cascades in organisms as diverse as yeast, *C. elegans,* or the mouse, relies on the principle that if two genes encode factors involved in the same functional pathway their co-haploinsufficiency should cause the same phenotype rather than fully inactivating either one of them. Accordingly, mice lacking one allele of *Htr1b* in osteoblasts and one allele of *Tph1* in gut cells develop the same high bone mass phenotype as either homozygous mutant mice [3]. Conversely, inactivating one allele of *Creb* is sufficient to normalize the high bone mass phenotype of the *Htr1b*-deficient mice [3]. These genetic and molecular evidences support the notion that Htr1b and CREB mediate the effect of circulating serotonin in osteoblasts (Fig. 7.2).

REGULATION OF SEROTONIN PRODUCTION IN GUT BY LRP5

As mentioned above, nutrients such as amino acids and glucose are known to affect the production of serotonin by gut cells as does the acidic pH of the stomach [27]. Although both stomach acidification and amino acid intake have been linked to the regulation of bone remodeling [67,68], there is as yet no demonstration that changes in blood serotonin levels are connected to these effects. Another pathway, however, has been unexpectedly linked to both serotonin and its effect on bone formation.

The turn of the second millennium has seen a major discovery in bone biology, namely the identification of a broadly expressed transmembrane molecule called low-density lipoprotein receptor-related protein 5 (Lrp5) as a major regulator of bone formation. Indeed, loss-of-function mutations in *Lrp5* cause osteoporosis pseudoglioma (OPPG, OMIM #259770) in humans, a pediatric disease, and gain-of-function mutations in *Lrp5* cause the high bone mass syndrome (HBM, OMIM #601884), a disorder most often appearing only in adolescents and persisting into adulthood [69–71]. Analysis of *Lrp5*-deficient mice revealed that this cell surface molecule affects exclusively bone formation through a positive effect on the proliferation of osteoblasts [72]. In agreement with the postnatal onset of the two human disorders linked to Lrp5, skeletogenesis is normal in *Lrp5*−/− mice and their low bone mass phenotype only develops postnatally [72]. These observations indicated that Lrp5 is an important regulator of bone mass. Moreover, because Lrp5 controls exclusively bone formation they inferred that elucidating how Lrp5 affects osteoblast proliferation could unravel a bone anabolic pathway and therefore have a major therapeutic impact for the treatment of bone loss diseases such as osteoporosis. It is thus not surprising that the elucidation of Lrp5 mode of action in bone became a major goal for many bone biology laboratories.

Lrp5 is one of the vertebrate homologues of the *Drosophila* gene *arrow* that acts as a co-receptor for Wingless, the drosophila homologue of the Wnt proteins [73,74]. It was therefore initially thought that Lrp5 could, if not would, also act as a Wnt co-receptor to achieve its positive effect on osteoblasts. This logical assumption is supported by both *in vitro* and *in vivo* data. In vertebrate cells Wnt signaling is mainly mediated by β-catenin which when translocated to the nucleus cooperates with Lef/Tcf transcription factors to activate gene expression [75,76]. In agreement with this canonical model, co-transfection of *Lrp5* increases the ability of Wnt proteins to enhance the activity of a Tcf-dependent promoter such as the TopFlash promoter in cell culture experiments [69,70,76]. Furthermore, the persistence of embryonic vascularization of the eye leading to early onset blindness, which is a second feature of the lack of Lrp5 signaling in OPPG patients as well as in *Lrp5*-deficient mice, is due to decreased Wnt7b/Lrp5-mediated programmed cell death [72,77]. Several experimental and clinical evidences, however, do not align with the notion that Lrp5 also acts as a regulator of bone formation via its activity on the canonical Wnt signaling pathway. First, there is no detectable bone abnormality at birth in *Lrp5*−/− mice or in OPPG and HBM patients [69–72] despite the fact that Wnts are expressed during skeletogenesis and, more generally, that all Wnts studied so far have a function during development [75]. Second, HBM patients that harbor gain-of-function mutations in *LRP5* do not develop tumors, yet this is a hallmark of increased Wnt signaling in most other organs [75]. Third, patients with inactivating mutations in SOST, a Wnt signaling inhibitor expressed in osteocytes, develop bone abnormalities different than HBM patients

[78–81]. Fourth and more directly, inactivation of canonical Wnt signaling in osteoblasts or in osteocytes or even in their embryonic progenitors does not cause a postnatal bone formation phenotype mimicking *Lrp5* inactivation [82–86]. As a matter of fact, β-catenin inactivation in either osteoblasts or osteocytes leads to a similar high bone mass phenotype caused by a decrease in OPG/RANKL-regulated bone resorption [85,87].

There are, instead, many similarities between the function of Lrp5 and the effect of gut-derived serotonin on osteoblasts. First, both the deletion of *Lrp5* and of *Tph1* cause a phenotype restricted to osteoblast proliferation [3]. Second, the molecular signature of this phenotype is similar; expression of regulators of cell proliferation *Cyclin D1*, *D2*, and *E1* is affected whereas expression of osteoblast differentiation (*Runx2*, *Osx*, *Atf4*) or osteoclast differentiation (*Osteoprotegerin*, *RankL*) markers is not [3]. Third, global inactivation of *Lrp5* or its deletion in gut cells only causes an increase in *Tph1* expression in enterochromaffin cells and thus raises blood serotonin levels; on the other hand, introducing an HBM gain-of-function in the *Lrp5* locus leads to a significant decrease in *Tph1* expression and circulating serotonin [3]. Fourth, and these are more direct evidence, decreasing blood serotonin levels either by using a low tryptophan diet or pharmacologically or genetically by inactivating one allele of *Tph1* in gut cells can normalize all aspects of the bone phenotype demonstrated by the *Lrp5*-deficient mice [3,88]. The specificity of this effect is demonstrated by the fact that no additional phenotype accompanies this normalization, for instance there is no change in bone resorption parameters, and by the persistence of the eye vascularization phenotype, which is known to be Wnt signaling dependent [3,77].

REGULATION OF BONE FORMATION BY SEROTONIN IN HUMANS

No matter how pertinent an animal model is in recapitulating the features of a disease or how valuable it appears to dissect a particular pathway, any finding of mouse genetics or animal-based research is always subject to validation in human biology. Accurately measuring circulating serotonin in human specimen is, however, a difficult task as it bears far more requirements than most commonly performed serological tests. Indeed, patients have to be abstained from tryptophan/serotonin-rich food (banana, avocado, plum, pineapple, walnut, turkey) and no coffee, tea, or chocolate should be taken for at least 48 hours before collection. In addition, many common medications such as aspirin, acetaminophen, fluorouracil, corticotropin, MAO inhibitors, phinezatin, catecholamines, reserpin, nicotine, caffein, heparin, or any vasodilatator may cause the release of serotonin and lead to altered circulating levels. Such treatments thus need to be discontinued for at least 5 days before blood collection. As for the quantification itself, measuring the levels of 5HIAA, serotonin's main metabolite, in the urine is poorly informative because it represents the combination of both central and gut-derived serotonin breakdown and therefore so does not reflect specific changes in peripheral serotonin levels. One is left with using blood draws as specimen. However, given the large quantity of serotonin stored in platelets and its release upon coagulation only poor platelet plasma isolated immediately after collection and devoid of any sign of hemolysis can be used.

In spite of these technical challenges, both direct and indirect clinical correlations have outlined the importance of the regulation of bone formation by gut-derived serotonin in humans. For instance, in a population-based sample of 275 women, serum serotonin levels were found to be inversely associated with body and spine areal bone mineral density (aBMD) as well as with femur neck total and trabecular volumetric bone mineral density (vBMD) [89]. More recently, the presence of a serotonin-producing tumor of the pancreas was correlated with a history of repeated fractures in a male patient diagnosed with severe osteoporosis [90]. Lastly, it has long been known that autistic children who display elevated blood serotonin levels also show a significant reduction in bone cortical thickness [91,92]. Although a growing number of studies have now shown that long-term use of serotonin reuptake inhibitors (SSRIs), a class of antidepressants that enhance serotonin signaling by decreasing the function of SERT, has deleterious consequences on bone mass it is unclear whether this pathology is caused by their influence on central or gut-derived serotonin signaling (see Chapter 16).

A second set of evidence linking bone formation and the levels of circulating serotonin originates from the analysis of patients with mutations in LRP5. Indeed, four independent groups have now demonstrated that OPPG patients, who harbor loss-of-function mutations in LRP5, have significantly increased levels of circulating serotonin [3,93—95]. On the other hand, analysis of cohorts of high bone mass syndrome patients from Europe and the United States that have different gain-of-function mutations in LRP5, T253I, and G171V, respectively, have revealed a decrease in circulating serotonin in these patients [3,96,97]. Notwithstanding that these studies are important because they further strengthen the notion of a functional link between Lrp5 and gut-derived serotonin, they support the notion that blood serotonin is a negative regulator of bone mass in humans, as it is in mice, and thereby suggest that directly and specifically inhibiting its synthesis in gut in humans could be a novel approach to treat osteoporosis.

MODULATION OF TPH1 ACTIVITY AS A NOVEL BONE ANABOLIC THERAPY

Several features underscore the therapeutic potential of blocking the synthesis of gut-derived serotonin to treat bone loss disorders. First and foremost, peripheral serotonin specifically targets osteoblasts and bone formation; hence, blocking its action would provide a much sought-after purely anabolic effect. Second, the clinical data presented above brought to light that gut-derived serotonin has the same effect on bone mass in humans and rodents. This notion implies that drugs targeting this pathway not only present a fair probability to be effective in humans but also that they can be quite reliably developed and tested in rodents. Third, that inactivating only one allele of Tph1 in gut cells is sufficient to protect mice from ovariectomy-induced bone loss [3,63] indicates that it is not necessary to completely block the synthesis of serotonin in gut to achieve a beneficial effect on bone mass. Given the other functions of serotonin and, for instance, the cardiovascular abnormalities of mice globally deficient in Tph1, this is a pivotal observation from a biomedical point of view.

In principle, decreasing the impact of gut-derived serotonin on osteoblasts can be achieved through two means: targeting its synthesis or targeting its signaling machinery via inactivation of its receptor. The latter strategy, which is one of the most usual in drug development, presents much uncertainty in this particular case. Indeed, inactivation of signaling by Htr1b, the receptor mediating serotonin activity in osteoblasts, has been shown to increase aggressiveness and preference for alcohol intake [98] as well as to increase the risk of cardiovascular adverse events as this receptor controls pulmonary vasoconstriction [15]. Thus, to elicit a positive effect on bone formation one would not only need to generate Htr1b-specific antagonists but also to find a mean to direct exclusively their activity to osteoblasts. If the former appears well within the reach of today's pharmacology, the latter, i.e. obtaining a very strict tropism for bone cells, might be more difficult to achieve. The second strategy involves decreasing the circulating levels of serotonin itself. Such a strategy, however, requires that only the synthesis of serotonin from gut cells, i.e. Tph1 levels or its activity, is inhibited. Indeed, generally inhibiting serotonin synthesis through feeding on a tryptophan-free diet or by inactivating both Tph1 in gut and Tph2 globally cause a low bone mass phenotype due to the dominant impact of central versus circulating serotonin on bone remodeling [54,99]. The main pharmacological challenge is therefore to succeed in targeting Tph1 activity without affecting the activity of Tph2. That these two proteins are more than 70% homologous has until now prevented the identification of a Tph1-specific inhibitor. In contrast, taking advantage of the fact that Tph2 is isolated from the general circulation by the blood—brain barrier, several compounds have been developed that can target Tph1 specifically because they remain peripheral. One of these compounds, LP533401, has been successfully tested for its ability to induce a bone anabolic effect [88,100].

LP533401 is a pyrimidine compound that binds near the Tph catalytic site on residues Tyr235 and Phe241, in the same region that is usually occupied by the BH4 cofactor [100,101] (Fig. 7.2). As a result, this compound is a potent inhibitor of both Tph1 and Tph2 activity and thereby of serotonin synthesis in general [100,101]. After oral administration, however, LP533401 is poorly absorbed and its penetration of the blood—brain barrier is negligible [101,102]. Hence, when this compound is administered orally, serotonin synthesis by enterochromaffin cells is robustly decreased whereas central serotonin levels are not affected [100,101].

In vivo, LP533401 given orally once a day decreases circulating levels of serotonin in a dose—response manner and causes a dose-dependent increase in bone mass. Consequently, mice or rats treated with LP533401 show a high bone mass phenotype reminiscent of the one observed in absence of *Tph1* or in high bone mass patients [100]. More importantly, this treatment can prevent bone loss and restore a normal bone mass in ovariectomized mice or rats, both in vertebrae and long bones, leading to significantly improved bone biomechanical properties [100]. A dose of LP533401 as low as 25 mg/kg/day is sufficient to reduce the level of circulating serotonin by 50% in mice [88]. Consistent with the fact that *Tph1* gut-specific haploinsufficient mice are protected from the bone loss caused by ovariectomy, this treatment is sufficient to increase bone-formation parameters while having no effect on hemostasis or gut motility [88,100]. Pharmacological inhibition of Tph1 is effective in both young (3-month-old) and aging (1-year-old) ovariectomized animals, the latter being a key feature given the most common onset and etiology of osteoporosis [88]. As predicted by the phenotype of the various *Lrp5* and *Tph1* genetic models the beneficial effect of Tph1 pharmacologic inhibition is solely due to enhanced bone formation, itself secondary to an increase in osteoblast numbers. As a matter of fact, the low bone mass phenotype of the *Lrp5*-deficient mice can be fully corrected by a treatment with LP533401 both at the cellular and molecular level [88]. In contrast, their eye phenotype, which is Wnt signaling dependent, is not rescued by decreasing serotonin levels [3].

Remarkably, serum serotonin levels are still low in mice treated with LP533401 even after the treatment has been discontinued for 6 weeks, and therefore their bone formation rate remains higher than in placebo-treated mice [88]. Also important is the fact that LP533401 therapy can be combined with a treatment with alendronate. Indeed, when mice are co-treated with the two drugs, they benefit from both their respective effects on bone formation and bone resorption as neither of them interferes with the activity of the other [88]. These two observations and the fact that Tph1 inhibition induces a strict anabolic effect highlight a potentially important difference with the treatment with intermittent PTH, which is for the present time the only available bone anabolic therapy [103—105]. On the one hand, the therapeutic window of a treatment with a Tph1 inhibitor could be longer than the one of intermittent PTH due its strict anabolic effect and the absence of a rebound effect requiring the use of an anti-resorptive treatment upon disruption of the treatment. On the other hand, antiresorptive treatments and use of Tph1 inhibitors could be administered simultaneously without loss of potency of either approach for a maximum benefit.

While promising, these positive results obtained in mice and rats still should be interpreted cautiously until clinical trials demonstrate that they can be reproduced in human. Yet, several observations already shed a positive light on the therapeutic potential of Tph1 inhibition. First, in terms of efficacy, the fact that high bone mass patients, who often have no more than a 50% decrease in serotonin levels, display an increase in bone mass sufficient to protect them from developing osteoporosis is consistent with the increase in bone mass observed in animals with LP533401-lowered serotonin levels [3,96,97]. Second, in terms of safety, Phase 2 trials evaluating the same type of Tph1 inhibitors for a different application and using doses more than 30 times higher than the dose sufficient to treat ovariectomy-induced bone loss in mice have already demonstrated a good tolerance and no dose-dependent toxicity of these compounds [106—108].

References

[1] Wei J, Ducy P. Co-dependence of bone and energy metabolisms. Arch Biochem Biophys 2010 Nov 1;503(1):35—40.

[2] Karsenty G, Oury F. Biology Without Walls: The Novel Endocrinology of Bone. Annu Rev Physiol 2011 Feb 15.

[3] Yadav VK, Ryu JH, Suda N, Tanaka KF, Gingrich JA, Schutz G, et al. Lrp5 controls bone formation by inhibiting serotonin synthesis in the duodenum. Cell 2008 Nov 28;135(5): 825—37.

[4] Rapport MM, Green AA, Page IH. Crystalline Serotonin. Science 1948 Sep 24;108(2804):329—30.

[5] Rapport MM, Green AA, Page IH. Serum vasoconstrictor, serotonin; isolation and characterization. J Biol Chem 1948 Dec;176(3):1243−51.

[6] Erspamer V, Asero B. Identification of enteramine, the specific hormone of the enterochromaffin cell system, as 5-hydroxy-tryptamine. Nature 1952 May 10;169(4306):800−1.

[7] Twarog BM, Page IH. Serotonin content of some mammalian tissues and urine and a method for its determination. Am J Physiol 1953 Oct;175(1):157−61.

[8] Mann JJ, McBride PA, Brown RP, Linnoila M, Leon AC, DeMeo M, et al. Relationship between central and peripheral serotonin indexes in depressed and suicidal psychiatric inpatients. Arch Gen Psychiatry 1992 Jun;49(6):442−6.

[9] Yuwiler A, Oldendorf WH, Geller E, Braun L. Effect of albumin binding and amino acid competition on tryptophan uptake into brain. J Neurochem 1977 May;28(5):1015−23.

[10] Grahame-Smith DG. Tryptophan hydroxylation in brain. Biochem Biophys Res Commun 1964 Aug 11;16(6):586−92.

[11] Lovenberg W, Jequier E, Sjoerdsma A. Tryptophan hydroxylation: measurement in pineal gland, brainstem, and carcinoid tumor. Science 1967 Jan 13;155(759):217−9.

[12] Henry JP, Sagne C, Bedet C, Gasnier B. The vesicular monoamine transporter: from chromaffin granule to brain. Neurochem Int 1998 Mar;32(3):227−46.

[13] Henry JP, Botton D, Sagne C, Isambert MF, Desnos C, Blanchard V, et al. Biochemistry and molecular biology of the vesicular monoamine transporter from chromaffin granules. J Exp Biol 1994 Nov;196:251−62.

[14] Nilsson O, Dahlstrom A, Geffard M, Ahlman H, Ericson LE. An improved immunocytochemical method for subcellular localization of serotonin in rat enterochromaffin cells. J Histochem Cytochem 1987 Mar;35(3):319−26.

[15] Berger M, Gray JA, Roth BL. The expanded biology of serotonin. Annu Rev Med 2009;60:355−66.

[16] Filip M, Bader M. Overview on 5-HT receptors and their role in physiology and pathology of the central nervous system. Pharmacol Rep 2009 Sep−Oct;61(5):761−77.

[17] Ahlman H, Nilsson. The gut as the largest endocrine organ in the body. Ann Oncol 2001;12(Suppl. 2):S63−8.

[18] Gershon MD, Tack J. The serotonin signaling system: from basic understanding to drug development for functional GI disorders. Gastroenterology 2007 Jan;132(1):397−414.

[19] Field BC, Chaudhri OB, Bloom SR. Bowels control brain: gut hormones and obesity. Nat Rev Endocrinol 2010 Aug;6(8):444−53.

[20] Drucker DJ. The role of gut hormones in glucose homeostasis. J Clin Invest 2007 Jan;117(1):24−32.

[21] Merchant JL. Tales from the crypts: regulatory peptides and cytokines in gastrointestinal homeostasis and disease. J Clin Invest 2007 Jan;117(1):6−12.

[22] Li HJ, Ray SK, Singh NK, Johnston B, Leiter AB. Basic helix−loop−helix transcription factors and enteroendocrine cell differentiation. Diabetes Obes Metab 2011 Oct;13(Suppl. 1):5−12.

[23] Thompson M, Fleming KA, Evans DJ, Fundele R, Surani MA, Wright NA. Gastric endocrine cells share a clonal origin with other gut cell lineages. Development 1990 Oct;110(2):477−81.

[24] Lee CS, Perreault N, Brestelli JE, Kaestner KH. Neurogenin 3 is essential for the proper specification of gastric enteroendocrine cells and the maintenance of gastric epithelial cell identity. Genes Dev 2002 Jun 15;16(12):1488−97.

[25] Branchek TA, Gershon MD. Time course of expression of neuropeptide Y, calcitonin gene-related peptide, and NADPH diaphorase activity in neurons of the developing murine bowel and the appearance of 5-hydroxytryptamine in mucosal enterochromaffin cells. J Comp Neurol 1989 Jul 8;285(2):262−73.

[26] Ahlman H. Gut neuroendocrine tumours. Wiad Lek 1997;50(Suppl. 1 Pt 1):4−9.

[27] Kidd M, Modlin IM, Gustafsson BI, Drozdov I, Hauso O, Pfragner R. Luminal regulation of normal and neoplastic human EC cell serotonin release is mediated by bile salts, amines, tastants, and olfactants. Am J Physiol Gastrointest Liver Physiol 2008 Aug;295(2):G260−72.

[28] Wald A, Back C, Bayless TM. Effect of caffeine on the human small intestine. Gastroenterology 1976 Nov;71(5):738−42.

[29] Peregrin AT, Ahlman H, Jodal M, Lundgren O. Involvement of serotonin and calcium channels in the intestinal fluid secretion evoked by bile salt and cholera toxin. Br J Pharmacol 1999 Jun;127(4):887−94.

[30] Barnett P. Somatostatin and somatostatin receptor physiology. Endocrine 2003 Apr;20(3):255−64.

[31] Hofland LJ, van Hagen PM, Lamberts SW. Functional role of somatostatin receptors in neuroendocrine and immune cells. Ann Med 1999 Oct;31(Suppl. 2):23−7.

[32] Mercado CP, Kilic F. Molecular mechanisms of SERT in platelets: regulation of plasma serotonin levels. Mol Interv 2010 Aug;10(4):231−41.

[33] Brenner B, Harney JT, Ahmed BA, Jeffus BC, Unal R, Mehta JL, et al. Plasma serotonin levels and the platelet serotonin transporter. J Neurochem 2007 Jul;102(1):206−15.

[34] Saier Jr MH. A functional-phylogenetic system for the classification of transport proteins. J Cell Biochem 1999; (Suppl. 32−33):84−94.

[35] Lee SL, Fanburg BL. Serotonin uptake by bovine pulmonary artery endothelial cells in culture. I. Characterization. Am J Physiol 1986 May;250(5 Pt 1):C761−5.

[36] Bonnin A, Levitt P. Fetal, maternal, and placental sources of serotonin and new implications for developmental programming of the brain. Neuroscience 2011 Dec 1;197:1−7.

[37] Talley NJ. Serotoninergic neuroenteric modulators. Lancet 2001 Dec 15;358(9298):2061−8.

[38] Wade PR, Chen J, Jaffe B, Kassem IS, Blakely RD, Gershon MD. Localization and function of a 5-HT transporter in crypt epithelia of the gastrointestinal tract. J Neurosci 1996 Apr 1;16(7):2352−64.

[39] Jonnakuty C, Gragnoli C. What do we know about serotonin? J Cell Physiol 2008 Nov;217(2):301−6.

[40] Gill RK, Pant N, Saksena S, Singla A, Nazir TM, Vohwinkel L, et al. Function, expression, and characterization of the serotonin transporter in the native human intestine. Am J Physiol Gastrointest Liver Physiol 2008 Jan;294(1):G254−62.

[41] Bliziotes M, McLoughlin S, Gunness M, Fumagalli F, Jones SR, Caron MG. Bone histomorphometric and biomechanical abnormalities in mice homozygous for deletion of the dopamine transporter gene. Bone 2000;26(1):15−9.

[42] Bliziotes MM, Eshleman AJ, Zhang XW, Wiren KM. Neurotransmitter action in osteoblasts: expression of a functional system for serotonin receptor activation and reuptake. Bone 2001 Nov;29(5):477−86.

[43] Warden SJ, Nelson IR, Fuchs RK, Bliziotes MM, Turner CH. Serotonin (5-hydroxytryptamine) transporter inhibition causes bone loss in adult mice independently of estrogen deficiency. Menopause 2008 Nov−Dec;15(6):1176−83.

[44] Warden SJ, Robling AG, Sanders MS, Bliziotes MM, Turner CH. Inhibition of the serotonin (5-hydroxytryptamine) transporter reduces bone accrual during growth. Endocrinology 2005 Feb;146(2):685−93.

[45] Sjoerdsma A, Palfreyman MG. History of serotonin and serotonin disorders. Ann NY Acad Sci 1990;600:1−7. discussion −8.

[46] Mann JJ. Role of the serotonergic system in the pathogenesis of major depression and suicidal behavior. Neuropsychopharmacology 1999 Aug;21(Suppl. 2):99S–105S.

[47] Zhou FC, Tao-Cheng JH, Segu L, Patel T, Wang Y. Serotonin transporters are located on the axons beyond the synaptic junctions: anatomical and functional evidence. Brain Res 1998 Sep 14;805(1–2):241–54.

[48] Haney EM, Chan BK, Diem SJ, Ensrud KE, Cauley JA, Barrett-Connor E, et al. Association of low bone mineral density with selective serotonin reuptake inhibitor use by older men. Arch Intern Med 2007 Jun 25;167(12):1246–51.

[49] Fuller RW, Wong DT. Serotonin uptake and serotonin uptake inhibition. Ann NY Acad Sci 1990;600:68–78; discussion 9–80.

[50] Sjoerdsma A. Serotonin. N Engl J Med 1959 Jul 23;261(4):181–8. contd.

[51] Walther DJ, Bader M. A unique central tryptophan hydroxylase isoform. Biochem Pharmacol 2003 Nov 1;66(9):1673–80.

[52] Walther DJ, Peter JU, Bashammakh S, Hortnagl H, Voits M, Fink H, et al. Synthesis of serotonin by a second tryptophan hydroxylase isoform. Science 2003 Jan 3;299(5603):76.

[53] Li Z, Chalazonitis A, Huang YY, Mann JJ, Margolis KG, Yang QM, et al. Essential roles of enteric neuronal serotonin in gastrointestinal motility and the development/survival of enteric dopaminergic neurons. J Neurosci 2011 Jun 15;31(24): 8998–9009.

[54] Yadav VK, Oury F, Suda N, Liu ZW, Gao XB, Confavreux C, et al. A serotonin-dependent mechanism explains the leptin regulation of bone mass, appetite, and energy expenditure. Cell 2009 Sep 4;138(5):976–89.

[55] Yadav VK, Oury F, Tanaka KF, Thomas T, Wang Y, Cremers S, et al. Leptin-dependent serotonin control of appetite: temporal specificity, transcriptional regulation, and therapeutic implications. J Exp Med 2011 Jan 17;208(1):41–52.

[56] Oury F, Karsenty G. Towards a serotonin-dependent leptin roadmap in the brain. Trends Endocrinol Metab 2011 Sep;22(9):382–7.

[57] Oury F, Yadav VK, Wang Y, Zhou B, Liu XS, Guo XE, et al. CREB mediates brain serotonin regulation of bone mass through its expression in ventromedial hypothalamic neurons. Genes Dev 2010 Oct 15;24(20):2330–42.

[58] Cote F, Thevenot E, Fligny C, Fromes Y, Darmon M, Ripoche MA, et al. Disruption of the nonneuronal tph1 gene demonstrates the importance of peripheral serotonin in cardiac function. Proc Natl Acad Sci USA 2003 Nov 11;100(23):13525–30.

[59] Walther DJ, Peter JU, Winter S, Holtje M, Paulmann N, Grohmann M, et al. Serotonylation of small GTPases is a signal transduction pathway that triggers platelet alpha-granule release. Cell 2003 Dec 26;115(7):851–62.

[60] Amireault P, Hatia S, Bayard E, Bernex F, Collet C, Callebert J, et al. Ineffective erythropoiesis with reduced red blood cell survival in serotonin-deficient mice. Proc Natl Acad Sci USA 2011 Aug 9;108(32):13141–6.

[61] Cote F, Fligny C, Bayard E, Launay JM, Gershon MD, Mallet J, et al. Maternal serotonin is crucial for murine embryonic development. Proc Natl Acad Sci USA 2007 Jan 2;104(1):329–34.

[62] Bonnin A, Goeden N, Chen K, Wilson ML, King J, Shih JC, et al. A transient placental source of serotonin for the fetal forebrain. Nature 2011 Apr 21;472(7343):347–50.

[63] Yadav VK, Ducy P. Lrp5 and bone formation: a serotonin-dependent pathway. Ann NY Acad Sci 2010 Mar;1192(1):103–9.

[64] Pytliak M, Vargova V, Mechirova V, Felsoci M. Serotonin receptors—from molecular biology to clinical applications. Physiol Res 2011;60(1):15–25.

[65] Kajimura D, Hinoi E, Ferron M, Kode A, Riley KJ, Zhou B, et al. Genetic determination of the cellular basis of the sympathetic regulation of bone mass accrual. J Exp Med 2011 Apr 11;208(4):841–51.

[66] Fu L, Patel MS, Bradley A, Wagner EF, Karsenty G. The molecular clock mediates leptin-regulated bone formation. Cell 2005 Sep 9;122(5):803–15.

[67] Schinke T, Schilling AF, Baranowsky A, Seitz S, Marshall RP, Linn T, et al. Impaired gastric acidification negatively affects calcium homeostasis and bone mass. Nat Med 2009 Jun;15(6):674–81.

[68] Elefteriou F, Benson MD, Sowa H, Starbuck M, Liu X, Ron D, et al. ATF4 mediation of NF1 functions in osteoblast reveals a nutritional basis for congenital skeletal dysplasiae. Cell Metab 2006 Dec;4(6):441–51.

[69] Gong Y, Slee RB, Fukai N, Rawadi G, Roman-Roman S, Reginato AM, et al. LDL receptor-related protein 5 (LRP5) affects bone accrual and eye development. Cell 2001;107(4):513–23.

[70] Boyden LM, Mao J, Belsky J, Mitzner L, Farhi A, Mitnick MA, et al. High bone density due to a mutation in LDL-receptor-related protein 5. N Engl J Med 2002;346(20):1513–21.

[71] Johnson ML, Gong G, Kimberling W, Recker SM, Kimmel DB, Recker RR. Linkage of a gene causing high bone mass to human chromosome 11(11q12-13). Am J Hum Genet 1997;60:1326–32.

[72] Kato M, Patel MS, Levasseur R, Lobov I, Chang BH, Glass 2nd DA, et al. Cbfa1-independent decrease in osteoblast proliferation, osteopenia, and persistent embryonic eye vascularization in mice deficient in Lrp5, a Wnt coreceptor. J Cell Biol 2002;157(2):303–14.

[73] Wehrli M, Dougan ST, Caldwell K, O'Keefe L, Schwartz S, Vaizel-Ohayon D. Arrow encodes an LDL-receptor-related protein essential for Wingless signalling. Nature 2000;407:527–30.

[74] Tamai K, Semenov M, Kato Y, Spokony R, Liu C, Katsuyama Y, et al. LDL-receptor-related proteins in Wnt signal transduction. Nature 2000;407:530–5.

[75] Logan CY, Nusse R. The Wnt signaling pathway in development and disease. Annu Rev Cell Dev Biol 2004;20:781–810.

[76] Mao J, Wang JY, Bo L, Pan W, Farr III GH, Flynn C, et al. Low-density lipoprotein receptor-related protein-5 binds to axin and regulates the canonical Wnt signaling pathway. Mol Cell 2001;7:801–9.

[77] Lobov IB, Rao S, Carroll TJ, Vallance JE, Ito M, Ondr JK, et al. WNT7b mediates macrophage-induced programmed cell death in patterning of the vasculature. Nature 2005 Sep 15;437(7057):417–21.

[78] Collette NM, Genetos DC, Murugesh D, Harland RM, Loots GG. Genetic evidence that SOST inhibits WNT signaling in the limb. Dev Biol 2010 Jun 15;342(2):169–79.

[79] Beighton P, Durr L, Hamersma H. The clinical features of sclerosteosis. A review of the manifestations in twenty-five affected individuals. Ann Intern Med 1976 Apr;84(4):393–7.

[80] Balemans W, Ebeling M, Patel N, Van Hul E, Olson P, Dioszegi M, et al. Increased bone density in sclerosteosis is due to the deficiency of a novel secreted protein (SOST). Hum Mol Genet 2001 Mar 1;10(5):537–43.

[81] Brunkow ME, Gardner JC, Van Ness J, Paeper BW, Kovacevich BR, Proll S, et al. Bone dysplasia sclerosteosis results from loss of the SOST gene product, a novel cystine knot-containing protein. Am J Hum Genet 2001 Mar;68(3): 577–89.

[82] Day TF, Guo X, Garrett-Beal L, Yang Y. Wnt/beta-catenin signaling in mesenchymal progenitors controls osteoblast and chondrocyte differentiation during vertebrate skeletogenesis. Dev Cell 2005 May;8(5):739–50.

[83] Hill TP, Spater D, Taketo MM, Birchmeier W, Hartmann C. Canonical Wnt/beta-catenin signaling prevents osteoblasts from differentiating into chondrocytes. Dev Cell 2005 May;8(5):727—38.

[84] Holmen SL, Giambernardi TA, Zylstra CR, Buckner-Berghuis BD, Resau JH, Hess JF, et al. Decreased BMD and limb deformities in mice carrying mutations in both Lrp5 and Lrp6. J Bone Miner Res 2004 Dec;19(12):2033—40.

[85] Glass 2nd DA, Bialek P, Ahn JD, Starbuck M, Patel MS, Clevers H, et al. Canonical Wnt signaling in differentiated osteoblasts controls osteoclast differentiation. Dev Cell 2005 May;8(5):751—64.

[86] Kramer I, Halleux C, Keller H, Pegurri M, Gooi JH, Weber PB, et al. Osteocyte Wnt/beta-catenin signaling is required for normal bone homeostasis. Mol Cell Biol 2010 Jun;30(12):3071—85.

[87] Kieslinger M, Folberth S, Dobreva G, Dorn T, Croci L, Erben R, et al. EBF2 regulates osteoblast-dependent differentiation of osteoclasts. Dev Cell 2005 Dec;9(6):757—67.

[88] Inose H, Zhou B, Yadav VK, Guo XE, Karsenty G, Ducy P. Efficacy of serotonin inhibition in mouse models of bone loss. J Bone Miner Res 2011 Sep;26(9):2002—11.

[89] Modder UI, Achenbach SJ, Amin S, Riggs BL, Melton 3rd LJ, Khosla S. Relation of serum serotonin levels to bone density and structural parameters in women. J Bone Miner Res 2010 Jul 13;25(2):415—22.

[90] Vilaca T, Yamamoto RM, Carvalho AB, Lazaretti-Castro M. Neuroendocrine tumor associated with severe osteoporosis in a male patient. Endocrine Reviews 2011;32:P3—136.

[91] Hanley HG, Stahl SM, Freedman DX. Hyperserotonemia and amine metabolites in autistic and retarded children. Arch Gen Psychiatry 1977 May;34(5):521—31.

[92] Hediger ML, England LJ, Molloy CA, Yu KF, Manning-Courtney P, Mills JL. Reduced bone cortical thickness in boys with autism or autism spectrum disorder. J Autism Dev Disord 2008 Sep 19;38:848—56.

[93] Yadav VK, Arantes HP, Barros ER, Lazaretti-Castro M, Ducy P. Genetic analysis of Lrp5 function in osteoblast progenitors. Calcif Tissue Int 2010 May;86(5):382—8.

[94] Saarinen A, Saukkonen T, Kivela T, Lahtinen U, Laine C, Somer M, et al. LDL receptor-related protein 5 (LRP5) mutations and osteoporosis, impaired glucose metabolism and hypercholesterolaemia. Clin Endocrinol (Oxf) 2009 Aug 5;72(4):481—8.

[95] Ramirez Rodriguez SP, Morton DH, Garcia Merino SA, Streeten EA. Elevated serum serotonin levels in patients with osteoporosis-pseudoglioma syndrome. Endocrine Reviews 2010;31:S1900.

[96] Frost M, Andersen T, Gossiel F, Hansen S, Bollerslev J, van Hul W, et al. Levels of serotonin, sclerostin, bone turnover markers as well as bone density and microarchitecture in patients with high-bone-mass phenotype due to a mutation in Lrp5. J Bone Miner Res 2011 Aug;26(8):1721—8.

[97] Frost M, Andersen TE, Yadav VK, Brixen K, Karsenty G, Kassem M. Patients with high bone mass phenotype due to Lrp5-T253I mutation have low plasma levels of serotonin. J Bone Min Res 2010;25(3):673—5.

[98] Saudou F, Amara DA, Dierich A, LeMeur M, Ramboz S, Segu L, et al. Enhanced aggressive behavior in mice lacking 5-HT1B receptor. Science 1994 Sep 23;265(5180):1875—8.

[99] Sibilia V, Pagani F, Lattuada N, Greco A, Guidobono F. Linking chronic tryptophan deficiency with impaired bone metabolism and reduced bone accrual in growing rats. J Cell Biochem 2009 Aug 1;107(5):890—8.

[100] Yadav VK, Balaji S, Suresh PS, Liu XS, Lu X, Li Z, et al. Pharmacological inhibition of gut-derived serotonin synthesis is a potential bone anabolic treatment for osteoporosis. Nat Med 2010 Mar;16(3):308—12.

[101] Shi ZC, Devasagayaraj A, Gu K, Jin H, Marinelli B, Samala L, et al. Modulation of peripheral serotonin levels by novel tryptophan hydroxylase inhibitors for the potential treatment of functional gastrointestinal disorders. J Med Chem 2008 Jul 10;51(13):3684—7.

[102] Liu Q, Yang Q, Sun W, Vogel P, Heydorn W, Yu XQ, et al. Discovery and characterization of novel tryptophan hydroxylase inhibitors that selectively inhibit serotonin synthesis in the gastrointestinal tract. J Pharmacol Exp Ther 2008 Apr;325(1):47—55.

[103] Girotra M, Rubin MR, Bilezikian JP. The use of parathyroid hormone in the treatment of osteoporosis. Rev Endocr Metab Disord 2006 Jun;7(1—2):113—21.

[104] Black DM, Greenspan SL, Ensrud KE, Palermo L, McGowan JA, Lang TF, et al. The effects of parathyroid hormone and alendronate alone or in combination in postmenopausal osteoporosis. N Engl J Med 2003 Sep 25;349(13):1207—15.

[105] Cosman F, Nieves J, Zion M, Woelfert L, Luckey M, Lindsay R. Daily and cyclic parathyroid hormone in women receiving alendronate. N Engl J Med 2005 Aug 11;353(6):566—75.

[106] Zambrowicz B, Brown P, Jackson JI, Frazier K, Clark E, Yang Q, et al. Serotonin biomaker levels correlate with clinical response in Phase 2 trial of LX1031, a novel serotonin synthesis inhibitor for non-constipating IBS. New Orleans, LA: Digestive Disease Week Meeting; 2010.

[107] Reagan-Shaw S, Nihal M, Ahmad N. Dose translation from animal to human studies revisited. FASEB J 2008 Mar;22(3):659—61.

[108] Brown PM, Drossman DA, Wood AJ, Cline GA, Frazier KS, Jackson JI, et al. The tryptophan hydroxylase inhibitor LX1031 shows clinical benefit in patients with nonconstipating irritable bowel syndrome. Gastroenterology 2011 Aug;141(2):507—16.

Skeletal Actions of Insulin

Ryan C. Riddle, PhD [1, 2], *Mathieu Ferron, PhD* [3], *Thomas L. Clemens, PhD* [1, 2]

[1] Johns Hopkins University School of Medicine, Baltimore, MD, USA [2] Baltimore Veterans Administration Medical Center, Baltimore, MD, USA [3] Columbia University, New York, NY, USA

INTRODUCTION

Insulin and the insulin-like growth factors (IGFs) are among the most familiar and widely studied growth factors. These related molecules evolved from a common precursor system comprised of a single receptor and multiple ligands that functioned in lower animals to enable a broad range of physiologic processes, including smell, food consumption, metabolism, growth, reproduction, and dormancy. In higher organisms, including mammals, the insulin and IGF ligands and their receptors evolved more circumscribed functions: IGFs are viewed as central to cell proliferation, survival, and organism growth, and insulin serves primarily in the regulation of fuel accumulation, storage, and energy expenditure. Such a simplistic paradigm, however, overlooks the fact that insulin and IGF-1 continue to exert overlapping roles in several physiologic processes. Indeed, recent studies have identified new skeletal actions of insulin, which suggest that insulin-responsive bone cells participate in the regulation of global energy homeostasis. Such findings raise new questions on the nature of the fuel sensing and processing mechanisms in bone and their relative importance to overall energy homeostasis in mammals. This chapter will review our current understanding of insulin's role in bone in the context of these recent findings and identify key areas where additional work is needed.

THE INSULIN/IGF FAMILY OF LIGANDS AND RECEPTORS

Insulin and insulin-like growth factors are evolutionarily conserved hormonal signaling molecules which arose in primitive eukaryotes, including ciliated protozoans and unicellular fungi [1,2]. In these more primitive species, a single IGF/IR appears to regulate both cell growth and metabolism. The *Caenorhabditis elegans daf-2* gene, for instance, encodes a protein that shares 35% sequence identity with the human insulin receptor (IR) and is the only member of the insulin receptor family present in the worm genome. Mutations in this gene give rise to *dauer* larvae with increased lifespan but reduced metabolic activity that is consistent with a role for *daf-2* in a metabolic regulatory pathway. Moreover, significant portions of *daf-2* mutants exhibit an arrest in larval development or embryonic lethality indicating a role in *C. elegans* development [3,4]. Similar functions have been ascribed to the *Drosophila* insulin receptor homologue, which regulates body size by promoting both cell growth and proliferation [5]. In addition, most *InsR* mutants in *Drosophila* are embryonic lethal.

During subsequent evolution, insulin/IGF-1 receptor genes and new ligands arose from duplication of the primitive precursors. In mammals, nine different genes encode insulin-like peptides. These include two nonallelic *Insulin* genes present in rodents, *Igf1*, *Igf2*, *Relaxin*, and four insulin-like peptides: *Insl3*, *Insl4*, *Insl5*, and *Insl6* [6]. Further complexity is added by the presence of four related receptors: insulin receptor, IGF-1 receptor, IGF-2 receptor, and IR-related receptor [6–10]. With the exception of the IGF-2 receptor (mannose-6-phosphate receptor), which appears to mediate IGF-2 clearance during embryogenesis [9], these receptors belong to a family of ligand-activated receptor tyrosine kinases. The ligand initiates signaling by binding to receptor homodimers composed of two identical α/β monomers (e.g. $IR_{\alpha\beta}/IR_{\alpha\beta}$) or heterodimers composed of two different receptor monomers (e.g. $IR_{\alpha\beta}/IGF\text{-}1R_{\alpha\beta}$) at the cell surface. This induces a conformational change that facilitates autophosphorylation and the engagement of downstream signaling components [11–13]. The major signaling pathways by which IR and IGF-1R exert their effects are shared. In particular, IRS proteins (IRS-1 and

IRS-2) act as key mediators that are recruited to the receptors by phosphotyrosine binding and pleckstrin homology domains [14,15]. The resulting tyrosine phosphorylation of IRS proteins in turn creates binding sites for SH2 domain containing proteins including PI3-kinase and the Grb2/Sos complex that facilitates MAP kinase activation.

Observations from gene knockout studies have begun to clarify the essential functions of the highly related IR and IGF-1R. Mice deficient for IR are born at term with slight growth retardation, but largely unimpaired embryonic development. However, death occurs within a few days of birth as a result of uncontrolled glucose metabolism, β-cell failure, and diabetic ketoacidosis [14,16]. Similar phenotypes are evident following the disruption of both *Ins1* and *Ins2* [17]. By contrast, mice lacking *Igf1* or *Igf1r* exhibit intrauterine growth retardation such that birth weight is 60% and 45% of normal, respectively [18–20]. The metabolic disturbances observed in *Igf1r*-null mice prior to perinatal lethality are considerably milder than those evident in *Insr* mutants, and is unlikely to be a cause of death [21]. These data led to the interpretation that IR primarily facilitates metabolic regulation while IGF-1R promotes cellular growth.

Results from several studies suggest that the two receptors also exert some overlapping functions. For example, *Igf1r/Igf2r* double mutants exhibit embryonic overgrowth (~130% of normal body weight) due to increased levels of circulating IGF-2 [22]. In this situation, it appears that IR fulfills a growth promoting function, as triple mutants are nonviable dwarfs [23]. Similarly, the levels of *Igf1r* expression are increased more than two-fold in IR-deficient mice, which enables the receptor to bind insulin and compensate for the loss of IR during embryonic growth [23]. Human studies further support the concept of partial functional overlap as mutations in the human *INSR* gene result in leprechaunism, a condition characterized by severe growth retardation in addition to the expected metabolic disturbances [24–26].

ACTIONS OF IGF-1 AND INSULIN IN OSTEOBLASTS

Before considering the new skeletal actions of insulin it is useful to review briefly the literature on insulin and IGF-1 action in bone. The most familiar action of IGF-1 is its ability to stimulate mesenchymal cell proliferation. The reduction in linear growth in the *Igf1* null mice described above is associated with a reduction in cell number and proliferation in chondrocytes and osteoblast precursors when examined by bromodeoxyuridine labeling [27]. Mitogenic effects of IGF-1 on osteoblasts have also been observed in *in vitro* studies which

demonstrated that growth factor stimulates an increase in the expression of the proto-oncogene *c-fos* [28]. IGF-1 is increasingly recognized as an important survival factor for osteoblasts. The growth factor activates the anti-apoptotic AKT and MAP kinase signaling pathways in osteoblasts [29], and neutralizating autocrine IGF-1 increases osteoblast apoptosis *in vitro* [30,31].

IGF-1 also exerts effects on differentiated osteoblast function. During the initial phases of differentiation of fetal rat calvarial osteoblasts *in vitro*, IGF-1 production increases and possibly serves to promote the progression of preosteoblast to mature osteoblast. IGF-1 expression then declines with the appearance of the differentiated osteoblast phenotype [32]. However, a second rise in IGF-1 expression occurs in association with osteoblast maturation, matrix synthesis, and mineralization. This second wave of IGF-1 production may account for the ability of IGF-1 to augment the synthesis of type I collagen and inhibit collagen degradation in differentiated fetal rat osteoblasts [33]. Studies in genetically altered mice underscore the importance of IGF-1 in the formation and maintenance of normal bone matrix. For example, targeted overexpression of IGF-1 accelerates new bone formation but also increases the pace at which matrix is mineralized [34]. In addition, osteoblast-specific disruption of IGF-1R causes a markedly impaired mineral apposition rate and an increase in mineralization lag time [35]. Interestingly, these genetic manipulations of IGF-1 action have their most dramatic effects during the pubertal growth spurt, which likely relates to an interaction between IGF-1 and sex steroids [36].

In keeping with its original name, somatomedin, IGF-1 is known to mediate many, but not all, of the effects of growth hormone on the skeleton. Linear bone growth is equally compromised in *Igf1*-null and *Ghr*-null mice, but combining the two mutations produces a much more severe phenotype [27], suggesting that growth hormone receptor (GHR) signaling is not entirely dispensable for normal growth plate development. Moreover, the impairment in postnatal bone mineral density has been reported to be more severe in *Igf1* null than *Ghr* null (*lit/lit*) mice [37], and GH administration increases bone formation rate in the *Igf1* mutants [38]. However, the severe disturbances in overall growth of these mice and problems with their reproductive hormone status complicate interpretation of these results. Indeed, more recent analysis using transgenic models has demonstrated that the loss of IGF-1R or IGF-1 neutralization impairs the ability of GH to stimulate osteoblast proliferation *in vitro*, and that expression of IGF-1R by osteoblasts is required for GH to increase osteoblast numbers *in vivo* [39].

Surprisingly little attention has been given to the skeletal actions of insulin, despite abundant circumstantial evidence for such a role. Osteoblasts express functional IR and exogenous insulin increases bone anabolic markers, including collagen synthesis [40], alkaline phosphatase production [41], and glucose uptake [42,43]. Moreover, patients with type I diabetes mellitus can develop early-onset osteopenia or osteoporosis [44,45] and have an increased risk of fragility fracture [46,47] as well as poor bone healing and regeneration after injury [48]. Localized insulin delivery accelerates healing in these models by enhancing osteogenesis [49]. Skeletal abnormalities are also observed in animal models of type I diabetes mellitus that exhibit bone loss [50,51] secondary to reduced bone formation [51–54]. However, defining and distinguishing the mechanisms of action of insulin in bone has been difficult because of the potential for crosstalk with IGF-1R and the metabolic disturbances and early postnatal death of *Insr*-null mice.

Initial analyses of bone mass in 6-month-old mice globally deficient for IR, but "rescued" from perinatal ketoacidosis by targeted re-expression of IR transgenes in the pancreas, liver, and brain (tTr-IR knockout mice [55]), indicated that insulin receptor signaling was not a major contributor to bone development as measurements of bone mineral density and osteoblast function were similar in the control and mutant mice [56]. Thus, it appeared that skeletal abnormalities evident in diabetic patients and animal models might be the result of detrimental effects of hyperglycemia or other metabolic disturbances on osteoblast function [57,58]. However, a recent re-analysis of the bone phenotype of these mice at early time points revealed a significant reduction in trabecular bone volume, which is in accordance with the phenotype of mice lacking IR specifically in the osteoblast [59].

Recent studies by Fulzele and colleagues [59] in mice selectively lacking the IR in osteoblasts suggest that insulin signaling is indeed required for normal bone acquisition. Loss of IR in osteoblasts reduced numbers of osteoblasts and decreased trabecular bone volume (Fig. 8.1). *In vitro*, IR-deficient osteoblasts proliferated poorly and failed to differentiate, while insulin stimulation of wild-type osteoblasts increased proliferation and enhanced matrix mineralization. Importantly, this phenotype was fundamentally different from that observed in mice deficient for IGF-1R in osteoblast. While IGF-1R mice also exhibited reduced trabecular bone volume, the numbers of osteoblasts were normal and the phenotype was instead accompanied by an osteomalacia-like defect in mineralization [35]. Interestingly, whereas insulin stimulation could partially rescue the effect of IGF-1R deficiency on matrix mineralization by osteoblasts [60], IGF-1 stimulation could not correct the impaired differentiation capacity of IR-deficient osteoblasts [59]. This may be related to the observation that IGF-1R reduces the sensitivity of osteoblasts to insulin, possibly via the formation of IR:IGF-1R hybrid receptors that are preferentially activated by IGF-1 [60].

The availability of primary osteoblasts lacking IGF-1 receptors enabled microarray profiling and the identification of two key insulin target genes [59]. Osteocalcin, a familiar gene to bone biologists (see below), was profoundly upregulated by insulin whereas Twist2, an inhibitor of the osteoblast transcription factor Runx2, was downregulated. Thus, insulin blocked the expression of an inhibitor of Runx2, the key regulator of osteocalcin and other genes required for osteoblast differentiation [61].

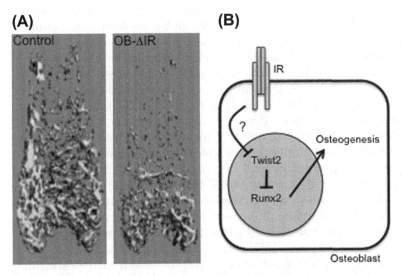

(A)

(B)

FIGURE 8.1 **Insulin signaling is required for normal bone acquisition.** (A) Computer renderings from micro-CT analysis of trabecular bone volume in the distal femur of 12-week-old mice lacking the insulin receptor specifically in osteoblasts (OB-ΔIR) and a littermate control. (B) Insulin receptor signaling regulates osteogenesis by inhibiting the expression of Twist2 a key regulator the Runx2, a transcription factor required for osteoblast differentiation. *Modified from Fulzele et al. [59].*

INSULIN SIGNALING IN THE OSTEOBLASTS REGULATES GLUCOSE METABOLISM

The concept that bone might participate in energy metabolism was first suggested over a decade ago when Ducy and colleagues [62] reported that fat-derived leptin altered bone mass through a hypothalamic—osteoblast endocrine loop. Nevertheless, the initial findings of hyperglycemia and weight gain in mice lacking the insulin receptor specifically in osteoblasts came as a surprise [59,63]. With age, the IR-deficient mice exhibit a generalized increase in peripheral adiposity and a reduction in energy expenditure. This alteration in body composition was accompanied by a defect in insulin production, as circulating insulin levels were reduced and islet morphology was altered, and the development of peripheral insulin resistance. Importantly, none of these metabolic abnormalities were observed in mice lacking the IGF-1R in the osteoblast [59].

Parallel studies ongoing in another lab produced a mouse with similar metabolic disturbances when lacking the insulin receptor in its osteoblasts [63], or when IR signaling was manipulated [64]. While profiling the mouse genome to identify osteoblast-specific hormones, Lee and colleagues [64] identified the *Esp* gene, encoding an unfamiliar protein tyrosine phosphatase, OST-PTP. Mice engineered to overexpress this gene in osteoblasts mirror the effect of disrupting the insulin receptor and become fat while developing hyperglycemia and hypoinsulinemia. Disrupting its expression resulted in the opposite phenotype. Using substrate trapping experiments this laboratory identified OST-PTP as an inhibitor of IR phosphorylation and downstream signaling [63] that functions similarly to a more familiar regulator of IR function, PTP-1B [65,66].

These *in vivo* studies together with the fact that co-culturing osteoblasts with β-cells or adipocytes induces an increase in the expression of insulin and adiponectin [64], respectively, indicated that the osteoblast secretes a circulating factor that contributes to metabolic regulation. As noted above, insulin is a potent stimulator of osteocalcin expression and while this factor was originally thought to be an extracellular matrix protein that inhibited skeletal mineralization [67], it exhibits several structural features found in classical hormones. Osteocalcin is synthesized as a prepro-molecule that is then processed in the endoplasmic reticulum. Before being secreted by osteoblasts, osteocalcin undergoes vitamin K-dependent carboxylation that confers the molecule with greater affinity for the bone matrix [68]. A small portion remains undercarboxylated and is secreted into the circulation [69], where it appears to act as a hormone.

In addition to the increase in bone formation originally noted by Ducy et al. [67], osteocalcin-null mice exhibit the marked disturbances in metabolism that would be expected if this molecule facilitates glucose metabolism [64]. By one month of age, the mutant mice already had larger fat depots, higher blood glucose levels, and reduced serum insulin levels. Insulin secretion, insulin sensitivity, and glucose tolerance were all impaired in the osteocalcin-null mice, with reduced levels of adiponectin being at least partially responsible for the reduced insulin sensitivity. Separate studies have now demonstrated that infusion of undercarboxylated osteocalcin via osmotic pump or daily injection improves glucose tolerance and protects mice from the deleterious effects of a high fat diet [70,71].

Several additional pieces of evidence indicated that alterations in the levels of circulating osteocalcin are indeed an underlying cause of the metabolic disturbances evident in mice lacking IR in osteoblasts. First, insulin stimulation of osteoblasts triggered the accumulation of undercarboxylated osteocalcin protein in conditioned media, and the osteoblast IR mutant mice had lower serum levels of the hormonal form of osteocalcin [59,63]. Second, infusion of undercarboxylated osteocalcin partially corrected the insulin resistance and glucose intolerance of the mutant mice [59]. Third, the metabolic disturbances evident in compound mutants lacking one allele of the insulin receptor in osteoblasts and one allele of osteocalcin mirror those of osteocalcin-null mice [63]. Taken together, these results suggest that IR signaling in osteoblasts regulates secretion of osteocalcin, which in turn acts in an endocrine fashion to regulate pancreatic insulin production and peripheral insulin responsiveness.

Additional support for this bone—pancreas endocrine loop is drawn from the recent identification of a putative osteocalcin receptor. GPCR6A is an orphan receptor that belongs to class C of the G-protein coupled receptor family that also includes glutamate receptors, γ-aminobutyric acid receptors, and the calcium-sensing receptor [72]. Expressed in skeletal muscle, kidney, liver, and pancreas, GPCR6A appears to sense extracellular calcium and amino acids [73] and also to be activated by osteocalcin [73]. Mice deficient for this receptor are osteopenic due to impaired osteoblast function [74] and also exhibit a metabolic syndrome compatible with the loss of osteocalcin action. Beginning at 12 weeks of age, the null mice exhibit an increase in body fat, which is accompanied by hyperglycemia, glucose intolerance, and the development of a fatty liver [75]. Further, the ability of osteocalcin to enhance insulin expression and secretion by the β-cell was ablated in GPCR6A null mice [76]. Thus, GPCR6A appears to represent at least one osteocalcin receptor, which mediates insulin secretory activity. The same receptor also appears to mediate osteocalcin's effects on testosterone production by testicular Leydig cells [77] and is required for full reproductive potency of male mice.

INSULIN SIGNALING REGULATES OSTEOCALCIN PRODUCTION AND BIOAVAILABILITY

In addition to controlling osteocalcin gene transcription, insulin signaling also appears to regulate the amount of this protein in the circulation. As noted above, insulin stimulation enhances the activity of Runx2 [59], a transcription factor originally identified by its ability to interact with the OSE2 site in the osteocalcin promoter and confer osteoblast specific expression [78]. However, regulation of osteocalcin expression by Runx2 may be more related to the ability of insulin to facilitate osteogenesis than its ability to stimulate production of the hormonal form of osteocalcin. In support of this idea, insulin stimulation did not regulate Runx2 mRNA on the same time scale that it regulated osteocalcin expression, and regulation of Runx2 activity by insulin appears to occur via an indirect mechanism involving Twist2 [59]. The fact that Runx2 expression was reduced in differentiating osteoblasts lacking the IR may actually be more related to the ability of Runx2 to auto-regulate its own expression during differentiation [79]. It is reasonable to assume that if osteocalcin acts as a hormone, there should be a more rapid mechanism to induce its expression in the osteoblast.

The transcription factor FoxO1 may facilitate such a function. FoxO proteins represent key transcriptional mediators of insulin action. Insulin suppresses the activity of FoxOs through the activation of AKT signaling and the subsequent phosphorylation of FoxO that results in its nuclear export [80,81]. FoxO1 is the mostly highly expressed isoform in the osteoblasts and its binding to the osteocalcin promoter suppresses osteocalcin expression [82,83]. Mice lacking FoxO1 specifically in the osteoblast had increased glucose tolerance, improved insulin sensitivity, and reduced body fat. As expected, serum levels of undercarboxylated osteocalcin were increased and genetic manipulation of the osteocalcin gene abolished the effects of FoxO1 deletion on glucose metabolism [83]. Additionally, deletion of one allele of FoxO1 in the osteoblast is sufficient to rescue the metabolic disturbances observed in osteoblast IR mutant mice [63].

Based on these observations, a working model has been proposed in which insulin signaling in the osteoblast inactivates FoxO1 to increase production of osteocalcin, which in turn stimulates increased insulin production in a positive feedback loop (Fig. 8.2). The transcription factor Atf4 may represent a molecular brake-point in this endocrine loop. In non-osseous cells, Atf4 protein is rapidly turned over, but the transcription factor accumulates in osteoblasts where it can drive osteoblast-specific gene expression [84,85]. Despite a reduction in bone mass, Atf4 global knockouts and osteoblast-specific mutants exhibit a metabolic phenotype compatible with enhanced osteocalcin endocrine function. The mutant mice are hypoglycemic with

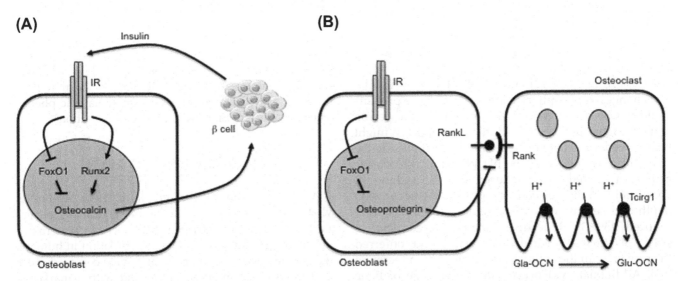

FIGURE 8.2 A feed-forward loop links insulin and osteocalcin. (A) Insulin signaling in the osteoblast increases osteocalcin transcription by suppressing the activity of FoxO1 and increasing the activity of Runx2. Osteocalcin, in turn, increases β-cell proliferation and the production and secretion of insulin. **(B)** Insulin-induced suppression of FoxO1 also leads to a decrease in the expression osteoprotegrin, which decreases the ratio of OPG to RANKL and in turn increases the expression of Tcirg1 in osteoclasts. Acidification of the resorption pit is sufficient to decarboxylate matrix-bound osteocalcin and allows it to enter the circulation. *Modified from Fulzele et al. [59] and Ferron et al. [63].*

TABLE 8.1   Metabolic Phenotypes of Mouse Mutants Associated with Insulin Signaling in Osteoblasts

Metabolic parameter	Insulin receptor**	Osteocalcin*	Esp/ OST-PTP*,**	FoxO1**	Atf4*,**
Bone mass	↓	↑	N.D.	↓	↓
Fat mass	↑	↑	↓	↓	↓
Random fed blood glucose	↑	↑	↓	↓	↓
Fasted blood glucose	↑	↑	↓	↓	↓
Serum insulin	↓	↓	↑	↑	↑
Glucose tolerance	↓	↓	↑	↑	↑
Insulin tolerance	↓	↓	↑	↑	↑
Energy expenditure	↓	↓	↑	↑	N.D.
Serum undercarboxylated osteocalcin	↓	KO	↑	↑	↑
Reference	59, 63	64, 67	64	82, 83	85, 86

Indicates a global mutant.
**Indicates an osteoblast-specific mutant.*
N.D. not determined.

improved glucose tolerance and insulin sensitivity relative to their control littermates. At the molecular level, the increase in serum undercarboxylated osteocalcin levels appears to be related to a reduction in *Esp* expression [86]. Since insulin can enhance the activity of Atf4 [87,88], this likely represents a mechanism for negative feedback. However, it is still unclear if this mechanism would exist in human osteoblasts, since *Esp* is a pseudogene in this species [89].

The ability of insulin to regulate the bioavailability of osteocalcin (i.e. its carboxylation status) may be related in part to the effects of the hormone on osteoclastic activity. Before being secreted, osteocalcin is γ-carboxylated at residues 17, 21, and 24 (residues 13, 17, and 20 in the mouse), which confers the protein with greater affinity for hydroxyapatite [68]. Since the expression of the factors necessary for carboxylation, γ-glutamyl carboxylase and Vkorc1, were not altered by insulin and changes in phosphorylation status of these proteins could not be detected after insulin stimulation, Ferron and colleagues [63] postulated that the osteoclast might be involved. Proteins can be decarboxylated outside the cell simply by lowering the pH [90], and osteoclastic activity appeared to be reduced in mice lacking IR specifically in the osteoblast, as osteoclastic erosion depth and serum cross-link C-telopeptide levels were reduced [59,63]. Indeed, incubating osteocalcin at pH 4.5 *in vitro* resulted in decarboxylation and conferred the protein with the ability to stimulate insulin secretion [63]. Additional evidence for the importance of bone resorption in decarboxylating osteocalcin was provided by a bone marrow transplant experiment in which hematopoietic cells from a mouse with osteopetrosis (*oc/oc*) conferred to otherwise wild-type mice an

osteopetrotic phenotype, a reduction in glucose tolerance, and led to a substantial decrease in the amount of undercarboxylated osteocalcin.

This hypothesis is further strengthened by the fact that osteoblasts lacking the IR exhibit higher levels of osteoprotegerin [59,63], which provides a mechanistic link between osteoblastic insulin signaling and osteoclast activity. However, two pieces of experimental evidence suggest that other osteoclast-independent mechanisms might also regulate osteocalcin carboxylation. First, insulin increased the accumulation of undercarboxylated osteocalcin in media conditioned by cultured osteoblasts, and a reduction in undercarboxylated osteocalcin was observed when the same experiment was performed using IR-deficient osteoblasts [59]. Second, in humans an oral glucose load that increases insulin secretion has clearly been demonstrated to suppress markers of bone resorption [91]. Table 8.1 provides a summary of the metabolic phenotypes of mouse models described in this section

FROM MOUSE TO MAN

A key question related to all of these studies is whether or to what extent they apply to humans, particularly in light of the striking differences in patterns of embryonic growth and metabolic regulation in humans and rodents. Rodents are born at a stage corresponding to 26 weeks of human gestation and with a markedly different body composition [92]. With regard to human bone growth and development, animal models may actually understate the role of insulin signaling. Mouse models [50–54] appear to replicate the deficits in bone mineral density and impaired fracture healing evident in diabetic patients [44–48]. However, insulin appears to be a fetal growth factor in humans. Humans lacking the IR are severely growth retarded [26,93], while the IR-deficient mice discussed above have relatively normal body size [16].

In terms of the influence of insulin signaling in the osteoblast on whole body metabolism in humans, a number of cross-sectional studies have now shown that total and/or undercarboxylated osteocalcin levels are negatively associated with body mass index, fat mass, insulin secretion, and insulin resistance in humans. In healthy men and men with metabolic syndrome, serum levels of osteocalcin are negatively correlated with fasting glucose, fasting insulin, and HOMA-IR, a representation of insulin resistance [94,95]. Untreated diabetics and prediabetics circulate decreased levels of the undercarboxylated form of osteocalcin, while higher serum levels were accompanied by higher HOMA-β, a representation of enhanced β-cell function [96]. In obese children, serum osteocalcin concentrations are significantly negatively related to leptin concentration and increased insulin resistance, but not to adiponectin [97]. Moreover, substantial weight loss in these children was associated with an increased serum osteocalcin level, improved insulin sensitivity, and decreased serum leptin levels. Thus, although these associations suggest a relationship between serum osteocalcin and energy metabolism, they do not address the possibility that osteocalcin directly mediates the changes.

In an attempt to more directly assess the effects of insulin on osteocalcin and bone turnover in humans, Basu and colleagues [98] performed a hyperinsulinemic–euglycemic clamp in healthy patients and measured its effect on serum levels of osteocalcin and other bone markers. Increasing insulin concentrations did not significantly alter circulating osteocalcin levels or other markers of bone turnover. However, measures of insulin sensitivity, including glucose disappearance rates, were positively correlated with serum levels of C-terminal telopeptide type 1 collagen, a bone resorption marker, suggesting that insulin might elicit factors that promote enhanced insulin sensitivity in the periphery.

PERSPECTIVES AND DIRECTIONS FOR FUTURE STUDIES

The studies described in this chapter are part of a larger emerging paradigm that implicates the skeleton as an integrator of energy metabolism. Bone and its cells should now be viewed as an insulin-responsive tissue that senses changes in whole body energy balance and

produces hormones that communicate information to other organs involved in energy production and usage. Given the size of the skeleton and its vast number of resident cells, the energy demands necessary to maintain skeletal integrity are likely to be large, particularly during periods of active bone formation and remodeling. Osteoblasts appear to have evolved mechanisms to survey fuel status and communicate metabolic demands to other metabolically active tissues. Osteocalcin likely represents the first of several osteoblast-derived hormones [99] that regulate metabolism and is sufficiently important to be regulated by insulin in a feed-forward endocrine loop. These skeletal, energy-managing pathways likely emerged in early terrestrial species when muscle and fat were evolving analogous pathways for fuel production, storage, and expenditure.

These discoveries raise important questions for additional studies. In particular, the metabolic demands and fuel utilizing machinery of the osteoblast lineage are relatively unexplored. Insulin stimulates glucose uptake by the osteoblast [42,43], but whether this is mediated by glucose transporter-1 or -4 is unknown. Do osteoblasts simply burn glucose or do bone cells also utilize lipids and amino acids as fuel? Can bone store fuel like muscle and fat and what role might marrow adipocytes play in this process? Additionally, determining whether our current repertoire of therapeutic agents for osteopenia, especially those that inhibit bone resorption, has effects on glucose homeostasis in humans will have important clinical implications. The answers to these questions will greatly expand our understanding of the basic biology of the skeleton and the actions of insulin. Moreover, they should have important implications for the diagnosis and management of patients with metabolic diseases, including osteoporosis and diabetes, and might lead to the development of therapeutic options that concurrently target both conditions.

Acknowledgments

This work was supported by a Career Development Award (RCR) and Merit Award (TLC) from the Veterans Administration. TLC is the recipient of a Research Career Scientist Award from the Veterans Administration.

References

[1] Le Roith D, Shiloach J, Roth J, Lesniak MA. Evolutionary origins of vertebrate hormones: substances similar to mammalian insulins are native to unicellular eukaryotes. Proc Natl Acad Sci USA 1980;77(10):6184–8.
[2] Chan SJ, Cao QP, Steiner DF. Evolution of the insulin superfamily: cloning of a hybrid insulin/insulin-like growth factor cDNA from amphioxus. Proc Natl Acad Sci USA 1990;87(23):9319–23.

[3] Kimura KD, Tissenbaum HA, Liu Y, Ruvkun G. daf-2, an insulin receptor-like gene that regulates longevity and diapause in Caenorhabditis elegans. Science 1997;277(5328):942–6.

[4] Tissenbaum HA, Ruvkun G. An insulin-like signaling pathway affects both longevity and reproduction in Caenorhabditis elegans. Genetics 1998;148(2):703–17.

[5] Chen C, Jack J, Garofalo RS. The Drosophila insulin receptor is required for normal growth. Endocrinology 1996;137(3):846–56.

[6] Nakae J, Kido Y, Accili D. Distinct and overlapping functions of insulin and IGF-I receptors. Endocrine Rev 2001;22(6):818–35.

[7] Ebina Y, Ellis L, Jarnagin K, Edery M, Graf L, Clauser E, et al. The human insulin receptor cDNA: the structural basis for hormone-activated transmembrane signalling. Cell 1985;40(4): 747–58.

[8] Ullrich A, Gray A, Tam AW, Yang-Feng T, Tsubokawa M, Collins C, et al. Insulin-like growth factor I receptor primary structure: comparison with insulin receptor suggests structural determinants that define functional specificity. EMBO J 1986;5(10):2503–12.

[9] Morgan DO, Edman JC, Standring DN, Fried VA, Smith MC, Roth RA, et al. Insulin-like growth factor II receptor as a multifunctional binding protein. Nature 1987;329(6137): 301–7.

[10] Shier P, Watt VM. Primary structure of a putative receptor for a ligand of the insulin family. J Biol Chem 1989;264(25):14605–8.

[11] Hubbard SR, Wei L, Ellis L, Hendrickson WA. Crystal structure of the tyrosine kinase domain of the human insulin receptor. Nature 1994;372(6508):746–54.

[12] Hubbard SR. Crystal structure of the activated insulin receptor tyrosine kinase in complex with peptide substrate and ATP analog. EMBO J 1997;16(18):5572–81.

[13] Schlessinger J. Cell signaling by receptor tyrosine kinases. Cell 2000;103(2):211–25.

[14] Taniguchi CM, Emanuelli B, Kahn CR. Critical nodes in signalling pathways: insights into insulin action. Nature reviews Mol Cell Biol 2006;7(2):85–96.

[15] White MF. IRS proteins and the common path to diabetes. Am J Physiol Endocrinol Metab 2002;283(3):E413–22.

[16] Accili D, Drago J, Lee EJ, Johnson MD, Cool MH, Salvatore P, et al. Early neonatal death in mice homozygous for a null allele of the insulin receptor gene. Nat Gen 1996;12(1):106–9.

[17] Duvillie B, Cordonnier N, Deltour L, Dandoy-Dron F, Itier JM, Monthioux E, et al. Phenotypic alterations in insulin-deficient mutant mice. Proc Natl Acad Sci USA 1997;94(10):5137–40.

[18] Baker J, Liu JP, Robertson EJ, Efstratiadis A. Role of insulin-like growth factors in embryonic and postnatal growth. Cell 1993;75(1):73–82.

[19] Liu JP, Baker J, Perkins AS, Robertson EJ, Efstratiadis A. Mice carrying null mutations of the genes encoding insulin-like growth factor I (Igf-1) and type 1 IGF receptor (Igf1r). Cell 1993;75(1):59–72.

[20] Powell-Braxton L, Hollingshead P, Warburton C, Dowd M, Pitts-Meek S, Dalton D, et al. IGF-I is required for normal embryonic growth in mice. Genes Dev 1993;7(12B):2609–17.

[21] Withers DJ, Burks DJ, Towery HH, Altamuro SL, Flint CL, White MF. Irs-2 coordinates Igf-1 receptor-mediated beta-cell development and peripheral insulin signalling. Nat Gen 1999;23(1):32–40.

[22] Ludwig T, Eggenschwiler J, Fisher P, D'Ercole AJ, Davenport ML, Efstratiadis A. Mouse mutants lacking the type 2 IGF receptor (IGF2R) are rescued from perinatal lethality in Igf2 and Igf1r null backgrounds. Dev Biol 1996;177(2):517–35.

[23] Louvi A, Accili D, Efstratiadis A. Growth-promoting interaction of IGF-II with the insulin receptor during mouse embryonic development. Dev Biol 1997;189(1):33–48.

[24] Krook A, Brueton L, O'Rahilly S. Homozygous nonsense mutation in the insulin receptor gene in infant with leprechaunism. Lancet 1993;342(8866):277–8.

[25] Kadowaki T, Bevins CL, Cama A, Ojamaa K, Marcus-Samuels B, Kadowaki H, et al. Two mutant alleles of the insulin receptor gene in a patient with extreme insulin resistance. Science 1988;240(4853):787–90.

[26] Wertheimer E, Lu SP, Backeljauw PF, Davenport ML, Taylor SI. Homozygous deletion of the human insulin receptor gene results in leprechaunism. Nat Gen 1993;5(1):71–3.

[27] Lupu F, Terwilliger JD, Lee K, Segre GV, Efstratiadis A. Roles of growth hormone and insulin-like growth factor 1 in mouse postnatal growth. Dev Biol 2001;229(1):141–62.

[28] Merriman HL, La Tour D, Linkhart TA, Mohan S, Baylink DJ, Strong DD. Insulin-like growth factor-I and insulin-like growth factor-II induce c-fos in mouse osteoblastic cells. Calc Tissue Int 1990;46(4):258–62.

[29] Grey A, Chen Q, Xu X, Callon K, Cornish J. Parallel phosphatidylinositol-3 kinase and p42/44 mitogen-activated protein kinase signaling pathways subserve the mitogenic and anti-apoptotic actions of insulin-like growth factor I in osteoblastic cells. Endocrinology 2003;144(11):4886–93.

[30] Hill PA, Tumber A, Meikle MC. Multiple extracellular signals promote osteoblast survival and apoptosis. Endocrinology 1997;138(9):3849–58.

[31] Tumber A, Meikle MC, Hill PA. Autocrine signals promote osteoblast survival in culture. J Endocrinol 2000;167(3): 383–90.

[32] Birnbaum RS, Bowsher RR, Wiren KM. Changes in IGF-I and -II expression and secretion during the proliferation and differentiation of normal rat osteoblasts. J Endocrinol 1995;144(2): 251–9.

[33] Rydziel S, Delany AM, Canalis E. Insulin-like growth factor I inhibits the transcription of collagenase 3 in osteoblast cultures. J Cell Biochem 1997;67(2):176–83.

[34] Zhao G, Monier-Faugere MC, Langub MC, Geng Z, Nakayama T, Pike JW, et al. Targeted overexpression of insulin-like growth factor I to osteoblasts of transgenic mice: increased trabecular bone volume without increased osteoblast proliferation. Endocrinology 2000;141(7):2674–82.

[35] Zhang M, Xuan S, Bouxsein ML, von Stechow D, Akeno N, Faugere MC, et al. Osteoblast-specific knockout of the insulin-like growth factor (IGF) receptor gene reveals an essential role of IGF signaling in bone matrix mineralization. J Biol Chem 2002;277(46):44005–12.

[36] Spelsberg TC, Subramaniam M, Riggs BL, Khosla S. The actions and interactions of sex steroids and growth factors/cytokines on the skeleton. Mol Endocrinol 1999;13(6):819–28.

[37] Mohan S, Richman C, Guo R, Amaar Y, Donahue LR, Wergedal J, et al. Insulin-like growth factor regulates peak bone mineral density in mice by both growth hormone-dependent and -independent mechanisms. Endocrinology 2003;144(3): 929–36.

[38] Bikle D, Majumdar S, Laib A, Powell-Braxton L, Rosen C, Beamer W, et al. The skeletal structure of insulin-like growth factor I-deficient mice. J Bone Miner Res 2001;16(12):2320–9.

[39] DiGirolamo DJ, Mukherjee A, Fulzele K, Gan Y, Cao X, Frank SJ, et al. Mode of growth hormone action in osteoblasts. J Biol Chem 2007;282(43):31666–74.

[40] Pun KK, Lau P, Ho PW. The characterization, regulation, and function of insulin receptors on osteoblast-like clonal osteosarcoma cell line. J Bone Miner Res 1989;4(6):853–62.

[41] Kream BE, Smith MD, Canalis E, Raisz LG. Characterization of the effect of insulin on collagen synthesis in fetal rat bone. Endocrinology 1985;116(1):296–302.

[42] Hahn TJ, Westbrook SL, Sullivan TL, Goodman WG, Halstead LR. Glucose transport in osteoblast-enriched bone explants: characterization and insulin regulation. J Bone Miner Res 1988;3(3):359–65.

[43] Ituarte EA, Halstead LR, Iida-Klein A, Ituarte HG, Hahn TJ. Glucose transport system in UMR-106-01 osteoblastic osteosarcoma cells: regulation by insulin. Calc Tissue Int 1989;45(1):27–33.

[44] Kemink SA, Hermus AR, Swinkels LM, Lutterman JA, Smals AG. Osteopenia in insulin-dependent diabetes mellitus; prevalence and aspects of pathophysiology. J Endocrinol Invest 2000;23(5):295–303.

[45] Thrailkill KM. Insulin-like growth factor-I in diabetes mellitus: its physiology, metabolic effects, and potential clinical utility. Diabetes Technol Ther 2000;2(1):69–80.

[46] Janghorbani M, Feskanich D, Willett WC, Hu F. Prospective study of diabetes and risk of hip fracture: the nurses' health study. Diabetes Care 2006;29(7):1573–8.

[47] Nicodemus KK, Folsom AR. Type 1 and type 2 diabetes and incident hip fractures in postmenopausal women. Diabetes Care 2001;24(7):1192–7.

[48] Loder RT. The influence of diabetes mellitus on the healing of closed fractures. Clin Orthop Relat Res 1988;(232)::210–6.

[49] Gandhi A, Beam HA, O'Connor JP, Parsons JR, Lin SS. The effects of local insulin delivery on diabetic fracture healing. Bone 2005;37(4):482–90.

[50] Herrero S, Calvo OM, Garcia-Moreno C, Martin E, San Roman JI, Martin M, et al. Low bone density with normal bone turnover in ovariectomized and streptozotocin-induced diabetic rats. Calc Tissue Int 1998;62(3):260–5.

[51] Verhaeghe J, van Herck E, Visser WJ, Suiker AM, Thomasset M, Einhorn TA, et al. Bone and mineral metabolism in BB rats with long-term diabetes. Decreased bone turnover and osteoporosis. Diabetes 1990;39(4):477–82.

[52] Goodman WG, Hori MT. Diminished bone formation in experimental diabetes. Relationship to osteoid maturation and mineralization. Diabetes 1984;33(9):825–31.

[53] Shires R, Teitelbaum SL, Bergfeld MA, Fallon MD, Slatopolsky E, Avioli LV. The effect of streptozotocin-induced chronic diabetes mellitus on bone and mineral homeostasis in the rat. J Lab Clin Med 1981;97(2):231–40.

[54] Verhaeghe J, Suiker AM, Visser WJ, Van Herck E, Van Bree R, Bouillon R. The effects of systemic insulin, insulin-like growth factor-I and growth hormone on bone growth and turnover in spontaneously diabetic BB rats. J Endocrinol 1992;134(3): 485–92.

[55] Okamoto H, Nakae J, Kitamura T, Park BC, Dragatsis I, Accili D. Transgenic rescue of insulin receptor-deficient mice. J Clin Invest 2004;114(2):214–23.

[56] Irwin R, Lin HV, Motyl KJ, McCabe LR. Normal bone density obtained in the absence of insulin receptor expression in bone. Endocrinology 2006;147(12):5760–7.

[57] Zayzafoon M, Stell C, Irwin R, McCabe LR. Extracellular glucose influences osteoblast differentiation and c-Jun expression. J Cell Biochem 2000;79(2):301–10.

[58] Botolin S, McCabe LR. Chronic hyperglycemia modulates osteoblast gene expression through osmotic and non-osmotic pathways. J Cell Biochem 2006;99(2):411–24.

[59] Fulzele K, Riddle RC, DiGirolamo DJ, Cao X, Wan C, Chen D, et al. Insulin receptor signaling in osteoblasts regulates postnatal bone acquisition and body composition. Cell 2010;142(2): 309–19.

[60] Fulzele K, DiGirolamo DJ, Liu Z, Xu J, Messina JL, Clemens TL. Disruption of the insulin-like growth factor type 1 receptor in osteoblasts enhances insulin signaling and action. J Biol Chem 2007;282(35):25649–58.

[61] Bialek P, Kern B, Yang X, Schrock M, Sosic D, Hong N, et al. A twist code determines the onset of osteoblast differentiation. Devel Cell 2004;6(3):423–35.

[62] Ducy P, Amling M, Takeda S, Priemel M, Schilling AF, Beil FT, et al. Leptin inhibits bone formation through a hypothalamic relay: a central control of bone mass. Cell 2000;100(2):197–207.

[63] Ferron M, Wei J, Yoshizawa T, Del Fattore A, DePinho RA, Teti A, et al. Insulin signaling in osteoblasts integrates bone remodeling and energy metabolism. Cell 2010;142(2):296–308.

[64] Lee NK, Sowa H, Hinoi E, Ferron M, Ahn JD, Confavreux C, et al. Endocrine regulation of energy metabolism by the skeleton. Cell 2007;130(3):456–69.

[65] Egawa K, Maegawa H, Shimizu S, Morino K, Nishio Y, Bryer-Ash M, et al. Protein-tyrosine phosphatase-1B negatively regulates insulin signaling in l6 myocytes and Fao hepatoma cells. J Biol Chem 2001;276(13):10207–11.

[66] Venable CL, Frevert EU, Kim YB, Fischer BM, Kamatkar S, Neel BG, et al. Overexpression of protein-tyrosine phosphatase-1B in adipocytes inhibits insulin-stimulated phosphoinositide 3-kinase activity without altering glucose transport or Akt/Protein kinase B activation. J Biol Chem 2000;275(24):18318–26.

[67] Ducy P, Desbois C, Boyce B, Pinero G, Story B, Dunstan C, et al. Increased bone formation in osteocalcin-deficient mice. Nature 1996;382(6590):448–52.

[68] Hauschka PV, Lian JB, Cole DE, Gundberg CM. Osteocalcin and matrix Gla protein: vitamin K-dependent proteins in bone. Physiol Rev 1989;69(3):990–1047.

[69] Delmas PD, Wilson DM, Mann KG, Riggs BL. Effect of renal function on plasma levels of bone Gla-protein. J Clin Endocrinol Metab 1983;57(5):1028–30.

[70] Ferron M, McKee MD, Levine RL, Ducy P, Karsenty G. Intermittent injections of osteocalcin improve glucose metabolism and prevent type 2 diabetes in mice. Bone 2011.

[71] Ferron M, Hinoi E, Karsenty G, Ducy P. Osteocalcin differentially regulates beta cell and adipocyte gene expression and affects the development of metabolic diseases in wild-type mice. Proc Natl Acad Sci USA 2008;105(13):5266–70.

[72] Wellendorph P, Brauner-Osborne H. Molecular cloning, expression, and sequence analysis of GPRC6A, a novel family C G-protein-coupled receptor. Gene 2004;335:37–46.

[73] Pi M, Faber P, Ekema G, Jackson PD, Ting A, Wang N, et al. Identification of a novel extracellular cation-sensing G-protein-coupled receptor. J Biol Chem 2005;280(48):40201–9.

[74] Pi M, Zhang L, Lei SF, Huang MZ, Zhu W, Zhang J, et al. Impaired osteoblast function in GPRC6A null mice. J Bone Miner Res 2010;25(5):1092–102.

[75] Pi M, Chen L, Huang MZ, Zhu W, Ringhofer B, Luo J, et al. GPRC6A null mice exhibit osteopenia, feminization and metabolic syndrome. PloS One 2008;3(12):e3858.

[76] Pi M, Wu Y, Quarles LD. GPRC6A mediates responses to osteocalcin in beta-cells in vitro and pancreas in vivo. J Bone Miner Res 2011;26(7):1680–3.

[77] Oury F, Sumara G, Sumara O, Ferron M, Chang H, Smith CE, et al. Endocrine regulation of male fertility by the skeleton. Cell 2011;144(5):796–809.

[78] Ducy P, Zhang R, Geoffroy V, Ridall AL, Karsenty G. Osf2/Cbfa1: a transcriptional activator of osteoblast differentiation. Cell 1997;89(5):747–54.

[79] Ducy P, Starbuck M, Priemel M, Shen J, Pinero G, Geoffroy V, et al. A Cbfa1-dependent genetic pathway controls bone formation beyond embryonic development. Genes Dev 1999;13(8):1025–36.

[80] Kops GJ, de Ruiter ND, De Vries-Smits AM, Powell DR, Bos JL, Burgering BM. Direct control of the Forkhead transcription factor AFX by protein kinase B. Nature 1999;398(6728):630–4.

[81] Brunet A, Bonni A, Zigmond MJ, Lin MZ, Juo P, Hu LS, et al. Akt promotes cell survival by phosphorylating and inhibiting a Forkhead transcription factor. Cell 1999;96(6):857−68.

[82] Rached MT, Kode A, Xu L, Yoshikawa Y, Paik JH, Depinho RA, et al. FoxO1 is a positive regulator of bone formation by favoring protein synthesis and resistance to oxidative stress in osteoblasts. Cell Metab 2010;11(2):147−60.

[83] Rached MT, Kode A, Silva BC, Jung DY, Gray S, Ong H, et al. FoxO1 expression in osteoblasts regulates glucose homeostasis through regulation of osteocalcin in mice. J Clin Invest 2010;120(1):357−68.

[84] Yang X, Karsenty G. ATF4, the osteoblast accumulation of which is determined post-translationally, can induce osteoblast-specific gene expression in non-osteoblastic cells. J Biol Chem 2004;279(45):47109−14.

[85] Yang X, Matsuda K, Bialek P, Jacquot S, Masuoka HC, Schinke T, et al. ATF4 is a substrate of RSK2 and an essential regulator of osteoblast biology; implication for Coffin−Lowry syndrome. Cell 2004;117(3):387−98.

[86] Yoshizawa T, Hinoi E, Jung DY, Kajimura D, Ferron M, Seo J, et al. The transcription factor ATF4 regulates glucose metabolism in mice through its expression in osteoblasts. J Clin Invest 2009;119(9):2807−17.

[87] Inageda K. Insulin modulates induction of glucose-regulated protein 78 during endoplasmic reticulum stress via augmentation of ATF4 expression in human neuroblastoma cells. FEBS Lett 2010;584(16):3649−54.

[88] Adams CM. Role of the transcription factor ATF4 in the anabolic actions of insulin and the anti-anabolic actions of glucocorticoids. J Biol Chem 2007;282(23):16744−53.

[89] Cousin W, Courseaux A, Ladoux A, Dani C, Peraldi P. Cloning of hOST-PTP: the only example of a protein-tyrosine-phosphatase the function of which has been lost between rodent and human. Biochem Biophys Res Com 2004;321(1):259−65.

[90] Engelke JA, Hale JE, Suttie JW, Price PA. Vitamin K-dependent carboxylase: utilization of decarboxylated bone Gla protein and matrix Gla protein as substrates. Biochim Biophys Acta 1991;1078(1):31−4.

[91] Clowes JA, Allen HC, Prentis DM, Eastell R, Blumsohn A. Octreotide abolishes the acute decrease in bone turnover in response to oral glucose. J Clin Endocrinol Metab 2003;88(10):4867−73.

[92] Widdowson EM. Chemical composition of newly born mammals. Nature 1950;166(4224):626−8.

[93] Takahashi Y, Kadowaki H, Momomura K, Fukushima Y, Orban T, Okai T, et al. A homozygous kinase-defective mutation in the insulin receptor gene in a patient with leprechaunism. Diabetologia 1997;40(4):412−20.

[94] Kindblom JM, Ohlsson C, Ljunggren O, Karlsson MK, Tivesten A, Smith U, et al. Plasma osteocalcin is inversely related to fat mass and plasma glucose in elderly Swedish men. J Bone Miner Res 2009;24(5):785−91.

[95] Yeap BB, Chubb SA, Flicker L, McCaul KA, Ebeling PR, Beilby JP, et al. Reduced serum total osteocalcin is associated with metabolic syndrome in older men via waist circumference, hyperglycemia, and triglyceride levels. Eur J Endocrinol 2010;163(2):265−72.

[96] Hwang YC, Jeong IK, Ahn KJ, Chung HY. The uncarboxylated form of osteocalcin is associated with improved glucose tolerance and enhanced beta-cell function in middle-aged male subjects. Diabetes Metab Res Rev 2009;25(8):768−72.

[97] Reinehr T, Roth CL. A new link between skeleton, obesity and insulin resistance: relationships between osteocalcin, leptin and insulin resistance in obese children before and after weight loss. Int J Obes (Lond) 2010;34(5):852−8.

[98] Basu R, Peterson J, Rizza R, Khosla S. Effects of physiological variations in circulating insulin levels on bone turnover in humans. J Clin Endocrinol Metab 2011;96(5):1450−5.

[99] Yoshikawa Y, Kode A, Xu L, Mosialou I, Silva BC, Ferron M, et al. Genetic evidence points to an osteocalcin-independent influence of osteoblasts on energy metabolism. J Bone Miner Res 2011;26(9):2012−25.

Transcriptional Regulation of the Endocrine Function of Bone

Stavroula Kousteni, PhD

Columbia University, New York, NY, USA

INTRODUCTION

During the last few years, the skeleton has been identified as a dynamic, interactive organ which receives and transmits regulatory signals from and to other tissues. These observations have expanded the homeostatic role of the skeleton beyond the regulation of bone growth and remodeling to at least two novel endocrine functions: as an important regulator of energy metabolism as well as male fertility. In its first endocrine function, the skeleton regulates energy metabolism by favoring β-cell proliferation, insulin secretion, insulin sensitivity, and energy expenditure [1–3]. In addition, it is a target of insulin signaling. Osteoblasts are the cells orchestrating these responses through the secretion of osteocalcin. In its under- or uncarboxylated form, osteocalcin acts as a hormone to promote hyperinsulinemia and improve insulin sensitivity, a combination that results in improved glucose tolerance and glucose metabolism. Several clinical studies have now come forward supporting the notion that osteocalcin is a marker of glucose tolerance [1,3–7]. In a tight regulatory mechanism, the skeleton signals not only to the pancreas and affects insulin signaling in other insulin-target tissues but insulin signaling is also operating in osteoblasts to regulate bone remodeling and, in turn, osteocalcin activity and its own, insulin, production by the pancreas [2]. Insulin acts on osteoblasts through the insulin receptor to suppress the activity of protein tyrosine phosphatase (OST-PTP), the product of *Esp*, the expression of which had been associated with decreased osteocalcin activity due to favoring of its carboxylation [1]. Reduced *Esp* expression, in turn, suppresses expression of the anti-osteoclastogenic cytokine osteoprotegerin and promotes bone resorption. The acidity of the resorptive environment decarboxylates osteocalcin to unleash its stimulatory effect on insulin production and glucose metabolism. In addition to its energy homeostatic properties, undercarboxylated osteocalcin favors male fertility by promoting testosterone synthesis and thus germ cell survival [8].

Like every endocrine organ, the skeleton not only regulates the function of other tissues. In a reciprocal and tightly controlled mechanism, bone endocrinology is also under the control of other organs. Such interactions serve either to maintain bone homeostasis and regulate bone mass accrual or to control and balance the endocrine functions of the skeleton in energy metabolism and male reproduction. Leptin is the first example of a hormone demonstrating the regulation of both the remodeling and endocrine functions of the skeleton by the fat–brain axis. Leptin inhibits the endocrine function of the skeleton in a three-step cascade that involves upregulation of sympathetic tone, sympathetic tone-mediated decrease in osteocalcin bioactivity resulting in decreased insulin expression, and secretion [9].

The role of leptin as a potent regulator of bone mass accrual through the sympathetic nervous system (SNS) was the first demonstration for central control of bone mass [10–14]. Leptin suppresses bone mass by enhancing sympathetic tone. Following these initial observations several studies support the central action of leptin on bone mass [15–19]. Subsequently, the mechanism of action of leptin signaling in the SNS brought to light another regulator of bone mass, serotonin. In a demonstration of an opposing and perhaps balancing regulation of bone mass accrual the brain and the gut exert opposite effects on the skeleton. Remarkably, the mediator of these effects is in both cases the same protein, serotonin. Brain-derived serotonin suppresses the SNS to promote bone mass accrual [20]. In addition, it is the target of leptin

Translational Endocrinology of Bone
DOI: http://dx.doi.org/10.1016/B978-0-12-415784-2.00009-9

which acts on the brain stem to control the synthesis of serotonin [20]. In contrast, serotonin produced by the enterochromaffin cells of the duodenum suppresses bone formation through direct actions on the osteoblasts and is a major regulator of bone formation in rodents and humans [21–24]. Serotonin does not cross the blood–brain barrier; hence, the two pools of serotonin may act independently of each other.

The intercommunication between the skeleton and its regulating or regulatory organs is corroborated by intricate transcriptional machinery that confers the specificity of the signals. The main mediators of this network are two transcription factors of the same family, CREB and ATF4, and a transcription factor with a well-established role in the regulation of energy metabolism in all glucose-regulating organs, FoxO1. More recently, another bone anabolic transcription factor, ΔFosB, has been implicated in the endocrine function of the skeleton.

FOXO1, A TRANSCRIPTIONAL MODULATOR OF THE ENDOCRINE FUNCTION OF THE SKELETON

FoxO1 is both a main transcriptional mediator of insulin signaling in glucose-regulating organs and a modulator of insulin production by the pancreas [25–30]. These properties establish a diverse role of FoxO1 in the control of metabolic homeostasis by affecting at least three important aspects of glucose metabolism: insulin production, insulin sensitivity, and hepatic glucose production [26,28,31,32]. Lately, FoxO1 has also been identified as an important transcriptional mediator of the endocrine function of the skeleton.

Studies in mice lacking *FoxO1* in osteoblasts have indicated a relationship between FoxO1 in the osteoblast and FoxO1 actions in the classical glucose-regulating organs. These mice show reduced blood glucose levels in both the fasting and the fed state and better disposal of glucose load and a marked improvement in glucose tolerance [33]. The cause of the hypoglycemia is two-fold: an increase in insulin production as well as an increase in insulin sensitivity. The increase in plasma insulin levels results from increased β-cell proliferation, higher islet cell numbers, greater islet size, and total β-cell mass in mice with osteoblast-specific deletion of *FoxO1*. Hyperinsulinemia was consistent with suppression of gluconeogenesis, a process inhibited by insulin in the liver, and was independent of any contributions from counter-regulatory hormones with anti-insulinemic activity such as glucagon or growth hormone. It was also independent of any potential actions of FoxO1 in the hypothalamus where it has been shown to regulate food intake and peripheral metabolism by

interacting with leptin signaling [34,35]. Despite hyperinsulinemia and improved insulin sensitivity, osteoblast-specific deletion of FoxO1 resulted in reduced gonadal fat pad weight [33]. Explaining, at least in part, the low gonadal fat weight, both energy expenditure and activity levels were increased whereas energy intake was not affected.

Another key feature of the phenotype of mice with osteoblast-specific inactivation of *FoxO1* is an increase in mitochondrial activity in muscle [27]. These animals demonstrate increased ATP/ADP ratio due to an increase in the ATP production concomitantly with a decrease in the levels of AMP. Further, expression of biomarkers in the oxidative phosphorylation metabolic pathway, which uses energy released by the oxidation of nutrients to produce ATP was also increased. Uncoupling protein 3 (*Ucp3*), muscle carnitine palmitoyl transferase I (*Cpt1b*), and pyruvate dehydrogenase kinase 4 (*Pdk4*) were all upregulated in the muscle of mutant mice. Similarly, there was upregulation of the mitochondrial respiratory chain proteins mitochondrial DNA-encoded (mtDNA-encoded) subunits: subunit 6 of NADH dehydrogenase (ND6, complex I) and subunit I of cytochrome *c* oxidase (COXI, complex IV). Thus, FoxO1, through its expression in osteoblasts, inhibits insulin sensitivity in muscle.

The observations linking FoxO1 and osteocalcin to energy metabolism raised the possibility that FoxO1 may be a transcriptional modulator of the activity or expression of osteocalcin. A comparison of the metabolic phenotypes of mice lacking *FoxO1* in osteoblasts with the metabolic phenotypes of gain- and loss-of-function mouse models of osteocalcin activity [1] suggested a functional relationship between FoxO1 and osteocalcin. Indeed, whereas the metabolic phenotype of mice lacking *FoxO1* in osteoblasts was identical to that of mice lacking *Esp*, and showing increased osteocalcin activity, it mirrored the phenotype of mice lacking *osteocalcin*. In agreement with these observations, *Esp* expression in bone was decreased and osteocalcin activity, measured by the percentage of its uncarboxylated and undercarboxylated form in the serum, was increased in mice lacking *FoxO1* in osteoblasts. A link between FoxO1 expression in osteoblasts and osteocalcin activity was demonstrated in heterozygous mice lacking one allele of *FoxO1* and one allele of *Esp*. These compound mutant mice had improved insulin sensitivity and glucose tolerance [33]. Likewise, removal of one allele of *osteocalcin* from mice lacking *FoxO1* from osteoblasts corrected the metabolic phenotype of improved glucose tolerance and insulin sensitivity that results from osteoblast-specific inactivation of *FoxO1*.

In terms of molecular interactions, FoxO1 suppresses osteocalcin activity by its ability to stimulate the expression of *Esp*. FoxO1 directly binds one of two FoxO1 binding sites, present at the −1098 site of the *Esp* first intron to stimulate its expression [33]. In addition to regulating osteocalcin activity through *Esp*, FoxO1 also suppresses *osteocalcin* expression, although to a lesser magnitude than regulation of *Esp* expression. The mechanism of this inhibitory effect on *osteocalcin* expression is presently unclear. Although FoxO1 binds to FoxO1-binding sites present in the promoter and first intron of the osteocalcin gene, suppressive effects of FoxO1 on transcription are in general not mediated by binding to consensus FoxO1 binding sites. Most frequently, those involve protein–protein interactions with other transcription factors, such as CREB, and inhibition of the activity of the FoxO1 transcriptional partner.

A broad spectrum of transcriptional alterations ensue the deletion of *FoxO1* in osteoblast. This is to be expected since through its expression in osteoblasts this transcription factor controls glucose levels and insulin production, b-cell proliferation, insulin sensitivity, and energy expenditure. Thus, consistent with higher insulin levels and greater insulin sensitivity, the expression of several insulin target genes in muscle, liver, and white adipose tissue is altered in mice lacking FoxO1 in osteoblasts. In the muscle, expression of *Ppargc1α* and its two target genes, *Nrf1* and *Mcad*, is increased in the muscle of *Foxo1ob−/−* mice as compared with WT animals. In the liver, expression of *Foxa2*, which regulates lipogenesis and ketogenesis during fasting, is increased whereas expression of *G6Pase* and *Pck1* is decreased, likely indicating that FoxO1, through its expression in osteoblasts, inhibits insulin sensitivity in the liver. In white adipose tissue, expression of the adipogenic gene *Cebpa* and two lipolytic genes, perilipin and triglyceride lipase (*Tgl*), whose expression is inhibited by insulin, was decreased in mice lacking FoxO1 in osteoblasts. Finally, expression and serum levels of the insulin-sensitizing hormone adiponectin [28] and its targets acyl-CoA oxidase, *Ppara*, and *Ucp2* are increased in these mice.

Thus, FoxO1 through its expression in osteoblasts controls glucose metabolism and energy expenditure, at least in part by regulating the activity of osteocalcin. These functions of FoxO1 result in indirect, perhaps insulin mediated, alteration in the transcriptional programs that control mitochondrial activity and insulin sensitivity in all insulin target tissues.

ATF4 IN SKELETAL REGULATION OF ENERGY HOMEOSTASIS

The transcriptional control of osteoblast differentiation and function involves many players, some broadly expressed and others with a more restricted expression. Thus, it is to be expected that in addition to the ubiquitously expressed FoxO1, cell-specific regulatory genes are involved in the process by which osteoblasts control energy metabolism. Activating transcription factor 4 (ATF4) is a transcription factor that accumulates predominantly in osteoblasts, where it regulates multiple functions linked to the maintenance of bone mass. Two observations in mice and humans prompted studies that led to its identification as a glucose-regulating factor. Mice lacking *Atf4* (*Atf4−/−* mice) have lower fat mass. Conversely, humans lacking the eukaryotic translation initiation factor 2 kinase (*EIF2AK3*), which enhances ATF4 translation during amino acid starvation or ER stress, are glucose intolerant and phosphorylation of eukaryotic translation initiation factor 2α (eIF2α) regulates glucose homeostasis [36–40].

Analysis of *Atf4−/−* mice showed a decrease in blood glucose levels that is secondary to an increase in circulating insulin levels, which resulted from an increase in insulin secretion suggesting that ATF4 inhibits insulin secretion [41]. Studies in the same mice also indicated that ATF4 suppresses insulin sensitivity in liver, fat, and muscle. The suppression of insulin sensitivity in the liver was demonstrated by the fact that gluconeogenesis was impaired and expression of phosphoenolpyruvate carboxykinase (*Pck1*) and glucose-6-phosphatase (*G6pase*), the two insulin target genes in the liver that are implicated in the process of gluconeogenesis was reduced in the absence of *Atf4*. Glycolysis was stimulated in the absence of *Atf4* as evidenced by altered expression of two key insulin targets in the liver, glucokinase (*Gck*) and pyruvate dehydrogenase kinase 4 (*Pdk4*). Furthermore, the expression of the transcription factor *Foxa2*, which regulates insulin sensitivity, was also increased in the liver of *Atf4−/−* mice. In the muscle, expression of medium-chain acyl-CoA dehydrogenase (*Mcad*), a maker of insulin sensitivity and phosphorylation of the insulin-activated kinase Akt, were both increased in *Atf4*-deficient mice. In white adipose tissue expression of *Pparγ*, a marker of insulin sensitivity in fat cells was also increased by *Atf4* deficiency indicating that *Atf4* deletion in all cells *in vivo* enhances insulin sensitivity also in the muscle and fat.

Several lines of evidence indicated that the energy-regulating properties of ATF4 occur through its expression in osteoblasts. First, insulin sensitivity is enhanced in the liver of *Atf4−/−* mice, but not in cultured hepatocytes from these mice. Second, mice overexpressing *Atf4* specifically in osteoblasts demonstrated a decrease in insulin secretion and were insulin insensitive. All the molecular markers of insulin sensitivity were altered in a manner mirroring that observed in the *Atf4−/−* mice. Third, overexpression of the *Atf4* transgene in osteoblasts corrected the metabolic phenotype of *Atf4*-deficient mice. Fourth, and more important, mice lacking ATF4 only in osteoblasts presented the same metabolic abnormalities as *Atf4*−/− mice. At the molecular level, ATF4 exerts its effects by directly binding to the promoter of Esp and favoring *Esp* expression in osteoblasts and thus decreasing the bioactivity of osteocalcin. This mode of molecular interaction was demonstrated *in vivo* genetically by showing that the metabolic phenotype of compound heterozygous mice lacking one allele of *Atf4* and one allele of *Esp* is identical to the phenotype of *Atf4*- or *Esp*-deficient mice.

Thus, ATF4 acts through osteoblasts to suppress insulin secretion and insulin sensitivity in the liver, fat, and muscle, and as a result to increase blood glucose levels. The parallel functions of FoxO1 and ATF4 pose the question of whether these two transcription factors, one ubiquitously expressed and the second one osteoblast-enriched, synergize to control aspects of energy metabolism through their expression in osteoblasts.

ΔFOSB RECIPROCALLY AFFECTS BONE MASS AND FAT ACCRUAL AND FAVORS INSULIN SENSITIVITY

ΔFosB is an activator protein (AP)-1 transcription factor that has been on the interface between bone mass accrual and fat metabolism. It is a naturally occurring alternatively spliced variant of FosB that lacks the 101 amino acids that encode the C-terminal transactivation domain of FosB due to the generation of a premature stop codon [42]. The less active ΔFosB competes with FosB for binding and consequently acts as an antagonist to FosB in most situations, although it retains some AP-1 transactivating potential [42–44]. Studies in mice overexpressing ΔFosB under the control of the enolase 2 promoter, which drives expression in bone, fat, and regions of the brain, exhibit both an increase in bone formation and a decrease in adipose mass [45]. The same mice demonstrated increases in fatty-acid oxidation and energy expenditure as well as increased insulin sensitivity and glucose tolerance [46]. These effects, however, were independent of expression of ΔFosB in either the osteoblasts or the adipocytes since targeted overexpression in either of these two cell types failed to induce changes in fat or in bone. Thus, the beneficial effect of ΔFosB on metabolic activity is not due to cell-autonomous effects of ΔFosB within adipocytes or osteoblasts.

CREB VERSUS ATF4 IN CENTRAL CONTROL OF BONE MASS: LEPTIN

A variety of locally produced as well as systemic growth factors and hormones are involved in the regulation of skeletal homeostasis; and, although the mechanism of action is not completely understood for all of them, it has been studied for several years. The novelty in the view of the skeleton as an endocrine organ is that it not only affects whole body endocrine functions but it is also regulated by extraskeletal signals. Fifteen years ago, this area of skeletal physiology was initiated by the finding that bone mass accrual can be controlled by the central nervous system (CNS). Interestingly, leptin, an adipokine charged with the role of suppressing appetite, was also found to be a potent inhibitor of bone mass accrual [5,9,22,25,26]. Indeed, studies in mice or humans lacking either leptin or its receptor show that they develop a high bone mass phenotype even though they are hypogonadic, a condition that tends to greatly increase bone resorption. Leptin delivers a double compromising signal to bone mass by concomitantly suppressing bone formation and increasing bone resorption. Both effects, on both bone accrual compartments, are mediated though centrally derived signals on osteoblasts. The mechanisms and the transcriptional functions that mediate the signal of leptin from the CNS to the bone cells have been deciphered and have brought into the limelight two transcription factors, one ubiquitously expressed and with multiple physiological functions, CREB, and one osteoblast enriched, ATF4.

cAMP response element binding (CREB) protein is a broadly expressed leucine zipper-containing transcription factor affecting differentiation and proliferation of multiple cell types. Although it acts in many different cellular contexts, CREB is a major regulator of multiple aspects of neurobiology, such as neuron survival, axon growth, and synaptic transmission [47,48]. These neurobiological functions of CREB agree well with what was found to be its ability to mediate some of the bone suppressing functions of leptin through the CNS. But how is it that CREB is brought into the roadmap of leptin central functions. There are two known pathways linking leptin signaling in the brain to the osteoblasts, the ultimate target cell of leptin. In the first pathway, leptin activates the sympathetic nervous system (SNS) which, in turn, signals through the β2-adrenergic receptor (Adrβ2) present in osteoblasts [11,13]. Relevant to that, β-blockers antagonizing Adrβ2 can cure osteoporosis in mice, rats, and humans [11,49]. In osteoblasts, sympathetic tone recruits several transcriptional regulators including components of the molecular clock, cMyc and CREB, to inhibit cell proliferation [12,50–54]. Via these actions leptin suppresses bone formation. In parallel, leptin-activated sympathetic tone also acts on osteoblasts to increase the expression of *RankL*, the most powerful osteoclastogenic cytokine; and thus favors bone resorption [13,55–57]. This sympathetic function is mediated by activation of protein kinase A (PKA) and subsequent phosphorylation (by PKA) and increase in the transactivation function of ATF4, the cell-specific CREB-related transcription factor essential for osteoblast differentiation and function [13]. As a result, ATF4 is recruited and directly binds to a CRE binding site in the promoter of *Rankl*, thus upregulating the expression of this osteoclastogenic factor. However, sympathetic regulation of *Rankl* expression by ATF4 is independent of its phosphorylation by RSK2, another kinase known to regulate ATF4 functions on osteoblast differentiation [58].

The second pathway by which leptin regulates bone mass accrual also affects bone resorption. However, through it leptin inhibits bone resorption. The mediator of this inhibitory action is the cocaine amphetamine regulated transcript (CART), a neuropeptide that is found in the brain and the general circulation [13]. CART expression in brain is increased by leptin, directly or indirectly; it is low in *ob/ob* mice and normal in *Adrb2−/−* mice [10]. *Cart−/−* mice have no overt phenotypic abnormalities but show a low bone mass phenotype which is solely attributed to increases in osteoclast formation and function [59]. CART is not expressed in osteoblasts or osteoclasts, *Cart−/−* bone cells show no cell-autonomous defects, and exogenous CART administration does not affect osteoclast formation. Yet, *Rankl* expression is increased in *Cart−/−* bones, suggesting that CART exerts its function by modulating *Rankl* signaling through the SNS. Thus, leptin controls bone resorption through, at least, two distinct and antagonistic pathways. On the one hand, sympathetic signaling via Adrb2 promotes osteoclast differentiation; on the other hand, CART inhibits it. Although both pathways regulate *Rankl* expression, the transcriptional mechanisms by which CART regulates bone resorption remain unknown in absence of a specific CART receptor.

CREB IN CENTRAL VERSUS LOCAL CONTROL OF BONE FORMATION: SEROTONIN

Central Actions

The role of CREB as a major transcriptional mediator of the effects of SNS on bone mass accrual was established with the identification of a second protein that has the ability to control bone remodeling through its actions in the brain, serotonin. Adding a level of complexity to its skeletal actions, CREB also confers a completely opposite effect on bone mass by its ability to also mediate the bone suppressing action of serotonin, when this is produced outside the brain and acts directly on osteoblasts.

Serotonin is a neuromediator made by brain stem neurons and is also a hormone synthesized by the enterochromaffin cells of the duodenum [60−62]. Remarkably, serotonin does not cross the blood−brain barrier; hence, the two pools of serotonin may act independently of each other [20,21]. Thus, serotonin is a rare example of a single molecule that exerts totally opposite effects on the same physiological function, depending on its site of synthesis. Consistent with the existence of two independent pools of serotonin, it exerts opposite influence on bone mass accrual depending on its site of synthesis. In the brain, it suppresses sympathetic tone activity and promotes osteoblast proliferation [20]. In contrast, serotonin produced by the gut is released in the circulation and acts as a hormone inhibiting osteoblast proliferation [21]. That each pool of serotonin affects bone mass through CREB also identified serotonin as a major transcriptional regulator of bone remodeling.

Brain serotonin signals through its Htr2c receptors expressed in the VMH nuclei to decrease sympathetic activity and to favor bone mass accrual by regulating both the bone forming and the osteoclast activating functions of osteoblasts [20]. This was demonstrated by two lines of experiments. First, VMH-specific gene inactivation of Htr2c receptors resulted in a severe low bone mass caused by a decrease in bone formation and an increase in bone resorption associated with increased sympathetic activity [20]. Second, compound mutant mice lacking one allele of *Tph2*, the enzyme responsible for serotonin synthesis in the brain stem, and one allele of *Htr2c* (*Tph2+/−;Htr2c+/−* mice) demonstrated the same low bone mass and high sympathetic activity phenotype as *Htr2c−/−* and *Tph2−/−* mice. In-depth molecular studies showed that in both hypothalamic nuclei serotonin fulfills its function through CamK-dependent activation of CREB and also through upregulation of *Creb* expression [21].

Htr2c is a G protein-coupled receptor using Ca^{2+} as a second messenger in a signal transduction pathway that also involves calcium-binding protein CaM [63,64]. CaM exerts its diverse functions by activation of the CaM kinases CaMKI, CaMKII, and CaMKIV [65−67]. CaMKI and CaMKIV become fully active only when phosphorylated by other kinases called CaMK kinases (CaMKKs), of which two are known: CaMKKα and CaMKKβ [68−72]. CaMKII, in contrast, is not phosphorylated by CaMKKβ [73]. Studies in neuronal cell lines showed that serotonin stimulates specifically phosphorylation of CaMKIV and, downstream of it, CREB on Ser 133. In addition, it increases the expression of *CaMKKβ*, *CaMKIV*, and *Creb* but not of *CaMKIIa* and *CaMKIIb*. Confirming these observations, serotonin induced phosphorylation of CaMKIV—and, subsequently, of CREB—in wild-type hypothalamic explants but not in explants obtained from mice lacking the *Htr2c* receptor in VMH neurons (*Htr2c−/−* mice).

Subsequent to these signaling events a series of genetic studies showed that the CaMK/CREB signaling module mediates the beneficial effects of brain-derived serotonin on bone mass accrual. First, inactivation of *CaMKKβ* or *CaMKIV* in *Sf1*-expressing neurons of the VMH nuclei resulted in a severe low bone mass phenotype that presented in both the vertebrae and long bones, and trabecular and cortical bones, and was due to a concomitant decrease in bone formation parameters and an increase in osteoclast number. The increase in osteoclast numbers translated into an increase in bone resorption, as measured by the increase in serum levels of CTx, a biomarker of bone resorption. Second, mutant mice lacking one allele of *Htr2c* and one allele of either *CaMKKβ* or *CaMKIV* (*Htr2c+/−; CaMKKβ$_{Sf1}$+/−* and *Htr2c+/−; CaMKIV$_{Sf1}$+/−* mice) in *Sf1*-expressing neurons demonstrated the same low bone mass phenotype that was observed in *Htr2c−/−, CaMKKβ$_{Sf1}$−/−,* or *CaMKIV$_{Sf1}$−/−* mice. These experiments provide genetic evidence that *CaMKKβ* and *CaMKIV* act downstream from serotonin signaling through *Htr2c* in *Sf1*-expressing neurons of the VMH nuclei to favor bone mass accrual. Finally, that CREB is a transcriptional mediator of serotonin regulation of bone mass accrual in VMH neurons was shown by deletion of *Creb* in VMH neurons (*Creb$_{Sf1}$−/−* mice). *Creb$_{Sf1}$−/−* mice demonstrated a marked decrease in bone mass, affecting vertebrae and long bones, and trabecular and cortical bones. This was due to a decrease in bone formation and an increase in bone resorption, as seen in mice lacking serotonin signaling or CaMKIV in VMH neurons. The similarities in the bone mass phenotypes of these various mouse mutant strains suggested that *Creb* lies downstream from the CaMK-dependent serotonin signaling in VMH neurons. This was indeed established in compound heterozygous mice lacking one allele of *Creb* in *Sf1*-expressing neurons of the VMH nuclei, and either one allele of *Htr2c* or one allele of *CaMKIV* in the same neurons. *Htr2c+/−; CrebSf1+/−* and *CaMKIVSf1+/−; CrebSf1+/−* mice had a low bone mass phenotype similar to the one seen in *Htr2c−/−* and *CaMKIVSf1−/−* mice and that was due to a decrease in bone formation along with a concomitant increase in bone resorption.

The genetic evidence demonstrated that brain-derived serotonin mediates its regulation of bone mass accrual through the activation of the transcription factor CREB in VMH neurons of the hypothalamus. Molecular biology experiments followed to identify the transcriptional targets and pathways that are controlled by *Creb* expression in VMH neurons and account for the function of serotonin. Microarray analyses in combination with observations in mice deficient in brain serotonin synthesis (*Tph2−/−*) or lacking the *Htr2c* serotonin receptor in the brain suggested that *Creb* suppresses the expression of tyrosine hydroxylase (*Th*), a rate-limiting enzyme of catecholamine synthesis, and butyrylcholinesterase (*Bche*), an enzyme inactivating acetylcholine, the main neurotransmitter of the parasympathetic nervous system [74,75] in VMH neurons [20]. This pattern of changes in gene expression is consistent with the fact that brain-derived serotonin favors bone mass accrual by decreasing the sympathetic tone; and reveal that serotonin regulates, in a Creb-dependent manner, catecholamine synthesis in VMH neurons to affect bone mass.

That brain serotonin controls bone mass by regulating sympathetic tone was established. That the transcriptional activity of CREB in VMH neurons is regulated by serotonin signaling was also established. What remained to be proven was that the sympathetic nervous system acts downstream from CREB in the VMH nuclei to regulate bone mass. This formal proof was obtained by studies in compound mutant mice lacking *Creb* in *Sf1*-expressing neurons of the VMH nuclei and one allele of *Adrβ2*, the adrenergic receptor used by the sympathetic nervous system to regulate bone mass [11]. Analysis of these animals showed that bone mass, bone formation, and bone resorption were indistinguishable from those of wild-type littermates thus suggesting that removal of the SNS signal in osteoblasts corrects the low bone mass phenotype of *Creb* inactivation in *Sf1*-expressing neurons.

Thus, CREB is a major transcriptional target of brain serotonin in VMH neurons and a transcriptional modulator of genes suppressing sympathetic tone to favor bone mass accrual.

Peripheral Actions

In contrast to the beneficial effects of brain serotonin, gut-derived serotonin decreases bone mass by hampering osteoblast proliferation [21]. The suppressing function of gut-derived serotonin in osteoblast proliferation is central to bone homeostasis because it directly applies to human diseases. Indeed, gut-derived serotonin is a mediator of Lrp5, a potent regulator of bone mass that controls bone formation by promoting osteoblast proliferation [83]. More important, alterations in the levels of serotonin produced by the enterochromaffin cells of the duodenum have been shown to account for the low bone formation phenotype of Lrp5 deficiency or the high bone mass phenotype of Lrp5 gain-of-function mutations not only in mice but also in humans. Circulating serotonin levels are inversely associated with body and spine aBMD, with femur neck total and trabecular vBMD as well as with bone volume, trabecular numbers, and trabecular thickness in women

[23]. In addition, and more to the point linking Lrp5 to suppression of serotonin suppression, serotonin levels decrease in patients with the high bone mass Lrp5 mutation [24]. That gain-of-function mutations in Lrp5 cause high bone mass [84–86] by increasing bone formation led to the hypothesis that inhibiting gut-derived serotonin synthesis may become a treatment for low bone mass diseases such as osteoporosis [22]. Thus, identification of the transcription factors that mediate gut-derived serotonin functions on osteoblasts has a direct therapeutic potential.

Remarkably, whereas brain-derived serotonin promotes bone mass by stimulating CREB phosphorylation in VMH neurons, gut-derived serotonin does exactly the opposite: it decreases bone mass by inhibiting phosphorylation and expression of CREB in osteoblasts. Cell-specific inactivation in mice of each of the three serotonin receptors expressed in osteoblasts identified Htr1b as the receptor transducing the inhibitory effect of gut-derived serotonin on osteoblast proliferation. This was performed by either global or osteoblast-specific deletion of Htr1b which in both mouse models resulted in a high bone mass phenotype, mirroring the cell and molecular changes caused by serotonin deficiency [21].

Htr1b is coupled to G(i)-type G proteins which can inhibit adenyl cyclase activity and thus suppress cAMP levels and PKA activity and also regulate Ca^{2+}/calmodulin-dependent kinase signaling [76]. Consistent with these actions of Htr1b in other cells, binding of serotonin to this receptor inhibits cAMP production and PKA-dependent phosphorylation of CREB at Ser133 in osteoblasts [21]. Serotonin-induced CREB inactivation abolishes binding of CREB to the promoter of CycD1, a known target of CREB [12]. In addition to suppressing CREB activity, serotonin appears to be decreasing Creb expression in vivo as determined by observations showing that Creb expression is decreased in the bones of mice lacking Lrp5, but increased in mice bearing the Lrp5 high bone mass mutation [21].

A series of genetic studies in simple and compound mutant mice were once more used to examine whether CREB is indeed the transcriptional mediator of serotonin signaling in osteoblasts. First, the requirement for CREB in osteoblast proliferation was established by osteoblast-specific inactivation of Creb which resulted in low bone mass due to low bone formation. This phenotype was caused by a decrease in osteoblast proliferation due to decreased expression of Cyclins D1, D2, and E1. Subsequently, removal of one allele of Creb only from osteoblasts of mice lacking one allele of Lrp5 reproduced the low bone formation/low bone mass phenotype observed in the Lrp5−/− mice that are characterized by increased levels of circulating serotonin. That Creb activity and expression is compromised in response to gut-derived serotonin was further established by demonstrating that removal of one allele of Creb, in an osteoblast-specific manner, from Htr1b−/− mice rescued the increase in bone formation and the high bone mass of these mutant mice.

These observations therefore indicate that osteoblasts are direct targets of gut-derived serotonin and that CREB is a major transcriptional mediator of serotonin signaling in osteoblasts.

CREB IN BONE REGULATION OF MALE REPRODUCTION

The role of the skeleton as an endocrine organ appears to be expanding beyond its energy homeostatic properties. Indeed, the spectrum of skeletal endocrine function has broadened to include the regulation of male fertility. Similar to the regulation of energy metabolism, osteoblasts induce testosterone production by the testes, but do not influence estrogen or testosterone production by the ovaries [8]. Analysis of cell-specific loss- (Ocn−/−) and gain-of-function (Esp−/−) models of osteocalcin activity revealed that the osteoblast-derived hormone osteocalcin, in its undercarboxylated form, performs this endocrine function by inducing testosterone synthesis and thus promoting germ cell survival. That it is specifically and only through its expression in osteoblasts that undercarboxylated osteocalcin promotes male fertility was demonstrated by the fact that inactivation of Esp, the gene suppressing osteocalcin activity by promoting its carboxylation, in Sertoli cells did not affect testis biology and male fertility. The relevance of this novel bone–testis axis identified in mice to human physiology was demonstrated in growing males [77]. In boys, at 4 to 20 years of age, serum testosterone correlated with total and undercarboxylated osteocalcin, suggesting that in human males this axis may be involved during rapid skeletal growth. In fact, during this phase, osteocalcin may further stimulate testicular testosterone production, which, in turn, contributes to an increase in bone size. The receptor mediating the reproductive action of osteocalcin was found to be a G protein-coupled receptor expressed in the Leydig cells of the testes, GPRc6A, but not in the ovaries [8].

The identification of GPRc6A as an osteocalcin receptor along with the fact that osteocalcin treatment of Leydig cells increased cAMP production suggested that CREB is the transcriptional effector of osteocalcin regulation of testosterone biosynthesis. Demonstrating the validity of this hypothesis in vivo, undercarboxylated osteocalcin favors CREB phosphorylation in Leydig cells. Furthermore, mice lacking Creb specifically in Leydig cells ($Creb_{Leydig}−/−$) showed a reduction in testis size and weight, in epididymides and seminal vesicle weight, in sperm count, and in circulating testosterone levels similar to those seen in mice lacking *Osteocalcin* or *Gprc6a* in Leydig cells. Establishing that CREB acts downstream of Gprc6a in Leydig cells to regulate male fertility, compound mutant mice lacking one copy of *Creb* and one copy of *Gprc6a* in Leydig cells demonstrated decreased fertility to an extent similar to that observed in $Creb_{Leydig}-/-$ or $Gprc6a_{Leydig}-/-$ male mice.

At the molecular level CREB mediates the effects of osteocalcin on male fertility by upregulating the expression of enzymes that are required for testosterone synthesis such as StAR, Cyp11a, Cyp17, and 3-β-hydroxysteroid dehydrogenase (3β-HSD). These transcriptional actions of CREB are due to its ability to bind to the promoter regions of *Cyp11a*, *3β-HSD*, and *StAR* [8,78]. On the other hand, testosterone aromatization is not affected as expression of Cyp19, the gene encoding the testosterone aromatase, or of HSD-17 is not altered in the loss- or gain-of-function models of osteocalcin or *Creb* activity. The osteocalcin-triggered increase in testosterone synthesis promotes germ cell survival by increasing expression of gonadotropin regulated testicular helicase (*Grth*), an essential regulator of spermatogenesis that inhibits germ cell apoptosis and the expression of which in germ cells and Leydig cells is regulated by testosterone [79–81]. GRTH, in turn, inhibits activation of the pro-apoptotic caspase 3, and favors expression of tACE, a protein favoring germ cell maturation [82]. Expression of *Grth* is also under the control of Creb in response to osteocalcin since it is decreased in mice with *Creb* inactivation in Leydig cells.

These observations identify CREB as a transcriptional mediator of osteocalcin regulation of testosterone biosynthesis in Leydig cells.

PERSPECTIVE

Ample genetic evidence and the combination of several mouse models have identified intricate transcriptional machinery that the skeleton utilizes to exert its two endocrine functions in energy metabolism and fertility. Conversely, in response to signals from other organs, transcriptional mediators are also inducing or mediating a network of interactions between different receptors and kinases that with specificity deliver either a beneficial or an adverse effect on mass accrual. These functional relationships between adipocytes, neurons, sympathetic tone, osteoblasts, and glucose-regulating organs illustrate *in vivo* the importance of the skeleton in the regulation of glucose homeostasis and provide an example of how critical the interplay is between

multiple organs in the establishment and regulation of major physiological functions in vertebrates.

References

[1] Lee NK, Sowa H, Hinoi E, Ferron M, Ahn JD, Confavreux C, et al. Endocrine regulation of energy metabolism by the skeleton. Cell 2007 August 10;130(3):456–69.

[2] Ferron M, Wei J, Yoshizawa T, Del FA, DePinho RA, Teti A, et al. Insulin signaling in osteoblasts integrates bone remodeling and energy metabolism. Cell 2010 July 23;142(2):296–308.

[3] Fulzele K, Riddle RC, Digirolamo DJ, Cao X, Wan C, Chen D, et al. Insulin receptor signaling in osteoblasts regulates postnatal bone acquisition and body composition. Cell 2010 July 23;142(2):309–19.

[4] Pittas AG, Harris SS, Eliades M, Stark P, Dawson-Hughes B. Association between serum osteocalcin and markers of metabolic phenotype. J Clin Endocrinol Metab 2009 March;94(3):827–32.

[5] Kindblom JM, Ohlsson C, Ljunggren O, Karlsson MK, Tivesten A, Smith U, et al. Plasma osteocalcin is inversely related to fat mass and plasma glucose in elderly Swedish men. J Bone Miner Res 2009 May;24(5):785–91.

[6] Kanazawa I, Yamaguchi T, Yamamoto M, Yamauchi M, Kurioka S, Yano S, et al. Serum osteocalcin level is associated with glucose metabolism and atherosclerosis parameters in type 2 diabetes mellitus. J Clin Endocrinol Metab 2009 January;94(1):45–9.

[7] Saleem U, Mosley Jr TH, Kullo IJ. Serum osteocalcin is associated with measures of insulin resistance, adipokine levels, and the presence of metabolic syndrome. Arterioscler Thromb Vasc Biol 2010 July;30(7):1474–8.

[8] Oury F, Sumara G, Sumara O, Ferron M, Chang H, Smith CE, et al. Endocrine regulation of male fertility by the skeleton. Cell 2011. In press.

[9] Hinoi E, Gao N, Jung DY, Yadav V, Yoshizawa T, Myers Jr MG, et al. The sympathetic tone mediates leptin's inhibition of insulin secretion by modulating osteocalcin bioactivity. J Cell Biol 2008 December 29;183(7):1235–42.

[10] Ducy P, Amling M, Takeda S, Priemel M, Schilling AF, Beil FT, et al. Leptin inhibits bone formation through a hypothalamic relay: a central control of bone mass. Cell 2000 January 21;100(2):197–207.

[11] Takeda S, Elefteriou F, Levasseur R, Liu X, Zhao L, Parker KL, et al. Leptin regulates bone formation via the sympathetic nervous system. Cell 2002 November 1;111(3):305–17.

[12] Fu L, Patel MS, Bradley A, Wagner EF, Karsenty G. The molecular clock mediates leptin-regulated bone formation. Cell 2005 September 9;122(5):803–15.

[13] Elefteriou F, Ahn JD, Takeda S, Starbuck M, Yang X, Liu X, et al. Leptin regulation of bone resorption by the sympathetic nervous system and CART. Nature 2005 March 24;434(7032):514–20.

[14] Shi Y, Oury F, Yadav VK, Wess J, Liu XS, Guo XE, et al. Signaling through the M(3) muscarinic receptor favors bone mass accrual by decreasing sympathetic activity. Cell Metab 2010 March 3;11(3):231–8.

[15] Pogoda P, Egermann M, Schnell JC, Priemel M, Schilling AF, Alini M, et al. Leptin inhibits bone formation not only in rodents, but also in sheep. J Bone Miner Res 2006 October;21(10):1591–9.

[16] Baldock PA, Sainsbury A, Allison S, Lin EJ, Couzens M, Boey D, et al. Hypothalamic control of bone formation: distinct actions of leptin and y2 receptor pathways. J Bone Miner Res 2005 October;20(10):1851–7.

[17] Sato S, Hanada R, Kimura A, Abe T, Matsumoto T, Iwasaki M, et al. Central control of bone remodeling by neuromedin U. Nat Med 2007 October;13(10):1234–40.

[18] Iwaniec UT, Boghossian S, Lapke PD, Turner RT, Kalra SP. Central leptin gene therapy corrects skeletal abnormalities in leptin-deficient ob/ob mice. Peptides 2007 May;28(5):1012–9.

[19] Beil FT, Barvencik F, Gebauer M, Beil B, Pogoda P, Rueger JM, et al. Effects of increased bone formation on fracture healing in mice. J Trauma 2011 April;70(4):857–62.

[20] Yadav VK, Oury F, Suda N, Liu ZW, Gao XB, Confavreux C, et al. A serotonin-dependent mechanism explains the leptin regulation of bone mass, appetite, and energy expenditure. Cell 2009 September 4;138(5):976–89.

[21] Yadav VK, Ryu JH, Suda N, Tanaka KF, Gingrich JA, Schutz G, et al. Lrp5 controls bone formation by inhibiting serotonin synthesis in the duodenum. Cell 2008 November 28;135(5):825–37.

[22] Yadav VK, Balaji S, Suresh PS, Liu XS, Lu X, Li Z, et al. Pharmacological inhibition of gut-derived serotonin synthesis is a potential bone anabolic treatment for osteoporosis. Nat Med 2010 March;16(3):308–12.

[23] Modder UI, Achenbach SJ, Amin S, Riggs BL, Melton III LJ, Khosla S. Relation of serum serotonin levels to bone density and structural parameters in women. J Bone Miner Res 2010 February;25(2):415–22.

[24] Frost M, Andersen T, Gossiel F, Hansen S, Bollerslev J, Van HW, et al. Levels of serotonin, sclerostin, bone turnover markers as well as bone density and microarchitecture in patients with high-bone-mass phenotype due to a mutation in Lrp5. J Bone Miner Res 2011 August;26(8):1721–8.

[25] Accili D, Arden KC. FoxOs at the crossroads of cellular metabolism, differentiation, and transformation. Cell 2004 May 14;117(4):421–6.

[26] Nakae J, Biggs III WH, Kitamura T, Cavenee WK, Wright CV, Arden KC, et al. Regulation of insulin action and pancreatic beta-cell function by mutated alleles of the gene encoding forkhead transcription factor Foxo1. Nat Genet 2002 October;32(2):245–53.

[27] Matsumoto M, Pocai A, Rossetti L, DePinho RA, Accili D. Impaired regulation of hepatic glucose production in mice lacking the forkhead transcription factor Foxo1 in liver. Cell Metab 2007 September;6(3):208–16.

[28] Puigserver P, Rhee J, Donovan J, Walkey CJ, Yoon JC, Oriente F, et al. Insulin-regulated hepatic gluconeogenesis through FOXO1-PGC-1alpha interaction. Nature 2003 May 29;423(6939):550–5.

[29] Nakae J, Kitamura T, Kitamura Y, Biggs III WH, Arden KC, Accili D. The forkhead transcription factor Foxo1 regulates adipocyte differentiation. Dev Cell 2003 January;4(1):119–29.

[30] Hribal ML, Nakae J, Kitamura T, Shutter JR, Accili D. Regulation of insulin-like growth factor-dependent myoblast differentiation by Foxo forkhead transcription factors. J Cell Biol 2003 August 18;162(4):535–41.

[31] Kitamura YI, Kitamura T, Kruse JP, Raum JC, Stein R, Gu W, et al. FoxO1 protects against pancreatic beta cell failure through NeuroD and MafA induction. Cell Metab 2005 September;2(3):153–63.

[32] Hashimoto N, Kido Y, Uchida T, Asahara S, Shigeyama Y, Matsuda T, et al. Ablation of PDK1 in pancreatic beta cells induces diabetes as a result of loss of beta cell mass. Nat Genet 2006 May;38(5):589–93.

[33] Rached MT, Kode A, Silva BC, Jung DY, Gray S, Ong H, et al. FoxO1 expression in osteoblasts regulates glucose homeostasis through regulation of osteocalcin in mice. J Clin Invest 2010 January 4;120(1):357–68.

[34] Kitamura T, Feng Y, Kitamura YI, Chua Jr SC, Xu AW, Barsh GS, et al. Forkhead protein FoxO1 mediates Agrp-dependent effects of leptin on food intake. Nat Med 2006 May;12(5):534–40.

[35] Yang G, Lim CY, Li C, Xiao X, Radda GK, Li C, et al. FoxO1 inhibits leptin regulation of pro-opiomelanocortin promoter activity by blocking STAT3 interaction with specificity protein 1. J Biol Chem 2009 February 6;284(6):3719–27.

[36] Delepine M, Nicolino M, Barrett T, Golamaully M, Lathrop GM, Julier C. EIF2AK3, encoding translation initiation factor 2-alpha kinase 3, is mutated in patients with Wolcott–Rallison syndrome. Nat Genet 2000 August;25(4):406–9.

[37] Harding HP, Zeng H, Zhang Y, Jungries R, Chung P, Plesken H, et al. Diabetes mellitus and exocrine pancreatic dysfunction in perk−/− mice reveals a role for translational control in secretory cell survival. Mol Cell 2001 June;7(6):1153–63.

[38] Scheuner D, Song B, McEwen E, Liu C, Laybutt R, Gillespie P, et al. Translational control is required for the unfolded protein response and in vivo glucose homeostasis. Mol Cell 2001 June;7(6):1165–76.

[39] Ron D, Walter P. Signal integration in the endoplasmic reticulum unfolded protein response. Nat Rev Mol Cell Biol 2007 July;8(7):519–29.

[40] Oyadomari S, Harding HP, Zhang Y, Oyadomari M, Ron D. Dephosphorylation of translation initiation factor 2alpha enhances glucose tolerance and attenuates hepatosteatosis in mice. Cell Metab 2008 June;7(6):520–32.

[41] Yoshizawa T, Hinoii E, Jung DY, Kajimura D, Ferron M, Seo J, et al. The transcription factor ATF4 regulates glucose metabolism through its expression in osteoblasts. J Clin Invest 2009;119(9).

[42] Nakabeppu Y, Nathans D. A naturally occurring truncated form of FosB that inhibits Fos/Jun transcriptional activity. Cell 1991 February 22;64(4):751–9.

[43] McClung CA, Nestler EJ. Regulation of gene expression and cocaine reward by CREB and DeltaFosB. Nat Neurosci 2003 November;6(11):1208–15.

[44] Sabatakos G, Rowe GC, Kveiborg M, Wu M, Neff L, Chiusaroli R, et al. Doubly truncated FosB isoform (Delta2-DeltaFosB) induces osteosclerosis in transgenic mice and modulates expression and phosphorylation of Smads in osteoblasts independent of intrinsic AP-1 activity. J Bone Miner Res 2008 May;23(5):584–95.

[45] Sabatakos G, Sims NA, Chen J, Aoki K, Kelz MB, Amling M, et al. Overexpression of DeltaFosB transcription factor(s) increases bone formation and inhibits adipogenesis. Nat Med 2000 September;6(9):985–90.

[46] Rowe GC, Choi CS, Neff L, Horne WC, Shulman GI, Baron R. Increased energy expenditure and insulin sensitivity in the high bone mass DeltaFosB transgenic mice. Endocrinology 2009 January;150(1):135–43.

[47] Wayman GA, Kaech S, Grant WF, Davare M, Impey S, Tokumitsu H, et al. Regulation of axonal extension and growth cone motility by calmodulin-dependent protein kinase I. J Neurosci 2004 April 14;24(15):3786–94.

[48] Ribar TJ, Rodriguiz RM, Khiroug L, Wetsel WC, Augustine GJ, Means AR. Cerebellar defects in Ca2+/calmodulin kinase IV-deficient mice. J Neurosci 2000 November 15;20(22):RC107.

[49] Bonnet N, Benhamou CL, Malaval L, Goncalves C, Vico L, Eder V, et al. Low dose beta-blocker prevents ovariectomy-induced bone loss in rats without affecting heart functions. J Cell Physiol 2008 December;217(3):819–27.

[50] Morse D, Sassone-Corsi P. Time after time: inputs to and outputs from the mammalian circadian oscillators. Trends Neurosci 2002 December;25(12):632–7.

[51] Okamura H, Miyake S, Sumi Y, Yamaguchi S, Yasui A, Muijtjens M, et al. Photic induction of mPer1 and mPer2 in cry-deficient mice lacking a biological clock. Science 1999 December 24;286(5449):2531–4.

[52] Teitelbaum SL, Ross FP. Genetic regulation of osteoclast development and function. Nat Rev Genet 2003 August;4(8):638–49.

[53] Zheng B, Albrecht U, Kaasik K, Sage M, Lu W, Vaishnav S, et al. Nonredundant roles of the mPer1 and mPer2 genes in the mammalian circadian clock. Cell 2001 June 1;105(5):683–94.

[54] Karsenty G, Kronenberg HM, Settembre C. Genetic control of bone formation. Annu Rev Cell Dev Biol 2009;25:629–48.

[55] Rejnmark L, Vestergaard P, Mosekilde L. Treatment with beta-blockers, ACE inhibitors, and calcium-channel blockers is associated with a reduced fracture risk: a nationwide case–control study. J Hypertens 2006 March;24(3):581–9.

[56] Schlienger RG, Kraenzlin ME, Jick SS, Meier CR. Use of beta-blockers and risk of fractures. JAMA 2004 September 15;292(11):1326–32.

[57] Turker S, Karatosun V, Gunal I. Beta-blockers increase bone mineral density. Clin Orthop Relat Res 2006 February;443:73–4.

[58] Yang X, Matsuda K, Bialek P, Jacquot S, Masuoka HC, Schinke T, et al. ATF4 is a substrate of RSK2 and an essential regulator of osteoblast biology; implication for Coffin–Lowry syndrome. Cell 2004 April 30;117(3):387–98.

[59] Asnicar MA, Smith DP, Yang DD, Heiman ML, Fox N, Chen YF, et al. Absence of cocaine- and amphetamine-regulated transcript results in obesity in mice fed a high caloric diet. Endocrinology 2001 October;142(10):4394–400.

[60] Goodrich JT, Bernd P, Sherman D, Gershon MD. Phylogeny of enteric serotonergic neurons. J Comp Neurol 1980 March 1;190(1):15–28.

[61] De-Miguel FF, Trueta C. Synaptic and extrasynaptic secretion of serotonin. Cell Mol Neurobiol 2005 March;25(2):297–312.

[62] Hoyer D, Clarke DE, Fozard JR, Hartig PR, Martin GR, Mylecharane EJ, et al. International Union of Pharmacology classification of receptors for 5-hydroxytryptamine (serotonin). Pharmacol Rev 1994 June;46(2):157–203.

[63] Fink KB, Gothert M. 5-HT receptor regulation of neurotransmitter release. Pharmacol Rev 2007 December;59(4):360–417.

[64] Drago A, Serretti A. Focus on HTR2C: a possible suggestion for genetic studies of complex disorders. Am J Med Genet B Neuropsychiatr Genet 2009 July 5;150B(5):601–37.

[65] Haribabu B, Hook SS, Selbert MA, Goldstein EG, Tomhave ED, Edelman AM, et al. Human calcium-calmodulin dependent protein kinase I: cDNA cloning, domain structure and activation by phosphorylation at threonine-177 by calcium-calmodulin dependent protein kinase I kinase. EMBO J 1995 August 1;14(15):3679–86.

[66] Schulman H, Heist K, Srinivasan M. Decoding Ca2+ signals to the nucleus by multifunctional CaM kinase. Prog Brain Res 1995;105:95–104.

[67] Tokumitsu H, Soderling TR. Requirements for calcium and calmodulin in the calmodulin kinase activation cascade. J Biol Chem 1996 March 8;271(10):5617–22.

[68] Bito H, Deisseroth K, Tsien RW. CREB phosphorylation and dephosphorylation: a Ca(2+)- and stimulus duration-dependent switch for hippocampal gene expression. Cell 1996 December 27;87(7):1203–14.

[69] Edelman AM, Mitchelhill KI, Selbert MA, Anderson KA, Hook SS, Stapleton D, et al. Multiple Ca(2+)-calmodulin-dependent protein kinase kinases from rat brain. Purification, regulation by Ca(2+)-calmodulin, and partial amino acid sequence. J Biol Chem 1996 May 3;271(18):10806–10.

[70] Corcoran EE, Means AR. Defining Ca2+/calmodulin-dependent protein kinase cascades in transcriptional regulation. J Biol Chem 2001 February 2;276(5):2975–8.

[71] Soderling TR, Stull JT. Structure and regulation of calcium-/calmodulin-dependent protein kinases. Chem Rev 2001 August; 101(8):2341–52.

[72] Tokumitsu H, Inuzuka H, Ishikawa Y, Kobayashi R. A single amino acid difference between alpha and beta Ca2+/calmodulin-dependent protein kinase kinase dictates sensitivity to the specific inhibitor, STO-609. J Biol Chem 2003 March 28;278(13):10908–13.

[73] Hook SS, Means AR. Ca(2+)/CaM-dependent kinases: from activation to function. Annu Rev Pharmacol Toxicol 2001;41:471–505.

[74] van Koppen CJ, Kaiser B. Regulation of muscarinic acetylcholine receptor signaling. Pharmacol Ther 2003 May;98(2):197–220.

[75] Nathanson NM. Synthesis, trafficking, and localization of muscarinic acetylcholine receptors. Pharmacol Ther 2008 July;119(1):33–43.

[76] Noda M, Higashida H, Aoki S, Wada K. Multiple signal transduction pathways mediated by 5-HT receptors. Mol Neurobiol 2004 February;29(1):31–9.

[77] Kirmani S, Atkinson EJ, Melton III LJ, Riggs BL, Amin S, Khosla S. Relationship of testosterone and osteocalcin levels during growth. J Bone Miner Res 2011 September;26(9):2212–6.

[78] Zhang X, Odom DT, Koo SH, Conkright MD, Canettieri G, Best J, et al. Genome-wide analysis of cAMP-response element binding protein occupancy, phosphorylation, and target gene activation in human tissues. Proc Natl Acad Sci USA 2005 March 22;102(12):4459–64.

[79] Dufau ML, Tsai-Morris CH. Gonadotropin-regulated testicular helicase (GRTH/DDX25): an essential regulator of spermatogenesis. Trends Endocrinol Metab 2007 October;18(8):314–20.

[80] Tsai-Morris CH, Sheng Y, Gutti R, Li J, Pickel J, Dufau ML. Gonadotropin-regulated testicular RNA helicase (GRTH/DDX25) gene: cell-specific expression and transcriptional regulation by androgen in transgenic mouse testis. J Cell Biochem 2010 April 15;109(6):1142–7.

[81] Tsai-Morris CH, Koh E, Sheng Y, Maeda Y, Gutti R, Namiki M, et al. Polymorphism of the GRTH/DDX25 gene in normal and infertile Japanese men: a missense mutation associated with loss of GRTH phosphorylation. Mol Hum Reprod 2007 December;13(12):887–92.

[82] Sheng Y, Tsai-Morris CH, Gutti R, Maeda Y, Dufau ML. Gonadotropin-regulated testicular RNA helicase (GRTH/Ddx25) is a transport protein involved in gene-specific mRNA export and protein translation during spermatogenesis. J Biol Chem 2006 November 17;281(46):35048–56.

[83] Kato M, Patel MS, Levasseur R, Lobov I, Chang BH, Glass DA, et al. Cbfa1-independent decrease in osteoblast proliferation, osteopenia, and persistent embryonic eye vascularization in mice deficient in Lrp5, a Wnt coreceptor. J Cell Biol 2002 April 15;157(2):303–14.

[84] Babij P, Zhao W, Small C, Kharode Y, Yaworsky PJ, Bouxsein ML, et al. High bone mass in mice expressing a mutant LRP5 gene. J Bone Miner Res 2003 Jun;18(6):960–74.

[85] Boyden LM, Mao J, Belsky J, Mitzner L, Farhi A, Mitnick MA, et al. High bone density due to a mutation in LDL-receptor-related protein 5. N Engl J Med 2002 May 16;346(20):1513–21.

[86] Little RD, Recker RR, Johnson ML. High bone density due to a mutation in LDL-receptor-related protein 5. N Engl J Med 2002 Sep 19;347(12):943–4.

10

Regulation of Bone Resorption by PPARγ

Wei Wei, Yihong Wan

University of Texas Southwestern Medical Center, Dallas, TX, USA

INTRODUCTION

Peroxisome proliferator-activated receptor γ (PPARγ) is a member of the nuclear receptor superfamily of transcription factors that can be activated by lipophilic ligands. It plays important roles in the regulation of a diverse array of physiological processes, including adipogenesis, lipid metabolism, insulin sensitivity, and inflammation [1,2]. Genetic mutations in PPARγ or deregulation of PPARγ function are associated with several human diseases including obesity, type 2 diabetes, lipodystrophy, and cancer. Pharmacologically, several synthetic PPARγ agonists have been developed as drugs that are either FDA approved or in clinical trials, such as rosiglitazone (Avandia) in the thiazolidinedione (TZD) class (Table 10.1) [3]. Since its discovery around 1994 [4–9], PPARγ has rapidly become one of the most intensively investigated nuclear receptors, and has been recognized as a master transcriptional regulator of energy metabolism. Recently, emerging evidence has revealed PPARγ as also an important regulator of skeletal homeostasis.

PPARγ is expressed as at least two isoforms, PPARγ1 and PPARγ2, which are encoded by the same gene via alternative promoter usage and subsequently differential mRNA splicing [4,10]. Compared to PPARγ1, PPARγ2 has 30 additional amino acids at the N-terminus and its location is mainly restricted to adipocyte, skeletal muscle, and liver, whereas PPARγ1 is more widely expressed in several tissues and cell types including adipocyte, macrophage, skeletal muscle, liver, spleen, intestine, kidney, and heart [11–13].

As a ligand-activated transcription factor, PPARγ forms a heterodimeric complex with the retinoid X receptor α (RXRα) and recruits coactivators to the PPAR response element (PPRE) in the promoters of its target genes, thereby inducing their transcription [1,2]. PPARγ functions as a metabolic switch of stem cell fate in both mesenchymal and hematopoietic lineages in bone [14]. Bone marrow mesenchymal stem cells have the capacity to differentiate into several lineages including osteoblast, adipocyte, and chondrocyte, depending on both extracellular cues and intrinsic signaling pathways [15]. PPARγ inhibits osteoblast differentiation by shifting towards adipocyte [16–19]. Consequently, PPARγ insufficiency in mice leads to high bone mass and diminished adipose tissue; whereas ligand activation of PPARγ in human and mice results in low bone mass and increased adiposity [16–19]. Similarly, the myeloid progenitors derived from hematopoietic stem cells (HSCs) also have the capacity to differentiate into several lineages including osteoclast and macrophage. PPARγ stimulates osteoclast differentiation by shifting away from mature macrophage [14,20]. Consequently, PPARγ deletion in the hematopoietic lineages in mice leads to a high bone mass due to decreased osteoclastogenesis and bone resorption [20]; whereas ligand activation of PPARγ in human and mice results in bone loss due to increased osteoclast function [20–22]. These findings unveil PPARγ as a transcriptional sensor that translates increased local concentration of ligands into an orchestrated set of cellular and metabolic responses. Hence, they identify PPARγ an important physiological regulator of both energy metabolism and skeletal homeostasis. This chapter will focus on the recent findings on the roles of PPARγ in osteoclastogenesis and bone resorption, as well as the underlying molecular mechanisms.

PPARγ EXPRESSION SPECIFIES OSTEOCLAST PROGENITOR

The multipotent hematopoietic stem cells in the adult bone marrow mainly differentiate into two lineages: lymphoid and myeloid. Lymphoid progenitors give

TABLE 10.1   Synthetic PPARγ Agonists on Market or in
              Clinical Trials

Company	Drug	Compound category	Phase
Takeda Pharmaceutical	Ciglitazone (INN)	TZDs*	Prototype
Daiichi Sankyo	Troglitazone (Rezulin, Resulin, Romozin)	TZDs	Withdrawn
MitsubishiTanabe Pharma	Netoglitazone	TZDs	Suspended
GlaxoSmithKline	Rosiglitazone (Avandia, Avandamet, Avandaryl)	TZDs	Marketed
Takeda Pharmaceutical	Pioglitazone (Actos, Glustin)	TZDs	Marketed
Dr. Reddy's Laboratories	Balaglitazone (DRF 2593)	TZDs	III
AstraZeneca	Tesaglitazar	Non-TZDs	Suspended
Bristol-Myers Squibb	Muraglitazar	Non-TZDs	Suspended
Metabolex	MBX-102	Non-TZDs	III
Hoffmann-La Roche	Aleglitazar (R1439)	Non-TZDs	III
Metabolex	MBX-2044	Non-TZDs	II
InteKrin Therapeutics	INT131	Non-TZDs	II
Plexxikon	Indeglitazar	Non-TZDs	II

TZDs: thiazolidinediones.

rise to T-lymphocytes, B-lymphocytes, and natural killer cells, which are associated with the adaptive immune system. Myeloid progenitors give rise to a diverse spectrum of cell types including erythrocytes, megakaryocytes, mast cells, granulocytes, and monocytes that can differentiate into macrophages or osteoclasts. Mature osteoclasts are large multinucleated cells formed by the fusion of macrophage precursors. They are located on the bone surfaces, associated with resorption pits, and responsible for removing the organic and inorganic components of bone [14,23,24]. The differentiation of osteoclasts from hematopoietic stem cells is controlled by the sequential action of a defined set of specific factors (Fig. 10.1).

Early on, the expression of PU.1, a member of the Ets family of transcription factors, commits hematopoietic stem cells to myeloid lineage or B-lymphoid lineage. In PU.1-deficient mice, both osteoclast and macrophage differentiation are blocked, this results in classical features of osteopetrosis, a high bone mass disease

caused by defective osteoclast function and bone resorption. Transplantation of bone marrow from wild--type (wt) mice rescues this osteopetrotic phenotype, as well as restores osteoclast and macrophage differentiation, which indicates that PU.1 functions intrinsically in hematopoietic cells [25,26]. However, PU.1 directs hematopoietic stem cells to either myeloid or B-lymphoid development [27], suggesting that it cooperates with other cell-type specific factors to specify macrophage/osteoclast lineage [28].

PPARγ is highly expressed in both monocyte/macrophage precursors and mature osteoclasts [20,29,30]. TRANSFAC transcription factor binding bioinformatics analysis predicts that the PU.1/Ets matrix is highly enriched in several PPARγ-binding regions specifically in macrophages but not in adipocytes. Chromatin immunoprecipitation and high-throughput sequencing (ChIP-seq) analysis demonstrates that PPARγ colocalizes with PU.1 in areas of open chromatin and histone acetylation, near a distinct set of immune genes [31]. This implicates that the combinatory action of PU.1 and PPARγ specifies macrophage lineage commitment away from other differentiation outcomes such as B-cell or adipocyte, and PPARγ expression is critical in osteoclast progenitor development from hematopoietic stem cells.

Our recent studies demonstrating that PPARγ deletion in mouse hematopoietic lineages causes osteoclast defects manifested as osteopetrosis and extramedullary hematopoiesis in the spleen provided the first evidence for the critical role of PPARγ in osteoclastogenesis [20]. Subsequently, using an inducible PPARγ-GFP reporter mouse model (PPARγ-tTA; TRE-H2BGFP) [32], we have found that osteoclast progenitors specifically reside in the PPARγ-expressing hematopoietic bone marrow cells (GFP+ cells) [33]. In vitro osteoclast colony formation assay reveals that osteoclastogenic potential is 140-fold enriched in PPARγ+ cells compared with PPARγ− cells. Imaging analysis shows that osteoclasts developed in vitro and in vivo are GFP+ cells. Microarray analysis of gene expression indicates that PPARγ+ population is enriched for stem/progenitor cells, and PPARγ expression specifically directs hematopoiesis towards monocyte/macrophage lineage but away from lymphoid or other myeloid lineages including megakaryocytes, erythrocytes, and mast cells [33]. A doxycycline pulse-chase strategy identifies the slow-cycling quiescent PPARγ-expressing hematopoietic bone marrow cells as the osteoclast progenitors. Furthermore, two PPARγ-tTA; TRE-cre-driven genetic models provided compelling in vivo functional evidence for the critical role of PPARγ in osteoclast progenitor and the entire osteoclast lineage: first, expressing a constitutively active Notch intracellular domain (NICD) in the PPARγ+ cells hinders osteoclast progenitor from

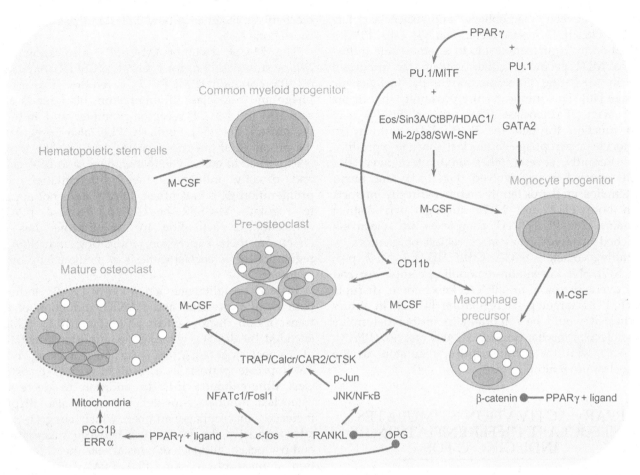

FIGURE 10.1 **A simplified model for PPARγ regulation of osteoclast differentiation.** During the M-CSF-mediated transition from hematopoietic stem cell (HSC) to common myeloid progenitor and then to monocyte progenitor, PPARγ functions in combination with PU.1 to upregulate the expression of GATA2 and promote monocyte/macrophage/osteoclast progenitor specification. In parallel, PPARγ also activates PU.1/MITF complex, which recruits other cofactors, such as Eos, Sin3A, CtBP, HDAC1, and Mi-2/p38/SWI-SNF, to facilitate the transition from common myeloid progenitor to monocyte progenitor. During the M-CSF and RANKL-mediated osteoclastogenesis, activation of PPARγ by its agonist, such as TZDs, accelerates osteoclast differentiation via several mechanisms including suppressing β-catenin protein level, inducing PGC1β and ERRα expression, potentiating c-fos transcription, and inhibiting the expression of OPG, which blocks RANKL signaling as a decoy receptor.

undergoing proliferation and consequently leading to fewer osteoclasts and a higher bone mass; second, DTA (diphtheria toxin attenuated)-mediated partial ablation of PPARγ+ cells also significantly reduces osteoclast number and bone resorption, resulting in a higher bone mass [33].

Mechanistic studies suggest that PPARγ, in combination with PU.1, promotes osteoclast progenitor commitment, at least in part, by directly binding to the promoter and activating the transcription of GATA2 [33]. The GATA family of zinc finger transcription factors is an important regulator of hematopoiesis. GATA2 is required to generate osteoclast progenitors [34,35], while GATA1 is dispensable for osteoclastogenesis but essential for erythropoiesis and megakaryocyte maturation [36–38]. Therefore, GATA2/GATA1 ratio in hematopoietic progenitors controls lineage divergence between osteoclasts and erythrocytes/megakaryocytes. We have found that this key GATA2/GATA1

ratio is significantly higher in the PPARγ+ cells compared to the PPARγ− cells. Chromatin-immunoprecipitation (ChIP) analyses demonstrate that PPARγ binds to three highly conserved PPREs in the GATA2 promoter specifically in PPARγ+ cells, leading to a higher level of histone acetylation at these regions [33]. These results indicate that PPARγ expression facilitates the specification of hematopoietic stem cell fate towards macrophage/osteoclast lineage but away from other myeloid and lymphoid lineages by transcriptionally activating GATA2 (Fig. 10.1).

As another PU.1 cofactor, microphthalmia-associated transcription factor (MITF), is also crucial to the early stage of osteoclast development (Fig. 10.1). Similar to PU.1, the MITF-deficient mice are osteopetrotic; while unlike PU.1, MITF-deficient mice exhibit intact macrophage differentiation but impaired osteoclast differentiation, which suggests that MITF functions downstream of PU.1 in osteoclast differentiation and regulates the balance between macrophage and osteoclast fate choices [26,39]. In mouse melanoma S91 cells, PPARγ activation by ciglitazone leads to a remarkable induction of MITF promoter activity, playing an important role in regulating differentiation in the melanocytic lineage [40]. This implicates the possibility that in the early stage of osteoclast differentiation, PPARγ may also function through the PU.1/MITF pathway in monocyte–macrophage–osteoclast lineage specification. Recently, several other modulators have also been reported to be involved (Fig. 10.1): zinc finger protein Eos, an Ikaros family member, directly interacts with both PU.1 and MITF through two distinct domains; Eos/PU.1/MITF complexes are selectively enriched at target genes in osteoclast progenitors by recruiting cofactors Sin3A, CtBP, HDAC1, Mi-2, p38, and SWI/SNF chromatin-remodeling complexes; and Eos overexpression or siRNA knockdown disrupts MITF/PU.1 target gene regulation [41,42]. In future studies, it would be important to further determine the molecular mechanisms for whether and how PPARγ interacts with these transcription regulators in the osteoclast progenitors.

PPARγ ACTIVATION STIMULATES OSTEOCLAST DIFFERENTIATION BY INDUCING C-FOS

Osteoclastogenesis is a multi-step process that requires osteoclast progenitor commitment [25,43], M-CSF (macrophage colony stimulating factor)-mediated osteoclast precursor proliferation [44], and RANKL (receptor activator of NFκB ligand)-mediated osteoclast differentiation [45–47]. In addition to the loss-of-function studies that show PPARγ deletion impairs osteoclastogenesis [20], gain-of-function studies reveal that rosiglitazone activation of PPARγ accelerates osteoclast differentiation *in vitro* and elevates bone resorption *in vivo* [20]. Together, these findings support the notion that PPARγ plays dual roles in osteoclastogenesis: PPARγ expression promotes osteoclast progenitor specification; and PPARγ ligand activation stimulates osteoclast differentiation. Consequently, the local availability of endogenous or synthetic PPARγ ligands functions as a molecular switch to modulate osteoclastogenesis and bone resorption. In line with this idea, it has been reported that aging is associated with an elevated expression of lipoxygenases and an increased production of oxidized lipids that can function as endogenous PPARγ agonists, such as 12-hydroxyeiscosatetraenoic acid (12-HETE), 15-HETE, 9-hydroxyoctadecadienoic acid (9-HODE), and 13-HODE [48–51]. Therefore, the discovery of PPARγ regulation of osteoclastogenesis provides critical

mechanistic insights in how TZDs and possibly aging cause bone loss.

The M-CSF receptor (M-CSFR), also known as colony stimulating factor 1 receptor (CSF1R), or cluster of differentiation 115 (CD115), is required for macrophage and osteoclast differentiation. PU.1 binds and activates the M-CSF receptor promoter and induces its transcription [52]. Similarly, PU.1 also upregulates the promoter of integrin α M (ITGAM, CD11b), which is expressed in monocyte, macrophage, and osteoclast, and directly influences their differentiation and proliferation [53]. In contrast, PPARγ does not appear to regulate M-CSFR or CD11b, because PPARγ deficiency or activation by rosiglitazone has no effect on their expression, indicating that PPARγ regulation of osteoclastogenesis is mediated by other factors.

Instead, rosiglitazone activation of PPARγ induces both basal expression and RANKL induction of the transcription factor c-fos [20] (Fig. 10.1). C-fos, encoded by the FOS gene, is an important mediator of osteoclastogenesis, and the mice lacking c-fos develop osteopetrosis as a result of a block in osteoclast differentiation [54]. In addition to decreased osteoclast number, c-fos-deficient mice also display increased macrophage number, which suggests that c-fos regulates the fate choice between macrophage and osteoclast, and lack of c-fos arrests the differentiation at macrophage stage [54]. PPARγ functions as a direct modulator of c-fos expression: PPARγ deficiency in hematopoietic lineages decreases c-fos mRNA levels; in RAW264.7 mouse macrophage cell line, the c-fos promoter can be upregulated with accumulating amounts of PPARγ/RXRα transcription complex, and further activated by the PPARγ agonist rosiglitazone. By using luciferase reporter assays and electrophoretic mobility shift assays, two conserved PPREs are identified in the c-fos promoter region. Furthermore, PPARγ regulation of c-fos occurs both before and after RANKL stimulation, suggesting that it accelerates both pre-osteoclast formation and osteoclast maturation by enhancing the levels of c-fos in both macrophage precursors and immature osteoclasts [20]. These findings have identified c-fos as a critical PPARγ target gene in macrophages and osteoclasts that contribute to the pro-osteoclastogenic effects of rosiglitazone.

PPARγ ACTIVATION STIMULATES OSTEOCLAST DIFFERENTIATION BY DOWNREGULATING β-CATENIN

β-catenin is an essential component transducing the canonical Wnt signaling. Wnt activation through this pathway results in inhibition of glycogen synthase kinase 3β (GSK-3β)-mediated β-catenin phosphorylation and thereby stabilization of β-catenin protein [55]. The Wnt/β-catenin pathway is an important regulator of skeletal physiology. β-catenin deletion in mesenchymal progenitors blocks osteoblast differentiation by shifting to chondrocyte formation [56,57]. β-catenin deletion in differentiated osteoblasts leads to osteopenia by reducing the expression of osteoprotegerin (OPG), a decoy RANKL receptor, thus indirectly elevating osteoclast formation [58,59]. Furthermore, Wnt/β-catenin activation enhances osteoblastogenesis and suppresses adipogenesis by inhibiting peroxisome proliferator-activated receptor γ (PPARγ) [60,61]. Therefore, β-catenin is required for osteoblast differentiation and modulates osteoblast function.

Despite the intense investigation of Wnt/β-catenin signaling in bone biology, previous studies mainly focused on its roles in osteoblasts; while its specific functions, if any, in osteoclasts have been unknown until our recent study. This is a clinically important question because neutralizing antibodies against Wnt antagonists may be promising new drugs for bone diseases. We have found that in osteoclastogenesis, β-catenin is induced during M-CSF-mediated quiescence-to-proliferation switch, but suppressed during RANKL-mediated proliferation-to-differentiation switch. Genetically, β-catenin deletion blocks osteoclast precursor proliferation, while β-catenin constitutive activation sustains proliferation but prevents osteoclast differentiation, both causing osteopetrosis. In contrast, β-catenin heterozygosity enhances osteoclast differentiation, causing osteoporosis. Biochemically, Wnt activation attenuates whereas Wnt inhibition stimulates osteoclastogenesis. Mechanistically, β-catenin activation increases GATA2/Evi1 expression but abolishes RANKL-induced c-Jun phosphorylation. Therefore, β-catenin exerts a pivotal biphasic and dosage-dependent regulation of osteoclastogenesis. Importantly, these findings suggest that Wnt activation-based drugs could be a more effective treatment for skeletal fragility than previously recognized because of their anabolic and anti-catabolic dual benefit [62]. Moreover, this discovery of the novel roles of β-catenin in osteoclastogenesis opens an exciting new path to future investigations of the ligands, receptors, signal transducers, and transcription factors that orchestrate the regulation of osteoclast physiology and pharmacology by the Wnt pathway.

PPARγ and Wnt signaling have been shown to be mutually inhibitory. For example, canonical or noncanonical Wnt signaling suppresses PPARγ to enhance osteoblastogenesis and reduces adipogenesis [61,63]. Reciprocally, PPARγ also suppresses β-catenin function

in various cell types, including MEFs and preadipocytes, to promote adipogenesis [64−66]. PPARγ activation decreases β-catenin protein levels via a proteasome-mediated and adenomatous polyposis coli (APC)-independent pathway in these mesenchymal cell types [67]. However, how PPARγ and Wnt signaling interact during osteoclastogenesis has been unknown until recently. We have found that rosiglitazone activations of PPARγ in macrophage precursors and osteoclasts also downregulate β-catenin protein level, leading to decreased cyclin D1 expression and attenuated precursor proliferation, thereby accelerating osteoclast differentiation [62]. This reveals that the pro-osteoclastogenic effects of PPARγ activation are also contributed by the suppression of Wnt/β-catenin signaling, hence the acceleration of the proliferation-to-differentiation switch (Fig. 10.1).

PPARγ ACTIVATION PROMOTES OSTEOCLASTOGENESIS BY ACTIVATING PGC1β AND ERRα

PPARγ activation of transcription depends on its ligand-mediated recruitment of co-activators; the functional diversity of PPARγ co-activators leads to its tissue-specific characteristics, adding another level of complexity to its gene and cell-specific transcriptional functions. Peroxisome proliferator-activated receptor γ co-activator 1β (PGC-1β), a transcriptional co-activator previously known to regulate energy metabolism by stimulating mitochondrial biogenesis and respiration of cells, has been recently identified as a critical regulator of osteoclastogenesis and an essential mediator of PPARγ-induced bone resorption [21,68] (Fig. 10.2). Mitochondria are required for osteoclast differentiation and activation, and become highly abundant during the transition from macrophage precursors to osteoclasts [68]. As one of the regulators of mitochondrial biogenesis, PGC-1β is highly induced by RANKL and further stimulated by rosiglitazone during osteoclast differentiation [21,68]. Interestingly, PGC1α, the prototype member of the PGC1 family of co-activators that has been more extensively investigated, is neither expressed nor induced during osteoclastogenesis, implicating a functional specificity for PGC1β in osteoclasts [21,68].

The PGC-1β induction by RANKL is proposed to be partially mediated by another important osteoclast transcription factor cAMP response element binding (CREB), which binds to putative CREB binding DNA elements in the PGC-1β promoter region [68,69]. PGC-1β deletion arrests the transition from macrophage precursors to young osteoclasts, accompanied by the inhibition of mitochondrial gene expression [68].

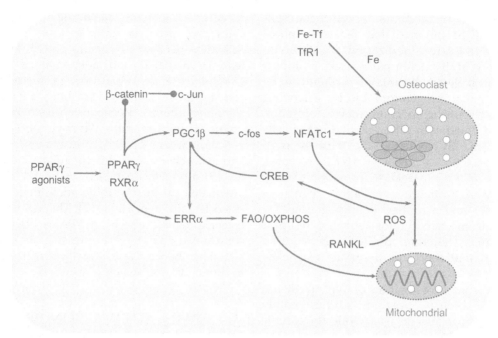

FIGURE 10.2 Rosiglitazone stimulates osteoclastogenesis via PPARγ/PGC1β/ERRα pathway. During RANKL-mediated osteoclast differentiation, rosiglitazone activation of PPARγ indirectly induces PGC1β expression by inhibiting β-catenin protein level, thus promoting both basal and c-jun-induced PGC1β transcription. On the one hand, PGC1β forms a positive feedback loop by functioning as a PPARγ co-activator to induce c-fos expression, stimulating osteoclastogenesis; on the other hand, PGC1β acts as a co-activator for ERRα, which is also induced by rosiglitazone, to induce mitochondrial genes involved in fatty acid β-oxidation (FAO) and oxidative phosphorylation (OXPHOS), promoting mitochondrial biogenesis and activation. Furthermore, TfR1-mediated iron uptake promotes osteoclastogenesis, and RANKL-activated ROS and CREB also induce PGC1β expression and mitochondria biogenesis. Importantly, the crosstalk among these signaling pathways synergistically promotes osteoclastogenesis. Therefore, rosiglitazone activates the PPARγ/PGC1β/ERRα transcriptional network to orchestrate the induction of both osteoclast differentiation and mitochondria biogenesis, which ultimately enhances osteoclast function and bone resorption.

Moreover, transferrin receptor protein 1 (TfR1) is also induced during osteoclast differentiation and stimulates osteoclastogenesis by promoting iron uptake; and TfR1 deletion inhibits the osteoclast formation [68]. There is a positive feedback regulation between TfR1/iron uptake and CREB/PGC-1β/mitochondria biogenesis: iron uptake by TfR1 stimulates mitochondrial activation; and the subsequent reactive oxygen species (ROS) accumulation leads to the transcriptional activation of PGC-1β by CREB, together promoting osteoclastogenesis [68].

PGC-1β also plays a key role in PPARγ activation of osteoclastogenesis and rosiglitazone-induced bone loss. Gain-of-function studies reveal that the induction of PGC1β during RANKL-initiated osteoclast differentiation is greatly potentiated by the PPARγ agonist rosiglitazone; PGC1β activation by rosiglitazone and RANKL is PPARγ dependent because it is severely impaired in the PPARγ−/− cells derived from the bone marrow of hematopoietic PPARγ knockout mice [21]. PGC1β promoter analysis by transient transfection and reporter analysis, in combination with chromatin immuno-precipitation (ChIP) and western blot analysis, suggests that PPARγ indirectly enhances PGC1β transcription by downregulating the β-catenin protein level, thereby attenuating the inhibitory effect of β-catenin on c-jun, which directly binds and robustly activates the PGC1β promoter at two conserved AP-1 (activator protein 1) sites [21]. In contrast to c-jun, c-fos exerts neither activity nor interference because it has no effect on either the basal or the c-jun-induced PGC1β promoter expression, suggesting that c-jun functions as homodimers herein [21]. As a result, PGC1β functions as a PPARγ co-activator to augment the rosiglitazone induction of its target genes during osteoclastogenesis [20,21].

Consistently, loss-of-function studies show that PGC1β is required for PPARγ stimulation of osteoclast differentiation and bone resorption *in vivo* and *in vitro* [21]. Targeted deletion of PGC1β in the hematopoietic lineage results in complete resistance to rosiglitazone-induced bone loss, and severe attenuation of rosiglitazone-stimulated osteoclastogenesis, resulting in a markedly reduced ability of rosiglitazone to potentiate the expression of RANKL-induced transcription factors (c-fos and NFATc1) and osteoclast function genes (TRAP, CAR2, and Calcr) [21].

Furthermore, another nuclear receptor ERRα (estrogen receptor-related receptor α) also participates in this pathway. ERRα, β, and γ (also known as

NR3B1, 2, and 3; nuclear receptor subfamily 3, group B, members 1, 2, and 3) belong to the ERR subgroup of the nuclear receptor superfamily of ligand-responsive transcription factors [70–72]. However, no natural ligand has been identified to date for any of the ERRs, thus they are referred to as orphan receptors [70–72]. ERRα is well known as an important regulator of energy metabolism [71,72]. PGC1β has been shown to function as a ligand-independent co-activator (or protein ligand) for ERRα to induce the expression of medium-chain acyl-CoA dehydrogenase (MCAD), a pivotal enzyme in mitochondrial fatty acid β-oxidation (FAO) [73]. PGC1β activation of ERRα also induces other mitochondrial target genes involved in the tricarboxylic acid (TCA) cycle and oxidative phosphorylation (OXPHOS), such as Ndg2 (Nur77 downstream gene 2), Aco2 (aconitase 2), IDH3a (isocitrate dehydrogenase 3), and ATP5b (ATP synthase 5b) [74].

Emerging evidence suggests that ERRα also controls skeletal homeostasis [70]. In addition to the numerous reports on the still controversial roles of ERRα in osteoblastogenesis, our recent study reveals that ERRα also regulates osteoclastogenesis [21]. We have found that rosiglitazone together with RANKL promote the expression of ERRα and its target genes regulating mitochondria biogenesis and fatty acid oxidation, including Ndg2, Aco2, IDH3a, ATP5b, MCAD, VLCAD, and SCAD [21]. This induction is completely abolished in PGC1β−/− differentiation cultures, demonstrating that it is PGC1β dependent [21]. Consistently, ERRα knockout mice exhibit a high bone mass and extramedullary hematopoiesis in the spleen owing to the decreased osteoclast number and bone resorption [21]. Together, these findings demonstrate that PPARγ promotes osteoclastogenesis by activating a transcription network that also comprises PGC1β and ERRα. PPARγ activation indirectly induces PGC1β expression by downregulating β-catenin, thus derepressing c-jun, which directly activates the PGC1β promoter; in turn, PGC1β functions as a PPARγ coactivator to stimulate the transcription of its target genes such as c-fos, thus promoting osteoclast differentiation. Complementarily, PGC1β also coordinates with ERRα to induce genes required for mitochondrial biogenesis and fatty acid oxidation, thereby activating osteoclast function. The concerted increase in osteoclast differentiation and function leads to the enhanced bone resorption (Fig. 10.2).

OTHER SIGNALING PATHWAYS THAT MAY INTERSECT WITH PPARγ DURING OSTEOCLASTOGENESIS

Recent studies have implicated new signaling pathways that may regulate PGC1β and PPARγ functions

in osteoclastogenesis. For example, G-protein-coupled receptor (GPCR)-kinase interacting protein-1 (GIT1) is a novel regulator of bone resorption by modulating osteoclast activity rather than osteoclast differentiation. GIT1-less mice show increased bone mass owing to impaired resorption function but unaltered osteoclast number. Consistently, upon stimulation with RANKL, phosphorylation of its downstream markers (JNK, ERK1/2, p-38, AKT, and IκBα) is unaffected by GIT1 deletion [75]. Instead, it is proposed that RANKL signaling triggers the tyrosine phosphorylation of GIT1 in a c-Src-dependent manner, which is required for podosome formation and osteoclast migration [75]. Interestingly, GIT1 has been shown to regulate mitochondrial biogenesis in the heart: compared with the wt mice, mitochondrial biogenesis in GIT1−/− mice is impaired, mitochondrial DNA is markedly reduced and expression of mitochondrial biogenesis-related genes, including PGC-1β, is also decreased [76]. Thus, in future studies, it will be interesting to examine whether GIT1 deletion also causes defects in mitochondrial biogenesis and PPARγ/PGC1β functions in osteoclasts; and, conversely, whether PPARγ and PGC1β regulate GIT1 activation upon RANKL stimulation.

Another example is phosphatidylinositol 3-kinase (PI3K). PI3K has been shown to coordinately activate the MEK/ERK and AKT/NFκB pathways to maintain osteoclast survival [77]. Recently, it was reported that PI3K also regulates mitochondrial homeostasis in human lung adenocarcinoma cells in part through PGC1β: suppressing PI3K activity selectively reduced both the mRNA and protein levels of PGC1β, but not PGC1α, leading to decreased expression of uncoupling protein 1, 2 (UCP1 and UCP2), and superoxide dismutase 2, reduced mitochondrial mass, and arrested cell growth; consistently, overexpression of PGC-1β partially reverses the alterations in mitochondrial function [78]. Thus, it will be important to examine whether PI3K also modulates mitochondrial activity and PPARγ/PGC1β functions in osteoclasts. Together, these evidences suggest that other pathways, such as GIT1 and PI3K, may also modulate mitochondrial functions and crosstalk with PPARγ/PGC-1β signaling during osteoclastogenesis.

Besides PGC1α and PGC1β, ERRα has also been reported to form a novel complex with PGC-1-related co-activator (PRC) to mediate the biogenesis of functional mitochondria. In three thyroid cell lines, FTC-133, XTC.UC1, and RO 82 W-1, ERRα requires PRC to directly activate transcription, leading to an increase in respiratory chain capacity and mitochondrial mass [79]. Similarly, it is worth exploring whether the ERRα/PRC complex also participates in RANKL-induced and PPARγ-stimulated osteoclast differentiation and mitochondrial activation.

In addition to the aforementioned roles of ERRα in promoting osteoclast differentiation and function by enhancing mitochondrial biogenesis and activation [21], it has been reported that ERRα is also required for osteoclast adhesion, spreading, and migration [80]. Osteoclasts are highly polarized cells that have the capability to adhere, spread, and migrate on the bone surface [23]. Several regulators have been identified to control this process, including tumor necrosis factor receptor-associated factor 6 (TRAF6), integrin subunits αv/β1/β3/β5, osteopontin (OPN), cluster of differentiation 44 (CD44), and c-src [80]. It is shown that ERRα is important for mature osteoclast adhesion and transmigration, as well as stabilization of podosome at the cell periphery: the expression of ERRα increases during in vitro osteoclast differentiation; inhibition of ERRα function decreases OPN and integrin β3 expression, as well as hinders osteoclast spreading and podosome belt formation in RAW264.7-derived osteoclasts [80]. In future studies, it will be interesting to investigate whether PPARγ also modulates the cytoskeleton functions in mature osteoclasts via the regulation of ERRα and other factors such as OPN and integrins.

Furthermore, as a member of the nuclear receptors, ERRα modulates the transcription of many other metabolic genes, which may also participate in osteoclast regulation. For example, ERRα stimulates the expression of PDK4 (pyruvate dehydrogenase kinases 4) by directly binding to the PDK4 promoter [81]. PDK4 has been recently reported to induce bone loss at unloading by promoting osteoclastogenesis: bone resorption is increased after unloading only in wt mice but not in PDK4 knockout mice; and the decreased osteoclastogenesis in PDK4 knockout mice results from both intrinsic differentiation defects in osteoclast precursors and reduced RANKL expression in osteoblasts [82]. In light of these findings, it will be interesting to further investigate whether PDK4 also contributes to the stimulation of osteoclastogenesis and bone resorption by the PPARγ/PGC1β/ERRα axis, especially in the context of disuse osteoporosis.

TZDs INDUCE BONE LOSS BY ACTIVATING BONE RESORPTION AND INHIBITING BONE FORMATION

The synthetic PPARγ agonists, thiazolidinediones (TZDs), also known as glitazones, are widely used for the management of diabetes mellitus type 2 (Table 10.1). Activation of PPARγ by TZDs improves insulin sensitivity in rodents and humans through a combination of metabolic actions, including partitioning of lipid stores and the regulation of metabolic and inflammatory mediators named adipokines. TZDs have also been implicated in the control of cell proliferation, atherosclerosis, macrophage function, and immunity [1,2]. The first prototypical compound of TZDs was ciglitazone, which was never used as a medication but sparked interest in the function of TZDs [83]. As an anti-diabetic and anti-inflammatory drug, troglitazone was the first oral TZD approved for use in treating non-insulin-dependent diabetes mellitus (NIDDM). However, due to the potential risk of drug-induced hepatitis, troglitazone was withdrawn from the US market in March 2000 [84]. Using isolated rat cardiomyocytes, netoglitazone (MCC-555) was identified to possess PPARγ agonist activity and display preclinical benefit, and thus was selected for further clinical development as a treatment of diabetes [85]. Because many patients treated with netoglitazone were unable to appropriately control blood sugar levels and were susceptible to serious complications such as retinopathy, neuropathy, and nephropathy, Mitsubishi Pharma suspended it in Japanese phase II trials in 2006. Currently, rosiglitazone (Avandia, Avandamet, Avandaryl) and pioglitazone (Actos, Glustin) are marketed, and balaglitazone (DRF 2593) is in phase III clinical trials (Table 10.1).

Drugs are often accompanied with side effects, and TZDs are no exceptions. Side effects of TZDs include weight gain, fluid retention, congestive heart failure, and bone fractures [86]. Increasing reports indicate that both rosiglitazone and pioglitazone are associated with a higher fracture risk: with 4 years of rosiglitazone treatments, 4360 type 2 diabetic patients in ADOPT (A Diabetes Outcome Progression Trial) showed an increased fracture risk in women [87]; similarly, pioglitazone has also been reported to have the same side effects [88,89]. A pooled safety evaluation of 19 studies on 8100 pioglitazone-treated patients compared with 7400 patients treated with a comparator drug indicates that 2.6% of the female pioglitazone recipients experienced a fracture compared with 1.7% of the women who received the comparator; there were no differences in fractures among men treated with pioglitazone (1.3%) versus men treated with comparator (1.5%) [88]. Interestingly, another clinical study reports that among the cohort of 84,339 patients (average age 59, 43% female), the patients treated with TZDs were associated with a 28% increased risk of peripheral fractures compared with the patients treated with a sulfonylurea control; pioglitazone was associated with more fractures in both men and women, whereas rosiglitazone was associated with more fractures in only women; moreover, pioglitazone was associated with a higher rate of fractures than rosiglitazone—therefore, it was concluded that both men and women who take TZDs could be at increased risk of fractures, and pioglitazone may be more strongly associated with fractures than rosiglitazone [90]. In the pioglitazone-treated patients, most of the fractures were located at the distal upper or lower limb; and reductions in bone mineral density at the lumbar spine and the hip were also reported [90]. Furthermore, by taking paired stored baseline and 12-month serum samples from 1605 participants (689 women, 916 men) in ADOPT, another recent study showed that CTX-1 (C-terminal telopeptide for type 1 collagen), a marker of bone resorption, was increased by 6.1% in the rosiglitazone group in women but not men; P1NP (procollagen type 1 N-propeptide) and bone alkaline phosphatase, two markers of bone formation, were decreased in both women and men. Therefore, it was concluded that excessive bone resorption may be an important mechanism contributing to the higher fracture risk in women taking TZDs, in addition to the diminished bone formation [22].

Recent studies using mouse models have provided mechanistic insights for how TZDs increase bone resorption—rosiglitazone promotes osteoclastogenesis and induces bone loss via a transcription network comprised of PPARγ, c-fos, PGC1β, and ERRα. During *in vitro* bone marrow osteoclast differentiation, rosiglitazone treatment promotes osteoclastogenesis by directly enhancing the mRNA expression of RANKL-induced transcription factor c-fos, leading to accelerated induction of osteoclast-specific genes, including TRAP (tartrate-resistant acid phosphatase type 5, Acp5), calcitonin receptor, carbonic anhydrase 2, cathepsin K, matrix metallopeptidase-9, and NFATc1. This pro-osteoclastogenic effect of rosiglitazone was completely abolished in PPARγ−/− bone marrow cells, demonstrating that they are PPARγ dependent [20]. Furthermore, rosiglitazone also upregulates the mRNA expression of PGC1β and ERRα, which induces genes involved in mitochondrial biogenesis and fatty acid oxidation, leading to osteoclast activation [21]. To evaluate the *in vivo* effects of long-term rosiglitazone treatment, mice were orally gavaged daily with rosiglitazone (10 mg/kg/day) or vehicle control for 6 weeks. The results show that rosiglitazone caused a significant increase in both bone resorption marker and osteoclast numbers in wt mice but not in hematopoietic PPARγ knockout mice, indicating that rosiglitazone-mediated osteoclast activation is largely hematopoietic cell autonomous [20].

During *in vitro* bone marrow osteoclast differentiation, rosiglitazone treatment also potentiates the induction of PGC1β by RANKL, implicating an important role of PGC1β in rosiglitazone stimulation of osteoclastogenesis. Indeed, although rosiglitazone highly stimulates the formation of multinucleated TRAP-positive mature osteoclasts in the wt differentiation culture, this effect is severely attenuated in the PGC1β−/− culture [21]. Consistently, PGC1β deletion prevents

rosiglitazone to potentiate the expression of RANKL-induced transcription factors (c-fos and NFATc1) and osteoclast function genes (TRAP, carbonic anhydrase 2, and calcitonin receptor) [21]. Furthermore, rosiglitazone in conjunction with RANKL promotes the mRNA expression of ERRα, thereby inducing the expression of ERRα target genes involved in mitochondrial biogenesis and fatty acid oxidation. These effects of rosiglitazone are PGC1β and ERRα dependent, because they were abolished in PGC1β−/− or ERRα−/− differentiation cultures. Like PPARγ, PGC1β is also required for rosiglitazone-induced bone resorption and bone loss in mice, because these effects were completely abolished in hematopoietic PGC1β knockout mice [21].

Due to the limitations of TZDs by side effects that include bone loss, weight gain, and fluid retention, a variety of non-TZD PPARγ agonists have been developed (Table 10.1). Unlike the full PPARγ agonist TZDs, INT131 is a highly potent, non-TZD, selective PPARγ modulator currently in phase II clinical trials for the treatment of type 2 diabetes mellitus [91]. As a selective PPARγ modulator, INT131 activates PPARγ with a maximal activity of about 10% of that of rosiglitazone and recruits selected co-activators with a maximal activity of about 20–25% of that of rosiglitazone, pioglitazone, and troglitazone; INT131 does not induce adipocyte differentiation or triglyceride accumulation in human and mouse pre-adipocytes *in vitro*, suggesting that INT131 has a desired, non-adipogenic effect [91]. Like INT131, MBX-102 is also a novel selective partial PPARγ agonist distinct from rosiglitazone, which displays anti-diabetic and insulin-sensitizing properties in rodent diabetic models; more importantly, long-term treatment of MBX-102 led to comparable efficacy compared with rosiglitazone while lacking the typical PPARγ side effects; MBX-102 induces less human adipocyte differentiation compared with rosiglitazone; in mesenchymal cells, MBX-102 does not inhibit the expression of osteoblastogenesis marker, and a high dose of MBX-102 can partly antagonize the rosiglitazone effect on osteoblast differentiation [92]. Interestingly, it is reported that different from the traditional PPARγ agonist, SR1664, a non-agonist PPARγ ligand that lacks classical PPARγ transcriptional agonism but still blocks PPARγ phosphorylation at Serine 273 by Cdk5 (cyclin-dependent kinase 5), exhibits potent anti-diabetic activity without causing fluid retention and weight gain; unlike rosiglitazone, SR1664 does not stimulate adipocyte differentiation or lipid accumulation, and does not affect the extent of calcification or the expression of osteoblast markers in MC3T3-E1 cells, suggesting that it may also eliminate the inhibition of bone formation seen with rosiglitazone [93,94]. However, it is unclear whether INT131, MBX-102, or

SR1664 treatment causes bone loss and increases bone resorption *in vivo*, in human or animal models. Therefore, these non-TZD PPARγ agonists are promising new diabetic drugs with fewer side effects, but comprehensive preclinical and clinical studies are required to fully examine their consequences on skeletal homeostasis.

Furthermore, unlike PPARγ agonists that induce bone loss via increasing bone resorption, PPARα agonists such as fenofibrate and wyeth 14643 directly inhibit osteoclast differentiation via blocking NFκB pathway [95,96]. Fenofibrate is currently used to treat hypercholesterolemia and hypertriglyceridemia. A recent study in ovariectomized rats indicates that fenofibrate could be beneficial for the skeleton [97]. In light of these findings, PPARα/γ dual agonists become a promising combination strategy for the treatment of type 2 diabetes mellitus to avoid a range of side effects. Among various dual PPARα/γ agonists, muraglitazar and tesaglitazar had completed phase III clinical trials, but had both been suspended in 2006 owing to safety concerns [98]. It has been reported that aleglitazar is a new, balanced, dual PPARα/γ agonist designed to minimize PPARγ-related side effects during the treatment of type 2 diabetes mellitus [99]. Similarly, indeglitazar is another drug on trial that has structural basis for PPAR pan-activity and partial agonistic response toward PPARγ; indeglitazar is less potent in promoting adipocyte differentiation and only partially effective in stimulating adiponectin gene expression compared with full PPARγ agonist rosiglitazone; evaluation *in vivo* confirmed the reduced adiponectin response in animal models of obesity and diabetes but revealed strong beneficial effects on glucose, triglycerides, cholesterol, body weight, and other metabolic parameters [100]. Nonetheless, preclinical evaluations on the pharmacological effects of these new compounds on bone mass, bone resorption, and bone formation are still needed to better predict how they affect bone safety in a clinical setting.

SYSTEMIC PPARγ ACTIVATION ENHANCES BONE RESORPTION BY BOTH OSTEOCLAST-AUTONOMOUS AND NON-AUTONOMOUS MECHANISMS

Osteoclastogenesis depends not only on the intrinsic differentiation potential of the osteoclast progenitors but also on the concentrations of various osteoclastogenic stimuli and modulators secreted by other cell types, some of which have also been shown to be regulated by PPARγ and TZDs. This indicates that the ultimate effects of TZDs on bone resorption are the sum of both their direct effects on osteoclast lineage and indirect effects from other cells and tissues.

Rankl and OPG

Encoded by tumor necrosis factor ligand superfamily member 11 gene (TNFSF11), RANKL, also known as osteoprotegerin ligand (OPGL), osteoclast differentiation factor (ODF), and TNF-related activation-induced cytokine (TRANCE), plays a key role in osteoclast differentiation. It is initially shown to be secreted from osteoblasts, but recently discovered to be predominantly secreted from osteocytes that are embedded in the bone matrix [101,102]. Its receptor RANK is highly expressed in both macrophage precursors and mature osteoclasts, and indispensable for the osteoclastogenic effects of RANKL [97]. As a decoy receptor for RANKL, osteoprotegerin (OPG) is capable of inhibiting osteoclast formation *in vitro* and bone resorption *in vivo* through blocking RANKL binding to RANK thus RANKL signaling [47,103].

It is reported that PPARγ regulates osteoclast differentiation by both acting on hematopoietic cells and influencing mesenchymal cells to control RANKL/OPG ratio. On the one hand, without changing RANK expression level, PPARγ deletion in hematopoietic lineages in the PPARγ$^{f/f}$-Tie2cre mice significantly reduces the number of tartrate-resistant acid phosphatase (TRAP) positive osteoclasts both *in vivo* and *in vitro* [20]. Importantly, bone marrow transplantation confirms that this is due to a hematopoietic cell-autonomous intrinsic defect in the RANKL-mediated osteoclast differentiation [20]. Furthermore, PPARγ deletion in hematopoietic lineage also substantially reduces RANKL induction of nuclear factor of activated T cells, cytoplasmic 1 (NFATc1), another key transcription factor that is critical for the late stage of osteoclast differentiation and maturation [20]. On the other hand, several clinical studies have shown that PPARγ agonists also affect OPG expression. It is reported that serum levels of OPG decreased in the pioglitazone-treated group, but were unchanged in the metformin group, after 24 weeks of treatment with pioglitazone or metformin in 67 type 2 diabetic patients [104]. A similar study also has shown that TZD treatment is associated with a decrease in plasma OPG levels, comparing 46 type 2 diabetic patients treated with TZDs with 152 type 2 diabetic patients receiving other oral anti-diabetes drugs [105]. In addition, rosiglitazone-induced bone resorption in aged mice has been reported to correlate with increased RANKL expression and thus RANKL/OPG ratio in bone [106]. These findings indicate that systemic PPARγ activation by its agonist increases osteoclastogenesis and bone resorption through not only osteoclast-autonomous differentiation enhancement, but also non-osteoclast-autonomous OPG reduction or RANKL induction, thereby an increased net availability of RANKL as the osteoclastogenic stimuli.

Wnt Antagonists: Sclerostin and Dkk1

In the adult skeletal system, osteocytes consist of 90–95% of all bone cells compared with 1–2% osteoclasts and 4–6% osteoblasts. Osteocytes have been shown to be the major cell type that secretes sclerostin (sost), a Wnt antagonist that has been shown to inhibit bone formation [107]. Our recent study reveals that suppression of Wnt signaling by β-catenin heterozygosity or synthetic Wnt inhibitors increases osteoclast differentiation and bone resorption [62]. This indicates that, as a Wnt antagonist, sclerostin may also enhance osteoclastogenesis. Genetic studies show that absence of sclerostin protein results in the high bone mass clinical disorder sclerosteosis. Consistently, sclerostin-transgenic mice exhibit bone loss and skeletal fragility [108]. Interestingly, it is reported that TZDs, including pioglitazone, rosiglitazone, and troglitazone, induce osteocyte apoptosis; apoptotic osteocytes express enhanced levels of sclerostin (sost) but not RANKL; and oestrogen prevents TZD-triggered osteocyte apoptosis and sclerostin induction [109]. Together, these findings suggest that TZD-induced bone resorption may be also partially mediated by the increased sclerostin expression as the result of osteocyte apoptosis.

Dickkopf-1 (DKK1) is another secreted inhibitor of Wnt signaling [110,111]. DKK1 has been shown to inhibit bone formation by suppressing osteoblastogenesis and promoting adipogenesis [112], and implicated to increase bone resorption by enhancing osteoclastogenesis [62]. In multiple myeloma patients, DKK1 derived from myeloma cells has also been reported to cause osteolytic lesions by diminishing bone formation and elevating bone resorption [113]. Interestingly, it is reported that rosiglitazone and pioglitazone rapidly increase DKK1 protein levels and secretion from both pre-adipocytes and mature adipocytes *in vitro*; and serum levels of DKK1 were also increased in several of the patients with type 2 diabetes after treatment with rosiglitazone for 90 days [114]. In light of these findings and the observation that TZDs also increase bone marrow adipogenesis, it will be important to determine whether TZD-induced bone resorption is also caused by an increase in DKK1 secretion.

PPARγ EFFECTS ON BONE RESORPTION ARE CONTEXT DEPENDENT

TZD-induced bone loss is attributable to the concerted decrease in bone formation and increase in bone resorption, both of which are required for the uncoupling of bone remodeling. However, the relative magnitude of these two effects varies among different studies, possibly because of the differences in the age and sex of the patients or experimental animals, the specific TZD compound used, and the dosage and duration of TZD treatment. This suggests that the regulation of bone homeostasis by PPARγ and TZDs is context dependent.

Aging and Metabolic State

Age plays an important role in influencing the effects of TZDs on bone turnover, a dynamic balance between bone resorption and bone formation. Over 60 years of age, this balance is compromised due to a progressive excess of bone resorption with a gradual decline in bone formation [115]. Rosiglitazone-induced bone loss in adult vs. old mice appears to associate with different changes in bone parameters: the bone loss in adult mice (6 months) is predominantly related to decreased osteoblast number and bone formation but sustained (thus relatively increased) bone resorption, while the bone loss in old mice (24 months) is predominantly related to increased osteoclast number and bone resorption without a concurrent elevation in bone formation [106]. Another study also supports this view: it shows that rosiglitazone-induced bone loss in ovariectomized rats resulted from enhanced bone resorption rather than inhibited bone formation [116]. This is further demonstrated in our recent investigation: 2 months of continuous rosiglitazone treatment in 8–10-month-old mice led to significantly increased osteoclast number and bone resorption [21]. It would be interesting to further delineate the mechanisms for how aging exerts such profound effects on bone and TZD-induced bone loss; to that end, several hypotheses have been proposed including aging-associated changes in oxidative stress and hormones.

This age-dependent regulation suggests that other metabolic states may also influence the effects of TZDs on bone. For example, epidemiological studies suggest that skeletal fragility is already increased in type 2 diabetes mellitus [117,118], potentially due to the inhibition of osteoblast differentiation and function by hyperglycemia-associated ROS (reactive oxygen species) accumulation and/or glucose toxicity [119–121]. Thus, rosiglitazone-induced bone loss may be exacerbated in diabetic patients compared with healthy individuals. An important question for future study is whether and how different metabolic states such as obesity, diabetes, and insulin resistance regulate the relative effects of TZDs on bone resorption versus bone formation.

HPG Axis

The metabolic landscape is shaped by an intricate network of neuronal and endocrine signaling pathways. The past decade has witnessed a series of ground-breaking discoveries revealing that bone remodeling is intimately connected to the central nervous system (CNS) [122]. A recent study has unveiled an unknown role for CNS PPARγ in the regulation of energy balance [123]: both acute and chronic activation of CNS PPARγ, by either TZDs or hypothalamic overexpression of a fusion protein consisting of PPARγ and the viral transcriptional activator VP16 (VP16-PPARγ), led to positive energy balance in rats, including cumulative food intake and body fat gain. Blocking the endogenous activation of CNS PPARγ with pharmacological antagonist GW9662 or reducing its expression with shRNA led to negative energy balance, restored leptin sensitivity in high fat diet-fed rats and blocked the hyperphagic response to oral TZD treatment [123]. These findings implicate that CNS PPARγ may also contribute to the regulation of bone mass and bone resorption by TZDs, potentially via the hypothalamic–pituitary–gonadal (HPG) relay.

Hormones in the HPG axis play important roles in maintaining bone homeostasis (Fig. 10.3). For example, follicle-stimulating hormone (FSH), derived from pituitary, has been proposed to regulate bone mass via several controversial and contradictory mechanisms. In perimenopausal women, increase of serum FSH, but not loss of estrogen, has been reported to better correlate with bone turnover and/or BMD across the menopause transition [124–126]. It has

been shown that FSH enhances osteoclastogenesis by activating MEK/Erk, NF-κB, and Akt; furthermore, FSHβ KO mice and FSH receptor (FSHR) KO mice are resistant to bone loss despite severe hypogonadism; and $FSH\beta+/-$ mice exhibit increased bone mass and decreased osteoclastic resorption with normal ovarian function, suggesting that the skeletal action of FSH is estrogen independent [127]. In contrast, two recent reports have provided opposing evidence. First, in a prospective clinical study, it has been found that suppression of FSH secretion by a GnRH agonist failed to reduce bone resorption markers in postmenopausal women [128]. Second, using FSH transgenic mice, it has been shown that FSH has dose-dependent anabolic (rather than catabolic) effects on bone, via an ovary-dependent and non-bone cell-autonomous mechanism [129]. PPARγ is highly expressed in the pituitary [130]. It has been reported that PPARγ and TZDs can alter the secretion and function of pituitary hormones. For example, pituitary-specific deletion of PPARγ increases luteinizing hormone (LH) levels in female mice, and decreases FSH levels in male mice [131]; and TZD activation of PPARγ inhibits LH secretion [132] and gonadotropin-releasing hormone (GnRH) signaling [131]. Together, these reports warrant future investigations on the hypothesis that TZDs may partially exert their effects on

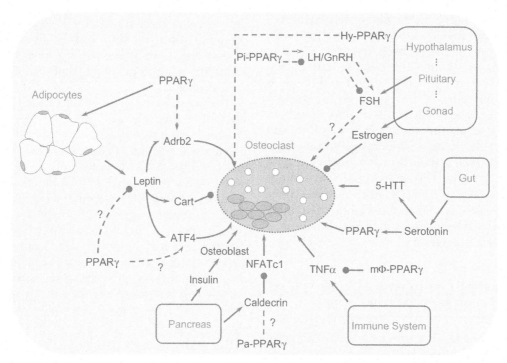

FIGURE 10.3 **PPARγ effects on bone resorption are context dependent.** The regulation of osteoclastogenesis by PPARγ and TZDs depends not only on cell-autonomous effects on osteoclast differentiation, but also on systemic effects via other tissues such as brain, pituitary, gonad, fat, gut, pancreas, and the immune system, by regulating the function of a complex network of neuronal, endocrine, and immunological signaling pathways (see text for details). Future studies are required to delineate whether and how this complex crosstalk modulates TZD actions in bone under a diverse physiological and pathological context.

bone resorption by regulating pituitary hormones such as LH, GnRH, and FSH.

Gonadal steroids such as estrogen are osteo-protective, and estrogen decline plays an important role in postmenopausal osteoporosis. First, estrogen is implied to decrease the osteoclastic resorption pit in bone by regulating several transcription factors (c-fos, c-jun, etc.) and inflammatory cytokines (IL-1RI, IL-1RII, etc.) [133]. Second, our recent study reveals that estrogen loss in mice by ovariectomy stimulates osteoclast progenitors to proliferate and differentiate; suggesting estrogen also inhibits osteoclastogenesis *in vivo* [33]. Third, estrogen has been shown to promote osteoclast apoptosis [134,135]. This suggests that estrogen antagonizes osteoclast differentiation and function, and potentially suppresses PPARγ-stimulated osteoclas-togenesis. Consistently, estrogen has been shown to be protective against TZD-induced bone loss. For example, TZD-induced bone loss is more significant in postmeno-pausal women [22,136,137]; and estrogen significantly reduces TZD-induced adipogenesis [138], osteocyte apoptosis, and sclerostin upregulation [139]. Interest-ingly, a recent study shows that TZDs (rosiglitazone or pioglitazone) also inhibit estrogen synthesis in human granulosa cells by interfering with androgen binding to aromatase, thus directly affecting estrogen production in human ovarian cells [140]. Together, these findings suggest another potential contributing mechanism for TZD-induced osteoclast activation and bone loss, which may involve the suppression of estrogen function and/or production. In future investigations, it would be important to further examine the *in vivo* effects of TZDs on estrogen synthesis and activity in animal models and in clinical trials.

Gut and Pancreas

It is reported that skeletal remodeling can also be modulated by a crosstalk between bone and gut (Fig. 10.3). First, evidence indicates that gut-derived serotonin (5-HT) can functionally inhibit bone forma-tion: the biosynthesis of the gut-derived serotonin depends on the rate-limiting enzyme tryptophan hydroxylase 1 (Tph1), which is suppressed by Lrp5 (LDL receptor-related protein 5); gut-specific activation of Lrp5, or inactivation of Tph1, increases bone mass and prevents ovariectomy-induced bone loss [124]. Moreover, it is shown that serotonin (5-HT) can enhance osteoclastogenesis *in vitro* through its transporter (5-HTT): serotonin treatment promotes osteoclast differ-entiation by activating NFκB; conversely, the 5-HTT inhibitor fluoxetine (Prozac) reduces osteoclast differen-tiation [141]. Intriguingly, PPARγ is found to respond to serotonin metabolism as a downstream receptor: sero-tonin metabolites act as endogenous PPARγ agonists to regulate macrophage function and adipogenesis; moreover, mutational analyses on receptor-mediated transcription and co-activator binding reveal that serotonin metabolites use distinct coregulator and/or heterodimer interfaces from the previously described fatty-acid metabolites [142]. Therefore, a provocative hypothesis is that gut-derived serotonin may inhibit bone formation and stimulate bone resorption, at least in part, via activation of PPARγ; and the effects of rosi-glitazone on bone may be also influenced by the endog-enous serum serotonin levels. LP533401, a novel small molecule inhibitor of Tph-1, has been shown to prevent and rescue osteoporosis in ovariectomized mice and rats [143]. Thus, inhibitors of Tph-1 or gut-derived serotonin may become a new class of bone anabolic and anti-cata-bolic drugs that can be used as a combination therapy to prevent TZD-induced bone loss in diabetic patients.

Similarly, skeletal homeostasis may be also modu-lated by a crosstalk between bone and pancreas (Fig. 10.3). Caldecrin/chymotrypsin C is a novel secre-tory-type serine protease that was originally isolated as a serum calcium-decreasing factor from the pancreas. Recent studies reveal that caldecrin inhibits osteoclasto-genesis by preventing a phospholipase C γ1-mediated Ca^{2+} oscillation—calcineurin—NFATc1 pathway, inde-pendent of its protease activity [144,145]. Conversely, the acidic environment in the bone resorption pit has been shown to be necessary for the decarboxylation and thus activation of osteocalcin [146], an endocrine hormone secreted from the osteoblast that can increase insulin secretion from the pancreas [128−131], suggest-ing that osteoclast activity also feeds back to pancreatic function. Future studies are required to answer several intriguing questions such as how PPARγ and TZDs regulate caldecrin expression in the pancreas, as well as whether TZD-induced bone resorption contributes to its beneficial effects on glucose metabolism and insulin sensitivity.

Energy Metabolism

PPARγ also takes part in the crosstalk between bone remodeling and energy metabolism (Fig. 10.3). It is first shown that leptin, an important adipose-derived hormone (adipokine), regulates not only energy metab-olism but also bone remodeling. Leptin modulates bone resorption via two distinct and antagonistic path-ways: on the one hand, leptin-activated sympathetic signaling functions through β-2-adrenergic receptor (Adrb2) on osteoblasts to increase RANKL secretion and thereby promote osteoclast differentiation; on the other hand, leptin increases the expression of the neuro-peptide cocaine amphetamine-regulated transcript (CART), which inhibits RANKL expression in osteoblast and thereby suppresses osteoclast differentiation and bone resorption [147]. The latter mechanism appears to be dominant because *ob/ob* mice that lack leptin display elevated bone resorption [147]. PPARγ and leptin have been suggested to be mutually inhibitory. *In vitro*, TZD activation of PPARγ represses leptin expression in differentiated 3T3-L1 adipocytes and primary rat adipocytes [148,149]; conversely, leptin downregulates PPARγ mRNA levels in primary human monocyte-derived macrophages, accompanied by a reduction in several of its target genes including ABCA1 [150]. *In vivo*, heterozygous PPARγ-deficient (PPARγ+/−) mice exhibits a higher serum leptin level than wt littermates [16]. PPARγ has also been shown to inhibit Adrb2 expression by directly binding and transcriptionally repressing the Adrb2 promoter in vascular smooth muscle cells (VMSCs): VMSC-selective PPARγ deletion is associated with increased Adrb2 response and enhanced sensitivity to Adrb2 agonists *in vivo*; conversely, ligand activation of PPARγ represses Adrb2 expression [151]. These findings suggest that TZD-induced bone loss may be also contributed by suppressing leptin function and the sympathetic tone. However, in terms of the regulation of osteoclastogenesis and bone resorption, how exactly PPARγ and TZDs intersect with leptin and CART signaling in the hypothalamus, as well as Adrb2 signaling in osteoblasts, is still an open question (Fig. 10.3).

Recent studies have revealed that ATF4 (activating transcription factor 4) plays an important role in the regulation of osteoclastogenesis in both osteoclast autonomous and non-autonomous manner. On the one hand, it is shown that ATF4 deletion severely inhibits osteoclast differentiation *in vitro* and *in vivo*; TRAP promoter-targeted ATF4 overexpression in the osteoclasts highly increases osteoclast differentiation and bone resorption; ATF4 is required for both M-CSF induction of RANK and RANKL induction of NFATc1 expression and MAPKs activation [152]. On the other hand, ATF4 has been reported also to stimulate osteoclastogenesis indirectly via osteoblasts: sympathetic tone signals in the osteoblasts not only to inhibit the phosphorylation of CREB (cAMP-responsive element-binding protein) and thus decrease osteoblast proliferation, but also to promote the phosphorylation of ATF4 and thus increase the expression of RANKL, which then stimulates osteoclast differentiation [153]. Provocatively, ATF4 expression can be induced by PPARγ agonist in breast cancer cell lines MCF-7 and MDA-MB-231 [154], implicating the possibility that PPARγ may also promote osteoclastogenesis by inducing ATF4 in osteoblast and/or osteoclasts. Together, these evidences suggest that PPARγ regulation of osteoclastogenesis and TZD-induced bone resorption may also crosstalk with the leptin/CART/Adrb2/CREB/ATF4 pathway via a complex signaling network, which remains to be delineated in the future investigations (Fig. 10.3).

Furthermore, a recent study reveals that insulin, secreted from the pancreas, signals through the insulin receptor on osteoblast to suppress OPG expression and thus enhance osteoclastogenesis and bone resorption [146] (Fig. 10.3). The acidic environment in the bone resorption pit, in turn, facilitates the decarboxylation, activation, and secretion of osteocalcin from the bone matrix, thereby forming a feed-forward loop to promote glucose metabolism by increasing insulin secretion, insulin sensitivity, and energy expenditure [146]. In light of the profound insulin-sensitizing effects of TZDs, a provocative question is that whether PPARγ/TZD activation of bone resorption is also partially contributed by its enhancement of insulin signaling in osteoblast.

Immune System

The effects of TZDs on osteoclastogenesis are also influenced by the immunologic state (Fig. 10.3). Numerous studies have shown that PPARγ and TZDs possess anti-inflammatory properties [24,120–122]. Inflammation and osteoclastogenesis are two highly integrated processes in certain bone diseases such as osteoarthritis (OA). Osteoarthritis is a common age-related disease that affects about 15% of the general population and 60% of people in the second half of their lifespan, with a higher prevalence in women compared to men [155]. Chondrocyte damage and deterioration is a critical event in osteoarthritis, and a number of chondrocyte macromolecules have been shown to have significant immunogenic properties. These components are released into the synovial fluid and are phagocyted by synovial lining macrophages, perpetuating the inflammation of the synovial membrane through the synthesis of pro-inflammatory mediators [155]. Human chondrocytes express predominantly PPARγ1 mRNA and the levels of PPARγ1 are decreased in osteoarthritis in comparison with normal chondrocytes, which indicates that inhibited PPARγ expression in osteoarthritis chondrocytes might reflect increased expression of inflammatory and catabolic factors [155]. Interleukin-1β (IL-1β) and tumor necrosis factor α (TNFα) are crucial regulators of inflammation and play a pivotal role in osteoarthritis. PPARγ ligands inhibit IL-1β-induced production of nitric oxide (NO) and matrix metalloproteinase 13 (MMP13) in human chondrocytes [155]. Consequently, agonists of PPARγ inhibit inflammation and reduce synthesis of cartilage degradation products both *in vitro* and *in vivo*, and reduce the development/progression of cartilage lesions in osteoarthritis animal models [155].

Osteoclastogenesis is also involved in the etiology of osteoarthritis. RANKL and its decoy receptor OPG are physiologically expressed in normal chondrocytes and synovial fibroblast. According to the subchondral bone mass, osteoarthritis can be distinguished into two subpopulations, low-OA and high-OA: in low-OA status, the OPG/RANKL ratio is low and osteoclastogenesis is continuously activated, resulting in excessive bone resorption and diminished subchondral bone thickness; while in high-OA status, the OPG/RANKL ratio is high and osteoclastogenesis is continuously inhibited, resulting in low bone resorption and normal subchondral bone thickness [156]. Importantly, growing evidence suggest that osteoclastogenesis can occur via non-canonical pathways in which RANKL can be substituted or potentiated by other growth factors including TNFα, LIGHT (TNFSF14), IL-6, TGFβ, APRIL, BAFF, NGF, IGF-I, or IGF-II [157–164]. Inhibition of bone resorption triggered by inflammatory stimuli such as TNFα is an important therapeutic approach to prevent the bone destruction occurring in inflammatory bone loss lesions. Although TZDs can stimulate RANKL-induced osteoclastogenesis [20,21,62], recent reports indicate that TZDs can inhibit TNFα-induced osteoclastogenesis (Fig. 10.3), in part by downregulating MCP-1 and NFATc1 expression [165–167]. Consequently, rosiglitazone inhibits inflammatory bone loss such as that induced in a rat model of experimental periodontitis [165]. Although more *in vivo* studies are required, these findings suggest that the anti-inflammatory effect of TZDs may be dominant over their pro-osteoclastogenic effect when the osteoclast stimuli originate from immune cell types activated by inflammatory cytokines. Thus, the physiologic and pathologic environment must be considered as a whole to understand the systemic effect of TZDs on bone resorption and skeletal integrity.

CONCLUSION

Emerging evidence reveals that PPARγ is a critical regulator of osteoclast differentiation and bone resorption by playing dual roles: the expression of PPARγ promotes osteoclast lineage specification; and the activation of PPARγ by agonists, such as the diabetic drug TZD, accelerates osteoclast differentiation by suppressing β-catenin while activating c-fos, PGC-1β, and ERRα. Furthermore, PPARγ regulation of bone resorption may be also influenced by non-osteoclast-autonomous effects of systemic TZD treatments, and dependent on the metabolic and immunological context. The future of TZD as a diabetic drug is currently tenuous mainly because of its cardiovascular side effects. Three independent metaanalyses have shown that TZDs are associated with an increased risk of myocardial ischemia [168]. These cardiovascular and skeletal side effects of TZDs suggest a need for alternative therapeutic strategies.

To this end, mechanistic understanding of cell type-specific gene regulation by PPARγ will facilitate the design of improved diabetic drugs, such as selective PPARγ regulators, which retain the insulin-sensitizing benefits but dampen the detrimental side effects. What is equally significant and promising, in light of the dual roles of PPARγ in suppressing bone formation and stimulating bone resorption, is that bone-specific PPARγ antagonists may represent a potential therapeutic strategy for the simultaneous anabolic and anti-catabolic treatment of skeletal fragility.

Acknowledgments

We thank all the investigators whose studies contributed to the understanding of PPARγ and TZD actions but could not be cited here because of space limitations. Y. Wan is a Virginia Murchison Linthicum Scholar in Medical Research. This work is supported by the University of Texas Southwestern Medical Center Endowed Scholar Startup Fund, a BD Biosciences Research Grant Award, CPRIT (RP100841), March of Dimes (#5-FY10-1), The Welch Foundation (I-1751), and NIH (R01 DK089113).

Conflict of Interest

The authors declare that they have no financial conflict of interest.

References

[1] Evans RM, Barish GD, Wang YX. PPARs and the complex journey to obesity. Nat Med 2004;10(4):355–61.

[2] Tontonoz P, Spiegelman BM. Fat and beyond: the diverse biology of PPARgamma. Annu Rev Biochem 2008;77:289–312.

[3] Jones D. Potential remains for PPAR-targeted drugs. Nat Rev Drug Discov 2010;9(9):668–9.

[4] Tontonoz P, Hu E, Graves RA, Budavari AI, Spiegelman BM. mPPAR gamma 2: tissue-specific regulator of an adipocyte enhancer. Genes Dev 1994;8(10):1224–34.

[5] Tontonoz P, Hu E, Spiegelman BM. Stimulation of adipogenesis in fibroblasts by PPAR gamma 2, a lipid-activated transcription factor. Cell 1994;79(7):1147–56.

[6] Chawla A, Schwarz EJ, Dimaculangan DD, Lazar MA. Peroxisome proliferator-activated receptor (PPAR) gamma: adipose-predominant expression and induction early in adipocyte differentiation. Endocrinology 1994;135(2):798–800.

[7] Kliewer SA, Forman BM, Blumberg B, Ong ES, Borgmeyer U, Mangelsdorf DJ, et al. Differential expression and activation of a family of murine peroxisome proliferator-activated receptors. Proc Natl Acad Sci USA 1994;91(15):7355–9.

[8] Zhu Y, Alvares K, Huang Q, Rao MS, Reddy JK. Cloning of a new member of the peroxisome proliferator-activated receptor gene family from mouse liver. J Biol Chem 1993;268(36):26817–20.

[9] Krey G, Keller H, Mahfoudi A, Medin J, Ozato K, Dreyer C, et al. Xenopus peroxisome proliferator activated receptors: genomic organization, response element recognition, heterodimer formation with retinoid X receptor and activation by fatty acids. J Steroid Biochem Mol Biol 1993;47(1–6):65–73.

[10] Zhu Y, Qi C, Korenberg JR, Chen XN, Noya D, Rao MS, et al. Structural organization of mouse peroxisome proliferator-activated receptor gamma (mPPAR gamma) gene: alternative promoter use and different splicing yield two mPPAR gamma isoforms. Proc Natl Acad Sci USA 1995;92(17):7921–5.

[11] Fajas L, Auboeuf D, Raspe E, Schoonjans K, Lefebvre AM, Saladin R, et al. The organization, promoter analysis, and expression of the human PPARgamma gene. J Biol Chem 1997;272(30):18779–89.

[12] Vidal-Puig A, Jimenez-Linan M, Lowell BB, Hamann A, Hu E, Spiegelman B, et al. Regulation of PPAR gamma gene expression by nutrition and obesity in rodents. J Clin Invest 1996;97(11):2553–61.

[13] Vidal-Puig AJ, Considine RV, Jimenez-Linan M, Werman A, Pories WJ, Caro JF, et al. Peroxisome proliferator-activated receptor gene expression in human tissues. Effects of obesity, weight loss, and regulation by insulin and glucocorticoids. J Clin Invest 1997;99(10):2416–22.

[14] Wan Y. PPARgamma in bone homeostasis. Trends Endocrinol Metab 2010;21(12):722–8.

[15] Pittenger MF, Mackay AM, Beck SC, Jaiswal RK, Douglas R, Mosca JD, et al. Multilineage potential of adult human mesenchymal stem cells. Science 1999;284(5411):143–7.

[16] Akune T, Ohba S, Kamekura S, Yamaguchi M, Chung UI, Kubota N, et al. PPARgamma insufficiency enhances osteogenesis through osteoblast formation from bone marrow progenitors. J Clin Invest 2004;113(6):846–55.

[17] Barak Y, Nelson MC, Ong ES, Jones YZ, Ruiz-Lozano P, Chien KR, et al. PPAR gamma is required for placental, cardiac, and adipose tissue development. Mol Cell 1999;4(4):585–95.

[18] Kubota N, Terauchi Y, Miki H, Tamemoto H, Yamauchi T, Komeda K, et al. PPAR gamma mediates high-fat diet-induced adipocyte hypertrophy and insulin resistance. Mol Cell 1999;4(4):597–609.

[19] Rosen ED, Sarraf P, Troy AE, Bradwin G, Moore K, Milstone DS, et al. PPAR gamma is required for the differentiation of adipose tissue in vivo and in vitro. Mol Cell 1999;4(4):611–7.

[20] Wan Y, Chong LW, Evans RM. PPAR-gamma regulates osteoclastogenesis in mice. Nat Med 2007;13(12):1496–503.

[21] Wei W, Wang X, Yang M, Smith LC, Dechow PC, Wan Y. PGC1beta mediates PPARgamma activation of osteoclastogenesis and rosiglitazone-induced bone loss. Cell Metab 2010;11(6):503–16.

[22] Zinman B, Haffner SM, Herman WH, Holman RR, Lachin JM, Kravitz BG, et al. Effect of rosiglitazone, metformin, and glyburide on bone biomarkers in patients with type 2 diabetes. J Clin Endocrinol Metab 2010;95(1):134–42.

[23] Novack DV, Teitelbaum SL. The osteoclast: friend or foe? Annu Rev Pathol 2008;3:457–84.

[24] Tolar J, Teitelbaum SL, Orchard PJ. Osteopetrosis. N Engl J Med 2004;351(27):2839–49.

[25] Tondravi MM, McKercher SR, Anderson K, Erdmann JM, Quiroz M, Maki R, et al. Osteopetrosis in mice lacking haematopoietic transcription factor PU.1. Nature 1997;386(6620):81–4.

[26] Edwards JR, Mundy GR. Advances in osteoclast biology: old findings and new insights from mouse models. Nat Rev Rheumatol 2011;7(4):235–43.

[27] Scott EW, Simon MC, Anastasi J, Singh H. Requirement of transcription factor PU.1 in the development of multiple hematopoietic lineages. Science 1994;265(5178):1573–7.

[28] Heinz S, Benner C, Spann N, Bertolino E, Lin YC, Laslo P, et al. Simple combinations of lineage-determining transcription factors prime cis-regulatory elements required for macrophage and B cell identities. Mol Cell 2010;38(4):576–89.

[29] Ricote M, Li AC, Willson TM, Kelly CJ, Glass CK. The peroxisome proliferator-activated receptor-gamma is a negative regulator of macrophage activation. Nature 1998;391(6662): 79–82.

[30] Tontonoz P, Nagy L, Alvarez JG, Thomazy VA, Evans RM. PPARgamma promotes monocyte/macrophage differentiation and uptake of oxidized LDL. Cell 1998;93(2):241–52.

[31] Lefterova MI, Steger DJ, Zhuo D, Qatanani M, Mullican SE, Tuteja G, et al. Cell-specific determinants of peroxisome proliferator-activated receptor gamma function in adipocytes and macrophages. Mol Cell Biol 2010;30(9):2078–89.

[32] Tang W, Zeve D, Suh JM, Bosnakovski D, Kyba M, Hammer RE, et al. White fat progenitor cells reside in the adipose vasculature. Science 2008;322(5901):583–6.

[33] Wei W, Zeve D, Wang X, Du Y, Tang W, Dechow PC, et al. Osteoclast progenitors reside in PPARγ-expressing bone marrow cell population. Mol Cell Biol 2011;31(23):4692–705.

[34] Tsai FY, Keller G, Kuo FC, Weiss M, Chen J, Rosenblatt M, et al. An early haematopoietic defect in mice lacking the transcription factor GATA-2. Nature 1994;371(6494):221–6.

[35] Yamane T, Kunisada T, Yamazaki H, Nakano T, Orkin SH, Hayashi SI. Sequential requirements for SCL/tal-1, GATA-2, macrophage colony-stimulating factor, and osteoclast differentiation factor/osteoprotegerin ligand in osteoclast development. Exp Hematol 2000;28(7):833–40.

[36] Fujiwara Y, Browne CP, Cunniff K, Goff SC, Orkin SH. Arrested development of embryonic red cell precursors in mouse embryos lacking transcription factor GATA-1. Proc Natl Acad Sci USA 1996;93(22):12355–8.

[37] Pevny L, Simon MC, Robertson E, Klein WH, Tsai SF, D'Agati V, et al. Erythroid differentiation in chimaeric mice blocked by a targeted mutation in the gene for transcription factor GATA-1. Nature 1991;349(6306):257–60.

[38] Shivdasani RA, Fujiwara Y, McDevitt MA, Orkin SH. A lineage-selective knockout establishes the critical role of transcription factor GATA-1 in megakaryocyte growth and platelet development. EMBO J 1997;16(13):3965–73.

[39] Hodgkinson CA, Moore KJ, Nakayama A, Steingrimsson E, Copeland NG, Jenkins NA, et al. Mutations at the mouse microphthalmia locus are associated with defects in a gene encoding a novel basic-helix-loop-helix-zipper protein. Cell 1993;74(2):395–404.

[40] Grabacka M, Placha W, Urbanska K, Laidler P, Plonka PM, Reiss K. PPAR gamma regulates MITF and beta-catenin expression and promotes a differentiated phenotype in mouse melanoma S91. Pigment Cell Melanoma Res 2008;21(3): 388–96.

[41] Hu R, Sharma SM, Bronisz A, Srinivasan R, Sankar U, Ostrowski MC. Eos, MITF, and PU.1 recruit corepressors to osteoclast-specific genes in committed myeloid progenitors. Mol Cell Biol 2007;27(11):4018–27.

[42] Sharma SM, Bronisz A, Hu R, Patel K, Mansky KC, Sif S, et al. MITF and PU.1 recruit p38 MAPK and NFATc1 to target genes during osteoclast differentiation. J Biol Chem 2007;282(21): 15921–9.

[43] Scheven BA, Visser JW, Nijweide PJ. In vitro osteoclast generation from different bone marrow fractions, including a highly enriched haematopoietic stem cell population. Nature 1986;321(6065):79–81.

[44] Yoshida H, Hayashi S, Kunisada T, Ogawa M, Nishikawa S, Okamura H, et al. The murine mutation osteopetrosis is in the coding region of the macrophage colony stimulating factor gene. Nature 1990;345(6274):442–4.

[45] Boyle WJ, Simonet WS, Lacey DL. Osteoclast differentiation and activation. Nature 2003;423(6937):337–42.

[46] Lacey DL, Timms E, Tan HL, Kelley MJ, Dunstan CR, Burgess T, et al. Osteoprotegerin ligand is a cytokine that regulates osteoclast differentiation and activation. Cell 1998; 93(2):165–76.

[47] Yasuda H, Shima N, Nakagawa N, Yamaguchi K, Kinosaki M, Mochizuki S, et al. Osteoclast differentiation factor is a ligand for osteoprotegerin/osteoclastogenesis-inhibitory factor and is identical to TRANCE/RANKL. Proc Natl Acad Sci USA 1998;95(7):3597–602.

[48] Almeida M, Ambrogini E, Han L, Manolagas SC, Jilka RL. Increased lipid oxidation causes oxidative stress, increased peroxisome proliferator-activated receptor-gamma expression, and diminished pro-osteogenic Wnt signaling in the skeleton. J Biol Chem 2009;284(40):27438–48.

[49] Funk CD, Chen XS, Johnson EN, Zhao L. Lipoxygenase genes and their targeted disruption. Prostaglandins Other Lipid Mediat 2002:68–9. 303–12.

[50] Nagy L, Tontonoz P, Alvarez JG, Chen H, Evans RM. Oxidized LDL regulates macrophage gene expression through ligand activation of PPARgamma. Cell 1998;93(2):229–40.

[51] Schild RL, Schaiff WT, Carlson MG, Cronbach EJ, Nelson DM, Sadovsky Y. The activity of PPAR gamma in primary human trophoblasts is enhanced by oxidized lipids. J Clin Endocrinol Metab 2002;87(3):1105–10.

[52] Zhang DE, Hetherington CJ, Chen HM, Tenen DG. The macrophage transcription factor PU.1 directs tissue-specific expression of the macrophage colony-stimulating factor receptor. Mol Cell Biol 1994;14(1):373–81.

[53] Pahl HL, Scheibe RJ, Zhang DE, Chen HM, Galson DL, Maki RA, et al. The proto-oncogene PU.1 regulates expression of the myeloid-specific CD11b promoter. J Biol Chem 1993; 268(7):5014–20.

[54] Grigoriadis AE, Wang ZQ, Cecchini MG, Hofstetter W, Felix R, Fleisch HA, et al. c-Fos: a key regulator of osteoclast-macrophage lineage determination and bone remodeling. Science 1994;266(5184):443–8.

[55] Logan CY, Nusse R. The Wnt signaling pathway in development and disease. Annu Rev Cell Dev Biol 2004;20:781–810.

[56] Day TF, Guo X, Garrett-Beal L, Yang Y. Wnt/beta-catenin signaling in mesenchymal progenitors controls osteoblast and chondrocyte differentiation during vertebrate skeletogenesis. Dev Cell 2005;8(5):739–50.

[57] Hill TP, Spater D, Taketo MM, Birchmeier W, Hartmann C. Canonical Wnt/beta-catenin signaling prevents osteoblasts from differentiating into chondrocytes. Dev Cell 2005;8(5):727–38.

[58] Glass 2nd DA, Bialek P, Ahn JD, Starbuck M, Patel MS, Clevers H, et al. Canonical Wnt signaling in differentiated osteoblasts controls osteoclast differentiation. Dev Cell 2005; 8(5):751–64.

[59] Holmen SL, Zylstra CR, Mukherjee A, Sigler RE, Faugere MC, Bouxsein ML, et al. Essential role of beta-catenin in postnatal bone acquisition. J Biol Chem 2005;280(22):21162–8.

[60] Bennett CN, Longo KA, Wright WS, Suva LJ, Lane TF, Hankenson KD, et al. Regulation of osteoblastogenesis and bone mass by Wnt10b. Proc Natl Acad Sci USA 2005; 102(9):3324–9.

[61] Kang S, Bennett CN, Gerin I, Rapp LA, Hankenson KD, Macdougald OA. Wnt signaling stimulates osteoblastogenesis of mesenchymal precursors by suppressing CCAAT/enhancer-binding protein alpha and peroxisome proliferator-activated receptor gamma. J Biol Chem 2007;282(19):14515–24.

[62] Wei W, Zeve D, Suh JM, Wang X, Du Y, Zerwekh JE, et al. Biphasic and dosage-dependent regulation of osteoclastogenesis by β-catenin. Mol Cell Biol 2011;31(23):4706–19.

[63] Takada I, Mihara M, Suzawa M, Ohtake F, Kobayashi S, Igarashi M, et al. A histone lysine methyltransferase activated by non-canonical Wnt signalling suppresses PPAR-gamma transactivation. Nat Cell Biol 2007;9(11):1273–85.

[64] Liu J, Farmer SR. Regulating the balance between peroxisome proliferator-activated receptor gamma and beta-catenin signaling during adipogenesis. A glycogen synthase kinase 3beta phosphorylation-defective mutant of beta-catenin inhibits expression of a subset of adipogenic genes. J Biol Chem 2004;279(43):45020–7.

[65] Liu J, Wang H, Zuo Y, Farmer SR. Functional interaction between peroxisome proliferator-activated receptor gamma and beta-catenin. Mol Cell Biol 2006;26(15):5827–37.

[66] Moldes M, Zuo Y, Morrison RF, Silva D, Park BH, Liu J, et al. Peroxisome-proliferator-activated receptor gamma suppresses Wnt/beta-catenin signalling during adipogenesis. Biochem J 2003;376(Pt 3):607–13.

[67] Sharma C, Pradeep A, Wong L, Rana A, Rana B. Peroxisome proliferator-activated receptor gamma activation can regulate beta-catenin levels via a proteasome-mediated and adenomatous polyposis coli-independent pathway. J Biol Chem 2004;279(34):35583–94.

[68] Ishii KA, Fumoto T, Iwai K, Takeshita S, Ito M, Shimohata N, et al. Coordination of PGC-1beta and iron uptake in mitochondrial biogenesis and osteoclast activation. Nat Med 2009;15(3):259–66.

[69] Sato K, Suematsu A, Nakashima T, Takemoto-Kimura S, Aoki K, Morishita Y, et al. Regulation of osteoclast differentiation and function by the CaMK-CREB pathway. Nat Med 2006;12(12): 1410–6.

[70] Gallet M, Vanacker JM. ERR receptors as potential targets in osteoporosis. Trends Endocrinol Metab 2010;21(10):637–41.

[71] Giguere V. Transcriptional control of energy homeostasis by the estrogen-related receptors. Endocr Rev 2008;29(6):677–96.

[72] Villena JA, Kralli A. ERRalpha: a metabolic function for the oldest orphan. Trends Endocrinol Metab 2008;19(8):269–76.

[73] Kamei Y, Ohizumi H, Fujitani Y, Nemoto T, Tanaka T, Takahashi N, et al. PPARgamma coactivator 1beta/ERR ligand 1 is an ERR protein ligand, whose expression induces a high-energy expenditure and antagonizes obesity. Proc Natl Acad Sci USA 2003;100(21):12378–83.

[74] Sonoda J, Laganiere J, Mehl IR, Barish GD, Chong LW, Li X, et al. Nuclear receptor ERR alpha and coactivator PGC-1 beta are effectors of IFN-gamma-induced host defense. Genes Dev 2007;21(15):1909–20.

[75] Menon P, Yin G, Smolock EM, Zuscik MJ, Yan C, Berk BC. GPCR kinase 2 interacting protein 1 (GIT1) regulates osteoclast function and bone mass. J Cell Physiol 2010;225(3):777–85.

[76] Pang J, Xu X, Getman MR, Shi X, Belmonte SL, Michaloski H, et al. G protein coupled receptor kinase 2 interacting protein 1 (GIT1) is a novel regulator of mitochondrial biogenesis in heart. J Mol Cell Cardiol 2011;51(5):769–76.

[77] Gingery A, Bradley E, Shaw A, Oursler MJ. Phosphatidylinositol 3-kinase coordinately activates the MEK/ERK and AKT/NFkappaB pathways to maintain osteoclast survival. J Cell Biochem 2003;89(1):165–79.

[78] Gao M, Wang J, Wang W, Liu J, Wong CW. Phosphatidylinositol 3-kinase affects mitochondrial function in part through inducing peroxisome proliferator-activated receptor gamma coactivator-1beta expression. Br J Pharmacol 2011;162(4):1000–8.

[79] Mirebeau-Prunier D, Le Pennec S, Jacques C, Gueguen N, Poirier J, Malthiery Y, et al. Estrogen-related receptor alpha and PGC-1-related coactivator constitute a novel complex mediating the biogenesis of functional mitochondria. FEBS J 2010; 277(3):713–25.

[80] Bonnelye E, Saltel F, Chabadel A, Zirngibl RA, Aubin JE, Jurdic P. Involvement of the orphan nuclear estrogen receptor-related receptor alpha in osteoclast adhesion and trans-migration. J Mol Endocrinol 2010;45(6):365–77.

[81] Zhang Y, Ma K, Sadana P, Chowdhury F, Gaillard S, Wang F, et al. Estrogen-related receptors stimulate pyruvate dehydrogenase kinase isoform 4 gene expression. J Biol Chem 2006;281(52):39897–906.

[82] Wang Y, Liu W, Masuyama R, Fukuyama R, Ito M, Zhang Q, et al. Pyruvate dehydrogenase kinase 4 induces bone loss at unloading by promoting osteoclastogenesis. Bone 2012;50(1):409–19.

[83] Pershadsingh HA, Szollosi J, Benson S, Hyun WC, Feuerstein BG, Kurtz TW. Effects of ciglitazone on blood pressure and intracellular calcium metabolism. Hypertension 1993;21(6 Pt 2):1020–3.

[84] Cohen JS. Risks of troglitazone apparent before approval in USA. Diabetologia 2006;49(6):1454–5.

[85] Liu LS, Tanaka H, Ishii S, Eckel J. The new antidiabetic drug MCC-555 acutely sensitizes insulin signaling in isolated cardiomyocytes. Endocrinology 1998;139(11):4531–9.

[86] McGuire DK, Inzucchi SE. New drugs for the treatment of diabetes mellitus: part I: thiazolidinediones and their evolving cardiovascular implications. Circulation 2008;117(3):440–9.

[87] Kahn SE, Haffner SM, Heise MA, Herman WH, Holman RR, Jones NP, et al. Glycemic durability of rosiglitazone, metformin, or glyburide monotherapy. N Engl J Med 2006;355(23):2427–43.

[88] Derosa G. Efficacy and tolerability of pioglitazone in patients with type 2 diabetes mellitus: comparison with other oral antihyperglycaemic agents. Drugs 2010;70(15):1945–61.

[89] Takeda. Observation of an increased incidence of fractures in female patients who received long-term treatment with ACTOS® (pioglitazone HCl) tablets for type 2 diabetes mellitus. (Letter to Health Care Providers), http://www.fda.gov/downloads/Safety/MedWatch/SafetyInformation/SafetyAlertsforHumanMedicalProducts/UCM153896.pdf; March 2007.

[90] Dormuth CR, Carney G, Carleton B, Bassett K, Wright JM. Thiazolidinediones and fractures in men and women. Arch Intern Med 2009;169(15):1395–402.

[91] Higgins LS, Mantzoros CS. The development of INT131 as a selective PPARgamma modulator: approach to a safer insulin sensitizer. PPAR Res 2008;2008:936906.

[92] Gregoire FM, Zhang F, Clarke HJ, Gustafson TA, Sears DD, Favelyukis S, et al. MBX-102/JNJ39659100, a novel peroxisome proliferator-activated receptor-ligand with weak transactivation activity retains antidiabetic properties in the absence of weight gain and edema. Mol Endocrinol 2009;23(7):975–88.

[93] Choi JH, Banks AS, Estall JL, Kajimura S, Bostrom P, Laznik D, et al. Anti-diabetic drugs inhibit obesity-linked phosphorylation of PPARgamma by Cdk5. Nature 2010;466(7305):451–6.

[94] Choi JH, Banks AS, Kamenecka TM, Busby SA, Chalmers MJ, Kumar N, et al. Antidiabetic actions of a non-agonist PPAR-gamma ligand blocking Cdk5-mediated phosphorylation. Nature 2011;477(7365):477–81.

[95] Chan BY, Gartland A, Wilson PJ, Buckley KA, Dillon JP, Fraser WD, et al. PPAR agonists modulate human osteoclast formation and activity in vitro. Bone 2007;40(1):149–59.

[96] Okamoto H, Iwamoto T, Kotake S, Momohara S, Yamanaka H, Kamatani N. Inhibition of NF-kappaB signaling by fenofibrate, a peroxisome proliferator-activated receptor-alpha ligand, presents a therapeutic strategy for rheumatoid arthritis. Clin Exp Rheumatol 2005;23(3):323–30.

[97] Stunes AK, Westbroek I, Gustafsson BI, Fossmark R, Waarsing JH, Eriksen EF, et al. The peroxisome proliferator-activated receptor (PPAR) alpha agonist fenofibrate maintains bone mass, while the PPAR gamma agonist pioglitazone exaggerates bone loss, in ovariectomized rats. BMC Endocr Disord 2011;11:11.

[98] Charbonnel B. PPAR-alpha and PPAR-gamma agonists for type 2 diabetes. Lancet 2009;374(9684):96–8.

[99] Henry RR, Lincoff AM, Mudaliar S, Rabbia M, Chognot C, Herz M. Effect of the dual peroxisome proliferator-activated receptor-alpha/gamma agonist aleglitazar on risk of cardiovascular disease in patients with type 2 diabetes (SYNCHRONY): a phase II, randomised, dose-ranging study. Lancet 2009;374(9684):126–35.

[100] Artis DR, Lin JJ, Zhang C, Wang W, Mehra U, Perreault M, et al. Scaffold-based discovery of indeglitazar, a PPAR pan-active anti-diabetic agent. Proc Natl Acad Sci USA 2009;106(1):262–7.

[101] Nakashima T, Hayashi M, Fukunaga T, Kurata K, Oh-Hora M, Feng JQ, et al. Evidence for osteocyte regulation of bone homeostasis through RANKL expression. Nat Med 2011;17(10):1231–4.

[102] Xiong J, Onal M, Jilka RL, Weinstein RS, Manolagas SC, O'Brien CA. Matrix-embedded cells control osteoclast formation. Nat Med 2011;17(10):1235–41.

[103] Simonet WS, Lacey DL, Dunstan CR, Kelley M, Chang MS, Luthy R, et al. Osteoprotegerin: a novel secreted protein involved in the regulation of bone density. Cell 1997;89(2):309–19.

[104] Park JS, Cho MH, Nam JS, Yoo JS, Ahn CW, Cha BS, et al. Effect of pioglitazone on serum concentrations of osteoprotegerin in patients with type 2 diabetes mellitus. Eur J Endocrinol 2011;164(1):69–74.

[105] Sultan A, Avignon A, Galtier F, Piot C, Mariano-Goulart D, Dupuy AM, et al. Osteoprotegerin, thiazolidinediones treatment, and silent myocardial ischemia in type 2 diabetic patients. Diabetes Care 2008;31(3):593–5.

[106] Lazarenko OP, Rzonca SO, Hogue WR, Swain FL, Suva LJ, Lecka-Czernik B. Rosiglitazone induces decreases in bone mass and strength that are reminiscent of aged bone. Endocrinology 2007;148(6):2669–80.

[107] Poole KE, van Bezooijen RL, Loveridge N, Hamersma H, Papapoulos SE, Lowik CW, et al. Sclerostin is a delayed secreted product of osteocytes that inhibits bone formation. FASEB J 2005;19(13):1842–4.

[108] Winkler DG, Sutherland MK, Geoghegan JC, Yu C, Hayes T, Skonier JE, et al. Osteocyte control of bone formation via sclerostin, a novel BMP antagonist. EMBO J 2003;22(23):6267–76.

[109] Kusu N, Laurikkala J, Imanishi M, Usui H, Konishi M, Miyake A, et al. Sclerostin is a novel secreted osteoclast-derived bone morphogenetic protein antagonist with unique ligand specificity. J Biol Chem 2003;278(26):24113–7.

[110] Glinka A, Wu W, Delius H, Monaghan AP, Blumenstock C, Niehrs C. Dickkopf-1 is a member of a new family of secreted proteins and functions in head induction. Nature 1998;391(6665):357–62.

[111] Mao B, Wu W, Li Y, Hoppe D, Stannek P, Glinka A, et al. LDL-receptor-related protein 6 is a receptor for Dickkopf proteins. Nature 2001;411(6835):321–5.

[112] Morvan F, Boulukos K, Clement-Lacroix P, Roman Roman S, Suc-Royer I, Vayssiere B, et al. Deletion of a single allele of the Dkk1 gene leads to an increase in bone formation and bone mass. J Bone Miner Res 2006;21(6):934–45.

[113] Tian E, Zhan F, Walker R, Rasmussen E, Ma Y, Barlogie B, et al. The role of the Wnt-signaling antagonist DKK1 in the development of osteolytic lesions in multiple myeloma. N Engl J Med 2003;349(26):2483–94.

[114] Gustafson B, Eliasson B, Smith U. Thiazolidinediones increase the wingless-type MMTV integration site family (WNT)

inhibitor Dickkopf-1 in adipocytes: a link with osteogenesis. Diabetologia 2010;53(3):536–40.

[115] Duque G. Bone and fat connection in aging bone. Curr Opin Rheumatol 2008;20(4):429–34.

[116] Sottile V, Seuwen K, Kneissel M. Enhanced marrow adipogenesis and bone resorption in estrogen-deprived rats treated with the PPARgamma agonist BRL49653 (rosiglitazone). Calcif Tissue Int 2004;75(4):329–37.

[117] Grey A. Thiazolidinedione-induced skeletal fragility—mechanisms and implications. Diabetes Obes Metab 2009;11(4):275–84.

[118] Strotmeyer ES, Cauley JA. Diabetes mellitus, bone mineral density, and fracture risk. Curr Opin Endocrinol Diabetes Obes 2007;14(6):429–35.

[119] McCabe LR. Understanding the pathology and mechanisms of type I diabetic bone loss. J Cell Biochem 2007;102(6):1343–57.

[120] de Paula FJ, Horowitz MC, Rosen CJ. Novel insights into the relationship between diabetes and osteoporosis. Diabetes Metab Res Rev 2010;26(8):622–30.

[121] Hamada Y, Fujii H, Fukagawa M. Role of oxidative stress in diabetic bone disorder. Bone 2009;1(Suppl. 45):S35–8.

[122] Karsenty G, Oury F. The central regulation of bone mass, the first link between bone remodeling and energy metabolism. J Clin Endocrinol Metab 2010;95(11):4795–801.

[123] Ryan KK, Li B, Grayson BE, Matter EK, Woods SC, Seeley RJ. A role for central nervous system PPAR-gamma in the regulation of energy balance. Nat Med 2011;17(5):623–6.

[124] Ebeling PR, Atley LM, Guthrie JR, Burger HG, Dennerstein L, Hopper JL, et al. Bone turnover markers and bone density across the menopausal transition. J Clin Endocrinol Metab 1996;81(9):3366–71.

[125] Sowers MR, Finkelstein JS, Ettinger B, Bondarenko I, Neer RM, Cauley JA, et al. The association of endogenous hormone concentrations and bone mineral density measures in pre- and perimenopausal women of four ethnic groups: SWAN. Osteoporos Int 2003;14(1):44–52.

[126] Sowers MR, Greendale GA, Bondarenko I, Finkelstein JS, Cauley JA, Neer RM, et al. Endogenous hormones and bone turnover markers in pre- and perimenopausal women: SWAN. Osteoporos Int 2003;14(3):191–7.

[127] Sun L, Peng Y, Sharrow AC, Iqbal J, Zhang Z, Papachristou DJ, et al. FSH directly regulates bone mass. Cell 2006;125(2):247–60.

[128] Drake MT, McCready LK, Hoey KA, Atkinson EJ, Khosla S. Effects of suppression of follicle-stimulating hormone secretion on bone resorption markers in postmenopausal women. J Clin Endocrinol Metab 2010;95(11):5063–8.

[129] Allan CM, Kalak R, Dunstan CR, McTavish KJ, Zhou H, Handelsman DJ, et al. Follicle-stimulating hormone increases bone mass in female mice. Proc Natl Acad Sci USA 2010; 107(52):22629–34.

[130] Bogazzi F, Russo D, Locci MT, Chifenti B, Ultimieri F, Raggi F, et al. Peroxisome proliferator-activated receptor (PPAR)gamma is highly expressed in normal human pituitary gland. J Endocrinol Invest 2005;28(10):899–904.

[131] Sharma S, Sharma PM, Mistry DS, Chang RJ, Olefsky JM, Mellon PL, et al. PPARG regulates gonadotropin-releasing hormone signaling in LbetaT2 cells in vitro and pituitary gonadotroph function in vivo in mice. Biol Reprod 2011; 84(3):466–75.

[132] Heaney AP, Fernando M, Melmed S. PPAR-gamma receptor ligands: novel therapy for pituitary adenomas. J Clin Invest 2003;111(9):1381–8.

[133] Krum SA. Direct transcriptional targets of sex steroid hormones in bone. J Cell Biochem 2011;112(2):401–8.

[134] Krum SA, Miranda-Carboni GA, Hauschka PV, Carroll JS, Lane TF, Freedman LP, et al. Estrogen protects bone by inducing Fas ligand in osteoblasts to regulate osteoclast survival. EMBO J 2008;27(3):535–45.

[135] Nakamura T, Imai Y, Matsumoto T, Sato S, Takeuchi K, Igarashi K, et al. Estrogen prevents bone loss via estrogen receptor alpha and induction of Fas ligand in osteoclasts. Cell 2007;130(5):811–23.

[136] Bilik D, McEwen LN, Brown MB, Pomeroy NE, Kim C, Asao K, et al. Thiazolidinediones and fractures: evidence from translating research into action for diabetes. J Clin Endocrinol Metab 2010;95(10):4560–5.

[137] Grey A, Bolland M, Gamble G, Wattie D, Horne A, Davidson J, et al. The peroxisome proliferator-activated receptor-gamma agonist rosiglitazone decreases bone formation and bone mineral density in healthy postmenopausal women: a randomized, controlled trial. J Clin Endocrinol Metab 2007;92(4): 1305–10.

[138] Benvenuti S, Cellai I, Luciani P, Deledda C, Saccardi R, Mazzanti B, et al. Androgens and estrogens prevent rosiglitazone-induced adipogenesis in human mesenchymal stem cells. J Endocrinol Invest 2012;35(4):365–71.

[139] Mabilleau G, Mieczkowska A, Edmonds ME. Thiazolidinediones induce osteocyte apoptosis and increase sclerostin expression. Diabet Med 2010;27(8):925–32.

[140] Seto-Young D, Avtanski D, Parikh G, Suwandhi P, Strizhevsky M, Araki T, et al. Rosiglitazone and pioglitazone inhibit estrogen synthesis in human granulosa cells by interfering with androgen binding to aromatase. Horm Metab Res 2011;43(4):250–6.

[141] Battaglino R, Fu J, Spate U, Ersoy U, Joe M, Sedaghat L, et al. Serotonin regulates osteoclast differentiation through its transporter. J Bone Miner Res 2004;19(9):1420–31.

[142] Waku T, Shiraki T, Oyama T, Maebara K, Nakamori R, Morikawa K. The nuclear receptor PPARgamma individually responds to serotonin- and fatty acid-metabolites. EMBO J 2010;29(19):3395–407.

[143] Yadav VK, Balaji S, Suresh PS, Liu XS, Lu X, Li Z, et al. Pharmacological inhibition of gut-derived serotonin synthesis is a potential bone anabolic treatment for osteoporosis. Nat Med 2010;16(3):308–12.

[144] Hasegawa H, Kido S, Tomomura M, Fujimoto K, Ohi M, Kiyomura M, et al. Serum calcium-decreasing factor, caldecrin, inhibits osteoclast differentiation by suppression of NFATc1 activity. J Biol Chem 2010;285(33):25448–57.

[145] Tomomura A, Yamada H, Fujimoto K, Inaba A, Katoh S. Determination of amino acid sequence responsible for suppression of bone resorption by serum calcium-decreasing factor (caldecrin). FEBS Lett 2001;508(3):454–8.

[146] Ferron M, Wei J, Yoshizawa T, Del Fattore A, DePinho RA, Teti A, et al. Insulin signaling in osteoblasts integrates bone remodeling and energy metabolism. Cell 2010;142(2):296–308.

[147] Elefteriou F, Ahn JD, Takeda S, Starbuck M, Yang X, Liu X, et al. Leptin regulation of bone resorption by the sympathetic nervous system and CART. Nature 2005;434(7032):514–20.

[148] De Vos P, Lefebvre AM, Miller SG, Guerre-Millo M, Wong K, Saladin R, et al. Thiazolidinediones repress ob gene expression in rodents via activation of peroxisome proliferator-activated receptor gamma. J Clin Invest 1996;98(4):1004–9.

[149] Kallen CB, Lazar MA. Antidiabetic thiazolidinediones inhibit leptin (ob) gene expression in 3T3-L1 adipocytes. Proc Natl Acad Sci USA 1996;93(12):5793–6.

[150] Cabrero A, Cubero M, Llaverias G, Alegret M, Sanchez R, Laguna JC, et al. Leptin down-regulates peroxisome proliferator-activated receptor gamma (PPAR-gamma) mRNA levels in primary human monocyte-derived macrophages. Mol Cell Biochem 2005;275(1–2):173–9.

[151] Chang L, Villacorta L, Zhang J, Garcia-Barrio MT, Yang K, Hamblin M, et al. Vascular smooth muscle cell-selective peroxisome proliferator-activated receptor-gamma deletion leads to hypotension. Circulation 2009;119(16):2161—9.

[152] Cao H, Yu S, Yao Z, Galson DL, Jiang Y, Zhang X, et al. Activating transcription factor 4 regulates osteoclast differentiation in mice. J Clin Invest 2010;120(8):2755—66.

[153] Kajimura D, Hinoi E, Ferron M, Kode A, Riley KJ, Zhou B, et al. Genetic determination of the cellular basis of the sympathetic regulation of bone mass accrual. J Exp Med 2011; 208(4):841—51.

[154] Zang C, Liu H, Bertz J, Possinger K, Koeffler HP, Elstner E, et al. Induction of endoplasmic reticulum stress response by TZD18, a novel dual ligand for peroxisome proliferator-activated receptor alpha/gamma, in human breast cancer cells. Mol Cancer Ther 2009;8(8):2296—307.

[155] Fahmi H, Martel-Pelletier J, Pelletier JP, Kapoor M. Peroxisome proliferator-activated receptor gamma in osteoarthritis. Mod Rheumatol 2011;21(1):1—9.

[156] Tat SK, Pelletier JP, Velasco CR, Padrines M, Martel-Pelletier J. New perspective in osteoarthritis: the OPG and RANKL system as a potential therapeutic target? Keio J Med 2009;58(1):29—40.

[157] Pfeilschifter J, Chenu C, Bird A, Mundy GR, Roodman GD. Interleukin-1 and tumor necrosis factor stimulate the formation of human osteoclastlike cells in vitro. J Bone Miner Res 1989;4(1):113—8.

[158] Kobayashi K, Takahashi N, Jimi E, Udagawa N, Takami M, Kotake S, et al. Tumor necrosis factor alpha stimulates osteoclast differentiation by a mechanism independent of the ODF/RANKL-RANK interaction. J Exp Med 2000;191(2): 275—86.

[159] Edwards JR, Sun SG, Locklin R, Shipman CM, Adamopoulos IE, Athanasou NA, et al. LIGHT (TNFSF14), a novel mediator of bone resorption, is elevated in rheumatoid arthritis. Arthritis Rheum 2006;54(5):1451—62.

[160] Ishimi Y, Miyaura C, Jin CH, Akatsu T, Abe E, Nakamura Y, et al. IL-6 is produced by osteoblasts and induces bone resorption. J Immunol 1990;145(10):3297—303.

[161] Tamura T, Udagawa N, Takahashi N, Miyaura C, Tanaka S, Yamada Y, et al. Soluble interleukin-6 receptor triggers osteoclast formation by interleukin 6. Proc Natl Acad Sci USA 1993;90(24):11924—8.

[162] Fujikawa Y, Sabokbar A, Neale SD, Itonaga I, Torisu T, Athanasou NA. The effect of macrophage-colony stimulating factor and other humoral factors (interleukin-1, -3, -6, and -11, tumor necrosis factor-alpha, and granulocyte macrophage-colony stimulating factor) on human osteoclast formation from circulating cells. Bone 2001;28(3). 261—7.

[163] Itonaga I, Sabokbar A, Sun SG, Kudo O, Danks L, Ferguson D, et al. Transforming growth factor-beta induces osteoclast formation in the absence of RANKL. Bone 2004;34(1):57—64.

[164] Hemingway F, Taylor R, Knowles HJ, Athanasou NA. RANKL-independent human osteoclast formation with APRIL, BAFF, NGF, IGF I and IGF II. Bone 2011;48(4):938—44.

[165] Hassumi MY, Silva-Filho VJ, Campos-Junior JC, Vieira SM, Cunha FQ, Alves PM, et al. PPAR-gamma agonist rosiglitazone prevents inflammatory periodontal bone loss by inhibiting osteoclastogenesis. Int Immunopharmacol 2009;9(10):1150—8.

[166] Hounoki H, Sugiyama E, Mohamed SG, Shinoda K, Taki H, Abdel-Aziz HO, et al. Activation of peroxisome proliferator-activated receptor gamma inhibits TNF-alpha-mediated osteoclast differentiation in human peripheral monocytes in part via suppression of monocyte chemoattractant protein-1 expression. Bone 2008;42(4):765—74.

[167] Yang CR, Lai CC. Thiazolidinediones inhibit TNF-alpha-mediated osteoclast differentiation of RAW264.7 macrophages and mouse bone marrow cells through downregulation of NFATc1. Shock 2010;33(6):662—7.

[168] Rosen CJ. Revisiting the rosiglitazone story—lessons learned. N Engl J Med 2010. 10.1056/NEJMp1008233.

11

From Gonads to Bone, and Back

Franck Oury, PhD

Columbia University, New York, NY, USA

INTRODUCTION

The sex steroid hormones estrogen and androgen have central roles in the control of sexual maturity and reproduction. While both males and females have all types of hormones present in their bodies, females produce the majority of two types of hormones, estrogens and progesterone, while males produce mainly androgens such as testosterone. Estrogens affect ovarian function and promote ovocyte maturation and ovulation. Testosterone promotes the development and function of the testes and stimulates spermatogenesis and germ cell survival.

In addition to their reproductive functions, sex steroid hormones are essential for skeletal development and the maintenance of bone health throughout adult life. Testosterone and estrogen influence positively the growth, maturation, and maintenance of the female and male skeleton [1–3]. Their effects are mediated by slow genomic mechanisms through nuclear hormonal receptors but also through fast non-genomic mechanisms by membrane-associated receptors and signaling cascades [2–4]. The biological importance of this regulation is best exemplified by the fact that gonadal failure triggers bone loss in both genders. Estrogen deficiencies at menopause in women and androgen decrease in elderly men are the major pathogenic factors in the development of osteoporosis [2,3,5–10].

The principle of mutual dependence between organs as an underlying notion of vertebrate physiology rejuvenated physiology. It is clear nowadays that there are crosstalks between the different organs in the regulation of whole organism physiology. In other words, our body is not simply an assembly of silos independent of each other. Instead, the organs need to communicate with each other to keep our body functional. Based on this notion, recent studies demonstrated that bone is not only a recipient for the hormonal input but the skeleton has emerged as an endocrine organ of major importance.

Multiple studies have shown that bone favors whole body glucose homeostasis and energy expenditure, both in mice and in humans [11–23]. These novel functions of bone are mediated by an osteoblast-specific secreted hormone, osteocalcin, that when undercarboxylated favors β-cell proliferation, insulin secretion, and insulin sensitivity in muscle, liver, and white adipose tissue [13,18,24]. Considering that most endocrine regulations are subjected to the same feedback loop mechanisms, the regulation of bone mass accrual by gonads suggests that bone, in its endocrine capacity, may affect the reproductive functions in one or both genders. Testing this hypothesis in mice, it was recently shown that osteocalcin regulates several aspects of male reproduction by favoring testosterone biosynthesis in testes [25]. This novel endocrine role of bone has also been recently supported by correlative data in human [26].

This chapter will review the concept of mutual dependence between the skeleton and gonads. It will also present the notion that disturbances in functional activity of bone cells and particularly for osteocalcin production and/or its receptor signaling may have ramifications not only for male fertility, but also for susceptibility to prostate cancer.

SEX STEROID HORMONES EFFECTS ON BONE PHYSIOLOGY

The integrity of the skeleton is maintained by the unique ability of bone to constantly renew itself through the coordinated action of two cell types: osteoclasts that resorb bone, followed by osteoblasts that form bone [27–30]. The concerted action of these two cell types defines bone modeling during childhood and remodeling during adulthood. Because of the essential role of the skeleton in locomotion, support, and protection of the body, this mechanism is critical for vertebrates. There are a number of diseases of bone that result from an imbalance between osteoblastic bone formation and osteoclastic bone resorption. The most frequent one, affecting nearly 45 million women worldwide, is osteoporosis, caused by a relative increase of bone resorption over bone formation [31,32].

The regulation of bone (re)modeling is complex and involves mechanical stimuli, locally produced factors, and hormones. Among these hormones, sex steroids play a crucial role during the bone growth spurts of puberty, and for the maintenance of bone mass. This notion is better illustrated by the fact that osteoporosis occurs most commonly in postmenopausal women as a result of a decrease in estrogen secretion by ovaries. Compared with women, men have greater bone strength, resulting in fewer fractures. However, recent studies have shown that there is a high incidence of loss of androgens in males following castration or a decrease in androgen levels related to aging [3,5,7,29,33—36].

SEX STEROID HORMONE REGULATION OF BONE GROWTH

Sex steroids play an important role in bone growth and the attainment of peak of bone mass. They are, at least in part, responsible for the skeletal gender differences in bone growth, which emerge during adolescence. Both adolescent boys and girls experience an increase in bone mineral acquisition during puberty, but they occur to a substantially greater extent in males than in females. Although skeletal size and volume are similar in pre-pubertal girls and boys [1,3,37—39], the sexual dimorphism in bone growth becomes apparent during puberty, with men reaching higher peak bone mass. The male skeleton is characterized by larger bone size and both a larger diameter and greater cortical thickness in long bone. The larger bone size in men confers significant biomechanical advantages and, at least in part, explains the lower incidence of fragility of fractures compared with women [31].

The skeletal gender differences are attributed to a stimulatory androgen action on periosteal bone formation in men versus an inhibitory estrogen-related action in women [2,4,39,40]. The role of androgens in growth of the male skeleton during puberty is supported by several observations. Androgen deficiency due to prepubertal hypogonadism is associated with low bone mineral density at puberty, while administration of testosterone before epiphyseal closure leads to increases in bone mass [41—43]. Moreover, in young adult men serum free testosterone is positively associated with cortical bone size [44]. However, recent findings have partly redefined the concept that androgens are the only factors involved in this process. A significant body of evidence points out the role of estrogen

action in men as well. In male mice, estrogen deficiency in addition to androgen withdrawal further reduces radial bone expansion during the early stages of puberty [1]. This could be explained by the presence of a local production of estrogens by conversion of testosterone. This notion is principally supported by the effects following an aromatase deficiency and/or estrogen resistance on skeletal growth during puberty [6,31,45]. Lastly, there is also evidence that androgens have effects on the peak of bone mass in women since an excess of androgen in women is associated with higher bone mineral density [46—48].

In addition to the sex steroid hormones several studies show that other hormones negatively regulated by estrogen, such as growth hormone (GH) and insulin-like growth factor 1 (IGF1), may further contribute to the development of the skeletal sexual dimorphism [1,49—51]. IGF1 levels are higher in male versus female during early puberty [49,52] and mice lacking GH receptor (GHR), IGF1, or both show a severe bone growth retardation [50]. Therefore, this evidence strongly suggests that skeletal dimorphism in bone growth cannot be only summarized to the end result of differences in sex steroid hormones secretion and action in males and females, but depends on a complex gender- and time-specific interaction between several factors [1].

SEX STEROID HORMONE REGULATION OF BONE MASS MAINTENANCE

Gonadal-derived sex steroid hormones are implicated in the maintenance of bone mass integrity during adulthood in the female and male skeleton; testosterone and estrogens are crucial determinants for maintaining bone homeostasis. Indeed, the absence or decrease of either testosterone or estrogen levels, with age or in gonadal dysfunction, leads to a decrease in bone mass and increases markedly the risk of osteoporosis [1,2,4,5,53—55].

Age-related Bone Loss in Females

As a matter of fact, estrogen deficiency is a major pathogenetic factor in the bone loss associated with the menopause and the development of osteoporosis in postmenopausal women. After menopause, bone resorption increases by 90% while bone formation also increases but only by 45% [31,56]. This difference between bone resorption and formation rate favors greater bone resorption, which leads to an accelerated bone loss during the first years after menopause. This rapid bone loss can be prevented by estrogen administration and characteristically results in an increase in bone mineral density during the first months of treatment [57–59].

Age-related Bone Loss in Males

Although osteoporosis more commonly affects women, men lose about half as much bone with aging as women, and suffer one third the number of fragility fractures as women [31,34]. Moreover, loss of androgens following castration in adult men or the administration of gonadotropin-releasing hormone agonist have a rapid bone loss with evidence of increased bone turnover [2,3,33,36]. Testosterone treatment effectively prevents bone loss in hypogonadal men, even at older age [43,60,61]. Taken together these observations demonstrate that hypogonadism and decrease in serum testosterone in men are important pathogenetic factors in male osteoporosis.

However, for a long time, it has been assumed that sex steroid hormones deficiency is a less significant cause of bone loss in men than in women. This notion was based on the fact that the majority of older men do not develop overt hypogonadism and the levels of total serum estrogens and testosterone decrease in men only slightly with normal aging. Several studies over the last decade have redefined this notion by showing that the lack of apparent age-related sex steroids deficiency in men is due to an increase (two-fold) of sex hormone binding globulin (SHBG) with aging in men [62–64]. SHBG is synthesized by the liver and binds with high avidity to testosterone and estrogens. Circulating sex steroids that are bound to SHBG are blocked in the bloodstream and have restricted access to target tissues. Therefore, there is not a change in serum total testosterone and estradiol but a decrease in free and bioavailable sex steroid hormone levels—although multiple groups have recently reported that in serum free or bioavailable sex steroids decrease with aging and that SHBG levels are inversely related to the bone density [63,65–68]. It remains unclear to what extent the association of an increase of SHBG with male skeletal aged-related bone loss might explain a decrease in sex steroid bioavailability [1].

Lastly, the dichotomy associating androgens and estrogens as pure "male" and "female" hormones, respectively, has been reconsidered recently [1]. This traditional concept has been challenged by series of evidences showing that estrogens may have a crucial role in the maintenance of bone mass accrual and skeletal homeostasis in elderly men [65,69–72]. Several studies reported that bone loss in aging men correlated even better with serum estradiol than testosterone [6,8,64,65,73]. It therefore appears that decreasing bioavailable estrogen levels in men play a significant role in mediating age-related bone loss in men similar to women [31,73].

In summary, these data suggest that the role of sex steroids in the maintenance of bone mass has a paramount importance but it appears more complex than initially anticipated. It is clear that age-related bone loss in women and men is not only due to deficiency in one or both sex steroid hormones (androgen/estrogens) but is a result of disturbances affecting a complex network regulating bone mass that remains to be further investigated.

ESTROGEN AND ANDROGEN MODE OF ACTION IN SKELETON

Estrogens

Estrogens actively suppress bone turnover and maintain balanced rates of bone formation and bone resorption. At the cellular level, estrogens affect the generation, lifespan, and functional activity of both osteoclasts and osteoblasts. They decrease osteoclast formation and activity, while increase osteoclast apoptosis [74,75]. The action of estrogens on osteoblasts is less clear and its investigation has produced conflicting results. While the majority of the studies indicate that estrogen suppresses osteoblast differentiation, in contrast some evidence suggests that estrogens may also increase osteoblast differentiation, proliferation, and function [3,76,77]. These opposing findings are most probably due to different potent actions of estrogen depending on the stage of osteoblast differentiation.

At the molecular level, estrogens decrease the production of cytokines inhibiting osteoclast apoptosis, such as IL-1, IL-6, TNFα, M-CSF, and downregulate the expression of NfκB-activated gene, a suppressor of apoptosis [2, 35, 74; 78–80]. In contrast, estrogens favor expression of TGF-β, a direct inhibitor of osteoclast activity and an activator of osteoclast apoptosis [81–83]. Estrogens can also directly suppress bone resorption. They enhance production of OPG and decrease RANKL expression by osteoblasts, an inhibitor and an activator of osteoclast activity, respectively [84]. Lastly, estrogens also suppress osteoclast formation by inducing osteoclast apoptosis through an activation of Fas/FasL signaling [9]. They favor the expression of *Fas Ligand* (*FasL*), a gene that belongs to the tumor necrosis factor (TNF) family, in osteoclasts and osteoblasts [9,85]. Therefore, estrogen action on bone is an important physiological mechanism to maintain bone mass during adulthood.

Androgens

Androgens have potent effects on osteoblast formation, and those are differential whether they act on trabecular or periosteal bone. While androgens maintain trabecular bone mass and integrity, they favor periosteal bone formation in men [3]. At the cellular level, testosterone increases the lifespan of osteoblasts by decreasing apoptosis, mainly through its action on IL-6 production [35,86]. Furthermore, androgens stimulate the proliferation of osteoblast progenitors and the differentiation of mature osteoblasts [35,87–89]. Molecular mechanisms of androgen action on bone cells are less well described than for estrogens. However, some evidence indicates that they favor osteoblast proliferation and differentiation by increasing TGF-β mRNA and responsiveness to FGF and IGF-II [2,81,82]. Androgens may also decrease osteoclast formation and bone resorption through increased production of OPG by osteoblasts [84]. The net result of these functions of testosterone is to favor bone formation (Fig. 11.1). Moreover, testosterone may influence different stages of osteoblast differentiation and may act on osteoblasts differentially from estrogen at various skeletal localizations. This last aspect of testosterone on bone formation is also important for the skeletal sexual dimorphism [39,90].

GENOMIC AND NON-GENOMIC SEX STEROID HORMONE SIGNALING IN BONE CELLS

Classical receptors for estrogens (ERs) or androgens (ARs) are expressed in osteoblasts, osteoclasts, osteocytes, and growth plate chondrocytes indicating that the sex steroid hormones may influence skeletal physiology, at least in part, by acting directly on bone cells [91–93]. Sex steroid receptors are present in an inactive form and are sequestered, within the cytoplasm, in a multi-protein complex by chaperon molecules (such as heat shock protein, Hsp90 and Hsp70). In the presence of the sex steroid hormones, the conformation of these complexes changes, resulting in a dissociation of the chaperon proteins and in a translocation of the receptor to the nucleus. The hormone-bound receptor dimerizes and binds with high affinity to specific DNA sequences (estrogen and androgen responsive elements, ERE and ARE, respectively) located in the regulatory elements of the target gene [4,94].

The analysis of ERα (αERKO), ERβ (βERKO), double ER (DERKO), and AR (ArKO) mutated mice showed

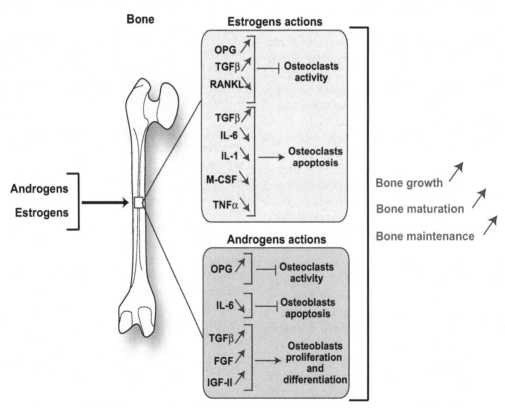

FIGURE 11.1 **Molecular mediators of sex steroid hormone action on bone cells.** Sex steroid hormones secreted by gonads play a crucial role during skeletal growth, maturation, and maintenance in both men and women. This figure summarizes the major targets of estrogens and androgens in bone cells. Their activation or repression is associated with effects on apoptosis and/or proliferation of osteoblasts and/or osteoclasts. Please see color plate section.

some skeletal abnormalities [95–100]. Yet, ER-deficient mouse models have been confounded by highly elevated levels of serum sex steroids, and the weakness of the phenotype by comparison to the one observed in estrogen-deficient mouse models [2,3,97]. In addition, it has been shown that sex steroid hormones may also act indirectly in the context of non-genomic sex steroid signaling. Androgens and estrogens can transmit anti-apoptotic effects on osteoblasts *in vitro* with a similar efficiency via either ARs or ERs, irrespective of whether the ligand is an androgen or an estrogen [35,87,89]. The non-genomic effects of sex steroid hormones are mediated through cell-surface receptors linked to intracellular signal transduction proteins [4,42,101]. The membrane-initiated steroid signaling results in the activation of conventional second messenger signal transduction cascades, including activation of protein kinase A (PKA), protein kinase C (PKC), cellular tyrosine kinases, MAPKs, PI3K, and Akt- and Src/Shc/ERK signaling [4,102,103]. In conclusion, taken together these data suggest that the mechanisms mediating estrogen and androgen function in the bone, via ERs and ARs, are not fully elucidated.

The Skeleton Talks to the Gonads

Recently, the view of bone as an assembly of inert calcified tubes, only characterized by its scaffolding functions, has considerably evolved to a much more dynamic picture of this tissue. Multiple studies have shown that bone is an endocrine organ favoring whole body glucose homeostasis and energy expenditure, both in mice and in humans [13,18]. These novel functions of bone are mediated by an osteoblast-specific secreted hormone called osteocalcin, which when undercarboxylated favors β-cell proliferation, insulin secretion, and insulin sensitivity in muscle, liver, and white adipose tissue. Remarkably, *Esp*, a gene encoding an intracellular tyrosine phosphatase called OST-PTP, exerts, through its osteoblast expression, metabolic functions opposite to those of osteocalcin [18]. It appeared that *Esp* inhibits the endocrine functions of osteocalcin by favoring, through an indirect mechanism, its carboxylation [18,104]. Exploring the molecular cascade regulating the expression and activity of this tyrosine phosphatase, it has been shown that insulin receptor is a substrate of OST-PTP in mice and human osteoblasts [13,24]. Further investigations have demonstrated that insulin signaling in osteoblasts favors glucose metabolism by increasing the undercarboxylated (active) form of osteocalcin in serum. Insulin signaling in osteoblasts activates osteoblast activity by a double inhibitory loop. The low pH (pH 4.5) generated by osteoclasts during bone resorption is necessary and sufficient to decarboxylate and by this way bio-activate osteocalcin present in the extracellular matrix of bone [13,24].

The hormonal functions of osteocalcin have raised multiple questions of great biological and medical importance. Chief among these was to elucidate the signaling events triggered by this hormone in target cells. A second question, with even broader implications, was to determine whether osteocalcin, like many other hormones, has functions in addition to those exerted on energy metabolism. The well-known regulation of bone remodeling by gonads provides an ideal setting to address the aforementioned question. As mentioned above, that menopause favors bone loss is well established. What this medical observation means biologically is that gonads, mostly through sex steroid hormones, affect the functions of bone cells, an aspect of bone physiology that has been discussed above. According to the general principle of feedback control, what the regulation of bone mass accrual by gonads also suggests is that bone may affect the reproductive functions in one or both genders. Verifying this hypothesis was of great conceptual importance as it would further enhance the emerging importance of bone as an endocrine organ.

The first hint that this hypothesis could be true came from *ex vivo* cell assays. Indeed, these studies showed that a factor secreted by osteoblasts but not by other cells of mesodermal origin could markedly increase testosterone production by testis explants and primary Leydig cells [25]. The effect of osteoblast supernatants was limited to males; osteoblasts did not stimulate testosterone or estrogens in females. Recently, this novel important role of osteoblasts has been verified *in vivo*. Using DTA_{osb} mice, an osteoblast-less mouse model, ablation of osteoblasts in adult mice profoundly affects circulating testosterone levels [105].

OSTEOCALCIN, A NEW PLAYER IN THE REGULATION OF TESTOSTERONE PRODUCTION

Since osteocalcin has an important role in the regulation of energy metabolism and glucose homeostasis, it was hypothesized that it may also affect testosterone production. Several experiments have confirmed this hypothesis *in vitro* and *ex vivo*. First, this hypothesis was verified by co-culture assays, since the supernatants of wild-type (wt) but not of *Osteocalcin*−/− osteoblasts in culture increased testosterone production by Leydig cells of the testes. Second, treating Leydig cells (primary and TM3 cells) with increasing amounts of undercarboxylated osteocalcin, the active form of the hormone, resulted in a dose-dependent increase in testosterone secretion. Third, injection of osteocalcin in wt mice

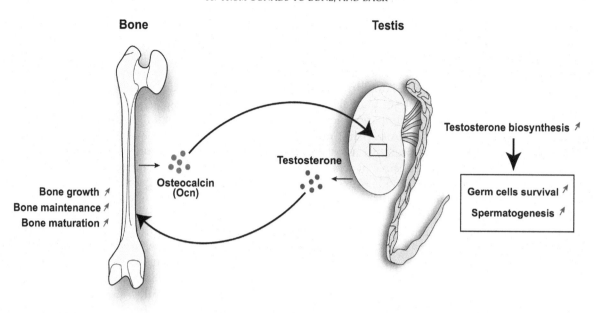

FIGURE 11.2   Mutual dependence between bone and gonads. The sex steroid hormone testosterone is a crucial determinant of bone growth during puberty, maturation, and maintenance of bone mass accrual. Osteocalcin, an osteoblast-derived hormone, regulates testosterone production by Leydig cells. Testosterone in testis favors spermatogenesis, sexual maturity, and germ cell survival. Please see color plate section.

increased significantly circulating levels of testosterone [25]. Lastly, administration of osteocalcin in mice lacking osteoblasts fully restored testosterone to normal serum levels [105].

Next, the role of osteocalcin in regulation of testosterone biosynthesis was also demonstrated *in vivo*, using *Osteocalcin*-deficient mice. This analysis was admittedly greatly helped by the fact that while female *Osteocalcin*−/− mice were normally fertile, the male mutant mice were rather poor breeders. The demonstration of a reproductive function of osteocalcin in male mice was greatly helped by the availability of both gain (*Esp*−/−) and loss-of-function (*Osteocalcin*−/−) mutations for osteocalcin functions [18]. *Osteocalcin*-deficient mice showed a decrease in testes, epidydimedes, and seminal vesicles weights; the opposite was seen in male *Esp*−/− mice. *Osteocalcin*−/− male mice showed a 50% decrease in sperm count, whereas *Esp*−/− male mice showed a 30% increase in this parameter. Moreover, Leydig cell maturation appeared to be halted in absence of *Osteocalcin*. These features suggested that osteocalcin could favor testosterone synthesis. Accordingly, testing this notion *in vivo*, it has been shown that circulating testosterone levels are low in *Osteocalcin*−/− and high in *Esp*−/− male mice [25]. Moreover, *Osteocalcin*- and *Gprc6a*-deficient male mice also have significantly increased levels of circulating estradiol, leading to a disturbance in testosterone/estradiol ratio. Lastly and more surprisingly, serum LH levels were higher in *Osteocalcin*−/− compare to wt male mice; suggesting a compensatory mechanism which is unlikely insufficient

to rescue the loss of function of the osteocalcin in regulation of testosterone production [25,106].

Taken together, these experiments established that osteocalcin is a bone-derived hormone favoring fertility in male mice by promoting testosterone production by Leydig cells (Fig. 11.2). In other words, it verified that, for at least one gender, there is an endocrine regulation of reproduction by the skeleton. It also suggested that there may be differences between males and females in the regulation of this function.

OSTEOCALCIN MODE OF ACTION IN LEYDIG CELLS

The identification of a novel hormone immediately raises the question of its mechanism of action. A prerequisite to answering this question was to identify the receptor to which this hormone would bind specifically on its target cells. The first step to address this question concerned the signal transduction pathway affected by osteocalcin in two target cells, the β-cell of the pancreas and the Leydig cell of the testis. This approach identified the production of cAMP as the only intracellular signaling event reproducibly triggered by osteocalcin in these two cell types, suggesting that the, or at least an, osteocalcin receptor would be a G protein coupled receptor (GPCR) linked to adenylate cyclase. Out of more than a hundred orphan GPCRs analyzed, 22 of them were more expressed in testes than in ovaries and only four were expressed predominantly, or only,

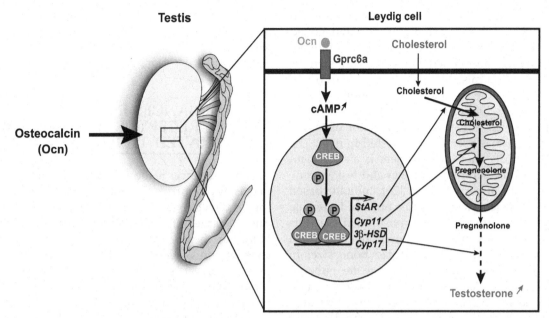

FIGURE 11.3   Bone endocrine regulation of testosterone biosynthesis. Osteocalcin, an osteoblast-derived hormone, regulates testosterone production in testis. Following osteocalcin binding to a G-couple receptor (Gprc6a) expressed in Leydig cells, cAMP production is increased leading to the activation of the transcription factor CREB (cAMP response element binding). CREB binds to the promoter regions and activates the expression of several genes encoding for the enzymes that are necessary for testosterone biosynthesis, such as *StAR*, *Cyp11a*, *3β-HSD*, and *Cyp17*. Steroidogenic acute regulatory protein (StAR) is crucial for transport of cholesterol to mitochondria where biosynthesis of steroids is initiated. *Cyp11a* encodes the cholesterol side-chain cleavage enzyme (P450scc) that catalyzes the first and rate-limiting step, which converts cholesterol to pregnenolone. *3β-HSD* and *Cyp17* encode two enzymes required during the conversion of pregnenolone to testosterone. Testosterone is a sex steroid hormone required for many aspects of testicular functions, for example germ cell survival and spermatogenesis. Please see color plate section.

in Leydig cells [25,106]. One of these four orphan GPCRs, Gprc6a, was a particularly good candidate to be an osteocalcin receptor since its inactivation in mice results in metabolic and reproduction phenotypes similar to those seen in *Osteocalcin*−/− mice [106]. The inactivation of *Gprc6a* in mice leads to an increase in adiposity, a decrease in muscle mass, and low circulating testosterone levels associated with an elevated estradiol serum levels in male mice [106]. Furthermore, it had been proposed that Gprc6a was a calcium sensing receptor, working better in the presence of osteocalcin [106]. In testing this hypothesis in mice, several criteria identified formally Gprc6a as an osteocalcin receptor present in Leydig cells. First, there is direct binding of osteocalcin to wt but not to *Gprc6a*-deficient Leydig cells; second, osteocalcin increases cAMP production in wt but not in *GPRc6a*-deficient Leydig cells; third, and more to the point, a Leydig cell-specific deletion of *GPRc6a* revealed a reproduction phenotype caused by low testosterone production similar, if not identical, to the one seen in the case of osteocalcin inactivation; fourth, in an even more convincing experiment, compound heterozygous mice lacking one copy of *Osteocalcin* and one copy of *Gprc6a* had a reproduction phenotype identical in all aspects to the one seen in *Osteocalcin*−/− or *Gprc6a*−/− mice [25,106]. Lastly, analyzing the role of osteocalcin in regulation of energy

metabolism, recent studies demonstrated that Gprc6a mediates responses to osteocalcin in β-cells *in vitro* and pancreas *in vivo* [107].

Investigating the identification of the downstream cascade mediated by Gprc6a as an osteocalcin receptor led to the demonstration that CREB is a transcriptional effector of osteocalcin regulation of testosterone biosynthesis. The activation of CREB by osteocalcin signaling favors the expression of key enzymes of testosterone biosynthetic pathway in Leydig cells, such as *StAR*, *Cyp11a*, *Cyp17*, and *3β-HSD* (Fig. 11.3). Interestingly, it does not affect the expression of the aromatase, responsible for estrogen synthesis [25]. The identification of an osteocalcin receptor now allows us to address many questions, and for instance to search for additional functions of osteocalcin. It also allows us to perform a more sophisticated dissection of the osteocalcin molecular mode of action in known, and yet to be identified, target cells.

CORRELATIVE OBSERVATION OF THE OSTEOCALCIN-DEPENDENT REGULATION OF TESTOSTERONE PRODUCTION IN HUMANS

Beyond bone biology, this novel endocrine role of the skeleton demonstrates how intimately connected are all the organs and the power of genetic manipulations in model organisms. When it comes to bone and gonad biology, these findings reveal a previously unknown regulation of a gonad-derived hormone, testosterone. An obvious question raised by this novel role of osteocalcin is whether the skeleton also regulates some aspects of the reproductive function in humans.

The function of osteocalcin as a regulator of testosterone production has been recently tested in men. The group of Dr. Khosla showed that there is a significant association between serum osteocalcin and testosterone levels during mid-puberty in men [26]. Initially, based on the effect of osteocalcin in males but not in female mice reproductive functions, they postulated that this axis may be most relevant during rapid skeletal growth in adolescent males to help maximize bone size. In testing this hypothesis in boys spanning the pubertal years of maximal skeletal growth, they observed that serum osteocalcin levels were significantly correlated with circulating testosterone levels, with a similar trend for undercarboxylated osteocalcin. As an internal control of bone formation they use another marker, serum PINP. No significant correlation between PINP levels and testosterone circulating levels were observed. These data underly the specificity between osteocalcin and testosterone and rule out the possibility that this correlation was the result of a non-specific association with bone formation. Lastly, serum osteocalcin or undercarboxylated osteocalcin levels were linked with periosteal circumference. However, adjusting this correlation to testosterone levels eliminated the association between osteocalcin and periosteal circumference of bone, suggesting that this relationship was mediated by testosterone. In summary, these data extended to humans the notion that osteocalcin is a new determinant in the regulation of testosterone biosynthesis. The correlation between the testosterone peak and osteocalcin level in adolescence in men suggests that osteocalcin may be most relevant during rapid skeletal growth in pubertal men [26]. In other words this correlative data in humans suggest that the bone–testis axis may act as a novel determinant of the skeletal sexual dimorphism at puberty.

Interestingly, the role of the bone–testis axis in the regulation of testosterone biosynthesis could be also associated to the age-related bone loss. In fact, it is well known that the decrease of circulating testosterone levels in men is always associated with an increase of estrogen and luteinizing hormone (LH), which cannot increase testosterone production [33]. There are also associated increases in body fat mass and decrease in sperm counts and sexual function [108]. All of these phenotypes are also present in Osteocalcin−/− mice. This observation would suggest that osteocalcin could be an anti-aging hormone. Clearly, however, this notion

needs to be tested in mice and humans and especially to assess the possible interactions between LH and osteocalcin in the control of testosterone biosynthesis by testes.

DISTURBANCES IN OSTEOCALCIN OR ITS RECEPTOR ACTIVITY ARE ASSOCIATED TO PROSTATE CANCER

Prostate cancer is the most frequent male malignancy in western countries. The mechanisms by which prostate cancer develops and progresses remain largely elusive due to a large number of factors involved in this process. However, there is increasing evidence showing that the contribution of genetic factors to the development of prostate cancer is larger than in other common human tumors [109–111]. Interestingly, there are links between prostate cancer and bone metabolism. Prostate cancer prevalently metastasizes to the bone and creates a common feature of osteosclerotic lesion with increased osteoblastic activity [112,113]. Skeletal metastases occur in more than 80% of cases of advanced-stage prostate cancer and they confer a high level of morbidity.

Recently, several studies point out the importance of using single nucleotide polymorphisms (SNPs) for identifying the prostate cancer diseases related to genetics causes. Polymorphism of Cyp17, androgen receptor, and glutathione S-transferase *pi* gene was reported to be associated with prostate cancer [114–117]. Based on this notion, a genome-wide association study in the Japanese population has recently identified the *GPRC6A* gene as a novel genetic locus associated with prostate cancer [111]. Moreover, several observations suggest that the *Osteocalcin* gene is also a susceptibility locus for the formation and progression of prostate cancer. A polymorphism with a single C→T base change, located in the promoter of the *Osteocalcin* gene (198 nucleotides upstream from exon1), has been identified [118]. This study showed that there is a significant difference in the distribution of the C/T polymorphism between control and prostate cancer patients. While no "CC" homozygotes are present in patients, both "CT" heterozygote and "TT" homozygote have a higher risk of prostate cancer.

In addition to genome-wide analyses, several recent observations support the notion that *GPRC6A* and *Osteocalcin* could be associated with prostate cancers. While *GPRC6A* is expressed at a low level in normal prostate tissue and cells, Dr. Quarley's group showed that in several human prostate cancer lines, as well as in human prostate cancer tissues, *GPRC6A* expression is markedly elevated [119]. These data could be related to the growing evidence that most of primary and metastatic cancers are associated with upregulation of several

GPCRs [120]. Next, to further demonstrate *in vivo* the implication of *GPRC6A* in cancer progression, they deleted *Gprc6a* gene in a mouse model of prostate cancer (TRAMP mice) [119,121]. Lack of *Gprc6a* in TRAMP mice resulted in a significant retardation in prostate cancer progression and an increase of over 40% of the lifespan of this compound mice compare to TRAMP mice with normal *Gprc6a*. Taken together, these data strongly support the association between disturbances of *Gprc6a* gene and a higher risk of prostate cancer. They also suggest that GPRC6A is a novel potential interesting target to regulate prostate cancer progression.

Osteocalcin is ectopically expressed in most malignant prostate epithelial cells in prostate cancers, which are preferably metastasized to bone [122–124]. Moreover, increased risks of advanced-stage and high-grade prostate cancer are linked with higher serum undercarboxylated osteocalcin/total osteocalcin ratio [125]. Therefore, a boost of the bioactive form of osteocalcin might be related to progression in prostate malignances.

Lastly, the notion that *GPRC6A* and *Osteocalcin* genes are related to prostate cancer progression in humans is also consistent with the fact that Osteocalcin−/− and Gprc6a−/− mice show a significant change in the testosterone/estradiol (T/E) ratio [25,106]. T/E is a crucial determinant in the development of benign and malignant prostate tumors associated with aging in men [126]. Disturbances in bone cell activity and more precisely in osteocalcin production by the skeleton is not only associated with fertility disorders in men but also with high risk of prostate cancer.

CONCLUSION

The functions of the skeleton are not all known yet, but the ones we do know demonstrate that skeleton physiology affects many more organs and functions than the skeleton itself. Conceptually, the regulation of energy metabolism and reproduction by bone suggest that the skeleton is an important member of an endocrine network affecting multiple functions of whole-organism physiology.

Interestingly, the "well-being" of various organs is reflected in several reproductive functions and ability to reproduce. Several metabolic disturbances may severely affect reproductive function. For example, it is well known that obesity is often associated with low sperm counts and reduced chance of pregnancy [108]. Conversely, poor nutrition or extreme physical activity can delay puberty and lead to infertility [127]. Multiple metabolic signals seem to act as gatekeepers of reproduction. In other words, in the absence of sufficient energy stores, our body will favor preferentially more vital functions than reproduction. Moreover, leptin (an adipocyte-derived hormone) and insulin (a pancreas-derived hormone actively involved in glucose metabolism) influence profoundly body weight, reproductive functions, and bone mass accrual [127,128]. More interestingly, both of them regulate osteocalcin bioactivity and functions. Therefore, all of this evidence supports the notion that there is a complex endocrine regulation-linked energy metabolism, bone mass accrual and reproduction (which need to be investigated further) and that osteocalcin may be one of them.

Following the identification of osteocalcin as a new determinant of several aspects in male reproductive functions, one of the most important questions to be answered is the relationship between LH and osteocalcin in the regulation of testosterone biosynthesis by Leydig cells in testis. Both of these hormones favor testosterone production, and both are coupled to stimulation of cAMP-dependent signaling cascades of androgen steroidogenesis in testis. However, *Osteocalcin*−/− mice have a high LH serum level in the face of low circulating testosterone levels. This observation indicates that LH is not sufficient to compensate the loss of function in testosterone production induced by the lack of osteocalcin in mice. This suggests that either osteocalcin acts downstream of LH or that it belongs to a second endocrine axis necessary for male fertility.

An obvious question raised by this novel endocrine role of bone in male fertility is to know whether osteocalcin also regulates some aspects of the reproductive function in humans. Recent correlative data from Dr. Khosla's group provide the first evidence that osteocalcin might function similarly in men by showing the role of osteocalcin in the regulation of testosterone peak during puberty in adolescent men [26]. However, a role of osteocalcin during aging needs also to be investigated in the future. As a matter of fact, aging is associated with a decrease in testosterone serum levels in men. This decrease is always associated with an increase of estrogen and LH, which cannot increase testosterone production. Furthermore, aging in men is linked with increases in body fat mass and decreases in bone mass, sperm counts, and sexual function. All these disorders observed in elderly men are also present in *Osteocalcin*−/− mice. Taken together these observations suggest that osteocalcin could be an anti-aging hormone. From a therapeutic point of view, all this evidence hints that osteocalcin may help to explain some sub- and/or infertility disorders in humans. Moreover, since osteocalcin injection in mice boosts testosterone production, osteocalcin or its receptor might be also viewed as a suitable treatment target for fertility disorders in men and also associated changes in aging men.

Lastly, genome-wide studies and associative data suggest that disturbances in osteocalcin production or in its receptor signaling might be linked to prostate cancers. Clearly, the rising frequency and the high level of morbidity of prostate cancers suffice to justify the importance in future research effort to uncover molecular bases of the appearance, development, and progression of prostate cancer related to osteocalcin or its receptor.

References

[1] Callewaert F, Boonen S, Vanderschueren D. Sex steroids and the male skeleton: a tale of two hormones. Trends Endocrinol Metab 2010a;21:89–95.

[2] Riggs BL, Khosla S, Melton, . 3rd LJ. Sex steroids and the construction and conservation of the adult skeleton. Endocr Rev 2002;23:279–302.

[3] Vanderschueren D, Vandenput L, Boonen S, Lindberg MK, Bouillon R, Ohlsson C. Androgens and bone. Endocr Rev 2004;25:389–425.

[4] Venken K, Callewaert F, Boonen S, Vanderschueren D. Sex hormones, their receptors and bone health. Osteoporos Int 2008;19:1517–25.

[5] Khosla S. Update in male osteoporosis. J Clin Endocrinol Metab 2010a;95:3–10.

[6] Khosla S. Update on estrogens and the skeleton. J Clin Endocrinol Metab 2010b;95:3569–77.

[7] Khosla S, Melton 3rd LJ, Atkinson EJ, O'Fallon WM. Relationship of serum sex steroid levels to longitudinal changes in bone density in young versus elderly men. J Clin Endocrinol Metab 2001;86:3555–61.

[8] Khosla S, Riggs BL. Pathophysiology of age-related bone loss and osteoporosis. Endocrinol Metab Clin North Am 2005;34:1015–30. xi.

[9] Nakamura T, Imai Y, Matsumoto T, Sato S, Takeuchi K, Igarashi K, et al. Estrogen prevents bone loss via estrogen receptor alpha and induction of Fas ligand in osteoclasts. Cell 2007;130:811–23.

[10] Riggs BL, O'Fallon WM, Muhs J, O'Connor MK, Kumar R, Melton 3rd LJ. Long-term effects of calcium supplementation on serum parathyroid hormone level, bone turnover, and bone loss in elderly women. J Bone Miner Res 1998;13:168–74.

[11] Aonuma H, Miyakoshi N, Hongo M, Kasukawa Y, Shimada Y. Low serum levels of undercarboxylated osteocalcin in postmenopausal osteoporotic women receiving an inhibitor of bone resorption. Tohoku J Exp Med 2009;218:201–5.

[12] Fernandez-Real JM, Izquierdo M, Ortega F, Gorostiaga E, Gomez-Ambrosi J, Moreno-Navarrete JM, et al. The relationship of serum osteocalcin concentration to insulin secretion, sensitivity, and disposal with hypocaloric diet and resistance training. J Clin Endocrinol Metab 2009;94:237–45.

[13] Ferron M, Wei J, Yoshizawa T, Del Fattore A, DePinho RA, Teti A, et al. Insulin signaling in osteoblasts integrates bone remodeling and energy metabolism. Cell 2010;142:296–308.

[14] Hwang YC, Jeong IK, Ahn KJ, Chung HY. The uncarboxylated form of osteocalcin is associated with improved glucose tolerance and enhanced beta-cell function in middle-aged male subjects. Diabetes Metab Res Rev 2009;25:768–72.

[15] Im JA, Yu BP, Jeon JY, Kim SH. Relationship between osteocalcin and glucose metabolism in postmenopausal women. Clin Chim Acta 2008;396:66–9.

[16] Kanazawa I, Yamaguchi T, Yamamoto M, Yamauchi M, Kurioka S, Yano S, et al. Serum osteocalcin level is associated with glucose metabolism and atherosclerosis parameters in type 2 diabetes mellitus. J Clin Endocrinol Metab 2009; 94:45–9.

[17] Kindblom JM, Ohlsson C, Ljunggren O, Karlsson MK, Tivesten A, Smith U, et al. Plasma osteocalcin is inversely related to fat mass and plasma glucose in elderly Swedish men. J Bone Miner Res 2009;24:785–91.

[18] Lee NK, Sowa H, Hinoi E, Ferron M, Ahn JD, Confavreux C, et al. Endocrine regulation of energy metabolism by the skeleton. Cell 2007;130:456–69.

[19] Levinger I, Zebaze R, Jerums G, Hare DL, Selig S, Seeman E. The effect of acute exercise on undercarboxylated osteocalcin in obese men. Osteoporos Int 2011;22(5):1621–6.

[20] Pittas AG, Harris SS, Eliades M, Stark P, Dawson-Hughes B. Association between serum osteocalcin and markers of metabolic phenotype. J Clin Endocrinol Metab 2009;94:827–32.

[21] Rached MT, Kode A, Xu L, Yoshikawa Y, Paik JH, Depinho RA, et al. FoxO1 is a positive regulator of bone formation by favoring protein synthesis and resistance to oxidative stress in osteoblasts. Cell Metab 2010;11:147–60.

[22] Winhofer Y, Handisurya A, Tura A, Bittighofer C, Klein K, Schneider B, et al. Osteocalcin is related to enhanced insulin secretion in gestational diabetes mellitus. Diabetes Care 2010;33:139–43.

[23] Yeap BB, Chubb SA, Flicker L, McCaul KA, Ebeling PR, Beilby JP, et al. Reduced serum total osteocalcin is associated with metabolic syndrome in older men via waist circumference, hyperglycemia, and triglyceride levels. Eur J Endocrinol 2010;163:265–72.

[24] Fulzele K, Riddle RC, DiGirolamo DJ, Cao X, Wan C, Chen D, et al. Insulin receptor signaling in osteoblasts regulates postnatal bone acquisition and body composition. Cell 2010; 142:309–19.

[25] Oury F, Sumara G, Sumara O, Ferron M, Chang H, Smith CE, et al. Endocrine regulation of male fertility by the skeleton. Cell 2011;144:796–809.

[26] Kirmani S, Atkinson EJ, Melton 3rd LJ, Riggs BL, Amin S, Khosla S. Relationship of testosterone and osteocalcin levels during growth. J Bone Miner Res 2011;26:2212–6.

[27] Harada S, Rodan GA. Control of osteoblast function and regulation of bone mass. Nature 2003;423:349–55.

[28] Karsenty G. Convergence between bone and energy homeostases: leptin regulation of bone mass. Cell Metab 2006;4:341–8.

[29] Rodan GA, Martin TJ. Therapeutic approaches to bone diseases. Science 2000;289:1508–14.

[30] Teitelbaum SL. Osteoclasts, integrins, and osteoporosis. J Bone Miner Metab 2000;18:344–9.

[31] Clarke BL, Khosla S. Physiology of bone loss. Radiol Clin North Am 2010;48:483–95.

[32] Raisz LG. Pathogenesis of osteoporosis: concepts, conflicts, and prospects. J Clin Invest 2005;115:3318–25.

[33] Kaufman JM, Vermeulen A. The decline of androgen levels in elderly men and its clinical and therapeutic implications. Endocr Rev 2005;26:833–76.

[34] Khosla S, Amin S, Orwoll E. Osteoporosis in men. Endocr Rev 2008;29:441–64.

[35] Manolagas SC, Kousteni S, Jilka RL. Sex steroids and bone. Recent Prog Horm Res 2002;57:385–409.

[36] Stepan JJ, Lachman M, Zverina J, Pacovsky V, Baylink DJ. Castrated men exhibit bone loss: effect of calcitonin treatment on biochemical indices of bone remodeling. J Clin Endocrinol Metab 1989;69:523–7.

[37] Kelly PJ, Twomey L, Sambrook PN, Eisman JA. Sex differences in peak adult bone mineral density. J Bone Miner Res 1990;5:1169–75.

[38] Kirmani S, Christen D, van Lenthe GH, Fischer PR, Bouxsein ML, McCready LK, et al. Bone structure at the distal radius during adolescent growth. J Bone Miner Res 2009;24:1033–42.

[39] Seeman E. Clinical review 137: sexual dimorphism in skeletal size, density, and strength. J Clin Endocrinol Metab 2001; 86:4576—84.

[40] Turner RT, Wakley GK, Hannon KS. Differential effects of androgens on cortical bone histomorphometry in gonadectomized male and female rats. J Orthop Res 1990;8:612—7.

[41] Bertelloni S, Baroncelli GI, Battini R, Perri G, Saggese G. Short-term effect of testosterone treatment on reduced bone density in boys with constitutional delay of puberty. J Bone Miner Res 1995;10:1488—95.

[42] Finkelstein JS, Klibanski A, Neer RM. A longitudinal evaluation of bone mineral density in adult men with histories of delayed puberty. J Clin Endocrinol Metab 1996;81:1152—5.

[43] Katznelson L, Finkelstein JS, Schoenfeld DA, Rosenthal DI, Anderson EJ, Klibanski A. Increase in bone density and lean body mass during testosterone administration in men with acquired hypogonadism. J Clin Endocrinol Metab 1996;81:4358—65.

[44] Lorentzon M, Swanson C, Andersson N, Mellstrom D, Ohlsson C. Free testosterone is a positive, whereas free estradiol is a negative, predictor of cortical bone size in young Swedish men: the GOOD study. J Bone Miner Res 2005;20:1334—41.

[45] Morishima A, Grumbach MM, Simpson ER, Fisher C, Qin K. Aromatase deficiency in male and female siblings caused by a novel mutation and the physiological role of estrogens. J Clin Endocrinol Metab 1995;80:3689—98.

[46] Buchanan JR, Myers C, Lloyd T, Leuenberger P, Demers LM. Determinants of peak trabecular bone density in women: the role of androgens, estrogen, and exercise. J Bone Miner Res 1988;3:673—80.

[47] Wei S, Jones G, Thomson R, Otahal P, Dwyer T, Venn A. Menstrual irregularity and bone mass in premenopausal women: cross-sectional associations with testosterone and SHBG. BMC Musculoskelet Disord 2010;11:288.

[48] Zborowski JV, Cauley JA, Talbott EO, Guzick DS, Winters SJ. Clinical Review 116: bone mineral density, androgens, and the polycystic ovary: the complex and controversial issue of androgenic influence in female bone. J Clin Endocrinol Metab 2000;85:3496—506.

[49] Callewaert F, Sinnesael M, Gielen E, Boonen S, Vanderschueren D. Skeletal sexual dimorphism: relative contribution of sex steroids, GH-IGF1, and mechanical loading. J Endocrinol 2010b;207:127—34.

[50] Lupu F, Terwilliger JD, Lee K, Segre GV, Efstratiadis A. Roles of growth hormone and insulin-like growth factor 1 in mouse postnatal growth. Dev Biol 2001;229:141—62.

[51] Venken K, Schuit F, Van Lommel L, Tsukamoto K, Kopchick JJ, Coschigano K, et al. Growth without growth hormone receptor: estradiol is a major growth hormone-independent regulator of hepatic IGF-I synthesis. J Bone Miner Res 2005;20:2138—49.

[52] Callewaert F, Venken K, Kopchick JJ, Torcasio A, van Lenthe GH, Boonen S, et al. Sexual dimorphism in cortical bone size and strength but not density is determined by independent and time-specific actions of sex steroids and IGF-1: evidence from pubertal mouse models. J Bone Miner Res 2010c; 25:617—26.

[53] Foresta C, Guarneri G, Scanelli G, Scandellari C. Osteoporosis in elderly men. Clin Endocrinol (Oxf) 1984;21:309—10.

[54] Reim NS, Breig B, Stahr K, Eberle J, Hoeflich A, Wolf E, et al. Cortical bone loss in androgen-deficient aged male rats is mainly caused by increased endocortical bone remodeling. J Bone Miner Res 2008;23:694—704.

[55] Vandenput L, Swinnen JV, Boonen S, Van Herck E, Erben RG, Bouillon R, et al. Role of the androgen receptor in skeletal homeostasis: the androgen-resistant testicular feminized male mouse model. J Bone Miner Res 2004;19:1462—70.

[56] Garnero P, Sornay-Rendu E, Chapuy MC, Delmas PD. Increased bone turnover in late postmenopausal women is a major determinant of osteoporosis. J Bone Miner Res 1996;11:337—49.

[57] Lindsay R, Hart DM, Aitken JM, MacDonald EB, Anderson JB, Clarke AC. Long-term prevention of postmenopausal osteoporosis by oestrogen. Evidence for an increased bone mass after delayed onset of oestrogen treatment. Lancet 1976; 1:1038—41.

[58] Lindsay R, Hart DM, Forrest C, Baird C. Prevention of spinal osteoporosis in oophorectomised women. Lancet 1980;2:1151—4.

[59] Stevenson JC, Cust MP, Gangar KF, Hillard TC, Lees B, Whitehead MI. Effects of transdermal versus oral hormone replacement therapy on bone density in spine and proximal femur in postmenopausal women. Lancet 1990;336:265—9.

[60] Behre HM, Kliesch S, Leifke E, Link TM, Nieschlag E. Long-term effect of testosterone therapy on bone mineral density in hypogonadal men. J Clin Endocrinol Metab 1997;82:2386—90.

[61] Wakley GK, Schutte Jr HD, Hannon KS, Turner RT. Androgen treatment prevents loss of cancellous bone in the orchidectomized rat. J Bone Miner Res 1991;6:325—30.

[62] Greendale GA, Edelstein S, Barrett-Connor E. Endogenous sex steroids and bone mineral density in older women and men: the Rancho Bernardo Study. J Bone Miner Res 1997;12:1833—43.

[63] Khosla S, Melton 3rd LJ, Atkinson EJ, O'Fallon WM, Klee GG, Riggs BL. Relationship of serum sex steroid levels and bone turnover markers with bone mineral density in men and women: a key role for bioavailable estrogen. J Clin Endocrinol Metab 1998;83:2266—74.

[64] Slemenda CW, Longcope C, Zhou L, Hui SL, Peacock M, Johnston CC. Sex steroids and bone mass in older men. Positive associations with serum estrogens and negative associations with androgens. J Clin Invest 1997;100:1755—9.

[65] Araujo AB, Travison TG, Leder BZ, McKinlay JB. Correlations between serum testosterone, estradiol, and sex hormone-binding globulin and bone mineral density in a diverse sample of men. J Clin Endocrinol Metab 2008;93:2135—41.

[66] Bjornerem A, Ahmed LA, Joakimsen RM, Berntsen GK, Fonnebo V, Jorgensen L, et al. A prospective study of sex steroids, sex hormone-binding globulin, and non-vertebral fractures in women and men: the Tromso Study. Eur J Endocrinol 2007;157:119—25.

[67] Mellstrom D, Vandenput L, Mallmin H, Holmberg AH, Lorentzon M, Oden A, et al. Older men with low serum estradiol and high serum SHBG have an increased risk of fractures. J Bone Miner Res 2008;23:1552—60.

[68] Orwoll E, Lambert LC, Marshall LM, Phipps K, Blank J, Barrett-Connor E, et al. Testosterone and estradiol among older men. J Clin Endocrinol Metab 2006;91:1336—44.

[69] Bouillon R, Bex M, Vanderschueren D, Boonen S. Estrogens are essential for male pubertal periosteal bone expansion. J Clin Endocrinol Metab 2004;89:6025—9.

[70] Mellstrom D, Johnell O, Ljunggren O, Eriksson AL, Lorentzon M, Mallmin H, et al. Free testosterone is an independent predictor of BMD and prevalent fractures in elderly men: MrOS Sweden. J Bone Miner Res 2006;21:529—35.

[71] Rochira V, Zirilli L, Madeo B, Aranda C, Caffagni G, Fabre B, et al. Skeletal effects of long-term estrogen and testosterone replacement treatment in a man with congenital aromatase deficiency: evidences of a priming effect of estrogen for sex steroids action on bone. Bone 2007;40:1662—8.

[72] van den Beld AW, de Jong FH, Grobbee DE, Pols HA, Lamberts SW. Measures of bioavailable serum testosterone and estradiol and their relationships with muscle strength, bone density, and body composition in elderly men. J Clin Endocrinol Metab 2000;85:3276—82.

[73] Gennari L, Khosla S, Bilezikian JP. Estrogen and fracture risk in men. J Bone Miner Res 2008;23:1548–51.

[74] Hughes DE, Dai A, Tiffee JC, Li HH, Mundy GR, Boyce BF. Estrogen promotes apoptosis of murine osteoclasts mediated by TGF-beta. Nat Med 1996;2:1132–6.

[75] Imai Y, Youn MY, Kondoh S, Nakamura T, Kouzmenko A, Matsumoto T, et al. Estrogens maintain bone mass by regulating expression of genes controlling function and life span in mature osteoclasts. Ann N Y Acad Sci 2009;1173(Suppl 1):E31–9.

[76] Majeska RJ, Ryaby JT, Einhorn TA. Direct modulation of osteoblastic activity with estrogen. J Bone Joint Surg Am 1994;76:713–21.

[77] Qu Q, Perala-Heape M, Kapanen A, Dahllund J, Salo J, Vaananen HK, et al. Estrogen enhances differentiation of osteoblasts in mouse bone marrow culture. Bone 1998;22:201–9.

[78] Jimi E, Ikebe T, Takahashi N, Hirata M, Suda T, Koga T. Interleukin-1 alpha activates an NF-kappaB-like factor in osteoclast-like cells. J Biol Chem 1996;271:4605–8.

[79] Pacifici R. Estrogen, cytokines, and pathogenesis of postmenopausal osteoporosis. J Bone Miner Res 1996;11:1043–51.

[80] Xing L, Boyce BF. Regulation of apoptosis in osteoclasts and osteoblastic cells. Biochem Biophys Res Commun 2005;328:709–20.

[81] Bodine PV, Riggs BL, Spelsberg TC. Regulation of c-fos expression and TGF-beta production by gonadal and adrenal androgens in normal human osteoblastic cells. J Steroid Biochem Mol Biol 1995;52:149–58.

[82] Gill RK, Turner RT, Wronski TJ, Bell NH. Orchiectomy markedly reduces the concentration of the three isoforms of transforming growth factor beta in rat bone, and reduction is prevented by testosterone. Endocrinology 1998;139:546–50.

[83] Tau KR, Hefferan TE, Waters KM, Robinson JA, Subramaniam M, Riggs BL, et al. Estrogen regulation of a transforming growth factor-beta inducible early gene that inhibits deoxyribonucleic acid synthesis in human osteoblasts. Endocrinology 1998;139:1346–53.

[84] Michael H, Harkonen PL, Vaananen HK, Hentunen TA. Estrogen and testosterone use different cellular pathways to inhibit osteoclastogenesis and bone resorption. J Bone Miner Res 2005;20:2224–32.

[85] Krum SA, Miranda-Carboni GA, Hauschka PV, Carroll JS, Lane TF, Freedman LP, et al. Estrogen protects bone by inducing Fas ligand in osteoblasts to regulate osteoclast survival. EMBO J 2008;27:535–45.

[86] Jilka RL, Hangoc G, Girasole G, Passeri G, Williams DC, Abrams JS, et al. Increased osteoclast development after estrogen loss: mediation by interleukin-6. Science 1992;257:88–91.

[87] Kasperk CH, Wergedal JE, Farley JR, Linkhart TA, Turner RT, Baylink DJ. Androgens directly stimulate proliferation of bone cells in vitro. Endocrinology 1989;124:1576–8.

[88] Kousteni S, Bellido T, Plotkin LI, O'Brien CA, Bodenner DL, Han L, et al. Nongenotropic, sex-nonspecific signaling through the estrogen or androgen receptors: dissociation from transcriptional activity. Cell 2001;104:719–30.

[89] Kousteni S, Chen JR, Bellido T, Han L, Ali AA, O'Brien CA, et al. Reversal of bone loss in mice by nongenotropic signaling of sex steroids. Science 2002;298:843–6.

[90] Seeman E. Pathogenesis of bone fragility in women and men. Lancet 2002;359:1841–50.

[91] Bord S, Horner A, Beavan S, Compston J. Estrogen receptors alpha and beta are differentially expressed in developing human bone. J Clin Endocrinol Metab 2001;86:2309–14.

[92] Noble B, Routledge J, Stevens H, Hughes I, Jacobson W. Androgen receptors in bone-forming tissue. Horm Res 1999;51:31–6.

[93] Vidal O, Kindblom LG, Ohlsson C. Expression and localization of estrogen receptor-beta in murine and human bone. J Bone Miner Res 1999;14:923–9.

[94] Tsai MJ, O'Malley BW. Molecular mechanisms of action of steroid/thyroid receptor superfamily members. Annu Rev Biochem 1994;63:451–86.

[95] Couse JF, Hewitt SC, Bunch DO, Sar M, Walker VR, Davis BJ, et al. Postnatal sex reversal of the ovaries in mice lacking estrogen receptors alpha and beta. Science 1999;286:2328–31.

[96] Couse JF, Korach KS. Estrogen receptor null mice: what have we learned and where will they lead us? Endocr Rev 1999;20:358–417.

[97] Lindberg MK, Alatalo SL, Halleen JM, Mohan S, Gustafsson JA, Ohlsson C. Estrogen receptor specificity in the regulation of the skeleton in female mice. J Endocrinol 2001;171:229–36.

[98] Oz OK, Zerwekh JE, Fisher C, Graves K, Nanu L, Millsaps R, et al. Bone has a sexually dimorphic response to aromatase deficiency. J Bone Miner Res 2000;15:507–14.

[99] Vidal O, Lindberg MK, Hollberg K, Baylink DJ, Andersson G, Lubahn DB, et al. Estrogen receptor specificity in the regulation of skeletal growth and maturation in male mice. Proc Natl Acad Sci USA 2000;97:5474–9.

[100] Callewaert F, Venken K, Ophoff J, De Gendt K, Torcasio A, van Lenthe GH, et al. Differential regulation of bone and body composition in male mice with combined inactivation of androgen and estrogen receptor-alpha. FASEB J 2009;23:232–40.

[101] Losel RM, Falkenstein E, Feuring M, Schultz A, Tillmann HC, Rossol-Haseroth K, et al. Nongenomic steroid action: controversies, questions, and answers. Physiol Rev 2003;83:965–1016.

[102] Migliaccio A, Castoria G, Di Domenico M, de Falco A, Bilancio A, Lombardi M, et al. Steroid-induced androgen receptor-oestradiol receptor beta-Src complex triggers prostate cancer cell proliferation. EMBO J 2000;19:5406–17.

[103] Song RX, McPherson RA, Adam L, Bao Y, Shupnik M, Kumar R, et al. Linkage of rapid estrogen action to MAPK activation by ERalpha-Shc association and Shc pathway activation. Mol Endocrinol 2002;16:116–27.

[104] Hinoi E, Gao N, Jung DY, Yadav V, Yoshizawa T, Myers Jr MG, et al. The sympathetic tone mediates leptin's inhibition of insulin secretion by modulating osteocalcin bioactivity. J Cell Biol 2008;183:1235–42.

[105] Yoshikawa Y, Kode A, Xu L, Mosialou I, Silva BC, Ferron M, et al. Genetic evidence points to an osteocalcin–independent influence of osteoblasts on energy metabolism. J Bone Miner Res 2011;26:2012–25.

[106] Pi M, Chen L, Huang MZ, Zhu W, Ringhofer B, Luo J, et al. GPRC6A null mice exhibit osteopenia, feminization and metabolic syndrome. PLoS One 2008;3:e3858.

[107] Pi M, Wu Y, Quarles LD. GPRC6A mediates responses to osteocalcin in beta-cells in vitro and pancreas in vivo. J Bone Miner Res 2011;26:1680–3.

[108] Mah PM, Wittert GA. Obesity and testicular function. Mol Cell Endocrinol 2010;316:180–6.

[109] Lichtenstein P, Holm NV, Verkasalo PK, Iliadou A, Kaprio J, Koskenvuo M, et al. Environmental and heritable factors in the causation of cancer—analyses of cohorts of twins from Sweden, Denmark, and Finland. N Engl J Med 2000;343:78–85.

[110] Schaid DJ. The complex genetic epidemiology of prostate cancer. Hum Mol Genet 13 Spec No 2004;1:R103–21.

[111] Takata R, Akamatsu S, Kubo M, Takahashi A, Hosono N, Kawaguchi T, et al. Genome-wide association study identifies

five new susceptibility loci for prostate cancer in the Japanese population. Nat Genet 2010;42:751—4.

[112] Goltzman D. Mechanisms of the development of osteoblastic metastases. Cancer 1997;80:1581—7.

[113] Sturge J, Caley MP, Waxman J. Bone metastasis in prostate cancer: emerging therapeutic strategies. Nat Rev Clin Oncol 2011;8:357—68.

[114] Chang BL, Zheng SL, Hawkins GA, Isaacs SD, Wiley KE, Turner A, et al. Polymorphic GGC repeats in the androgen receptor gene are associated with hereditary and sporadic prostate cancer risk. Hum Genet 2002;110:122—9.

[115] Habuchi T, Liqing Z, Suzuki T, Sasaki R, Tsuchiya N, Tachiki H, et al. Increased risk of prostate cancer and benign prostatic hyperplasia associated with a CYP17 gene polymorphism with a gene dosage effect. Cancer Res 2000;60:5710—3.

[116] Ho GY, Knapp M, Freije D, Nelson WG, Smith JR, Carpten JD, et al. Transmission/disequilibrium tests of androgen receptor and glutathione S-transferase pi variants in prostate cancer families. Int J Cancer 2002;98:938—42.

[117] Thomas G, Jacobs KB, Yeager M, Kraft P, Wacholder S, Orr N, et al. Multiple loci identified in a genome-wide association study of prostate cancer. Nat Genet 2008;40:310—5.

[118] Wu HC, Lin CC, Chen WC, Chen HY, Tsai FJ. Osteocalcin gene HindIII C/T polymorphism is a biomarker for prostate cancer and responsiveness to hormone therapy. Eur Urol 2003; 43:197—200.

[119] Pi M, Quarles LD. GPRC6A regulates prostate cancer progression. Prostate 2012 Mar;72(4):399—409.

[120] Li S, Huang S, Peng SB. Overexpression of G protein-coupled receptors in cancer cells: involvement in tumor progression. Int J Oncol 2005;27:1329—39.

[121] Greenberg NM, DeMayo F, Finegold MJ, Medina D, Tilley WD, Aspinall JO, et al. Prostate cancer in a transgenic mouse. Proc Natl Acad Sci USA 1995;92:3439—43.

[122] Gardner TA, Lee SJ, Lee SD, Li X, Shirakawa T, Kwon DD, et al. Differential expression of osteocalcin during the metastatic progression of prostate cancer. Oncol Rep 2009;21:903—8.

[123] Levedakou EN, Strohmeyer TG, Effert PJ, Liu ET. Expression of the matrix Gla protein in urogenital malignancies. Int J Cancer 1992;52:534—7.

[124] Yeung F, Law WK, Yeh CH, Westendorf JJ, Zhang Y, Wang R, et al. Regulation of human osteocalcin promoter in hormone-independent human prostate cancer cells. J Biol Chem 2002;277:2468—76.

[125] Nimptsch K, Rohrmann S, Nieters A, Linseisen J. Serum undercarboxylated osteocalcin as biomarker of vitamin K intake and risk of prostate cancer: a nested case—control study in the Heidelberg cohort of the European prospective investigation into cancer and nutrition. Cancer Epidemiol Biomarkers Prev 2009;18:49—56.

[126] Ellem SJ, Risbridger GP. Aromatase and regulating the estrogen:androgen ratio in the prostate gland. J Steroid Biochem Mol Biol 2010;118:246—51.

[127] Ahima RS. No Kiss1ng by leptin during puberty? J Clin Invest 2010;121:34—6.

[128] Tena-Sempere M, Barreiro ML. Leptin in male reproduction: the testis paradigm. Mol Cell Endocrinol 2002;188:9—13.

Regulation of Phosphate Metabolism by FGF23

Beate Lanske, Michael Densmore, Mohammed S. Razzaque

Harvard School of Dental Medicine, Boston, MA, USA

INTRODUCTION

Phosphate has multiple roles, from skeletal mineralization to cellular biochemistry, and optimal phosphate balance in the body is critical to health. Insufficient levels of phosphate disrupt a multitude of physiological processes, whereas excessive levels are toxic and cause or exacerbate several diseases, including cardiovascular calcification. Bone is a repository of phosphate, and research conducted in the last decade has revealed an even more active role for bone in phosphate homeostasis. Not only is bone a phosphate storage system, it also functions as an endocrine organ that secretes one of the three key hormonal factors in the complex, highly integrated, regulatory network that controls homeostatic balance of phosphate and calcium in the body. Fibroblast growth factor 23 (FGF23) is produced in osteoblasts and osteocytes [1] and released into the bloodstream to target the kidneys and parathyroid glands where it affects phosphate metabolism in the kidney and gene transcription in both organs. In turn, the parathyroid gland and kidney produce parathyroid hormone (PTH) and active vitamin D, which regulate FGF23 production. Thus, the three hormones control each other's' activity in order to maintain homeostatic balance of serum phosphate [2]. FGF23 is the focus of this chapter. First, however, a necessary introduction to phosphate metabolism, including key organs and hormonal factors, is presented. We also give an overview of FGF biology in order to place FGF23 in an evolutionary and physiological context. The major section of this chapter explains what we know about FGF23 (and its required co-factor Klotho), its role in phosphate homeostasis and disease, and how it interacts with the other key factors in the phosphate regulatory network. We also present an overview of some of the possible roles of FGF23 in other organs and disease processes. (Note that there is a more detailed discussion of these diseases in a separate chapter.) We conclude with a summary of what we know about FGF23 and what remains to be discovered about this biologically important molecule.

PHOSPHATE METABOLISM

Phosphate is widely distributed in the body, with more than 80% of total phosphate sequestered in bone and teeth in the form of apatite. The remaining phosphate is mostly present in various soft tissues, including skeletal muscle. Less than 0.1% of phosphate is present in extracellular fluids or within cells [3–6]. Intracellular phosphate ions are required for critical physiological activity, including energy production and enzyme activation by phosphorylation [7]. Adequate phosphate is controlled by interactions among the intestine, kidney, and bone (Fig. 12.1) [4,8–11]. Phosphate absorption takes place mostly in the small intestine [12]. The sodium-dependent phosphate (NaPi) co-transporter, NaPi-2b, in the luminal side of the intestinal cells is primarily responsible for intestinal phosphate absorption. The transport activity of intestinal NaPi-2b is influenced by 1,25-dihydroxyvitamin D and dietary phosphate [13]. For instance, 1,25-dihydroxyvitamin D increases the expression of intestinal NaPi-2b protein in order to enhance intestinal phosphate absorption. The importance of NaPi-2b has been demonstrated in *NaPi-2b−/−* mice where phosphate absorption decreases by 50% after acute administration of phosphate in comparison with wild-type mice [14]. However, the human relevance of *NaPi-2b−/−* mice is not clear, since loss-of-function mutations in the human NaPi-2b gene did not lead to significantly altered phosphate balance [15].

Renal tubular epithelial phosphate reabsorption is accomplished by sodium-dependent phosphate uptake through the NaPi2a and NaPi2c transporters; PTH has a major influence on integration and retrieval of the NaPi2a transporter located on the apical membrane of the proximal tubular epithelial cells [16,17]. PTH suppresses NaPi-dependent phosphate reabsorption in

Translational Endocrinology of Bone
DOI: http://dx.doi.org/10.1016/B978-0-12-415784-2.00012-9

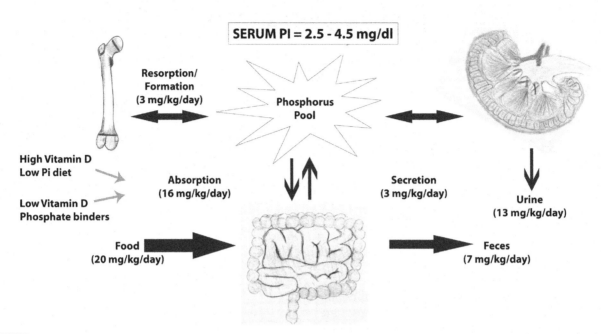

FIGURE 12.1 **Phosphate homeostasis.** The human body has 15–20 M of phosphate under healthy conditions. The amount of phosphate is a balance between intake and excretion in the intestines and kidneys. The level of phosphate in the serum is 2.5–4.5 mg/dl and this level is maintained by the constant interchange of phosphate between the serum and bone. The skeleton contains the bulk of the phosphate in the body, accounting for 80–90% of the total amount. Phosphate is transferred between bone and serum at a rate of about 3 mg per kilogram of body weight per day (3 mg/kg/day) as bone forms and is reabsorbed to balance bone strength and serum phosphate levels. Phosphate is abundant in the diet, with the average adult ingesting about 20 mg per kg of body weight. The intestine absorbs 55–80% of this intake. Around 16 mg/kg/day are absorbed in the proximal intestine while the digestive process eliminates 3 mg/kg/day. Approximately 7 mg/kg/day phosphate is excreted in the feces. The kidneys contribute to phosphate balance by regulating how much phosphate is excreted in the urine or reabsorbed into the serum. Under normal conditions, approximately 13 mg/kg/day, the equivalent of the amount taken in by the intestines, is excreted in the urine. Please see color plate section.

order to increase urinary phosphate excretion [16,17]. Recent studies have shown that bone-derived FGF23 and kidney-derived Klotho can also suppress sodium phosphate co-transporter activities [18–21]. However, the exact mechanism by which the FGF23–Klotho system affects the functionality of the transporters in the kidney is not completely clear, and further research is required to explain the underlying mechanism [22,23].

In addition to intestine and kidney, bone plays a major role in phosphate metabolism. Not only does it act as an endocrine organ in the regulation of mineral ion homeostasis as we describe later, it is the major repository of phosphate in the body. Phosphate, in combination with calcium, forms the hydroxyapatite required for bone mineralization. The skeleton is being continuously remodeled, releasing and taking in phosphate in a relatively balanced fashion. The remodeling process is typically activated in response to mechanical strain or bone damage as the body works to maintain proper skeletal strength and integrity. Osteoblastic and osteoclastic activities through the activation of the Rankl–Rank system delicately control bone remodeling. Stromal cells on the bone surface are stimulated to express a surface protein calledreceptor activator of nuclear factor κ B

ligand (Rankl). This protein binds with another surface protein called receptor activator of nuclear factor κ B (Rank) on circulating osteoclast progenitor cells, inducing them to differentiate into mature osteoclasts that break down bone. In addition, the stromal cells can also downregulate the expression of osteoprotegerin (OPG), a decoy receptor for Rankl, which would otherwise block the Rankl–Rank binding between the stromal and progenitor cells [24]. Thus, the relative balance of Rankl and OPG can also influence the remodeling process.

Bone remodeling can also occur when the mineral ion concentration in the blood falls below normal values. When serum phosphate levels fall irrespective of etiologies, additional phosphate is released into the serum by increased bone resorption, a process that is mostly regulated by PTH and vitamin D. PTH acts directly on stromal cells to stimulate Rankl expression and reduce expression of OPG [25,26], while vitamin D stimulates osteoclast differentiation and activity [27]. Moreover, as we describe in the following sections, PTH and vitamin D are also hormonal factors that can induce FGF23 production in bone to regulate serum phosphate levels and thus indirectly regulate bone resorption.

FGF BIOLOGY

FGF23 is a member of the FGF of signaling molecules. Almost all FGFs are secreted paracrine signals that target specific tyrosine kinase receptors (FGFRs) to perform their actions. A few, including FGF23, act in an endocrine fashion as hormonal regulators. There are also a small number of intracrine FGFs that are not secreted and act intracellularly. The genes that encode FGFs have a deep evolutionary history in metazoans and are of particular importance in vertebrates which consequently have the largest number of FGFs. In this section we briefly describe the structure, mechanism, actions, regulation, and evolution of these important molecules.

Mammalian FGFs

There are 22 known *Fgf* genes in the mouse and human genome. These are organized into seven subfamilies based on their structure and evolutionary history. The first FGFs to be identified, FGF1 and FGF2, were isolated from the brain and pituitary and were used as mitogens for fibroblasts in culture, hence the family name. Additional family members were identified by their mitogenic properties in cultures and by homology-based PCR or genomic database searches. A few were identified by their roles in hereditary diseases, including FGF23 [28–33]. All FGFs have a core sequence of approximately 120 amino acids. There are also four conserved structural motifs that align with the three modes in which FGFs act: intracrine, paracrine, and endocrine [29].

Intracrine FGFs are the earliest members of the FGFs and are represented as a single family of four genes in mammals: *Fgf11*, *Fgf12*, *Fgf13*, and *Fgf14*. These FGFs have a heparin binding sequence in addition to the core sequence but have no secreted signal sequence. Thus, these FGFs are not secreted and act intracellularly. They have only one known physiological role: to regulate electrical sensitivity in neurons by interacting with the intracellular domains of voltage-gated sodium channels [34].

Paracrine FGFs make up the majority of FGFs in mammals. An early gene duplication, followed by a series of genome duplications in vertebrates, led to five subfamilies of paracrine FGFs (see Table 12.1 for a list of paracrine FGF subfamilies and genes) [28]. The original duplicate gene had acquired a cleavable secreted signal sequence which allowed this form of FGF to be secreted. Four of the five families retain this feature. Paracrine FGFs require heparin sulfate proteoglycans (HSPG) as a co-factor in order to bind efficiently with their receptors. HSPGs are produced by all cells and their presence on neighboring cells limits the range of activity for secreted paracrine FGFs. Paracrine FGFs have a wide range of roles in embryonic development where they are important regulators in patterning and morphogenesis [30].

Another gene duplication that occurred early in the evolution of vertebrates produced the subfamily of *endocrine* FGFs: *Fgf15/19*, *Fgf21*, and *Fgf23* [28]. This type of FGF is only found in vertebrates and they are important regulators of physiological activity. These FGFs lost the ability to properly bind with heparin during evolution (see "FGF23 Biology," below) and this is the key adaptation that allowed these molecules to become circulating, hormonal factors since they were no longer immediately bound to nearby cells. They still require a co-factor for efficient binding to their receptors, however. But instead of HSPG, they now use a different protein family called Klotho that has two forms, α-Klotho and β-Klotho.

Klotho is a membrane protein and is bound to the surface of the cells that produce it. This limits the action of the endocrine FGFs to cells that express the type of Klotho required for receptor binding. FGF23, which is a key hormone in regulating phosphate homeostasis, is secreted by osteoblasts and osteocytes and targets cells in the parathyroid and kidney that express a form of Klotho called α-Klotho. The remaining endocrine FGFs, 19 and 21, use the other form of Klotho, β-Klotho, to bind their receptors and target the tissues where they act to regulate glucose metabolism and bile acid production.

Mammalian FGF Receptors

Mammals have four fibroblast growth factor receptors (FGFR) that co-evolved with the FGFs. These genes (*Fgfr1–Fgfr4*) encode a transmembrane protein with a tyrosine kinase intracellular domain and an extracellular domain with three immunoglobulin (Ig) domains [28]. FGF ligands bind to the second and third IGg domains with their co-factors (HSPG or Klotho) to activate the signaling pathways in the targeted cells. Alternate splicing of these two domains creates variants in three of the four FGFRs, increasing the number of functional receptors to seven. Table 12.1 lists the specific matches between FGFs and FGFR variants. The binding of the FGF ligand to a pair of FGFRs results in a receptor dimer that activates the tyrosine kinases through mutual phosphorylation.

Generic FGF Signaling

All FGFs, including FGF23, activate a common set of pathways when they bind to their receptors. We briefly describe FGF signaling and regulation in this section [35]. A more detailed and specific description of FGF23 binding and signaling is presented in the section "FGF23 Biology," below.

TABLE 12.1   FGF Superfamily

Subfamily	Member	FGFR1b	FGFR1c	FGFR2b	FGFR2c	FGFR3b	FGFR3c	FGFR4
				Receptor binding				
FGF1	FGF1	x	x	x	x	x	x	x
	FGF2	x	x		x		x	x
FGF4	FGF4		x		x		x	x
	FGF5		x					
	FGF6		x		x			x
FGF7	FGF3	x		x				
	FGF7			x				
	FGF10	x		x				
	FGF22			x				
FGF8	FGF8						x	x
	FGF17				x		x	x
	FGF18				x		x	x
FGF9	FGF9				x	x	x	x
	FGF16							x
	FGF20		x	x	x		x	
FGF11	FGF11							
	FGF12							
	FGF13							
	FGF14							
FGF19	FGF15/19		x					x
	FGF21		x					x
	FGF23		x				x	x

Members of the FGF superfamily are grouped by subfamily and receptor binding specificity for each member is indicated. Subfamilies are grouped by mode of activity. Top: paracrine FGFs. Middle: intracrine FGFs. Bottom: endocrine FGFs.

Once an FGF ligand and co-factor bind to two FGFRs to form the receptor dimer, the activated tyrosine kinases can initiate a signaling pathway [36]. FGFs activate common pathways, including RAS–RAF–MAPK, PI₃K–AKT, PLCγ–PKC, and STAT. The MAPK and AKT pathways are activated via a scaffold of proteins that assembles around the tyrosine kinases while the PLCγ–PKC and STAT are directly activated by the kinases. The MAPK pathway, which includes MEK and ERK1/2 as downstream components, is the most important of the FGF signaling pathways and is commonly used by FGF23. There is also crosstalk among the FGF pathways and pathways of other important signaling proteins such as Wnt and BMP [37,38].

FGF signaling is regulated in several ways [36]. Sulfatases can modify HSPG, for example, and reduce or eliminate its FGFR binding capacity. Enzymes that affect Klotho expression and stability exert a similar regulatory effect on the endocrine FGFs. Another mechanism to regulate FGF binding is to block the ligand. "Similar expression to FGF" (SEF) is a transmembrane protein that associates with FGFRs to negatively regulate FGF activity. FGFRL1 is a potential regulator in that it may act as a decoy receptor and sequester the FGF ligands, preventing them from activating FGFRs. Once an FGF ligand binds an FGFR and the active dimer is produced, the downstream signaling mechanisms can be disrupted. Typically, these internal regulators disrupt the scaffold required for the MAPK and AKT pathways or dephosphorylate key signaling components in a pathway. Interestingly, some of the internal regulators are stimulated by FGF signaling to self-modulate its effects.

FGF23 AND PHOSPHATE METABOLISM

In the previous section, we described the overall biology and evolution of FGFs including FGF23. In this section we focus on FG23 and its central role in phosphate metabolism (Fig. 12.2). First, we describe the specific biology of FGF23, including its requirement for Klotho as a co-factor, and how these two work together to regulate systemic phosphate levels. We then describe how FGF23 works with its key partners PTH and vitamin D to form a regulatory network to maintain a balanced mineral homeostasis.

FGF23 Biology

FGF23 is a 251aa, secreted protein that belongs to the FGF19 subfamily of endocrine FGFs. Its NH2-terminus carries a 25aa signal peptide followed by a well-conserved core area found in all FGF ligands which contain the FGFR binding domain. As described above, endocrine FGFs have a conformation change in this core region which reduces heparin binding affinity [39]. This conformational change prevents the secreted ligand from being bound by heparin in nearby cells and thus allows the ligands to circulate and act as endocrine hormones. To compensate for the loss of heparin binding capacity, the COOH-terminus of FGF23 has a unique sequence that contains a Klotho binding site [40]. Thus the α-form of Klotho acts as a replacement co-factor for HSPG.

FGF23 is mostly expressed in brain and bone, but lower levels have also been found in the thymus, small intestine, heart, liver, thyroid/parathyroid, and skeletal muscle [41]. The active form of FGF23 is a large 30 kDa protein that functions as a phosphaturic hormone. It contains a number of glycosylation sites (71S, 96M, 129S, and 178T). Uridine diphosphate-N-acetyl-alpha-D-galactosamine:polypeptide N-acetylgalactosaminyl-transferase 3 (GALNT3) has been shown to O-glycosylate

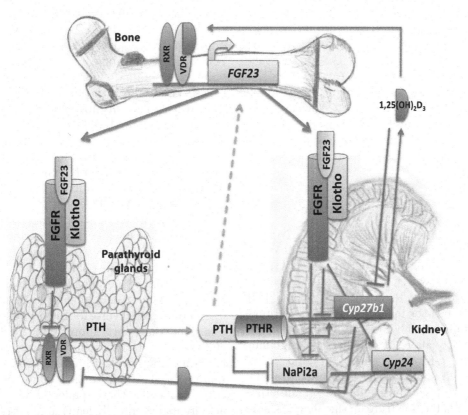

FIGURE 12.2 The bone, kidney, and parathyroid gland axis. FGF23 from bone, PTH from the parathyroid glands, and vitamin D from the kidneys regulate phosphate serum levels and each other. PTH is produced in the parathyroid glands and targets the kidney to increase phosphate wasting by downregulating the sodium transporter, NaPi2a. It also increases the production of active vitamin D by upregulating Cyp27b1 which converts 25(OH) vitamin D to its active form (1,25(OH)$_2$D$_3$). 1,25(OH)$_2$D$_3$ downregulates PTH production in a negative feedback loop to regulate PTH activity. 1,25(OH)$_2$D$_3$ stimulates FGF23 production in the bone which also targets the kidney to reduce NaPi2a activities, thereby increasing urinary phosphate wasting. In addition, FGF23 suppresses active vitamin D production in the kidney by downregulating Cyp27b1 and upregulating Cyp24, a hydroxylase that catabolizes 1,25(OH)$_2$D$_3$. This forms a second negative feedback loop in the phosphate regulatory network. Finally, PTH and FGF23 mutually regulate each other to form the third feedback loop. PTH stimulates FGF23 production in bone while FGF23 suppresses PTH in the parathyroid glands. Klotho is an important member of the network since it is required for FGF23 binding and signaling. Presence of Klotho in the parathyroid glands and kidneys allows FGF23 to specifically target these organs to maintain physiologic phosphate balance. Please see color plate section.

FGF23, thereby preventing proteolytic processing and allowing secretion of intact FGF23. Mutations in GALNT3 lead to enhanced degradation of FGF23, causing tumoral calcinosis [42−47]. The full-length protein is cleaved at position ^{176}RXXR^{179} by an unknown subtilisin-like proconvertase into 18 kDa N-terminal and 12 kDa C-terminal inactive fragments as part of its regulation. Missense mutations found at this cleavage site in humans have been shown to result in an accumulation of the active full-length FGF23 protein that results in uncontrolled renal phosphate wasting and ultimately rickets [23].

It was recently shown that iron has a role in FGF23 activity, and thus in phosphate metabolism [48]. It has been observed that reduced serum iron levels in ADHR patients are associated with increased serum FGF23. It was found that iron deficiencies in both healthy and transgenic mice with an ADHR phenotype led to increased expression of FGF23. However, the normal regulation of active FGF23 by cleavage has been compromised in ADHR patients due to a mutation in the cleavage site. Therefore, unlike healthy individuals, ADHR patients have no counterbalance for the increase in active FGF23 in the face of lower levels of iron and the subsequent build-up of active FGF23 that causes the clinical manifestations of the disease. This research also showed that the iron deficiency stimulates activation of a transcription factor, HIF1α, which is followed by the increase in transcription of FGF23. However, further research is needed to determine the molecular mechanism by which iron affects FGF23 production.

FGF23-Klotho and Phosphate Regulation

FGF23 favors phosphate renal excretion, in other words it acts as a phosphatonin. In vitro studies suggested that FGF23 binds to FGFR1c, FGFR3c, and FGFR4 [18,49−52]. However, in vivo studies failed to show that FGF23 binds with FGFR3 and FGFR4 [53], thus identifying FGFR1c as the target receptor. As previously noted, the interaction between FGF23 and FGFR1c and subsequent activation of downstream signaling networks requires α-Klotho. FGF23 can bind to its receptor complex with high affinity only in the presence of α-Klotho. FGF23-Klotho causes the FGFR1c dimerization and activation of the downstream signaling cascades described in the previous section. In particular, studies have shown that the FGF23−Klotho−FGFR1c complex recruits a number of phosphoproteins, including FGF receptor substrate-2α (FRS2α), to activate the extracellular signal-regulated kinase 1/2 (ERK1/2) pathway [54,55].

Klotho Co-receptor

Klotho is a 130-kDa membrane protein [56,57] with two extracellular domains (KL1 and KL2) that can be cleaved from the plasma membrane by disintegrin and metalloproteinases (ADAM-10 and ADAM-17) [58] releasing the extracellular domains into circulation. Klotho is primarily expressed in the kidney (distal convoluted tubules), in the brain (choroid plexus epithelium), and in the parathyroid glands [59]. The limited expression of membrane-bound Klotho restricts the activity of circulating FGF23 to these specific tissues. FGF23 targets the kidney, using locally expressed Klotho in order to increase urinary phosphate excretion by suppressing the functions of NaPi2a and NaPi2c co-transporters [18,20,60]. The mechanism for reduction in renal NaPi co-transporter activity by the FGF23−Klotho system is not yet clear. A recent study detected low levels of Klotho expression in the proximal tubules and thus raising a possibility of downregulation of Napi2a by direct action of the FGF23−Klotho system [21].

FGF23 and Phosphate

The ability of FGF23 to reduce serum phosphate levels has been observed both in human and animal studies [19,23,45,61−63]. For example, in autosomal dominant hypophosphatemic rickets (ADHR) patients, FGF23 activity is increased by gain-of-function mutations in the human FGF23 gene. The increased activity is associated with hypophosphatemia caused by excessive urinary loss of phosphate [23]. Similarly, reduced serum phosphate levels in patients with autosomal recessive hypophosphatemic rickets (ARHR) or with X-linked hypophosphatemia (XLH) are also attributed to increased activity of FGF23 [64,65]. Phosphate wasting is also observed in transgenic mice that overexpress human FGF23 [66−69].

The effect of FGF23 is confirmed by genetically eliminating the functions of Fgf23 from mice. The loss of FGF23 function results in reduced phosphate excretion, leading to hyperphosphatemia [68−70]. More importantly, restoring the function of FGF23 in Fgf23−/− mice, either by genetic manipulation or by therapeutic intervention, can reverse the hyperphosphatemia to hypophosphatemia, clearly showing the phosphate regulating ability of FGF23 in vivo [69]. Moreover, the hyperphosphatemia and ectopic calcification observed in Fgf23−/− mice mimics the clinical features of familial tumoral calcinosis (FTC) patients. These patients have reduced FGF23 activity that eventually leads to hyperphosphatemia and ectopic calcification [63,69]. As mentioned before, changes in proper glycosylation of the FGF23 protein due to either a mutation in the glycosylation site or lack of GALNT3 activity were shown to lead to enhanced proteolysis of the FGF23 protein, rendering it non-functional [46]. FGF23 acts on the kidney to promote phosphate wasting and this is modulated by the NaPi2a transporter. Two studies with transgenic mice demonstrated this mechanism. NaPi2a expression in Fgf23−/− and Klotho−/−

mice is highly upregulated. When *NaPi2a−/−* mice are crossed with *Fgf23−/−* or *Klotho−/−* mice to ablate this transporter, the hyperphosphatemia is reversed to hypophosphatemia in *Fgf23−/−/NaPi2a−/−* and *Klotho−/−/NaPi2a−/−* mice [60,71].

FGF23 and Klotho

The requirement for Klotho in FGF23-mediated phosphate metabolism has been convincingly demonstrated in various animal models. Wild-type mice challenged with bioactive FGF23 protein have significantly reduced serum phosphate levels. However, FGF23 is unable to exert its phosphate lowering effects in mice that lack Klotho such as *Klotho−/−* mice or *Fgf23−/−/ Klotho−/−* mice [62]. Hyp mutant mice that have a deletion mutation of the *Phex* (*phosphate regulating gene with homologies to endopeptidases on the X chromosome*) gene are a model for X-linked hypophosphatemia. Genetically eliminating Klotho from *Hyp* mice results in hyperphosphatemia, even though the *Hyp/Klotho−/−* double mutant mice have extremely high serum levels of Fgf23 [62,72]. Eliminating Klotho expression from *FGF23* transgenic mice reverses their hypophosphatemia to hyperphosphatemia, clearly suggesting the *in vivo* importance of Klotho in FGF23-mediated phosphate metabolism [73]. The requirement for Klotho by FGF23 to function has also been demonstrated in human studies. A homozygous loss-of-function mutation in the human Klotho gene results in high levels of FGF23 and severe hyperphosphatemia in a patient with tumoral calcinosis [45].

The identification of the indispensable role of Klotho in FGF23 activity has not only increased our understanding of the physiological regulation of phosphate metabolism [39,74,75], but it has also explained the pathogenesis of diseases associated with dysregulation of the FGF23−Klotho system [4,76]. The overlapping phenotypes of *Fgf23−/−*, *Klotho−/−* and *Fgf23−/−/- Klotho−/−* mice clearly suggest that a limited number of molecules form the biological network to coordinately regulate mineral ion balance [19], and one such important molecule is PTH.

FGF23 and PTH

Parathyroid hormone (PTH) is an 84 amino acid protein produced in the parathyroid glands in response to low levels of serum calcium. Secreted PTH targets bone and kidney in order to raise the level of serum calcium. The parathyroid glands monitor calcium levels via a membrane bound protein, the calcium-sensor receptor (CaR) which activates a $PIP_3−IP_3$ pathway that increases intracellular Ca^{2+} and promotes cleavage of PTH to an inactive form [2]. Lower serum calcium

levels reduce CaR signaling and allow active PTH to be secreted. PTH binds to the PTHR1, a seven transmembrane G-protein coupled receptor, to activate the PKA, PKC, and MAPK pathways in kidney and bone, two of the primary organs for maintaining mineral ion homeostasis [77]. In addition to serum calcium, PTH is regulated by vitamin D which suppresses PTH expression and parathyroid hyperplasia [78−80]. More recent findings show that FGF23 also suppresses PTH production (see below).

In the Kidney

Both PTH and FGF23 target the same renal co-transporters to reduce serum phosphate. PTH causes the internalization of the two sodium-phosphate co-transporters, NaPi2a and NaPi2c, which, in turn, leads to urinary phosphate wasting. Circulating FGF23 targets the proximal tubular epithelial cells to decrease phosphate reabsorption by suppressing expression of *NaPi2a* and *NaPi2c*, although the exact mechanism by which FGF23 downregulates these genes is still unclear. Interestingly, low levels of *Klotho* are also detected in proximal renal tubular epithelial cells [21], raising the possibility of direct effects of FGF23 on these transporters.

Furthermore, FGF23 reduces production of the active form of vitamin D, 1,25-dihydroxyvitamin D_3 $(1,25(OH)_2D_3)$, in the renal proximal tubules by suppressing the expression of $1\alpha(OH)$ase (Cyp27b1) which converts the inactive form to the active form [81]. Furthermore, FGF23 enhances expression of 25-hydroxyvitamin D3-24-hydroxylase (Cyp24), which then catabolizes $1,25(OH)_2D_3$ [81]. (See next section for more details.) Conversely, vitamin D is a potent stimulator of *Fgf23* expression in bone. FGF23 thus regulates its own production in a negative feedback loop by reducing active vitamin D production in the kidney. PTH, in contrast, induces production of active vitamin D in the kidney by upregulating $1\alpha(OH)$ase (Cyp27b1) which, in turn, suppresses PTH synthesis as a negative feedback loop. Hence, both FGF23 and PTH use renal vitamin D to regulate their own production but by exerting opposite actions upon vitamin D production. To compensate for this, the two factors also directly regulate each other.

Mutual Regulation of FGF23 and PTH

The roles of PTH and vitamin D in calcium homeostasis were worked out well before the full regulatory network for phosphate homeostasis was understood. We now know that PTH and FGF23 also control each other's expression directly as well as indirectly in order to form a negative feedback loop as part of this network (Fig. 12.2). This regulatory network is crucial since failure to properly modulate the activities of FGF23 and PTH leads to severe health consequences due to deregulation of phosphate metabolism, as seen in chronic kidney disease (CKD).

FGF23 and PTH directly regulate each other in a negative feedback loop whereby PTH stimulates FGF23 production and FGF23 suppresses PTH. The effect of PTH on serum FGF23 was first observed in mouse models of hyperparathyroidism where FGF23 levels were positively correlated with those of PTH but inversely with phosphate levels [82]. Later it was discovered that activation of the PTH receptor in bone via the PKA signaling pathway suppresses the Wnt inhibitor sclerostin, allowing Wnt to increase *Fgf23* transcription [83]. The PKA pathway may also act directly to increase transcription of *Fgf23* in bone. Conversely, the possibility that FGF23 might regulate PTH was hypothesized when it was found that Klotho and FRFR1c are both expressed in the parathyroid glands [84]. *In vivo* experiments showed that FGF23 activated the MAPK (MEK-ERK1/2) pathway in the parathyroid glands to suppress PTH. *In vitro* experiments showed that FGF23 also acts to increase 1α(OH)ase in bovine parathyroid cells, further suppressing PTH [85]. Both of these studies confirm a direct role for FGF23 in regulating PTH.

Using Disease Models to Study FGF23–PTH

The use of disease models to explore FGF23 and PTH interactions has provided a better understanding of how they function together, but equally important, how they function independently. While FGF23 acts on the parathyroid glands to suppress PTH production, it has been noted that PTH levels rise significantly in CKD patients, resulting in secondary hyperparathyroidism. This occurs despite the presence of very high levels of serum FGF23 in these patients, indicating that some sort of resistance to FGF23 develops over time. One study used the *Hyp* mouse model for X-linked hypophosphatemic rickets (XLH) to determine the role of PTH in the biochemical changes associated with this disease [86]. These mice mimic much of the phenotype of XLH patients, including severe hypophosphatemia due to defective renal reabsorption, elevated serum alkaline phosphatase, high levels of serum FGF23, and bone mineralization defects. Moreover, these mice have low-normal serum vitamin D levels when the opposite would be expected since they are hypophosphatemic. These mice were crossed with *PTH−/−* mice in order to eliminate PTH expression. Removing PTH led to hyperphosphatemia, severe hypocalcemia and, ultimately, early death. These biochemical effects and shortened survival could be reversed by administering exogenous PTH [87]. These results indicate that the high levels of PTH in *Hyp* mice are a response to the low serum calcium that is a result of the suppression of active vitamin D production by FGF23.

Ffg23−/− and *Klotho−/−* mice are another model used to study the relationship between FGF23 and PTH. FGF23 activity is eliminated in these mice and the actions of PTH can be studied in isolation from the systemic effects of FGF23. *Ffg23−/−* and *Klotho−/−* mice exhibit identical aging-like phenotypes that include soft tissue calcification and skeletal anomalies, accompanied by high serum levels of calcium, phosphate, and vitamin D. The high serum levels of phosphate are similar to those seen in CKD patients. However, PTH levels in these mice are almost undetectable, whereas the levels in patients with CKD are abnormally high. This key difference provided a unique experimental model to study altered serum mineral levels with different systemic hormonal conditions. In one study, *Ffg23−/−* mice were crossed with *PTH−/−* mice to ablate PTH expression in these mice [87]. Complete removal of PTH function resulted in lower levels of vitamin D and normal levels of calcium. The overall condition of the mice, including soft tissue and bone morphology, was also improved, although survival was not affected by this genetic manipulation of PTH functions. Surprisingly, these changes were seen even though serum phosphate levels were not reduced and, in fact, were even higher in the double mutant. These results suggested that some of the physical effects that result from the loss of FGF23 are caused by abnormal vitamin D and calcium levels mediated by PTH [87].

Ffg23−/− and *Klotho−/−* mice were used to determine how FGF23 may or may not affect PTH functions on bone [88]. This is a clinically important issue, as PTH is administered therapeutically to patients with osteoporosis. The study focused on the effects of intermittent administration of PTH since this regimen has an anabolic effect on bone that increases bone mass. The purpose of the study was to determine if FGF23–Klotho signaling is required to mediate these anabolic responses. The results showed that administration of PTH has similar effects on bone mass, bone mass density, and the activity of osteoblastic genes in *Ffg23−/−*, *Klotho−/−*, and wild-type mice. These observations indicate that although FGF23–Klotho signaling acts as a negative regulator of PTH, the signaling does not modulate the anabolic effects of PTH on bone, thus confirming the therapeutic benefits of intermittent PTH irrespective of FGF23 functions. Interestingly, a study to determine the effect of FGF23 on the catabolic effects of PTH suggests that FGF23 does affect this function of PTH. Long term, continuous administration of PTH reduces bone mass. When *FGF23−/−* mice were infused with PTH through osmotic pumps over a 3-week period, the reduction in bone was significantly increased. This would indicate that FGF23 might exert a protective effect against the long-term effects of PTH on bone [87].

FGF23 and Vitamin D

In the previous section, the role of vitamin D as an intermediary for mutual regulation of FGF23 and PTH was described. In this section, a more comprehensive view of vitamin D, FGF23, and the systemic effects of vitamin D are reviewed. The focus here is on the role that vitamin D plays in mineral homeostasis and bone metabolism but this metabolite has a more extensive role in physiology and health [81]. This magnifies the importance of vitamin D deregulation that occurs when FGF23 levels are not adequately maintained. Vitamin D is a multifunctional protein, and can suppress cell growth and regulate apoptosis. These activities have important implications for tumor growth and progression. Vitamin D also modulates immune response, affects blood pressure, and is important for proper function in the muscular and nervous systems [81].

The active metabolite of vitamin D is formed in the renal proximal tubules from its precursor through hydroxylation by the enzyme $1\alpha(OH)$ase (Cyp27b1) to form $1,25(OH)_2D_3$ [81]. Both FGF23 and PTH affect renal $1\alpha(OH)$ase expression to control $1,25(OH)_2D_3$ production as part of their individual and mutual regulation. $1,25(OH)_2D_3$ induces expression of both FGF23 and Klotho which increases urinary phosphate excretion to reduce serum phosphate levels. A marked increase in renal *$1\alpha(OH)$ase* gene expression accompanied by high serum $1,25(OH)_2D_3$ levels is observed in both *Fgf23−/−* and *Klotho−/−* mice [19]. These elevated serum $1,25(OH)_2D_3$ levels are associated with organ atrophy, soft tissue, and vascular calcifications in both *Fgf23−/−* and *Klotho−/−* mice. These abnormalities are due to the effects of $1,25(OH)_2D_3$ on the intestine to increase calcium and phosphate absorption [19,89,90]. This was demonstrated in studies in which vitamin D actions were eliminated from *Fgf23−/−* and *Klotho−/−* mice by generating *Fgf23−/−/1α(OH)ase−/−* and *Klotho−/−/1α(OH)ase−/−* mice. Both serum calcium and serum phosphate levels are reduced in *Fgf23−/−/ 1α(OH)ase−/−* and *Klotho−/−/1α(OH)ase−/−* mice, completely eliminating the extensive vascular and ectopic calcifications [60,70]. These observations thus confirm the role of vitamin D in contributing to these pathologies.

It is highly relevant that serum Fgf23 levels are extremely elevated in *Klotho−/−* mice, while undetectable in *Klotho−/−/1α(OH)ase−/−* mice. This indicates that vitamin D is a potent inducer of FGF23 since blocking vitamin D synthesis completely reverses FGF23 serum levels [91]. Moreover, it has been reported that mice deficient in vitamin D activity, such as in VDR−/− or *1α(OH)ase−/−* mice, have undetectable serum Fgf23 levels, again confirming that active vitamin D is a potent stimulator of Fgf23 production. This is consistent with studies that have shown that $1,25(OH)_2D_3$ can induce the expression of FGF23 in osteocytes through a vitamin D response element (VDRE) that is present in the FGF23 promoter [92]. However, it must be noted that FGF23 levels are also regulated by phosphate and/or calcium levels in the absence of vitamin D. It has been shown that FGF23 levels increase in *VDR−/−* mice that are placed on a rescue diet to restore mineral levels [93].

Additional mouse genetic studies have shown that the presence of high serum $1,25(OH)_2D_3$ in the absence of high serum phosphate is not as detrimental to the animal as previously believed. Mice lacking both *Klotho* and *Napi2a* (*Klotho−/−/NaPi2a−/−*) or both *Fgf23* and *NaPi2a* (*Fgf23−/−/NaPi2a−/−*) do not develop soft tissue calcifications or organ atrophy despite their very high serum $1,25(OH)_2D_3$ and calcium levels [60,71,91]. This implies the existence of a $1,25(OH)_2D_3$-independent calcification process that might be driven by the elevated serum levels of phosphate [60,91]. One needs to consider, however, that mouse models of hyperphosphatemia, such as *PTH−/−* mice with low serum calcium and $1,25(OH)_2D_3$, do not develop any calcifications, emphasizing that it is a combination of the effects of $1,25(OH)_2D_3$ and mineral ions that is responsible for the pathology [87]. The studies presented above show the importance of keeping a balanced mineral ion homeostasis in the body and that hormones such as PTH, FGF23, Klotho, and vitamin D are necessary to maintain such equilibrium.

FGF23: EMERGING ROLES IN DISEASE PROCESSES

Recent basic research and clinical studies have suggested potential roles for FGF23 in disease processes involving the cardiovascular, renal, and other systems. Generally, the roles of FGF23 in these diseases are implied by data associating FGF23 with a disease phenotype underlying mechanisms that have not been determined. Questions regarding possible roles for FGF23 in disease processes are very important since the answers may provide novel avenues for monitoring prognosis and influencing the course of treatment. In this section we review some of the recent studies in order to illustrate the potential role of FGF23 independent of phosphate metabolism.

Kidney

FGF23 targets the kidney as part of its major role in phosphate homeostasis so it is no surprise that research into potential functions of FGF23 beyond mineral homeostasis would include renal disease models.

Mouse models for CKD have been used to help dissect the interrelated physiological functions of FGF23 and PTH as detailed earlier [87,88]. Two additional studies have probed the possible direct roles of FGF23 in other kidney diseases: autosomal dominant polycystic kidney disease (ADPKD) and kidney transplant mortality.

ADPKD is caused by mutations in the polycystin-1 gene (Pkd1). FGF23 levels were found to be abnormal in ADPKD patients while PTH and vitamin D levels remained normal [94]. The high FGF23 levels were not associated with phosphate retention as they are in CKD so this observation appears to be specifically associated with ADPKD. The reasons for these elevated levels are not clear as is their clinical relevance. The Pkd1 gene is highly expressed in osteoblasts and osteocytes where FGF23 is expressed and studies have shown that Pkd1 affects bone metabolism. Thus it is possible that the mutation in Pkd1 may alter FGF23 synthesis and production, although the possibility of epiphenomenon could not be ruled out at this stage.

Heart

Researchers have also been looking at the potential effects of FGF23 on the cardiovascular system. These studies include research exploring the roles for FGF23 in the risk for developing left ventricular hypertrophy (LVH) and in cardiac-related mortality in general. LVH is associated with increased mortality in CKD patients as well as the general population [95]. Since elevated FGF23 is associated with mortality in CKD patients [96,97], a study was performed on a cohort ($n = 795$) consisting of elderly residents (over 70 years old) with additional analysis of a sub-cohort ($n = 164$) with reduced renal function, found that elevated FGF23 levels are positively associated with left ventricular mass index and an increased risk for LVH. Importantly, this relationship was independent of other known LVH risk factors such as hypertension. However, as the authors of the study correctly point out, whether FGF23 could directly increase in cardiac mass is as yet unknown. FGF23 is expressed in low levels in the heart during embryonic development [70,98]. The authors suggest that if FGF23 is still expressed in adults, something that has not been proven to date, the elevated levels may be a result of an increased cardiac workload in patients with renal disease. Or, FGF23 could act directly on the heart since some studies suggest that α-Klotho may be expressed in heart tissue [99]. However, the results of this study need to be complemented by additional studies in order to resolve possible confounding factors such as deregulated mineral homeostasis and factors omitted in the study such as 1,25(OH)$_2$D$_3$.

A more recent study of FGF23 and LVH [100] confirmed a relationship between FGF23 and the risk of LVH in CKD patients. In accord with the human studies, both in vitro and mouse model studies showed that FGF23 could directly induce cardiac hypertrophy independent of Klotho. These results are provocative but need additional research to decisively establish the role of FGF23 in cardiac hypertrophy.

There have been several recent clinical studies that examined the possibility that FGF23 is either a risk factor or marker in cardiovascular disease [101–103]. High serum levels of FGF23 have already been noted as a predictor for coronary disease in patients with mild chronic kidney disease [97,104] and these studies were undertaken to determine if FGF23 is also a factor in populations without underlying renal disease. Each study involved a different cohort and different time frames so, not surprisingly, the results are not consistent. The first study used a cohort consisting of 1024 patients with underlying coronary disease, some with moderate kidney disease [101]. The patients were followed for 6 years and the results indicated that high FGF23 levels are associated with mortality and coronary events. A second study also found a similar possible link [103]. A cohort consisting of 659 70–79-year-old women was studied for 4 years. A little more than half were classified as physically disabled while the remaining women were selected from the least disabled in the same community. The third study used a cohort of 1259 men aged 40 to 75 years at the beginning of the study [102]. The selected men had no history of coronary disease prior to the start of the 10-year study period. The results of this study showed no association between FGF23 levels and risk for non-fatal or fatal coronary incidents. It is obvious that more investigation is needed to resolve the contradictory results from different cohorts. At this point it is not clear if the association between FGF23 and cardiovascular disease is direct, or is incidental to pre-existing conditions.

Vascular Tissue

In addition to cardiovascular disease, FGF23 and Klotho have been associated with vascular calcifications. Human vascular tissue has been analyzed for expression of FGF23, Klotho, and FGFRs as part of ongoing research to find evidence for a possible direct role for FGF23 in heart and vascular diseases [105]. The results indicated that Klotho, FGFR1, and FGFR3 were expressed in aortic tissue. FGF23 and FGFR4, the other known receptor for FGF23 in addition to FGFR1c, were not detected. Interestingly, the research also showed that expression levels of two genes that cleave Klotho to create a circulating form, ADAM17 and IL-10, correlated to levels of Klotho expression, raising the possibility that vascular tissue may be an additional source of humoral Klotho. The potential functions for

FGF23—Klotho on vascular tissue remodeling needs further experimental validation.

SUMMARY

FGF23 was isolated and associated with phosphate metabolism disorders in three nearly simultaneous studies, published in early 2000 [23,41,106]. In the decade since its discovery, we have learned much about FGF23 and how it works with other hormonal factors to maintain mineral ion balance in the body. We know how it evolved, how it functions as a generic FGF ligand and how it functions uniquely as an endocrine FGF. We have learned much about its role as a phosphatonin and how it interacts with its co-factor, Klotho, and two partner hormones to regulate phosphate homeostasis. Moreover, we now have a better understanding of how it functions in some specific diseases such as rickets and CKD.

Despite the progress made to date, there is much more to learn about this important multifunction protein. The complex interactions among FGF23, PTH, and vitamin D are such that questions still remain about the precise action of these factors in both healthy and diseased states. Since all three factors act systemically, it is therefore often difficult to dissociate individual from mutual functions. Also, FGF23 has poorly understood roles in diseases affecting various organ systems that may be independent of its role in mineral ion homeostasis. Many of these potential roles are circumstantial and the underlying mechanisms, if any, need to be defined. The questions that remain about the regulation and actions of FGF23 have high clinical relevance. Further discoveries may lead to better diagnostic, prognostic, and therapeutic applications for FGF23.

Acknowledgments

We would like to thank Insa Mannstadt for illustrating the tissues in Figs 12.1 and 12.2.

References

[1] Liu S, Guo R, Simpson LG, Xiao ZS, Burnham CE, Quarles LD. Regulation of fibroblastic growth factor 23 expression but not degradation by PHEX. J Biol Chem 2003 Sep 26;278(39):37419—26.

[2] Bergwitz C, Juppner H. Regulation of phosphate homeostasis by PTH, vitamin D, and FGF23. Annu Rev Med 2010;61:91—104.

[3] Gaasbeek A, Meinders AE. Hypophosphatemia: an update on its etiology and treatment. Am J Med 2005 Oct;118(10):1094—101.

[4] Razzaque MS. The FGF23-Klotho axis: endocrine regulation of phosphate homeostasis. Nat Rev Endocrinol 2009 Nov;5(11):611—9.

[5] Iotti S, Lodi R, Gottardi G, Zaniol P, Barbiroli B. Inorganic phosphate is transported into mitochondria in the absence of ATP biosynthesis: an in vivo 31P NMR study in the human skeletal muscle. Biochem Biophys Res Commun 1996 Aug 5;225(1):191—4.

[6] Hutson SM, Williams GD, Berkich DA, LaNoue KF, Briggs RW. A 31P NMR study of mitochondrial inorganic phosphate visibility: effects of Ca2+, Mn2+, and the pH gradient. Biochemistry 1992 Feb 11;31(5):1322—30.

[7] KEGG (Kyoto Encyclopedia of Genes and Genomes), http://wwwgenomejp/dbgetbin/www_bfind_sub?mode=bfind&mode=bfind&max_hit=1000&serv=kegg&dbkey=reaction&keywords=phosphate&page=.

[8] Drezner M. Phosphorus homeostasis and related disorders. In: Bilezikian J, Raisz L, Rodan G, editors. Principles in Bone Biology. 2nd ed. New York: Academic Press; 2002. p. 321—38.

[9] Econs MJ. New insights into the pathogenesis of inherited phosphate wasting disorders. Bone 1999;25(1):131—5.

[10] Miyamoto K, Ito M, Segawa H, Kuwahata M. Molecular targets of hyperphosphataemia in chronic renal failure. Nephrol Dial Transplant 2003 Jun;18(Suppl. 3:iii):79—80.

[11] Quarles LD. FGF23, PHEX, and MEPE regulation of phosphate homeostasis and skeletal mineralization. Am J Physiol Endocrinol Metab 2003 Jul;285(1):E1—9.

[12] Marks J, Debnam ES, Unwin RJ. Phosphate homeostasis and the renal-gastrointestinal axis. Am J Physiol Renal Physiol 2010 August 1;299(2):F285—96.

[13] Hattenhauer O, Traebert M, Murer H, Biber J. Regulation of small intestinal Na-Pi type IIb cotransporter by dietary phosphate intake. Am J Physiol Gastrointest Liver Physiol 1999 October 1;277(4):G756—62.

[14] Sabbagh Y, O'Brien SP, Song W, Boulanger JH, Stockmann A, Arbeeny C, et al. Intestinal npt2b plays a major role in phosphate absorption and homeostasis. J Am Soc Nephrol 2009 Nov;20(11):2348—58.

[15] Corut A, Senyigit A, Ugur SA, Altin S, Ozcelik U, Calisir H, et al. Mutations in SLC34A2 cause pulmonary alveolar microlithiasis and are possibly associated with testicular microlithiasis. Am J Hum Genet 2006;79(4):650—6.

[16] Tenenhouse HS. Regulation of phosphorus homeostasis by the type iia na/phosphate cotransporter. Annu Rev Nutr 2005; 25:197—214.

[17] Murer H, Forster I, Hilfiker H, Pfister M, Kaissling B, Lotscher M, et al. Cellular/molecular control of renal Na/Pi-cotransport. Kidney Int Suppl 1998;65:S2—10.

[18] Gattineni J, Bates C, Twombley K, Dwarakanath V, Robinson ML, Goetz R, et al. FGF23 decreases renal NaPi-2a and NaPi-2c expression and induces hypophosphatemia in vivo predominantly via FGF receptor 1. Am J Physiol Renal Physiol 2009 Aug;297(2):F282—91.

[19] Nakatani T, Sarraj B, Ohnishi M, Densmore MJ, Taguchi T, Goetz R, et al. In vivo genetic evidence for klotho-dependent, fibroblast growth factor 23 (Fgf23)-mediated regulation of systemic phosphate homeostasis. FASEB J 2009 Feb; 23(2):433—41.

[20] Miyamoto K, Ito M, Kuwahata M, Kato S, Segawa H. Inhibition of intestinal sodium-dependent inorganic phosphate transport by fibroblast growth factor 23. Ther Apher Dial 2005 Aug;9(4):331—5.

[21] Hu MC, Shi M, Zhang J, Pastor J, Nakatani T, Lanske B, et al. Klotho: a novel phosphaturic substance acting as an autocrine enzyme in the renal proximal tubule. FASEB J 2010 Sep; 24(9):3438—50.

[22] Yamashita T, Yoshitake H, Tsuji K, Kawaguchi N, Nabeshima Y, Noda M. Retardation in bone resorption after bone marrow ablation in klotho mutant mice. Endocrinology 2000 Jan;141(1):438—45.

[23] ADHR_Consortium. Autosomal dominant hypophosphataemic rickets is associated with mutations in FGF23. The ADHR Consortium. Nat Genet 2000;26(3):345—8.

[24] Simonet WS, Lacey DL, Dunstan CR, Kelley M, Chang MS, Luthy R, et al. Osteoprotegerin: a novel secreted protein

involved in the regulation of bone density. Cell. 1997 Apr 18;89(2):309—19.

[25] Kondo H, Guo J, Bringhurst FR. Cyclic adenosine monophosphate/protein kinase A mediates parathyroid hormone/parathyroid hormone-related protein receptor regulation of osteoclastogenesis and expression of RANKL and osteoprotegerin mRNAs by marrow stromal cells. J Bone Miner Res 2002 Sep;17(9):1667—79.

[26] Ma YL, Cain RL, Halladay DL, Yang X, Zeng Q, Miles RR, et al. Catabolic effects of continuous human PTH (1-38) in vivo is associated with sustained stimulation of RANKL and inhibition of osteoprotegerin and gene-associated bone formation. Endocrinology 2001 Sep;142(9):4047—54.

[27] Baldock PA, Thomas GP, Hodge JM, Baker SU, Dressel U, O'Loughlin PD, et al. Vitamin D action and regulation of bone remodeling: suppression of osteoclastogenesis by the mature osteoblast. J Bone Miner Res 2006 Oct;21(10):1618—26.

[28] Itoh N, Ornitz DM. Evolution of the Fgf and Fgfr gene families. Trends Genet. 2004 Nov;20(11):563—9.

[29] Hormone-like Itoh N. (endocrine) Fgfs: their evolutionary history and roles in development, metabolism, and disease. Cell Tissue Res 2010 Oct;342(1):1—11.

[30] Itoh N. The Fgf families in humans, mice, and zebrafish: their evolutionary processes and roles in development, metabolism, and disease. Biol Pharm Bull 2007 Oct;30(10):1819—25.

[31] Itoh N, Ornitz DM. Functional evolutionary history of the mouse Fgf gene family. Dev Dyn 2008 Jan;237(1):18—27.

[32] Krejci P, Prochazkova J, Bryja V, Kozubik A, Wilcox WR. Molecular pathology of the fibroblast growth factor family. Hum Mutat 2009 Sep;30(9):1245—55.

[33] Beenken A, Mohammadi M. The FGF family: biology, pathophysiology and therapy. Nat Rev Drug Discov 2009 Mar;8(3):235—53.

[34] Goldfarb M, Schoorlemmer J, Williams A, Diwakar S, Wang Q, Huang X, et al. Fibroblast growth factor homologous factors control neuronal excitability through modulation of voltage-gated sodium channels. Neuron 2007 Aug 2;55(3):449—63.

[35] Pownall ME, Isaacs HV. FGF Signaling in Vertebrates. Morgan & Claypool Life Sciences; 2010.

[36] Pownall ME, Isaac J. FGF Signalling in Vertebrate Development. Morgan & Claypool Life Sciences; 2010.

[37] Katoh M. Cross-talk of WNT and FGF signaling pathways at GSK3beta to regulate beta-catenin and SNAIL signaling cascades. Cancer Biol Ther 2006 Sep;5(9):1059—64.

[38] Boswell BA, Lein PJ, Musil LS. Cross-talk between fibroblast growth factor and bone morphogenetic proteins regulates gap junction-mediated intercellular communication in lens cells. Mol Biol Cell 2008 Jun;19(6):2631—41.

[39] Goetz R, Beenken A, Ibrahimi OA, Kalinina J, Olsen SK, Eliseenkova AV, et al. Molecular insights into the klotho-dependent, endocrine mode of action of fibroblast growth factor 19 subfamily members. Mol Cell Biol. 2007 May;27(9):3417—28.

[40] Yamashita T. Structural and biochemical properties of fibroblast growth factor 23. Ther Apher Dial 2005 Aug;9(4):313—8.

[41] Shimada T, Mizutani S, Muto T, Yoneya T, Hino R, Takeda S, et al. Cloning and characterization of FGF23 as a causative factor of tumor-induced osteomalacia. Proc Natl Acad Sci USA 2001 May 22;98(11):6500—5.

[42] Ichikawa S, Lyles KW, Econs MJ. A novel GALNT3 mutation in a pseudoautosomal dominant form of tumoral calcinosis: evidence that the disorder is autosomal recessive. J Clin Endocrinol Metab 2005 Apr;90(4):2420—3.

[43] Ichikawa S, Imel EA, Sorenson AH, Severe R, Knudson P, Harris GJ, et al. Tumoral calcinosis presenting with eyelid calcifications due to novel missense mutations in the glycosyl transferase domain of the GALNT3 gene. J Clin Endocrinol Metab 2006 Nov;91(11):4472—5.

[44] Ichikawa S, Guigonis V, Imel EA, Courouble M, Heissat S, Henley JD, et al. Novel GALNT3 mutations causing hyperostosis-hyperphosphatemia syndrome result in low intact fibroblast growth factor 23 concentrations. J Clin Endocrinol Metab 2007 May;92(5):1943—7.

[45] Ichikawa S, Imel EA, Kreiter ML, Yu X, Mackenzie DS, Sorenson AH, et al. A homozygous missense mutation in human KLOTHO causes severe tumoral calcinosis. J Clin Invest 2007 Sep;117(9):2684—91.

[46] Ichikawa S, Sorenson AH, Austin AM, Mackenzie DS, Fritz TA, Moh A, et al. Ablation of the Galnt3 gene leads to low-circulating intact fibroblast growth factor 23 (Fgf23) concentrations and hyperphosphatemia despite increased Fgf23 expression. Endocrinology 2009 Jun;150(6):2543—50.

[47] Ichikawa S, Baujat G, Seyahi A, Garoufali AG, Imel EA, Padgett LR, et al. Clinical variability of familial tumoral calcinosis caused by novel GALNT3 mutations. Am J Med Genet A 2010 Apr;152A(4):896—903.

[48] Farrow EG, Yu X, Summers LJ, Davis SI, Fleet JC, Allen MR, et al. Iron deficiency drives an autosomal dominant hypophosphatemic rickets (ADHR) phenotype in fibroblast growth factor-23 (Fgf23) knock-in mice. Proc Natl Acad Sci USA 2011 Oct 17.

[49] Eswarakumar VP, Lax I, Schlessinger J. Cellular signaling by fibroblast growth factor receptors. Cytokine Growth Factor Rev 2005 Apr;16(2):139—49.

[50] Mohammadi M, Olsen SK, Ibrahimi OA. Structural basis for fibroblast growth factor receptor activation. Cytokine Growth Factor Rev 2005 Apr;16(2):107—37.

[51] Kurosu H, Ogawa Y, Miyoshi M, Yamamoto M, Nandi A, Rosenblatt KP, et al. Regulation of fibroblast growth factor-23 signaling by klotho. J Biol Chem 2006 Mar 10;281(10):6120—3.

[52] Urakawa I, Yamazaki Y, Shimada T, Iijima K, Hasegawa H, Okawa K, et al. Klotho converts canonical FGF receptor into a specific receptor for FGF23. Nature 2006 Dec 7;444(7120):770—4.

[53] Liu S, Vierthaler L, Tang W, Zhou J, Quarles LD. FGFR3 and FGFR4 do not mediate renal effects of FGF23. J Am Soc Nephrol 2008 Dec;19(12):2342—50.

[54] Kuro-o M. Klotho as a regulator of fibroblast growth factor signaling and phosphate/calcium metabolism. Curr Opin Nephrol Hypertens 2006 Jul;15(4):437—41.

[55] Medici D, Razzaque MS, Deluca S, Rector TL, Hou B, Kang K, et al. FGF-23—Klotho signaling stimulates proliferation and prevents vitamin D-induced apoptosis. J Cell Biol 2008 Aug 11;182(3):459—65.

[56] Nabeshima Y. The discovery of alpha-Klotho and FGF23 unveiled new insight into calcium and phosphate homeostasis. Cell Mol Life Sci 2008 Oct;65(20):3218—30.

[57] Kuro-o M, Matsumura Y, Aizawa H, Kawaguchi H, Suga T, Utsugi T, et al. Mutation of the mouse klotho gene leads to a syndrome resembling ageing. Nature 1997 Nov 6;390(6655):45—51.

[58] Chen CD, Podvin S, Gillespie E, Leeman SE, Abraham CR. Insulin stimulates the cleavage and release of the extracellular domain of Klotho by ADAM10 and ADAM17. Proc Natl Acad Sci USA 2007 Dec 11;104(50):19796—801.

[59] Matsumura Y, Aizawa H, Shiraki-Iida T, Nagai R, Kuro-o M, Nabeshima Y. Identification of the human klotho gene and its two transcripts encoding membrane and secreted klotho protein. Biochem Biophys Res Commun 1998 Jan 26; 242(3):626—30.

[60] Ohnishi M, Nakatani T, Lanske B, Razzaque MS. In vivo genetic evidence for suppressing vascular and soft-tissue calcification through the reduction of serum phosphate levels, even in the

presence of high serum calcium and 1,25-dihydroxyvitamin D levels. Circ Cardiovasc Genet 2009 Dec;2(6):583—90.

[61] Ohnishi M, Razzaque MS. Dietary and genetic evidence for phosphate toxicity accelerating mammalian aging. FASEB J 2010 Sep;24(9):3562—71.

[62] Nakatani T, Ohnishi M, Razzaque MS. Inactivation of klotho function induces hyperphosphatemia even in presence of high serum fibroblast growth factor 23 levels in a genetically engineered hypophosphatemic (Hyp) mouse model. FASEB J 2009 Nov;23(11):3702—11.

[63] Benet-Pages A, Orlik P, Strom TM, Lorenz-Depiereux B. An FGF23 missense mutation causes familial tumoral calcinosis with hyperphosphatemia. Hum Mol Genet 2005 Feb 1;14(3):385—90.

[64] HYP_Consortium. A gene (PEX) with homologies to endopeptidases is mutated in patients with X-linked hypophosphatemic rickets. Nature Genet 1995;11:130—6.

[65] Lorenz-Depiereux B, Bastepe M, Benet-Pages A, Amyere M, Wagenstaller J, Muller-Barth U, et al. DMP1 mutations in autosomal recessive hypophosphatemia implicate a bone matrix protein in the regulation of phosphate homeostasis. Nat Genet 2006 Nov;38(11):1248—50.

[66] Bai X, Miao D, Li J, Goltzman D, Karaplis AC. Transgenic mice overexpressing human fibroblast growth factor 23 (R176Q) delineate a putative role for parathyroid hormone in renal phosphate wasting disorders. Endocrinology 2004 Nov; 145(11):5269—79.

[67] Larsson T, Marsell R, Schipani E, Ohlsson C, Ljunggren O, Tenenhouse HS, et al. Transgenic mice expressing fibroblast growth factor 23 under the control of the alpha1(I) collagen promoter exhibit growth retardation, osteomalacia, and disturbed phosphate homeostasis. Endocrinology 2004 Jul; 145(7):3087—94.

[68] Shimada T, Kakitani M, Yamazaki Y, Hasegawa H, Takeuchi Y, Fujita T, et al. Targeted ablation of Fgf23 demonstrates an essential physiological role of FGF23 in phosphate and vitamin D metabolism. J Clin Invest 2004 Feb;113(4):561—8.

[69] DeLuca S, Sitara D, Kang K, Marsell R, Jonsson K, Taguchi T, et al. Amelioration of the premature ageing-like features of Fgf-23 knockout mice by genetically restoring the systemic actions of FGF-23. J Pathol 2008 Nov;216(3):345—55.

[70] Sitara D, Razzaque MS, Hesse M, Yoganathan S, Taguchi T, Erben RG, et al. Homozygous ablation of fibroblast growth factor-23 results in hyperphosphatemia and impaired skeletogenesis, and reverses hypophosphatemia in Phex-deficient mice. Matrix Biol 2004 Nov;23(7):421—32.

[71] Sitara D, Kim S, Razzaque MS, Bergwitz C, Taguchi T, Schuler C, et al. Genetic evidence of serum phosphate-independent functions of FGF-23 on bone. PLoS Genet 2008;4(8):e1000154.

[72] Razzaque MS. Therapeutic potential of klotho-FGF23 fusion polypeptides: WO2009095372. Expert Opin Ther Pat 2010 Jul;20(7):981—5.

[73] Bai X, Dinghong Q, Miao D, Goltzman D, Karaplis AC. Klotho ablation converts the biochemical and skeletal alterations in FGF23 (R176Q) transgenic mice to a Klotho-deficient phenotype. Am J Physiol Endocrinol Metab 2009 Jan;296(1):E79—88.

[74] Goetz R, Nakada Y, Hu MC, Kurosu H, Wang L, Nakatani T, et al. Isolated C-terminal tail of FGF23 alleviates hypophosphatemia by inhibiting FGF23-FGFR-Klotho complex formation. Proc Natl Acad Sci USA 2010 Jan 5;107(1):407—12.

[75] Razzaque MS. FGF23-mediated regulation of systemic phosphate homeostasis: is Klotho an essential player? Am J Physiol Renal Physiol 2009 Mar;296(3):F470—6.

[76] Lanske B, Razzaque MS. Mineral metabolism and aging: the fibroblast growth factor 23 enigma. Curr Opin Nephrol Hypertens 2007 Jul;16(4):311—8.

[77] Juppner H, Abou-Samra AB, Freeman M, Kong XF, Schipani E, Richards J, et al. A G protein-linked receptor for parathyroid hormone and parathyroid hormone-related peptide. Science 1991 Nov 15;254(5034):1024—6.

[78] Silver J, Naveh-Many T, Mayer H, Schmelzer HJ, Popovtzer MM. Regulation by vitamin D metabolites of parathyroid hormone gene transcription in vivo in the rat. J Clin Invest 1986 Nov;78(5):1296—301.

[79] Silver J, Russell J, Sherwood LM. Regulation by vitamin D metabolites of messenger ribonucleic acid for preproparathyroid hormone in isolated bovine parathyroid cells. Proc Natl Acad Sci USA 1985 Jun;82(12):4270—3.

[80] Silver J, Sela SB, Naveh-Many T. Regulation of parathyroid cell proliferation. Curr Opin Nephrol Hypertens 1997 Jul;6(4): 321—6.

[81] Dusso AS, Brown AJ, Slatopolsky E, Vitamin D. Am J Physiol Renal Physiol 2005 Jul;289(1):F8—28.

[82] Kawata T, Imanishi Y, Kobayashi K, Miki T, Arnold A, Inaba M, et al. Parathyroid hormone regulates fibroblast growth factor-23 in a mouse model of primary hyperparathyroidism. J Am Soc Nephrol 2007 Oct;18(10):2683—8.

[83] Rhee Y, Bivi N, Farrow E, Lezcano V, Plotkin LI, White KE, et al. Parathyroid hormone receptor signaling in osteocytes increases the expression of fibroblast growth factor-23 in vitro and in vivo. Bone 2011 Jun 25.

[84] Ben-Dov IZ, Galitzer H, Lavi-Moshayoff V, Goetz R, Kuro-o M, Mohammadi M, et al. The parathyroid is a target organ for FGF23 in rats. J Clin Invest 2007 Dec;117(12):4003—8.

[85] Krajisnik T, Bjorklund P, Marsell R, Ljunggren O, Akerstrom G, Jonsson KB, et al. Fibroblast growth factor-23 regulates parathyroid hormone and 1alpha-hydroxylase expression in cultured bovine parathyroid cells. J Endocrinol 2007 Oct;195(1):125—31.

[86] Bai X, Miao D, Goltzman D, Karaplis AC. Early lethality in Hyp mice with targeted deletion of Pth gene. Endocrinology 2007 Oct;148(10):4974—83.

[87] Yuan Q, Sitara D, Sato T, Densmore M, Saito H, Schuler C, et al. PTH ablation ameliorates the anomalies of Fgf23-deficient mice by suppressing the elevated vitamin D and calcium levels. Endocrinology 2011 Nov;152(11):4053—61.

[88] Yuan Q, Sato T, Densmore M, Saito H, Schuler C, Erben RG, et al. Fgf23/Klotho signaling is not essential for the phosphaturic and anabolic functions of PTH. J Bone Miner Res 2011 May 16.

[89] Tsujikawa H, Kurotaki Y, Fujimori T, Fukuda K, Nabeshima Y. Klotho, a gene related to a syndrome resembling human premature aging, functions in a negative regulatory circuit of vitamin D endocrine system. Mol Endocrinol 2003 Dec;17(12): 2393—403.

[90] Memon F, El-Abbadi M, Nakatani T, Taguchi T, Lanske B, Razzaque MS. Does Fgf23-klotho activity influence vascular and soft tissue calcification through regulating mineral ion metabolism? Kidney Int 2008 Sep;74(5):566—70.

[91] Ohnishi M, Nakatani T, Lanske B, Razzaque MS. Reversal of mineral ion homeostasis and soft-tissue calcification of klotho knockout mice by deletion of vitamin D 1alpha-hydroxylase. Kidney Int 2009 Jun;75(11):1166—72.

[92] Liu S, Tang W, Zhou J, Stubbs JR, Luo Q, Pi M, et al. Fibroblast growth factor 23 is a counter-regulatory phosphaturic hormone for vitamin D. J Am Soc Nephrol 2006 May;17(5):1305—15.

[93] Yu X, Sabbagh Y, Davis SI, Demay MB, White KE. Genetic dissection of phosphate- and vitamin D-mediated regulation of circulating Fgf23 concentrations. Bone 2005 Jun;36(6):971—7.

[94] Pavik I, Jaeger P, Kistler AD, Poster D, Krauer F, Cavelti-Weder C, et al. Patients with autosomal dominant polycystic kidney disease have elevated fibroblast growth factor 23 levels and a renal leak of phosphate. Kidney Int 2011 Jan;79(2):234—40.

[95] Levy D, Garrison RJ, Savage DD, Kannel WB, Castelli WP. Prognostic implications of echocardiographically determined left ventricular mass in the Framingham Heart Study. N Engl J Med 1990 May 31;322(22):1561–6.

[96] Mirza MA, Larsson A, Melhus H, Lind L, Larsson TE. Serum intact FGF23 associate with left ventricular mass, hypertrophy and geometry in an elderly population. Atherosclerosis 2009 Dec;207(2):546–51.

[97] Gutierrez OM, Mannstadt M, Isakova T, Rauh-Hain JA, Tamez H, Shah A, et al. Fibroblast growth factor 23 and mortality among patients undergoing hemodialysis. N Engl J Med 2008 August 7;359(6):584–92.

[98] Weber TJ, Liu S, Indridason OS, Quarles LD. Serum FGF23 levels in normal and disordered phosphorus homeostasis. J Bone Miner Res 2003 Jul;18(7):1227–34.

[99] Takeshita K, Fujimori T, Kurotaki Y, Honjo H, Tsujikawa H, Yasui K, et al. Sinoatrial node dysfunction and early unexpected death of mice with a defect of klotho gene expression. Circulation 2004 Apr 13;109(14):1776–82.

[100] Faul C, Amaral AP, Oskouei B, Hu MC, Sloan A, Isakova T, et al. FGF23 induces left ventricular hypertrophy. J Clin Invest 2011 Nov 1;121(11):4393–408.

[101] Parker BD, Schurgers LJ, Brandenburg VM, Christenson RH, Vermeer C, Ketteler M, et al. The associations of fibroblast growth factor 23 and uncarboxylated matrix Gla protein with mortality in coronary artery disease: the Heart and Soul Study. Ann Intern Med 2010 May 18;152(10):640–8.

[102] Taylor EN, Rimm EB, Stampfer MJ, Curhan GC. Plasma fibroblast growth factor 23, parathyroid hormone, phosphorus, and risk of coronary heart disease. Am Heart J 2011 May;161(5):956–62.

[103] Dalal M, Sun K, Cappola AR, Ferrucci L, Crasto C, Fried LP, et al. Relationship of serum fibroblast growth factor 23 with cardiovascular disease in older community-dwelling women. Eur J Endocrinol 2011 Nov;165(5):797–803.

[104] Jean G, Terrat JC, Vanel T, Hurot JM, Lorriaux C, Mayor B, et al. High levels of serum fibroblast growth factor (FGF)-23 are associated with increased mortality in long haemodialysis patients. Nephrol Dial Transplant 2009 Sep;24(9):2792–6.

[105] Donate-Correa J, Mora-Fernandez C, Martinez-Sanz R, Muros-de-Fuentes M, Perez H, Meneses-Perez B, et al. Expression of FGF23/KLOTHO system in human vascular tissue. Int J Cardiol 2011 Sep 24.

[106] Yamashita T, Yoshioka M, Itoh N. Identification of a novel fibroblast growth factor, FGF-23, preferentially expressed in the ventrolateral thalamic nucleus of the brain. Biochem Biophys Res Commun 2000;277(2):494–8.

Clinical Aspects of Fibroblast Growth Factor 23

Seiji Fukumoto
University of Tokyo Hospital, Tokyo, Japan

INTRODUCTION

Electrolytes have several important roles in normal physiology and abnormal electrolytes levels cause several pathological manifestations. For example, hypocalcemia induces tetany, numbness and seizure, and hypercalcemia can result in constipation, consciousness disturbance, and renal impairment. In addition, hyperphosphatemia is a risk factor for ectopic calcification, and hypophosphatemia underlies most forms of rickets/osteomalacia. These facts imply that there must be some mechanisms to maintain circulatory levels of mineral ions in certain ranges to avoid these adverse events. It has been well known that two calciotropic hormones, parathyroid hormone (PTH) and 1,25-dihydroxyvitamin D [1,25(OH)$_2$D], work to increase serum calcium level and are essential for the regulation of serum calcium. On the other hand, it had been unclear whether there is a specific phosphotropic hormone because both PTH and 1,25(OH)$_2$D affect serum phosphate levels. Fibroblast growth factor 23 (FGF23) has been shown to play major roles in the regulation of serum phosphate level. FGF23 is produced by bone and binds to Klotho—FGF receptor complex in kidney [1–3]. FGF23 inhibits phosphate reabsorption in renal proximal tubules by suppressing the expression of type 2a and 2c sodium-phosphate co-transporters. FGF23 also decreases circulatory 1,25(OH)$_2$D level by decreasing the expression of 25-hydroxyvitamin D-1α-hydroxylase and also enhancing the expression of 25-hydroxyvitamin D-24-hydroxylase (see Chapter 12) [4]. In addition, FGF23 has been reported to inhibit the production and secretion of PTH [5,6]. Therefore, it is now believed that FGF23 works as a phosphotropic hormone. In this chapter, clinical findings concerning FGF23 in humans are summarized and discussed.

HYPOPHOSPHATEMIC DISEASES

Phosphate Metabolism and Rickets/Osteomalacia

Bone is a hard tissue produced by the deposition of hydroxyapatite crystal on matrix proteins secreted by osteoblasts. Rickets and osteomalacia are diseases characterized by impaired mineralization of bone extracellular matrix. Therefore, unmineralized osteoid increases and mineralized bone decreases in rickets and osteomalacia making bone soften. Rickets develops during childhood before the closure of growth plates. Growth retardation and bone deformity are major features of rickets. On the other hand, osteomalacia which develops in adults causes muscle weakness and bone pain. Because of these symptoms, it is not uncommon that patients with osteomalacia are misdiagnosed with neurological or muscular diseases. While rickets and osteomalacia develop in different ages, these diseases share the same etiologies. The causes of rickets and osteomalacia are quite variable. However, hypophosphatemia underlies most cases of rickets and osteomalacia (Table 13.1). Rickets/osteomalacia without hypophosphatemia is observed in patients with hypophosphatasia caused by mutations in *tissue non-specific alkaline phosphatase* gene or patients receiving drugs that inhibit mineralization of bone. Some patients with vitamin D deficiency also can show rickets with hypocalcemia and normophosphatemia [7].

Serum phosphate level is maintained by intestinal phosphate absorption, renal phosphate handling, and dynamic equilibrium between serum phosphate and phosphate in bone or intracellular space. Of these, renal handling of phosphate is the most important determinant of serum phosphate level. Eighty to ninety percent of phosphate filtered from glomeruli is reabsorbed in renal tubules and most of this tubular phosphate

TABLE 13.1　Causes of Rickets and Osteomalacia

Impaired mineralization
　Hypophosphatasia
　　Infantile hypophosphatasia (OMIM #241500)
　　Childhood hypophosphatasia (OMIM #241510)
　　Adult hypophosphatasia (OMIM #146300)
　Drugs such as aluminum and etidronate

Hypophosphatemia
　Impaired actions of vitamin D metabolites
　　Vitamin D deficiency
　　Vitamin D hydroxylation-deficient rickets, type 1A (OMIM #264700)
　　Vitamin D-dependent rickets, type 2A (OMIM #277440)
　　Drugs such as diphenylhydantoin
　Proximal tubular damage
　　Hereditary hypophosphatemic rickets with hypercalcemia (OMIM #241530)
　　Dent's disease 1 (OMIM #300009)
　　Fanconi syndrome
　　Renal tubular acidosis
　　Drugs such as ifosphamide, adefovir dipivoxil, valpronic acid and deferasirox
　FGF23-related hypophosphatemic rickets/osteomalacia
　　X-linked dominant hypophosphatemic rickets (XLHR) (OMIM #307800)
　　Autosomal dominant hypophosphatemic rickets (ADHR) (OMIM #193100)
　　Autosomal recessive hypophosphatemic rickets 1 (ADHR1) (OMIM #241520)
　　Autosomal recessive hypophosphatemic rickets 2 (ADHR2) (OMIM #613312)
　　Tumor-induced rickets/osteomalacia
　　Hypophosphatemic rickets/osteomalacia associated with McCune-Albright syndrome/fibrous dysplasia
　　Hypophosphatemic rickets/osteomalacia by saccharated ferric oxide or iron polymaltose
　　Hypophosphatemic rickets associated with Schimmelpenning-Feuerstein-Mims syndrome (OMIM % 163200)
　　Phosphate depletion

reabsorption occurs in proximal tubules. Type 2a and 2c sodium-phosphate co-transporters are physiological mediators of this phosphate reabsorption in proximal tubules. It has been known that PTH reduces serum phosphate level by suppressing the expression of these sodium-phosphate co-transporters in the brush border membrane of proximal tubules [8]. FGF23 was also shown to decrease the expression of type 2a and 2c sodium-phosphate co-transporters and reduce serum phosphate level [4].

Identification of FGF23 and Development of Assays for FGF23

FGF23 was identified in 2000 as a responsible gene for autosomal dominant hypophosphatemic rickets

(ADHR: OMIM #193100) [9]. Almost simultaneously, FGF23 was identified by homology to FGF15 in mice and also as a responsible humoral factor for tumor-induced osteomalacia (TIO) [10,11]. ADHR and TIO are diseases characterized by impaired proximal tubular phosphate reabsorption. In addition, hypophosphatemia usually enhances $1,25(OH)_2D$ production and increases circulatory level of $1,25(OH)_2D$. However, $1,25(OH)_2D$ remains to be low to low normal in patients with ADHR or TIO indicating that $1,25(OH)_2D$ levels in these diseases are inappropriately low for hypophosphatemia. The impaired proximal tubular phosphate reabsorption and inappropriately suppressed level of $1,25(OH)_2D$ are explained by excessive FGF23 activity.

The FGF23 gene produces a 251 amino acid-long peptide [10]. N-terminal 24 amino acids compose a signal peptide and there is an FGF homology region with other members of the FGF family in the N-terminal portion of the secreted protein. There are 22 members of the FGF family in humans and these family members are characterized by the FGF homology region with β-trefoil structure [12]. These 22 FGF family members are divided into several subfamilies. FGF23 belongs to the FGF19 subfamily together with FGF19 and FGF21. A part of the FGF23 protein is proteolytically cleaved between ^{179}Arg and ^{180}Ser by enzymes that recognize the ^{176}Arg-X-X-^{179}Arg motif [13−15]. This cleavage is proposed to occur either before or during the process of secretion of FGF23 [15]. While full-length FGF23 protein reduces serum phosphate and $1,25(OH)_2D$ levels, the processed N-terminal and C-terminal fragments do not have biological activity to reduce serum phosphate [14]. This is confirmed by the finding that FGF23 uses its N-terminal FGF homology region for the association with FGF receptor and C-terminal region for binding to Klotho [16]. Rather, the excess C-terminal fragment of FGF23 was reported to inhibit the activity of full-length FGF23 [17]. FGF19 subfamily members are known to work as systemic factors while many other FGF family members are local factors [18]. Therefore, FGF19 family members are called hormone-like FGFs or endocrine FGFs [19,20].

Following the cloning of FGF23 and the demonstration of its functions, several assay methods for FGF23 have been developed [21−24]. Intact assays use two kinds of antibodies that recognize the N-terminal and C-terminal portions of the processing site of FGF23. In contrast, the C-terminal assay uses two polyclonal antibodies against the C-terminal region of the cleavage site. The intact assays recognize only full-length FGF23 while the C-terminal assay detects both full-length and the processed C-terminal fragment of FGF23. There seem to be some differences in the performance of these assays [21,22]. In addition, the measured values could be quite different in some circumstances depending on assays used as described below. However, the assays for FGF23 made it clear that there is intact FGF23 in normal circulation and therefore FGF23 is working as a physiological humoral factor [24]. These assays also greatly contributed to define diseases caused by aberrant actions of FGF23 as shown below.

Autosomal Dominant Hypophosphatemic Rickets (ADHR) and Tumor-induced Osteomalacia (TIO)

Mutations so far reported in patients with ADHR replace either [176]Arg or [179]Arg with other amino acids, thus destroying the consensus R-X-X-R motif [9,25]. These results suggested that the mutant FGF23 proteins in patients with ADHR escape the processing between [179]Arg and [180]Ser. *In vitro* experiments actually revealed that the mutant FGF23 proteins were resistant to the processing between [179]Arg and [180]Ser [14,15,26]. Because only full-length FGF23 has biological activity to induce hypophosphatemia as mentioned above, the resistance to the processing of the mutant FGF23 protein was considered to increase the circulating level of biologically active full-length FGF23 and result in excess activity of FGF23.

However, the precise mechanism of the development of hypophosphatemic rickets in patients with ADHR remains to be clarified. FGF23 works as a physiological regulator of serum phosphate concentration and FGF23 levels in patients with some hypophosphatemic diseases such as Fanconi's syndrome and vitamin D deficiency are rather low (Fig. 13.1) [27]. These results indicate that the production and release of FGF23 must be tightly regulated. If this regulatory mechanism of FGF23 production and FGF23 levels remains intact in patients with ADHR, it is anticipated

that circulatory concentration of FGF23 and therefore serum phosphate become normal even though they harbor one mutant allele of *FGF23* [15]. Actually, it is known that hypophosphatemia disappears in some patients with ADHR by natural course and it was reported that FGF23 inversely correlated with phosphate level in these patients [28]. Therefore, despite the existence of mutations in the *FGF23* gene causing ADHR, FGF23 and phosphate levels can be maintained within the reference ranges at least in some patients and in some conditions. It is also known that some ADHR patients present with the disease as adult-onset hypophosphatemic osteomalacia rather than hypophosphatemic rickets early in life [29]. Collectively, these results indicate that mutations in *FGF23* found in patients with ADHR do not necessarily cause high circulatory FGF23 levels and hypophosphatemia, and that some other accompanying factor(s) is/are necessary for the development of ADHR. Recently, it was reported that iron deficiency increases FGF23 levels in a mouse model of ADHR [30]. It was also described that serum iron was negatively correlated with FGF23 levels in patients with ADHR [31]. It remains to be clarified whether iron deficiency is the only and universal cause of excess FGF23 activity in patients with ADHR and how iron deficiency elevates circulatory FGF23 levels in these patients.

TIO is a paraneoplastic syndrome usually caused by slow-growing mesenchymal tumors. Patients with TIO often complain of severe muscle weakness and bone pain that impair the quality of life of the affected patients. In addition, the diagnosis of this disease is often delayed due to insidious onset and slow progress of the symptoms. Some patients with TIO are misdiagnosed with neuromuscular diseases or metastatic bone disease from their symptoms and multiple uptakes on bone scintigraphy obtained for the evaluation of bone pain, respectively. TIO is cured by complete removal of the responsible tumors indicating that those tumors are producing humoral factor(s) that causes impaired proximal tubular phosphate reabsorption and hypophosphatemia. After the cloning of FGF23, it was shown that FGF23 levels were elevated in most patients with TIO (Fig. 13.1) and rapidly decreased after the removal of the responsible tumors with a half-life of about 30–60 minutes [24,27,32]. These results indicate that FGF23 measurement is useful for both the diagnosis and the follow-up of patients with TIO.

Most responsible tumors for TIO are pathologically classified as phosphaturic mesenchymal tumor, mixed connective tissue variant (PMTMCT), and present in bone or soft tissues [33]. It is also reported that some other tumors including prostatic carcinoma and oat cell carcinoma of the lung can cause TIO [34]. However,

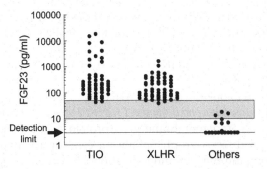

FIGURE 13.1 FGF23 levels in patients with chronic hypophosphatemia. While FGF23 was high in most patients with FGF23-related hypophosphatemic diseases such as tumor-induced osteomalacia (TIO) and X-linked dominant hypophosphatemic rickets (XLHR), it was rather low in patients from other causes including vitamin D deficiency, Fanconi's syndrome, and ectopic adrenocorticotropic hormone syndrome. *From Fukumoto and Shimizu [27].*

it is not clear why these tumors can produce FGF23. It is not uncommon that tumors causing TIO are small and difficult to be detected. Several diagnostic methods have been used to find the responsible tumors for TIO such as magnetic resonance imaging survey, octreotide scintigraphy, and positron emission tomography [35—39]. However, none of these methods can definitely prove that the detected tumors are actually causing TIO by producing FGF23. Venous sampling for FGF23 may be useful for both the identification of the causative tumors and the confirmation that the detected tumors are responsible for TIO [40—44].

In addition to FGF23, several humoral factors including secreted frizzled-related protein 4 (sFRP4), matrix extracellular phosphoglycoprotein (MEPE), and FGF7 were shown to either inhibit phosphate transport *in vitro* or induce hypophosphatemia *in vivo* [45—47]. MEPE was also reported to inhibit mineralization of bone [47]. However, none of these factors has been shown to be elevated in patients with TIO. Therefore, FGF23 seems to be the primary humoral factor causing TIO while it is still possible that other factors like sFRP4, MEPE, and FGF7 work together with FGF23 in the development of TIO.

X-linked Dominant Hypophosphatemic Rickets (XLHR: OMIM #307800)

XLHR is a prototype of vitamin D-resistant rickets which is not cured by a physiological dose of native vitamin D. The responsible gene for XLHR was identified by positional cloning and named *phosphate-regulating gene with homologies to endopeptidases on the X chromosome (PHEX)* [48]. PHEX protein is composed of 749 amino acids and belongs to a family of metalloen-dopeptidases with a single membrane-spanning region. Nearly 300 mutations in the *PHEX* gene are deposited in a database (http://www.phexdb.mcgill.ca/) [49]. Because a nonsense mutation in codon 20, and some deletion and insertion mutations were reported to cause XLHR, these mutations found in patients with *PHEX* are considered to be inactivating ones. Even before the identification of *PHEX*, several studies suggested that impaired renal tubular phosphate reabsorption and XLHR are caused by a humoral factor. For instance, renal transplantation from a healthy donor to a patient with XLHR did not cure phosphate wasting [50]. In addition, *Hyp* mouse is a murine homologue of XLHR and 3'-region of *Phex* is deleted in *Hyp* [51]. Parabiosis between *Hyp* and wild-type mice induced hypophosphatemia and phosphate wasting in wild-type mice suggesting that some humoral factor caused these changes [52]. Furthermore, crosstransplantation of kidneys from wild-type mice to *Hyp* did not correct

hypophosphatemia while transfer of kidneys from *Hyp* mice to wild-type did not cause hypophosphatemia [53]. These results indicate that there is no intrinsic defect of phosphate handling in kidneys of *Hyp* mice. After the identification of FGF23, it was shown that circulatory FGF23 levels were elevated in most patients with XLHR and also in *Hyp* mice (Fig. 13.1) [23,24,54]. It was also reported that the expression of FGF23 was enhanced in bone of *Hyp* mice [54,55]. These results indicate that inactivating mutations in *PHEX/Phex* cause enhanced expression of FGF23 in bone resulting in hypophosphatemic rickets/osteomalacia. Genetically engineered animal models also support the notion that deficient action of Phex in osteoblasts/osteocytes underlies *Hyp*. Deletion of both *FGF23* alleles in *Hyp* mice increased serum phosphate level [56]. In addition, conditional deletion of *Phex* in osteoblasts/osteocytes in the mouse induced hypophosphatemia and high circulatory FGF23 levels without increased sFRP4 or MEPE [54]. Therefore, FGF23 seems to be the primary humoral factor inducing hypophosphatemia in *Hyp* mice and patients with XLHR. However, it is not entirely clear how inactivating mutations in *PHEX/Phex* result in enhanced expression of FGF23 in bone.

Autosomal Recessive Hypophosphatemic Rickets 1 (ARHR1: OMIM #241520) and Autosomal Recessive Hypophosphatemic Rickets 2 (ARHR2: OMIM #613312)

Patients with ARHR1 or ARHR2 show similar clinical and biochemical features to those of patients with XLHR. The responsible gene for ARHR1 is *dentin matrix protein 1 (DMP1)* [57,58]. DMP1 is a matrix protein found mainly in bone and teeth. DMP1 was reported to transduce signals by binding to cell surface integrin [59]. DMP1 was also reported to work as a transcriptional factor [60]. While the precise mechanism is not clear, FGF23 was shown to be overexpressed in osteocytes of *DMP1*-null mice [57]. Circulatory FGF23 levels are elevated in patients with ARHR1 and *DMP1*-null mice indicating that ARHR1 is caused by excess activity of FGF23 [48,49].

The responsible gene for ARHR2 is *ectonucleotide pyrophosphatase/phosphodiesterase 1 (ENPP1)* [61,62]. ENPP1 is a type II transmembrane glycoprotein and an enzyme that produces pyrophosphate on cell surface which is a strong inhibitor of mineralization. However, it is possible that ENPP1 has some other roles than producing pyrophosphate. Inactivating mutations of *ENPP1* have been known to cause generalized arterial calcification of infancy (GACI), a potentially fatal disease [63,64]. This phenotype was considered to be explained by reduced pyrophosphate level. Probably because serum phosphate decreases with age, the phenotypes of GACI regress with time. Some patients with mutations in the *ENPP1* gene later develop hypophosphatemic rickets with high FGF23 levels. It was reported that the same mutation in the *ENPP1* gene can cause both GACI and hypophosphatemic rickets [62]. However, it is not yet explained how mutations in the *ENPP1* gene result in high FGF23 levels and why the mutations in one gene cause both enhanced ectopic calcification in vascular tissues and impaired mineralization in bone. Tiptoe walking mouse (ttw) is a model of ossification of posterior longitudinal ligament. This mouse is known to have a mutation in the *Enpp1* gene [65]. It was reported that one patient with a mutation in the *ENPP1* gene had both hypophosphatemic rickets with high FGF23 levels and widespread ossification of posterior longitudinal ligament [66]. It is possible that mutations in the *ENPP1* gene cause several phenotypes depending on age and other confounding factors of the affected patients.

Iron and Hypophosphatemic Diseases

Some drugs can cause hypophosphatemic diseases by several mechanisms. There are many formulations of iron and some specific preparations of iron are used in each country. It was reported that intravenous administration of saccharated ferric oxide in patients with iron deficiency anemia caused hypophosphatemic osteomalacia especially in Japan [67]. This hypophosphatemia was proposed to be caused by proximal tubular damage caused by this drug [67]. However, it was revealed that FGF23 levels were high in hypophosphatemic patients receiving intravenous administration of saccharated ferric oxide [68]. In addition, the cessation of saccharated ferric oxide corrected both high FGF23 and hypophosphatemia. In contrast, intravenous administration of the dextrin citrate—iron (III) complex did not cause high FGF23 or hypophosphatemia [68]. Hypophosphatemia and high FGF23 levels were also reported in patients receiving intravenous administration of iron polymaltose [69]. Especially, a single administration of iron polymaltose increased FGF23 and decreased renal tubular phosphate reabsorption and lowered serum phosphate in patients with iron deficiency anemia [70]. These results indicate that intravenous administration of some formulations of iron can cause hypophosphatemia by increasing circulating levels of FGF23. However, it is not clear why only some formulations of intravenous iron can increase FGF23 concentrations. As mentioned above, iron depletion rather than iron administration was shown to increase FGF23 levels in model mice of ADHR and there was a negative correlation between serum iron and FGF23 in patients with

ADHR [30,31]. These apparently contradictory results are not explained at the moment.

Other Hypophosphatemic Diseases

McCune—Albright syndrome (MAS: OMIM #174800) is caused by activating mutations in a gene coding α subunit of Gs protein. MAS is characterized clinically by the classic triad of polyostotic fibrous dysplasia (POFD), cafe-au-lait skin pigmentation, and precocious puberty. About 50% of patients with MAS present with hypophosphatemic rickets/osteomalacia. It was reported that FGF23 was elevated in patients with McCune—Albright syndrome who had renal phosphate wasting and correlated with the disease burden [71]. It was also shown that FGF23 was produced by bone including lesions affected by fibrous dysplasia [71]. These results suggest that cells in fibrous dysplasia produce FGF23 and induce hypophosphatemic diseases. However, it is not established whether fibrous dysplasia tissue is the only source of FGF23 in patients with MAS.

High FGF23 in hypophosphatemic patients was also reported in several other rare diseases. Schimmelpenning—Feuerstein—Mims syndrome (OMIM %163200) (linear sebaceous nevus syndrome) is characterized by craniofacial sebaceous nevi that appear along the lines of Blaschko. While the responsible gene for this disease has not been identified, it is thought to be caused by mosaicism of a certain lethal gene [72]. FGF23 was shown to be high in hypophosphatemic patients with this syndrome [73]. However, it has not been established whether the nevi are the source of FGF23 in these patients. Osteoglophonic dysplasia (OMIM #166250) is caused by activating mutations in *FGF receptor 1 (FGFR1)*. Patients with osteoglophonic dysplasia show craniosynostosis, rhizomelic dwarfism, and nonossifying bone lesions. Some patients with osteoglophonic dysplasia show hypophosphatemia and high FGF23 [74]. Nonossifying bone lesions are postulated to be the source of FGF23 in these patients and signaling through FGFR1 may be the mechanism of FGF23 overproduction. Jansen-type metaphyseal chondrodysplasia (OMIM #156400) is caused by activating mutations in *parathyroid hormone 1 receptor (PTH1R)*. A patient with Jansen-type chondrodysplasia was reported to show both hypophosphatemia and high FGF23 levels [75]. Finally, a patient with hypophosphatemic rickets and hyperparathyroidism due to parathyroid hyperplasia was found to have a chromosomal translocation with a breakpoint adjacent to *Klotho*. While the mechanism is not clear, circulating FGF23 levels were elevated in this patient indicating that FGF23 was contributing to the development of hypophosphatemia [76]. In summary, there are several rare diseases in which high FGF23 is the postulated cause of hypophosphatemia.

However, the precise mechanisms of high FGF23 in these diseases are largely unknown. Evaluation of circulating FGF23 levels seems to be useful for the differential diagnosis of these FGF23-related hypophosphatemic diseases and other causes of hypophosphatemia.

TREATMENT OF FGF23-RELATED HYPOPHOSPHATEMIC DISEASES

The above-mentioned hypophosphatemic diseases are caused by excess activity of FGF23. Neutral phosphate and active vitamin D_3 are the current standard medical treatment for these diseases. However, these medications can induce several complications including hypercalcemia, hypercalciuria, nephrocalcinosis, nephrolithiasis, diarrhea, and secondary—tertiary hyperparathyroidism. Therefore, periodic monitoring of serum and urinary biochemical parameters are mandatory during treatment with these medications [77]. In addition, these drugs further increased FGF23 levels [78].

Therefore, it is possible that the inhibition of FGF23 activity is an alternate method for treating these diseases. Several studies were reported using *Hyp* mouse as a model of FGF23-related hypophosphatemic rickets/osteomalacia. Some anti-FGF23 antibodies were shown to induce hyperphosphatemia and high 1,25(OH)$_2$D when injected into wild-type mice indicating that these antibodies can inhibit the activity of endogenous FGF23 [16]. These antibodies increased serum phosphate and 1,25(OH)$_2$D also in *Hyp* mice [79]. Once weekly injections of these antibodies for several weeks were reported to correct hypomineralization of bone, disorganized growth plate, and enhance longitudinal growth of long bones [79]. Furthermore, grip strength and spontaneous movement of *Hyp* mice increased by these antibodies while it was not entirely clear what this spontaneous movement represented [80]. FGF23 activates mitogen-activated kinase signaling after binding to the Klotho—FGF receptor complex. It was shown that an inhibitor of MEK increased serum phosphate and 1,25(OH)$_2$D in *Hyp* mice [81]. Furthermore, the C-terminal fragment of FGF23 was also shown to inhibit the activity of full-length FGF23 and increase serum phosphate in wild-type rats [17]. Therefore, it is possible that FGF23 activity can be inhibited by several methods and the inhibition of FGF23 activity seems to be promising as a new therapeutic maneuver for FGF23-related hypophosphatemic diseases. However, long-term efficiency of these methods is not clear at the moment. In addition, while mitogen-activated kinase can be involved in many cellular processes, it has not been established how the activity of administered drug can be limited to the signaling by FGF23 in the case of the inhibition of this kinase. Furthermore, there are no reports about the utility of these methods in humans. More studies are necessary to establish the therapeutic methods to inhibit the activity of FGF23.

TUMORAL CALCINOSIS

FGF23 is a physiological regulator of serum phosphate and 1,25(OH)$_2$D levels. Therefore, the impaired activity of FGF23 also results in deranged levels of phosphate and 1,25(OH)$_2$D. Tumoral calcinosis is characterized by ectopic calcification especially around large joints. Tumoral calcinosis is most commonly observed in patients with end-stage renal disease in whom increased calcium x phosphate product promotes ectopic calcification. However, there are several kinds of tumoral calcinosis observed in patients with normal renal function. Hyperphosphatemia with enhanced proximal tubular phosphate reabsorption and high 1,25(OH)$_2$D level are typical features of hyperphosphatemic familial tumoral calcinosis (HFTC: OMIM #211900) [82]. Because these biochemical findings are exact opposites of those in patients with FGF23-related hypophosphatemic diseases, it was anticipated that HFTC is caused by impaired actions of FGF23. Three genes, *UDP-N-acetyl-alpha-D-galactosamine: polypeptide N-acetylgalactosaminyltransferase 3 (GALNT3)*, *FGF23*, and *Klotho* have been identified as responsible genes for this autosomal recessive disease [83—85].

GALNT3 was identified using a linkage analysis as a responsible gene for HFTC. GALNT3 is an enzyme that transfers N-acetyl galactosamine from a sugar donor UDP-N-acetylgalactosamine to Ser or Thr residue as an initial step of mucin-type O-linked glycosylation. There are 20 kinds of GALNTs and these enzymes are considered to have different tissue distribution and substrate specificity [86]. Several mutations of *GALNT3* were identified in patients with HFTC [85,87—101]. It was reported that FGF23 levels measured by the C-terminal assay were quite high in patients with HFTC caused by mutations in the *GALNT3* gene [85]. Therefore, impaired activity of FGF23 was initially considered to be unlikely as a mechanism of hyperphosphatemia in these patients. Yet, it is clear that FGF23 in these patients measured by the intact assay is rather low [89—91,94,95,99]. Because the C-terminal assay detects both full-length FGF23 and the processed C-terminal fragment of FGF23, these results suggest that there is a large amount of C-terminal fragment of FGF23, but only a little, if any, full-length FGF23 in these patients implying that O-linked glycosylation is somehow involved in the regulation of the processing of FGF23 protein. Actually, Western blot analysis of plasma from patients with mutations in *GALNT3* indicated the presence of increased amount of FGF23 fragments [90]. These results also indicate that

FGF23 values measured by the intact assay and the C-terminal assay can be discrepant.

Analysis of posttranslational FGF23 modifications indicated that FGF23 has three O-linked glycans [90]. In addition, GALNT3 was shown to mediate the attachment of N-acetylgalactosamine to [178]Thr and prevent the processing of FGF23 protein between [179]Arg and [180]Ser [102]. Therefore, patients with inactivating mutations in GALNT3 gene were considered to produce aberrant FGF23 protein which is susceptible for the processing between [179]Arg and [180]Ser. In vitro study indicated that silencing GALNT3 expression enhanced the proteolytic processing of FGF23 protein [90]. This results in decreased full length of FGF23 and causes deficient actions of FGF23. While the detailed regulatory mechanisms of FGF23 production remain to be clarified, it is likely that the resultant hyperphosphatemia and high $1,25(OH)_2D$ stimulate FGF23 production and further increase the level of FGF23 fragments [103]. However, it is not known why the deficient action of GALNT3 cannot be compensated by other GALNTs. Actually, many diseases are caused by mutations in genes involved in the process of glycosylation and are collectively called congenital disorders of glycosylation (CDG). While mucin-type O-glycosylation is the most frequent posttranslational modification of proteins, HFTC by mutations in GALNT3 is the only so far known disease in this type of O-glycosylation [104]. Partial redundancy of substrate specificity of 20 GALNT proteins is a possible cause of the rarity of the disease in mucin-type O-linked glycosylation.

Hyperphosphatemia is also observed in patients with hyperostosis—hyperphosphatemia syndrome. This syndrome is characterized by hyperphosphatemia and cortical hyperostosis. HFTC and hyperphosphatemia—hyperostosis syndrome can be found in the same family with mutations in the GALNT3 gene [93]. Therefore, these two diseases are considered to be allelic disorders [105].

Several mutations in the FGF23 gene were also reported to be responsible for HFTC [83,106—112]. FGF23 levels measured in these patients show a similar pattern to those in patients with mutations in the GALNT3 gene. FGF23 measured by C-terminal assay is very high while FGF23 by intact assay is rather low [106,111]. When mutant FGF23 protein was expressed in vitro, it was reported that the mutant full-length FGF23 was retained in the Golgi complex while the C-terminal fragment of FGF23 was secreted [83]. These results agree with the clinical findings of FGF23 levels in patients with HFTC caused by mutations in the FGF23 gene. On the other hand, enhanced proteolytic cleavage of mutant FGF23, probably because of a defect in O-linked glycosylation, was also reported [107,113]. Therefore it is possible that mutations in FGF23 cause

low intact FGF23 by different mechanisms. Considering these results, there are two possibilities to explain the high C-terminal fragment of FGF23. One is that mutations in FGF23 cause susceptibility for the processing between [179]Arg and [180]Ser and results in a high C-terminal fragment as discussed in the case of mutations in GALNT3. However, it is unknown whether all the mutations of FGF23 reported in patients with HFTC cause similar susceptibility for the processing. The other possibility is that these mutations cause only impaired secretion of full-length FGF23 without affecting the stability of FGF23 protein. Because a certain amount of circulatory FGF23 seems to be present in the processed form [24], the enhanced expression of FGF23 and the impaired secretion of full-length FGF23 are expected to result in a high C-terminal fragment. As enhanced expression of FGF23 is likely in the presence of hyperphosphatemia and high $1,25(OH)_2D$ as discussed previously, it is possible that the latter possibility is actually working. However, these two possibilities are not necessarily mutually exclusive. In any case, the impaired secretion of full-length FGF23 seems to be the cause of insufficient actions of FGF23 in patients with HFTC by mutations in FGF23.

One patient with a homozygous mutation in the Klotho gene was reported to show severe tumoral calcinosis [84]. Because Klotho works as a co-receptor for FGF23, this mutation was considered to induce resistance to FGF23. Actually, FGF23 levels measured by both C-terminal and intact assays were high in this patient [84]. This patient also showed primary hyperparathyroidism by parathyroid hyperplasia. While Klotho is expressed in parathyroid glands and FGF23 suppresses PTH production and secretion in vivo and in vitro [5,6], it is unknown whether primary hyperparathyroidism in this patient is the direct consequence of impaired actions of FGF23 on parathyroid glands.

In addition to HFTC, there is a disease called normophosphatemic familial tumoral calcinosis (NFTC: OMIM #610455). The responsible gene of NFTC was identified to be sterile alpha motif domain-containing protein 9 (SAMD9) [114]. SAMD9 was shown to be induced by interferon-γ and reduce the expression of early growth response-1 [115]. However, the precise mechanism of the development of NFTC remains to be clarified.

CHRONIC KIDNEY DISEASE—MINERAL AND BONE DISORDER (CKD—MBD)

Results mentioned above suggest that circulatory FGF23 levels are regulated by serum phosphate. For example, FGF23 levels are low in hypophosphatemic patients with Fanconi's syndrome and vitamin D deficiency (Fig. 13.1) [27]. In addition, FGF23 rapidly decreases sometimes to undetectable levels after complete removal of responsible tumors for TIO indicating that the expression of endogenous FGF23 in bone is suppressed in these patients [44]. Furthermore, FGF23 measured by C-terminal assay is high in patients with HFTC by mutations in *GALNT3* and *FGF23* genes and FGF23 levels by both C-terminal and intact assay are high in a patient with a mutation in *Klotho* [84,89−91,94,95,99,106,111]. The most frequent case of hyperphosphatemia is CKD. Therefore, it is reasonable to expect that FGF23 is high in patients with CKD. After the development of assays for FGF23, it was actually reported that FGF23 was high in patients with CKD and sometimes extremely high in patients with end-stage renal disease (ESRD) [116−118]. However, the mechanism of high FGF23 in patients with CKD is not fully understood. It was reported that 1,25(OH)$_2$D stimulated FGF23 production and increased FGF23 levels while 1,25(OH)$_2$D is rather low in patients with CKD [103,119]. It was also reported that FGF23 levels correlated with serum phosphate, calcium, calcium x phosphate product, and PTH in patients with ESRD [116]. PTH was shown to be able to stimulate FGF23 production in several studies [120−122] while discrepant results were also reported [123,124]. Therefore, it is possible that PTH contributes to the high FGF23 levels in patients with CKD at least in part. It remains to be established whether phosphate and calcium can directly stimulate FGF23 production. The expression of *Klotho* was reported to be decreased in the kidneys of patients with CKD and this reduction of Klotho was proposed to be a possible cause of high FGF23 [125,126]. In addition, it was recently reported that the development of increased FGF23 level preceded that of overproduction of FGF23 in bone in a model animal of CKD [127]. Therefore, there may be several mechanisms of the increased FGF23 level in patients with CKD.

FGF23 is a hormone working on kidney to regulate phosphate and vitamin D metabolism. Therefore, the next question is to determine what is FGF23 doing in patients with impaired renal function? The kidney plays important roles in the regulation of mineral and bone metabolism. Traditionally, secondary hyperparathyroidism associated with the impaired renal function was considered to be important in the development of renal osteodystrophy (ROD). Specifically, impaired urinary phosphate excretion by reduced nephron mass causes hyperphosphatemia. Hyperphosphatemia together with reduced kidney mass suppresses 1,25(OH)$_2$D production which results in hypocalcemia. Together, hyperphosphatemia, low 1,25(OH)$_2$D, and hypocalcemia contribute to the development of secondary hyperparathyroidism and continuously high PTH causes osteitis fibrosa, one type of ROD

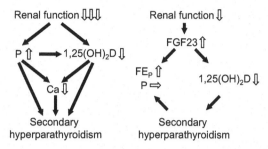

FIGURE 13.2 Pathogenesis of secondary hyperparathyroidism in patients with chronic kidney disease (CKD). Secondary hyperparathyroidism has been considered to be caused by hyperphosphatemia, low 1,25(OH)$_2$D and hypocalcemia (the left panel). Recent studies indicate that FGF23 starts to increase early in the progression of CKD. In CKD patients with remaining renal function, FGF23 reduces 1,25(OH)$_2$D and contributes to the development of secondary hyperparathyroidism. At the same time, FGF23 together with PTH works to inhibit proximal tubular phosphate reabsorption and increase fractional excretion of phosphate (FE$_{Pi}$), thus preventing the development of hyperphosphatemia (the right panel).

(Fig. 13.2). Recently, the new concept of CKD−MBD has been developed. CKD−MBD is defined as a systemic disorder of mineral and bone metabolism due to CKD manifested by either one or a combination of the following: abnormalities of calcium, phosphorus, PTH, or vitamin D metabolism; abnormalities in bone turnover, mineralization, volume, linear growth, or strength; or vascular or other soft-tissue calcification [128].

Because FGF23 regulates vitamin D metabolism and FGF23 is high in patients with CKD, the role of FGF23 in the development of CKD−MBD has been investigated in several studies. In a cross-sectional study investigating the development of hyperphosphatemia, high PTH, and high FGF23 in patients with CKD, it was shown that the increase of FGF23 appeared before the rise of PTH and phosphate [129]. For example, almost half of patients with estimated glomerular filtration rate (eGFR) between 60 and 69 ml/min/1.73 m^2 showed high FGF23 while less than a quarter of these patients had high PTH [129]. In addition, another cross-sectional study indicated that 1,25(OH)$_2$D gradually decreased and fractional excretion of phosphate (FE$_{Pi}$) increased as GFR declined [130]. This increased FE$_{Pi}$ was considered to work to prevent the development of hyperphosphatemia. In addition, the increase of FE$_{Pi}$ was shown to be associated with PTH and FGF23, and the reduction of 1,25(OH)$_2$D was described to be correlated with FGF23 [130]. Furthermore, inhibition of FGF23 activity by neutralizing anti-FGF23 antibodies increased serum 1,25(OH)$_2$D and phosphate, and reduced FE$_{Pi}$ in a model rat of early CKD [131]. Collectively, these studies indicate that FGF23, which starts to increase early in the progression of CKD, reduces 1,25(OH)$_2$D and contributes to the development of later secondary hyperparathyroidism. At the same time, FGF23 seems to work to inhibit proximal tubular phosphate reabsorption and increase FE$_{Pi}$, thus preventing the development of hyperphosphatemia (Fig. 13.2). These results indicate that FGF23 in patients with CKD is biologically active and a clinical study showed that most circulatory FGF23 was full length in patients undergoing peritoneal dialysis [132]. These results also suggest that high FGF23 in patients with CKD cannot be explained by impaired excretion of FGF23 into urine because it is unlikely that FGF23 accumulates in patients with eGFR of more than 60 ml/min/1.73 m^2.

In addition, FGF23 is active in patients who received renal transplantation. Posttransplantation hypophosphatemia associated with renal phosphate wasting is a very frequent complication. This hypophosphatemia has been considered to be caused by PTH. However, several studies indicated that FGF23 is also contributing to the development of hypophosphatemia after renal transplantation [133–135]. It was reported that FGF23 gradually decreased after renal transplantation and reached the comparable level for renal function after several months [135]. However, it is not known why FGF23 does not decrease more rapidly after renal transplantation.

FGF23 can inhibit proximal tubular phosphate reabsorption and decrease 1,25(OH)$_2$D level in patients with preserved renal function. However, FGF23 cannot work in patients with ESRD while FGF23 is sometimes quite high in these patients. One of the possible roles of FGF23 in patients with ESRD is to suppress PTH secretion [5,6]. However, there is a positive correlation between PTH and FGF23 in patients with ESRD [116]. In addition, the expression of Klotho and FGFR1 was reported to be decreased in patients with ESRD suggesting the existence of a resistance to FGF23 in these patients [136,137]. On the other hand, it was also reported that Klotho expression was enhanced in uremic rats [138]. Therefore, further studies are necessary to establish the importance of FGF23 in the regulation of PTH secretion in patients with ESRD.

It has recently been reported that FGF23 induced left ventricular hypertrophy [139]. FGF23 activated calcineurin signaling pathway in a Klotho-independent manner in rat cardiomyocytes [139]. In addition, it was also shown that *Klotho* mice with very high levels of FGF23 showed cardiac hypertrophy and the inhibitor of FGFR attenuated left ventricular hypertrophy in a model animal of CKD [139]. These results are quite important considering that many epidemiological studies show association of high FGF23 levels with various adverse events as shown below. However, these results also raise several questions. Since basic FGF (FGF2) was also shown to induce expression of hypertrophic genes in cardiomyocytes [139], hypertrophic effect does not seem to be a specific function of FGF23.

Therefore, it is likely that some other FGFs may show similar effects if their circulatory levels become high enough. It is possible that it is only FGF23 that can be quite high in patients with CKD as a systemic factor, thereby the association between FGF23 and left ventricular hypertrophy remains intriguing. On the other hand, it was shown that FGF23 uses its N-terminal FGF homology region for the association with FGFR1 and C-terminal unique domain for binding to Klotho. Because of this, FGF23 requires both the N-terminal and C-terminal regions for its physiological effects and the tissue distribution of Klotho has been considered to determine the tissue-specific effects of FGF23 [16]. However, if FGF23 can transduce signals without Klotho, then FGF23 might activate signaling pathways in many organs in patients with ESRD. It is unknown whether this is actually the case and what the consequences of signaling by FGF23 are in these patients. In addition, it is unknown how high FGF23 should be to induce cardiac hypertrophy. Furthermore, some other accompanying factors besides high FGF23 may be necessary to cause ventricular hypertrophy in a clinical setting as it is not known whether patients with high FGF23 such as TIO show cardiac hypertrophy or not. Further studies will clarify these issues and also examine effects of inhibiting FGF23 actions in the state of CKD.

FGF23 IN EPIDEMIOLOGICAL STUDIES

In the past several years, many epidemiological studies examining the association of FGF23 levels with several adverse events especially in patients with CKD have been published. One of the most influential reports indicated that patients with higher FGF23 levels among subjects starting hemodialysis showed worse mortality in the next one year [140]. Especially, this association was significant even after adjustment with various compounding factors including serum phosphate level. Similarly, higher FGF23 was reported to be associated with worse mortality in patients undergoing dialysis, patients with CKD, kidney transplantation recipients, and also in patients with stable coronary artery disease [141–146]. Only 22% of the subjects studied by Parker et al. had estimated GFR of less than 60 ml/min/1.73 m^2 [144]. Therefore, these studies suggest that higher FGF23 is associated with worse survival even in subjects with preserved renal function. On the other hand, a couple of studies indicated that FGF23 levels were not associated with mortality [147,148].

Similarly, many reports indicated the association of FGF23 levels with cardiovascular events or indices in subjects with various renal functions. In patients undergoing dialysis, FGF23 was shown to correlate with arterial calcification of hands, calcification score of total body evaluated by X-ray, left ventricular hypertrophy by echocardiography, intima-media thickness of carotid artery, calcification index of aorta or coronary artery evaluated by computed tomography, and past history of coronary artery disease [147,149—156]. FGF23 was also reported to be associated with left ventricular mass index, cardiovascular events, Gensini score by coronary arteriography, impaired flow-mediated vaso-dilation, and vascular calcification by computed tomography in patients with CKD [143,157—163]. Even in the general population, FGF23 was shown to be associated with impaired endothelium-dependent and independent vasodilatation, systemic arteriosclerosis evaluated by magnetic resonance imaging, left ventricular mass index, lower ejection fraction, and cardiovascular events while some of these subjects should have CKD [164—168]. However, again these associations are not observed in all studies. It was reported that FGF23 level was not associated with coronary artery calcification by computed tomography and coronary artery events [168—170].

In addition, FGF23 was also shown to be associated with diseases of bone and kidney. High FGF23 was reported to correlate with the decrease of bone mineral density in lumbar spine and femoral neck in patients who received renal transplantation [171]. FGF23 was also shown to associate with lower femoral neck bone mineral density and fracture risk of lumbar spine, femoral neck, and non-vertebral bone [172,173]. Again, negative association of FGF23 with bone mineral density of lumbar spine and femoral neck was also reported in patients undergoing dialysis [174]. BMD of the thoracic spine was also reported not to correlate with FGF23 in patients with CKD [163]. In addition, high FGF23 was shown to be associated with improved indices of skeletal mineralization in pediatric patients on peritoneal dialysis [175]. Higher FGF23 was shown to be associated with the progression of CKD, induction of dialysis, and impaired function of transplanted kidney [141,143,145,176—178].

Collectively, these epidemiological studies seem to indicate that higher FGF23 is associated with unfavorable events in cardiovascular, skeletal, and renal systems, and increased mortality. There are several interpretations of these findings. As discussed in the previous section, FGF23 may be able to transduce signals in a Klotho-independent manner and directly affect cardiovascular, skeletal, and renal systems. However, the association of FGF23 and various events is also reported in patients with preserved renal function in whom circulatory FGF23 is not so high. In these patients, it is unlikely that FGF23 affects various tissues

considering the low affinity of FGF23 to various canonical FGF receptors [3,179]. Therefore, the reason why FGF23 level is associated with various adverse events may be different depending on the renal function and FGF23 levels of the subjects. Another possibility is that FGF23 is a sensitive marker of some changes in our body that affect several organs. More studies are necessary to show whether high FGF23 is the cause or result of various events described above.

FUTURE DIRECTION

FGF23 was cloned in 2000 and has been established as a hormone regulating phosphate and vitamin D metabolism since then. In addition, several diseases seem to be caused by aberrant functions of FGF23 thereby making a new classification of disorders of phosphate metabolism possible. Still, many important questions about FGF23 remain unanswered. For example, the detailed mechanisms of the regulation of FGF23 production remain largely unknown. Therefore, it is not understood how mutations in PHEX, DMP1, and ENPP1 result in overproduction of FGF23 and it is impossible at the moment to precisely regulate the production of FGF23. In addition, we do not know how FGF23 actually works. While FGF23 was shown to activate several intracellular signaling pathways, it has not been directly shown how these signals actually regulate phosphate and vitamin D metabolism. Clinically, it is important to understand why there are associations between FGF23 and various adverse events, and what happens if we can decrease FGF23 levels and suppress FGF23 activity especially in patients with CKD. Answering these questions may lead to better treatment for diseases with deranged mineral and bone metabolism.

References

[1] Kurosu H, Ogawa Y, Miyoshi M, Yamamoto M, Nandi A, Rosenblatt KP, et al. Regulation of fibroblast growth factor-23 signaling by klotho. J Biol Chem 2006;281(10):6120—3.
[2] Liu S, Zhou J, Tang W, Jiang X, Rowe DW, Quarles LD. Pathogenic role of Fgf23 in Hyp mice. Am J Physiol Endocrinol Metab 2006;291(1):E38—49.
[3] Urakawa I, Yamazaki Y, Shimada T, Iijima K, Hasegawa H, Okawa K, et al. Klotho converts canonical FGF receptor into a specific receptor for FGF23. Nature 2006;444(7120):770—4.
[4] Shimada T, Hasegawa H, Yamazaki Y, Muto T, Hino R, Takeuchi Y, et al. FGF-23 is a potent regulator of vitamin D metabolism and phosphate homeostasis. J Bone Miner Res 2004;19(3):429—35.
[5] Ben-Dov IZ, Galitzer H, Lavi-Moshayoff V, Goetz R, Kuro-o M, Mohammadi M, et al. The parathyroid is a target organ for FGF23 in rats. J Clin Invest 2007;117(12):4003—8.

[6] Krajisnik T, Bjorklund P, Marsell R, Ljunggren O, Akerstrom G, Jonsson KB, et al. Fibroblast growth factor-23 regulates parathyroid hormone and 1{alpha}-hydroxylase expression in cultured bovine parathyroid cells. J Endocrinol 2007;195(1): 125–31.

[7] Chehade H, Girardin E, Rosato L, Cachat F, Cotting J, Perez MH. Acute life-threatening presentation of vitamin D deficiency rickets. J Clin Endocrinol Metab 2011; 96(9):2681–3.

[8] Miyamoto K, Segawa H, Ito M, Kuwahata M. Physiological regulation of renal sodium-dependent phosphate cotransporters. Jpn J Physiol 2004;54(2):93–102.

[9] ADHR Consortium. Autosomal dominant hypophosphataemic rickets is associated with mutations in FGF23. Nat Genet 2000;26(3):345–8.

[10] Shimada T, Mizutani S, Muto T, Yoneya T, Hino R, Takeda S, et al. Cloning and characterization of FGF23 as a causative factor of tumor-induced osteomalacia. Proc Natl Acad Sci USA 2001;98(11):6500–5.

[11] Yamashita T, Yoshioka M, Itoh N. Identification of a novel fibroblast growth factor, FGF-23, preferentially expressed in the ventrolateral thalamic nucleus of the brain. Biochem Biophys Res Commun 2000;277(2):494–8.

[12] Itoh N, Ornitz DM. Evolution of the *Fgf* and *Fgfr* gene families. Trends Genet 2004;20(11):563–9.

[13] Benet-Pages A, Lorenz-Depiereux B, Zischka H, White KE, Econs MJ, Strom TM. FGF23 is processed by proprotein convertases but not by PHEX. Bone 2004;35(2):455–62.

[14] Shimada T, Muto T, Urakawa I, Yoneya T, Yamazaki Y, Okawa K, et al. Mutant FGF-23 responsible for autosomal dominant hypophosphatemic rickets is resistant to proteolytic cleavage and causes hypophosphatemia in vivo. Endocrinology 2002;143(8):3179–82.

[15] White KE, Carn G, Lorenz-Depiereux B, Benet-Pages A, Strom TM, Econs MJ. Autosomal-dominant hypophosphatemic rickets (ADHR) mutations stabilize FGF-23. Kidney Int 2001;60(6):2079–86.

[16] Yamazaki Y, Tamada T, Kasai N, Urakawa I, Aono Y, Hasegawa H, et al. Anti-FGF23 neutralizing antibodies show the physiological role and structural features of FGF23. J Bone Miner Res 2008;23(9):1509–18.

[17] Goetz R, Nakada Y, Hu MC, Kurosu H, Wang L, Nakatani T, et al. Isolated C-terminal tail of FGF23 alleviates hypophosphatemia by inhibiting FGF23–FGFR–Klotho complex formation. Proc Natl Acad Sci USA 2010;107(1):407–12.

[18] Moore DD. Sister act. Science 2007;316(5830):1436–8.

[19] Itoh N. Hormone-like (endocrine) Fgfs: their evolutionary history and roles in development, metabolism, and disease. Cell Tissue Res 2010;342(1):1–11.

[20] Long YC, Kharitonenkov A. Hormone-like fibroblast growth factors and metabolic regulation. Biochim Biophys Acta 2011;1812(7):791–5.

[21] Imel EA, Peacock M, Pitukcheewanont P, Heller HJ, Ward LM, Shulman D, et al. Sensitivity of fibroblast growth factor 23 measurements in tumor-induced osteomalacia. J Clin Endocrinol Metab 2006;91(6):2055–61.

[22] Ito N, Fukumoto S, Takeuchi Y, Yasuda T, Hasegawa Y, Takemoto F, et al. Comparison of two assays for fibroblast growth factor (FGF)-23. J Bone Miner Metab 2005;23(6):435–40.

[23] Jonsson KB, Zahradnik R, Larsson T, White KE, Sugimoto T, Imanishi Y, et al. Fibroblast growth factor 23 in oncogenic osteomalacia and X-linked hypophosphatemia. N Engl J Med 2003;348(17):1656–63.

[24] Yamazaki Y, Okazaki R, Shibata M, Hasegawa Y, Satoh K, Tajima T, et al. Increased circulatory level of biologically active full-length FGF-23 in patients with hypophosphatemic rickets/osteomalacia. J Clin Endocrinol Metab 2002;87(11):4957–60.

[25] Gribaa M, Younes M, Bouyacoub Y, Korbaa W, Ben Charfeddine I, Touzi M, et al. An autosomal dominant hypophosphatemic rickets phenotype in a Tunisian family caused by a new FGF23 missense mutation. J Bone Miner Metab 2010;28(1):111–5.

[26] Bai XY, Miao D, Goltzman D, Karaplis AC. The autosomal dominant hypophosphatemic rickets R176Q mutation in fibroblast growth factor 23 resists proteolytic cleavage and enhances in vivo biological potency. J Biol Chem 2003;278(11):9843–9.

[27] Fukumoto S, Shimizu Y. Fibroblast growth factor 23 as a phosphotropic hormone and beyond. J Bone Miner Metab 2011;29(5):507–14.

[28] Imel EA, Hui SL, Econs MJ. FGF23 concentrations vary with disease status in autosomal dominant hypophosphatemic rickets. J Bone Miner Res 2007;22(4):520–6.

[29] Econs MJ, McEnery PT. Autosomal dominant hypophosphatemic rickets/osteomalacia: clinical characterization of a novel renal phosphate-wasting disorder. J Clin Endocrinol Metab 1997;82(2):674–81.

[30] Farrow EG, Yu X, Summers LJ, Davis SI, Fleet JC, Allen MR, et al. Iron deficiency drives an autosomal dominant hypophosphatemic rickets (ADHR) phenotype in fibroblast growth factor-23 (Fgf23) knock-in mice. Proc Natl Acad Sci USA 2011.

[31] Imel EA, Peacock M, Gray AK, Padgett LR, Hui SL, Econs MJ. Iron modifies plasma FGF23 differently in autosomal dominant hypophosphatemic rickets and healthy humans. J Clin Endocrinol Metab 2011;96(11):3541–9.

[32] Khosravi A, Cutler CM, Kelly MH, Chang R, Royal RE, Sherry RM, et al. Determination of the elimination half-life of fibroblast growth factor-23. J Clin Endocrinol Metab 2007; 92(6):2374–7.

[33] Folpe AL, Fanburg-Smith JC, Billings SD, Bisceglia M, Bertoni F, Cho JY, et al. Most osteomalacia-associated mesenchymal tumors are a single histopathologic entity: an analysis of 32 cases and a comprehensive review of the literature. Am J Surg Pathol 2004;28(1):1–30.

[34] Drezner MK. Tumor-induced osteomalacia. In: Favus MJ, editor. Primer on the Metabolic Bone Diseases and Disorders of Mineral Metabolism. 4th ed. Philadelphia: Lippincott Williams & Wilkins; 1999. p. 331–7.

[35] Dupond JL, Mahammedi H, Prie D, Collin F, Gil H, Blagosklonov O, et al. Oncogenic osteomalacia: diagnostic importance of fibroblast growth factor 23 and F-18 fluorodeoxyglucose PET/CT scan for the diagnosis and follow-up in one case. Bone 2005;36(3):375–8.

[36] Fukumoto S, Takeuchi Y, Nagano A, Fujita T. Diagnostic utility of magnetic resonance imaging skeletal survey in a patient with oncogenic osteomalacia. Bone 1999;25(3):375–7.

[37] Hesse E, Moessinger E, Rosenthal H, Laenger F, Brabant G, Petrich T, et al. Oncogenic osteomalacia: exact tumor localization by co-registration of positron emission and computed tomography. J Bone Miner Res 2007;22(1):158–62.

[38] Jan de Beur SM, Streeten EA, Civelek AC, McCarthy EF, Uribe L, Marx SJ, et al. Localisation of mesenchymal tumours by somatostatin receptor imaging. Lancet 2002;359(9308): 761–3.

[39] Seufert J, Ebert K, Muller J, Eulert J, Hendrich C, Werner E, et al. Octreotide therapy for tumor-induced osteomalacia. N Engl J Med 2001;345(26):1883–8.

[40] Andreopoulou P, Dumitrescu CE, Kelly MH, Brillante BA, Peck CM, Wodajo FM, et al. Selective venous catheterization for the localization of phosphaturic mesenchymal tumors. J Bone Miner Res 2011;26(6):1295–302.

[41] Ito N, Shimizu Y, Suzuki H, Saito T, Okamoto T, Hori M, et al. Clinical utility of systemic venous sampling of FGF23 for identifying tumours responsible for tumour-induced osteomalacia. J Intern Med 2010;268(4):390–4.

[42] Nasu T, Kurisu S, Matsuno S, Tatsumi K, Kakimoto T, Kobayashi M, et al. Tumor-induced hypophosphatemic osteomalacia diagnosed by the combinatory procedures of magnetic resonance imaging and venous sampling for FGF23. Intern Med 2008;47(10):957–61.

[43] Ogura E, Kageyama K, Fukumoto S, Yagihashi N, Fukuda Y, Kikuchi T, et al. Development of tumor-induced osteomalacia in a subcutaneous tumor, defined by venous blood sampling of fibroblast growth factor-23. Intern Med 2008; 47(7):637–41.

[44] Takeuchi Y, Suzuki H, Ogura S, Imai R, Yamazaki Y, Yamashita T, et al. Venous sampling for fibroblast growth factor-23 confirms preoperative diagnosis of tumor-induced osteomalacia. J Clin Endocrinol Metab 2004;89(8):3979–82.

[45] Berndt T, Craig TA, Bowe AE, Vassiliadis J, Reczek D, Finnegan R, et al. Secreted frizzled-related protein 4 is a potent tumor-derived phosphaturic agent. J Clin Invest 2003;112(5):785–94.

[46] Carpenter TO, Ellis BK, Insogna KL, Philbrick WM, Sterpka J, Shimkets R. Fibroblast growth factor 7: an inhibitor of phosphate transport derived from oncogenic osteomalacia-causing tumors. J Clin Endocrinol Metab 2005;90(2):1012–20.

[47] Rowe PS, Kumagai Y, Gutierrez G, Garrett IR, Blacher R, Rosen D, et al. MEPE has the properties of an osteoblastic phosphatonin and minhibin. Bone 2004;34(2):303–19.

[48] The Hyp Consortium. A gene (PEX) with homologies to endopeptidases is mutated in patients with X-linked hypophosphatemic rickets. Nat Genet 1995;11(2):130–6.

[49] Sabbagh Y, Jones AO, Tenenhouse HS. PHEXdb, a locus-specific database for mutations causing X-linked hypophosphatemia. Hum Mutat 2000;16(1):1–6.

[50] Morgan JM, Hawley WL, Chenoweth AI, Retan WJ, Diethelm AG. Renal transplantation in hypophosphatemia with vitamin D-resistant rickets. Arch Intern Med 1974; 134(3):549–52.

[51] Beck L, Soumounou Y, Martel J, Krishnamurthy G, Gauthier C, Goodyer CG, et al. Pex/PEX tissue distribution and evidence for a deletion in the 3′ region of the Pex gene in X-linked hypophosphatemic mice. J Clin Invest 1997;99(6):1200–9.

[52] Meyer Jr RA, Meyer MH, Gray RW. Parabiosis suggests a humoral factor is involved in X-linked hypophosphatemia in mice. J Bone Miner Res 1989;4(4):493–500.

[53] Nesbitt T, Coffman TM, Griffiths R, Drezner MK. Cross-transplantation of kidneys in normal and Hyp mice. Evidence that the Hyp mouse phenotype is unrelated to an intrinsic renal defect. J Clin Invest 1992;89(5):1453–9.

[54] Yuan B, Takaiwa M, Clemens TL, Feng JQ, Kumar R, Rowe PS, et al. Aberrant Phex function in osteoblasts and osteocytes alone underlies murine X-linked hypophosphatemia. J Clin Invest 2008;118(2):722–34.

[55] Liu S, Guo R, Simpson LG, Xiao ZS, Burnham CE, Quarles LD. Regulation of fibroblastic growth factor 23 expression but not degradation by PHEX. J Biol Chem 2003;278(39):37419–26.

[56] Sitara D, Razzaque MS, Hesse M, Yoganathan S, Taguchi T, Erben RG, et al. Homozygous ablation of fibroblast growth factor-23 results in hyperphosphatemia and impaired skeletogenesis, and reverses hypophosphatemia in Phex-deficient mice. Matrix Biol 2004;23(7):421–32.

[57] Feng JQ, Ward LM, Liu S, Lu Y, Xie Y, Yuan B, et al. Loss of DMP1 causes rickets and osteomalacia and identifies a role for

osteocytes in mineral metabolism. Nat Genet 2006;38(11): 1310–5.

[58] Lorenz-Depiereux B, Bastepe M, Benet-Pages A, Amyere M, Wagenstaller J, Muller-Barth U, et al. DMP1 mutations in autosomal recessive hypophosphatemia implicate a bone matrix protein in the regulation of phosphate homeostasis. Nat Genet 2006;38(11):1248–50.

[59] Wu H, Teng PN, Jayaraman T, Onishi S, Li J, Bannon L, et al. Dentin matrix protein 1 (DMP1) signals via cell surface integrin. J Biol Chem 2011;286(34):29462–9.

[60] Narayanan K, Gajjeraman S, Ramachandran A, Hao J, George A. Dentin matrix protein 1 regulates dentin sialophosphoprotein gene transcription during early odontoblast differentiation. J Biol Chem 2006;281(28):19064–71.

[61] Levy-Litan V, Hershkovitz E, Avizov L, Leventhal N, Bercovich D, Chalifa-Caspi V, et al. Autosomal-recessive hypophosphatemic rickets is associated with an inactivation mutation in the ENPP1 gene. Am J Hum Genet 2010;86(2): 273–8.

[62] Lorenz-Depiereux B, Schnabel D, Tiosano D, Hausler G, Strom TM. Loss-of-function ENPP1 mutations cause both generalized arterial calcification of infancy and autosomal-recessive hypophosphatemic rickets. Am J Hum Genet 2010;86(2):267–72.

[63] Ruf N, Uhlenberg B, Terkeltaub R, Nurnberg P, Rutsch F. The mutational spectrum of ENPP1 as arising after the analysis of 23 unrelated patients with generalized arterial calcification of infancy (GACI). Hum Mutat 2005;25(1):98.

[64] Rutsch F, Boyer P, Nitschke Y, Ruf N, Lorenz-Depierieux B, Wittkampf T, et al. Hypophosphatemia, hyperphosphaturia, and bisphosphonate treatment are associated with survival beyond infancy in generalized arterial calcification of infancy. Circ Cardiovasc Genet 2008;1(2):133–40.

[65] Okawa A, Nakamura I, Goto S, Moriya H, Nakamura Y, Ikegawa S. Mutation in Npps in a mouse model of ossification of the posterior longitudinal ligament of the spine. Nat Genet 1998;19(3):271–3.

[66] Saito T, Shimizu Y, Hori M, Taguchi M, Igarashi T, Fukumoto S, et al. A patient with hypophosphatemic rickets and ossification of posterior longitudinal ligament caused by a novel homozygous mutation in ENPP1 gene. Bone 2011;49(4):913–6.

[67] Sato K, Shiraki M. Saccharated ferric oxide-induced osteomalacia in Japan: iron-induced osteopathy due to nephropathy. Endocr J 1998;45(4):431–9.

[68] Shimizu Y, Tada Y, Yamauchi M, Okamoto T, Suzuki H, Ito N, et al. Hypophosphatemia induced by intravenous administration of saccharated ferric oxide—another form of FGF23-related hypophosphatemia. Bone 2009;45(4):814–6.

[69] Schouten BJ, Doogue MP, Soule SG, Hunt PJ. Iron polymaltose-induced FGF23 elevation complicated by hypophosphataemic osteomalacia. Ann Clin Biochem 2009;46(Pt 2):167–9.

[70] Schouten BJ, Hunt PJ, Livesey JH, Frampton CM, Soule SG. FGF23 elevation and hypophosphatemia after intravenous iron polymaltose: a prospective study. J Clin Endocrinol Metab 2009;94(7):2332–7.

[71] Riminucci M, Collins MT, Fedarko NS, Cherman N, Corsi A, White KE, et al. FGF-23 in fibrous dysplasia of bone and its relationship to renal phosphate wasting. J Clin Invest 2003;112(5):683–92.

[72] Rijntjes-Jacobs EG, Lopriore E, Steggerda SJ, Kant SG, Walther FJ. Discordance for Schimmelpenning—Feuerstein—Mims syndrome in monochorionic twins supports the concept of a postzygotic mutation. Am J Med Genet A 2010; 152A(11):2816–9.

[73] Hoffman WH, Jueppner HW, Deyoung BR, O'Dorisio MS, Given KS. Elevated fibroblast growth factor-23 in hypophosphatemic linear nevus sebaceous syndrome. Am J Med Genet A 2005;134(3):233–6.

[74] White KE, Cabral JM, Davis SI, Fishburn T, Evans WE, Ichikawa S, et al. Mutations that cause osteoglophonic dysplasia define novel roles for FGFR1 in bone elongation. Am J Hum Genet 2005;76(2):361–7.

[75] Brown WW, Juppner H, Langman CB, Price H, Farrow EG, White KE, et al. Hypophosphatemia with elevations in serum fibroblast growth factor 23 in a child with Jansen's metaphyseal chondrodysplasia. J Clin Endocrinol Metab 2009; 94(1):17–20.

[76] Brownstein CA, Adler F, Nelson-Williams C, Iijima J, Li P, Imura A, et al. A translocation causing increased alpha-klotho level results in hypophosphatemic rickets and hyperparathyroidism. Proc Natl Acad Sci USA 2008;105(9):3455–60.

[77] Carpenter TO, Imel EA, Holm IA. Jan de Beur SM, Insogna KL. A clinician's guide to X-linked hypophosphatemia. J Bone Miner Res 2011;26(7):1381–8.

[78] Carpenter TO, Insogna KL, Zhang JH, Ellis B, Nieman S, Simpson C, et al. Circulating levels of soluble klotho and FGF23 in X-linked hypophosphatemia: circadian variance, effects of treatment, and relationship to parathyroid status. J Clin Endocrinol Metab 2010;95(11):E352–7.

[79] Aono Y, Yamazaki Y, Yasutake J, Kawata T, Hasegawa H, Urakawa I, et al. Therapeutic effects of anti-FGF23 antibodies in hypophosphatemic rickets/osteomalacia. J Bone Miner Res 2009;24(11):1879–88.

[80] Aono Y, Hasegawa H, Yamazaki Y, Shimada T, Fujita T, Yamashita T, et al. Anti-FGF23 neutralizing antibodies ameliorate muscle weakness and decreased spontaneous movement of Hyp mice. J Bone Miner Res 2011;26(4):803–10.

[81] Ranch D, Zhang MY, Portale AA, Perwad F. Fibroblast growth factor 23 regulates renal 1,25-dihydroxyvitamin D and phosphate metabolism via the MAP kinase signaling pathway in Hyp mice. J Bone Miner Res 2011;26(8):1883–90.

[82] Lyles KW, Halsey DL, Friedman NE, Lobauch B. Correlations of serum concentrations of 1,25-dihydroxyvitamin D, phosphorus, and parathyroid hormone in tumoral calcinosis. J Clin Endocrinol Metab 1988;67(1):88–92.

[83] Benet-Pages A, Orlik P, Strom TM, Lorenz-Depiereux B. An FGF23 missense mutation causes familial tumoral calcinosis with hyperphosphatemia. Hum Mol Genet 2005;14(3):385–90.

[84] Ichikawa S, Imel EA, Kreiter ML, Yu X, Mackenzie DS, Sorenson AH, et al. A homozygous missense mutation in human KLOTHO causes severe tumoral calcinosis. J Clin Invest 2007;117(9):2684–91.

[85] Topaz O, Shurman DL, Bergman R, Indelman M, Ratajczak P, Mizrachi M, et al. Mutations in GALNT3, encoding a protein involved in O-linked glycosylation, cause familial tumoral calcinosis. Nat Genet 2004;36(6):579–81.

[86] Gram Schjoldager KT, Vester-Christensen MB, Goth CK, Petersen TN, Brunak S, Bennett EP, et al. A systematic study of site-specific GalNAc-Type O-glycosylation modulating proprotein convertase processing. J Biol Chem 2011;286(46):40122–32.

[87] Barbieri AM, Filopanti M, Bua G, Beck-Peccoz P. Two novel nonsense mutations in GALNT3 gene are responsible for familial tumoral calcinosis. J Hum Genet 2007;52(5):464–8.

[88] Campagnoli MF, Pucci A, Garelli E, Carando A, Defilippi C, Lala R, et al. Familial tumoral calcinosis and testicular microlithiasis associated with a new mutation of GALNT3 in a white family. J Clin Pathol 2006;59(4):440–2.

[89] Dumitrescu CE, Kelly MH, Khosravi A, Hart TC, Brahim J, White KE, et al. A case of familial tumoral calcinosis/hyperostosis–hyperphosphatemia syndrome due to a compound heterozygous mutation in GALNT3 demonstrating new phenotypic features. Osteoporos Int 2009;20(7):1273–8.

[90] Frishberg Y, Ito N, Rinat C, Yamazaki Y, Feinstein S, Urakawa I, et al. Hyperostosis–hyperphosphatemia syndrome: a congenital disorder of O-glycosylation associated with augmented processing of fibroblast growth factor 23. J Bone Miner Res 2007;22(2):235–42.

[91] Garringer HJ, Fisher C, Larsson TE, Davis SI, Koller DL, Cullen MJ, et al. The role of mutant UDP-N-acetyl-alpha-D-galactosamine-polypeptide N-acetylgalactosaminyltransferase 3 in regulating serum intact fibroblast growth factor 23 and matrix extracellular phosphoglycoprotein in heritable tumoral calcinosis. J Clin Endocrinol Metab 2006; 91(10):4037–42.

[92] Garringer HJ, Mortazavi SM, Esteghamat F, Malekpour M, Boztepe H, Tanakol R, et al. Two novel GALNT3 mutations in familial tumoral calcinosis. Am J Med Genet A 2007; 143(20):2390–6.

[93] Ichikawa S, Baujat G, Seyahi A, Garoufali AG, Imel EA, Padgett LR, et al. Clinical variability of familial tumoral calcinosis caused by novel GALNT3 mutations. Am J Med Genet A 2010;152A(4):896–903.

[94] Ichikawa S, Guigonis V, Imel EA, Courouble M, Heissat S, Henley JD, et al. Novel GALNT3 mutations causing hyperostosis–hyperphosphatemia syndrome result in low intact fibroblast growth factor 23 concentrations. J Clin Endocrinol Metab 2007;92(5):1943–7.

[95] Ichikawa S, Imel EA, Sorenson AH, Severe R, Knudson P, Harris GJ, et al. Tumoral calcinosis presenting with eyelid calcifications due to novel missense mutations in the glycosyl transferase domain of the GALNT3 gene. J Clin Endocrinol Metab 2006;91(11):4472–5.

[96] Ichikawa S, Lyles KW, Econs MJ. A novel GALNT3 mutation in a pseudoautosomal dominant form of tumoral calcinosis: evidence that the disorder is autosomal recessive. J Clin Endocrinol Metab 2005;90(4):2420–3.

[97] Joseph L, Hing SN, Presneau N, O'Donnell P, Diss T, Idowu BD, et al. Familial tumoral calcinosis and hyperostosis–hyperphosphataemia syndrome are different manifestations of the same disease: novel missense mutations in GALNT3. Skeletal Radiol 2010;39(1):63–8.

[98] Laleye A, Alao MJ, Gbessi G, Adjagba M, Marche M, Coupry I, et al. Tumoral calcinosis due to GALNT3 C.516-2A >T mutation in a black African family. Genet Couns 2008;19(2):183–92.

[99] Olauson H, Krajisnik T, Larsson C, Lindberg B, Larsson TE. A novel missense mutation in GALNT3 causing hyperostosis–hyperphosphataemia syndrome. Eur J Endocrinol 2008;158(6):929–34.

[100] Specktor P, Cooper JG, Indelman M, Sprecher E. Hyperphosphatemic familial tumoral calcinosis caused by a mutation in GALNT3 in a European kindred. J Hum Genet 2006; 51(5):487–90.

[101] Yancovitch A, Hershkovitz D, Indelman M, Galloway P, Whiteford M, Sprecher E, et al. Novel mutations in GALNT3 causing hyperphosphatemic familial tumoral calcinosis. J Bone Miner Metab 2011;29(5):621–5.

[102] Kato K, Jeanneau C, Tarp MA, Benet-Pages A, Lorenz-Depiereux B, Bennett EP, et al. Polypeptide GalNAc-transferase T3 and familial tumoral calcinosis. Secretion of fibroblast growth factor 23 requires O-glycosylation. J Biol Chem 2006;281(27):18370–7.

[103] Saito H, Maeda A, Ohtomo S, Hirata M, Kusano K, Kato S, et al. Circulating FGF-23 is regulated by 1alpha,25-dihydroxyvitamin D3 and phosphorus in vivo. J Biol Chem 2005;280(4):2543–9.

[104] Jaeken J, Hennet T, Matthijs G, Freeze HH. CDG nomenclature: time for a change!. Biochim Biophys Acta 2009;1792(9):825–6.

[105] Frishberg Y, Topaz O, Bergman R, Behar D, Fisher D, Gordon D, et al. Identification of a recurrent mutation in GALNT3 demonstrates that hyperostosis–hyperphosphatemia syndrome and familial tumoral calcinosis are allelic disorders. J Mol Med (Berl) 2005;83(1):33–8.

[106] Araya K, Fukumoto S, Backenroth R, Takeuchi Y, Nakayama K, Ito N, et al. A novel mutation in fibroblast growth factor 23 gene as a cause of tumoral calcinosis. J Clin Endocrinol Metab 2005;90(10):5523–7.

[107] Bergwitz C, Banerjee S, Abu-Zahra H, Kaji H, Miyauchi A, Sugimoto T, et al. Defective O-glycosylation due to a novel homozygous S129P mutation is associated with lack of fibroblast growth factor 23 secretion and tumoral calcinosis. J Clin Endocrinol Metab 2009;94(11):4267–74.

[108] Chefetz I, Heller R, Galli-Tsinopoulou A, Richard G, Wollnik B, Indelman M, et al. A novel homozygous missense mutation in FGF23 causes familial tumoral calcinosis associated with disseminated visceral calcification. Hum Genet 2005;118(2): 261–6.

[109] Garringer HJ, Malekpour M, Esteghamat F, Mortazavi SM, Davis SI, Farrow EG, et al. Molecular genetic and biochemical analyses of FGF23 mutations in familial tumoral calcinosis. Am J Physiol Endocrinol Metab 2008;295(4):E929–37.

[110] Lammoglia JJ, Mericq V. Familial tumoral calcinosis caused by a novel FGF23 mutation: response to induction of tubular renal acidosis with acetazolamide and the non-calcium phosphate binder sevelamer. Horm Res 2009;71(3):178–84.

[111] Larsson T, Yu X, Davis SI, Draman MS, Mooney SD, Cullen MJ, et al. A novel recessive mutation in fibroblast growth factor-23 causes familial tumoral calcinosis. J Clin Endocrinol Metab 2005;90(4):2424–7.

[112] Masi L, Gozzini A, Franchi A, Campanacci D, Amedei A, Falchetti A, et al. A novel recessive mutation of fibroblast growth factor-23 in tumoral calcinosis. J Bone Joint Surg Am 2009;91(5):1190–8.

[113] Larsson T, Davis SI, Garringer HJ, Mooney SD, Draman MS, Cullen MJ, et al. Fibroblast growth factor-23 mutants causing familial tumoral calcinosis are differentially processed. Endocrinology 2005;146(9):3883–91.

[114] Topaz O, Indelman M, Chefetz I, Geiger D, Metzker A, Altschuler Y, et al. A deleterious mutation in SAMD9 causes normophosphatemic familial tumoral calcinosis. Am J Hum Genet 2006;79(4):759–64.

[115] Hershkovitz D, Gross Y, Nahum S, Yehezkel S, Sarig O, Uitto J, et al. Functional characterization of SAMD9, a protein deficient in normophosphatemic familial tumoral calcinosis. J Invest Dermatol 2011;131(3):662–9.

[116] Larsson T, Nisbeth U, Ljunggren O, Juppner H, Jonsson KB. Circulating concentration of FGF-23 increases as renal function declines in patients with chronic kidney disease, but does not change in response to variation in phosphate intake in healthy volunteers. Kidney Int 2003;64(6):2272–9.

[117] Shigematsu T, Kazama JJ, Yamashita T, Fukumoto S, Hosoya T, Gejyo F, et al. Possible involvement of circulating fibroblast growth factor 23 in the development of secondary hyperparathyroidism associated with renal insufficiency. Am J Kidney Dis 2004;44(2):250–6.

[118] Weber TJ, Liu S, Indridason OS, Quarles LD. Serum FGF23 levels in normal and disordered phosphorus homeostasis. J Bone Miner Res 2003;18(7):1227–34.

[119] Shimada T, Yamazaki Y, Takahashi M, Hasegawa H, Urakawa I, Oshima T, et al. Vitamin D receptor-independent FGF23 actions in regulating phosphate and vitamin D metabolism. Am J Physiol Renal Physiol 2005;289(5): F1088–95.

[120] Lavi-Moshayoff V, Wasserman G, Meir T, Silver J, Naveh-Many T. PTH increases FGF23 gene expression and mediates the high-FGF23 levels of experimental kidney failure: a bone parathyroid feedback loop. Am J Physiol Renal Physiol 2010;299(4):F882–9.

[121] Lopez I, Rodriguez-Ortiz ME, Almaden Y, Guerrero F, de Oca AM, Pineda C, et al. Direct and indirect effects of parathyroid hormone on circulating levels of fibroblast growth factor 23 in vivo. Kidney Int 2011;80(5):475–82.

[122] Rhee Y, Bivi N, Farrow E, Lezcano V, Plotkin LI, White KE, et al. Parathyroid hormone receptor signaling in osteocytes increases the expression of fibroblast growth factor-23 in vitro and in vivo. Bone 2011;49(4):636–43.

[123] Saji F, Shigematsu T, Sakaguchi T, Ohya M, Orita H, Maeda Y, et al. Fibroblast growth factor 23 production in bone is directly regulated by 1{alpha},25-dihydroxyvitamin D, but not PTH. Am J Physiol Renal Physiol 2010;299(5):F1212–7.

[124] Samadfam R, Richard C, Nguyen-Yamamoto L, Bolivar I, Goltzman D. Bone formation regulates circulating concentrations of fibroblast growth factor 23. Endocrinology 2009;150(11):4835–45.

[125] John GB, Cheng CY, Kuro-o M. Role of Klotho in aging, phosphate metabolism, and CKD. Am J Kidney Dis 2011; 58(1):127–34.

[126] Koh N, Fujimori T, Nishiguchi S, Tamori A, Shiomi S, Nakatani T, et al. Severely reduced production of klotho in human chronic renal failure kidney. Biochem Biophys Res Commun 2001;280(4):1015–20.

[127] Stubbs JR, He N, Idiculla A, Gillihan R, Liu S, David V, et al. Longitudinal evaluation of FGF23 changes and mineral metabolism abnormalities in a mouse model of chronic kidney disease. J Bone Miner Res 2012. in press.

[128] Moe S, Drueke T, Cunningham J, Goodman W, Martin K, Olgaard K, et al. Definition, evaluation, and classification of renal osteodystrophy: a position statement from Kidney Disease: Improving Global Outcomes (KDIGO). Kidney Int 2006;69(11):1945–53.

[129] Isakova T, Wahl P, Vargas GS, Gutierrez OM, Scialla J, Xie H, et al. Fibroblast growth factor 23 is elevated before parathyroid hormone and phosphate in chronic kidney disease. Kidney Int 2011;79(12):1370–8.

[130] Gutierrez O, Isakova T, Rhee E, Shah A, Holmes J, Collerone G, et al. Fibroblast growth factor-23 mitigates hyperphosphatemia but accentuates calcitriol deficiency in chronic kidney disease. J Am Soc Nephrol 2005;16(7):2205–15.

[131] Hasegawa H, Nagano N, Urakawa I, Yamazaki Y, Iijima K, Fujita T, et al. Direct evidence for a causative role of FGF23 in the abnormal renal phosphate handling and vitamin D metabolism in rats with early-stage chronic kidney disease. Kidney Int 2010;78(10):975–80.

[132] Shimada T, Urakawa I, Isakova T, Yamazaki Y, Epstein M, Wesseling-Perry K, et al. Circulating fibroblast growth factor 23 in patients with end-stage renal disease treated by peritoneal dialysis is intact and biologically active. J Clin Endocrinol Metab 2010;95(2):578–85.

[133] Bhan I, Shah A, Holmes J, Isakova T, Gutierrez O, Burnett SA, et al. Post-transplant hypophosphatemia: Tertiary "Hyper-Phosphatoninism"? Kidney Int 2006;70(8):1486–94.

[134] Evenepoel P, Naesens M, Claes K, Kuypers D, Vanrenterghem Y. Tertiary "hyperphosphatoninism"

accentuates hypophosphatemia and suppresses calcitriol levels in renal transplant recipients. Am J Transplant 2007;7(5):1193−200.

[135] Kawarazaki H, Shibagaki Y, Fukumoto S, Kido R, Ando K, Nakajima I, et al. Natural history of mineral and bone disorders after living-donor kidney transplantation: a one-year prospective observational study. Ther Apher Dial 2011;15(5):481−7.

[136] Komaba H, Goto S, Fujii H, Hamada Y, Kobayashi A, Shibuya K, et al. Depressed expression of Klotho and FGF receptor 1 in hyperplastic parathyroid glands from uremic patients. Kidney Int 2010;77(3):232−8.

[137] Krajisnik T, Olauson H, Mirza MA, Hellman P, Akerstrom G, Westin G, et al. Parathyroid Klotho and FGF-receptor 1 expression decline with renal function in hyperparathyroid patients with chronic kidney disease and kidney transplant recipients. Kidney Int 2010;78(10):1024−32.

[138] Hofman-Bang J, Martuseviciene G, Santini MA, Olgaard K, Lewin E. Increased parathyroid expression of klotho in uremic rats. Kidney Int 2010;78(11):1119−27.

[139] Faul C, Amaral AP, Oskouei B, Hu MC, Sloan A, Isakova T, et al. FGF23 induces left ventricular hypertrophy. J Clin Invest 2011;121(11):4393−408.

[140] Gutierrez OM, Mannstadt M, Isakova T, Rauh-Hain JA, Tamez H, Shah A, et al. Fibroblast growth factor 23 and mortality among patients undergoing hemodialysis. N Engl J Med 2008;359(6):584−92.

[141] Isakova T, Xie H, Yang W, Xie D, Anderson AH, Scialla J, et al. Fibroblast growth factor 23 and risks of mortality and end-stage renal disease in patients with chronic kidney disease. JAMA 2011;305(23):2432−9.

[142] Jean G, Terrat JC, Vanel T, Hurot JM, Lorriaux C, Mayor B, et al. High levels of serum fibroblast growth factor (FGF)-23 are associated with increased mortality in long haemodialysis patients. Nephrol Dial Transplant 2009;24(9):2792−6.

[143] Kendrick J, Cheung AK, Kaufman JS, Greene T, Roberts WL, Smits G, et al. FGF-23 associates with death, cardiovascular events, and initiation of chronic dialysis. J Am Soc Nephrol 2011;22(10):1913−22.

[144] Parker BD, Schurgers LJ, Brandenburg VM, Christenson RH, Vermeer C, Ketteler M, et al. The associations of fibroblast growth factor 23 and uncarboxylated matrix Gla protein with mortality in coronary artery disease: the Heart and Soul Study. Ann Intern Med 2010;152(10):640−8.

[145] Wolf M, Molnar MZ, Amaral AP, Czira ME, Rudas A, Ujszaszi A, et al. Elevated fibroblast growth factor 23 is a risk factor for kidney transplant loss and mortality. J Am Soc Nephrol 2011;22(5):956−66.

[146] Holden RM, Beseau D, Booth SL, Adams MA, Garland JS, Morton RA, et al. FGF-23 is associated with cardiac troponin T and mortality in hemodialysis patients. Hemodial Int 2012;16(1):53−8.

[147] Hsu HJ, Wu MS. Fibroblast growth factor 23: a possible cause of left ventricular hypertrophy in hemodialysis patients. Am J Med Sci 2009;337(2):116−22.

[148] Olauson H, Qureshi AR, Miyamoto T, Barany P, Heimburger O, Lindholm B, et al. Relation between serum fibroblast growth factor-23 level and mortality in incident dialysis patients: are gender and cardiovascular disease confounding the relationship? Nephrol Dial Transplant 2010;25(9):3033−8.

[149] Balci M, Kirkpantur A, Gulbay M, Gurbuz OA. Plasma fibroblast growth factor-23 levels are independently associated with carotid artery atherosclerosis in maintenance hemodialysis patients. Hemodial Int 2010;14(4):425−32.

[150] Coen G, De Paolis P, Ballanti P, Pierantozzi A, Pisano S, Sardella D, et al. Peripheral artery calcifications evaluated by

histology correlate to those detected by CT: relationships with fetuin-A and FGF-23. J Nephrol 2011;24(3):313−21.

[151] Inaba M, Okuno S, Imanishi Y, Yamada S, Shioi A, Yamakawa T, et al. Role of fibroblast growth factor-23 in peripheral vascular calcification in non-diabetic and diabetic hemodialysis patients. Osteoporos Int 2006;17(10):1506−13.

[152] Jean G, Bresson E, Terrat JC, Vanel T, Hurot JM, Lorriaux C, et al. Peripheral vascular calcification in long-haemodialysis patients: associated factors and survival consequences. Nephrol Dial Transplant 2009;24(3):948−55.

[153] Kirkpantur A, Balci M, Gurbuz OA, Afsar B, Canbakan B, Akdemir R, et al. Serum fibroblast growth factor-23 (FGF-23) levels are independently associated with left ventricular mass and myocardial performance index in maintenance haemossdialysis patients. Nephrol Dial Transplant 2011; 26(4):1346−54.

[154] Nasrallah MM, El-Shehaby AR, Salem MM, Osman NA, El Sheikh E, Sharaf El Din UA. Fibroblast growth factor-23 (FGF-23) is independently correlated to aortic calcification in haemodialysis patients. Nephrol Dial Transplant 2010;25(8):2679−85.

[155] Negishi K, Kobayashi M, Ochiai I, Yamazaki Y, Hasegawa H, Yamashita T, et al. Association between fibroblast growth factor 23 and left ventricular hypertrophy in maintenance hemodialysis patients. Comparison with B-type natriuretic peptide and cardiac troponin T. Circ J 2010;74(12):2734−40.

[156] Srivaths PR, Goldstein SL, Silverstein DM, Krishnamurthy R, Brewer ED, Elevated FGF. 23 and phosphorus are associated with coronary calcification in hemodialysis patients. Pediatr Nephrol 2011;26(6):945−51.

[157] Gutierrez OM, Januzzi JL, Isakova T, Laliberte K, Smith K, Collerone G, et al. Fibroblast growth factor 23 and left ventricular hypertrophy in chronic kidney disease. Circulation 2009;119(19):2545−52.

[158] Kanbay M, Nicoleta M, Selcoki Y, Ikizek M, Aydin M, Eryonucu B, et al. Fibroblast growth factor 23 and fetuin A are independent predictors for the coronary artery disease extent in mild chronic kidney disease. Clin J Am Soc Nephrol 2010;5(10):1780−6.

[159] Peiskerova M, Kalousova M, Kratochvilova M, Dusilova-Sulkova S, Uhrova J, Bandur S, et al. Fibroblast growth factor 23 and matrix-metalloproteinases in patients with chronic kidney disease: are they associated with cardiovascular disease? Kidney Blood Press Res 2009;32(4):276−83.

[160] Seiler S, Reichart B, Roth D, Seibert E, Fliser D, Heine GH. FGF-23 and future cardiovascular events in patients with chronic kidney disease before initiation of dialysis treatment. Nephrol Dial Transplant 2010;25(12):3983−9.

[161] Stevens KK, McQuarrie EP, Sands W, Hillyard DZ, Patel RK, Mark PB, et al. Fibroblast growth factor 23 predicts left ventricular mass and induces cell adhesion molecule formation. Int J Nephrol 2011;2011:297070.

[162] Yilmaz MI, Sonmez A, Saglam M, Yaman H, Kilic S, Demirkaya E, et al. FGF-23 and vascular dysfunction in patients with stage 3 and 4 chronic kidney disease. Kidney Int 2010;78(7):679−85.

[163] Desjardins L, Liabeuf S, Renard C, Lenglet A, Lemke HD, Choukroun G, et al. FGF23 is independently associated with vascular calcification but not bone mineral density in patients at various CKD stages. Osteoporos Int 2012. in press.

[164] Dalal M, Sun K, Cappola AR, Ferrucci L, Crasto C, Fried LP, et al. Relationship of serum fibroblast growth factor 23 with cardiovascular disease in older community-dwelling women. Eur J Endocrinol 2011;165(5):797−803.

[165] Mirza MA, Hansen T, Johansson L, Ahlstrom H, Larsson A, Lind L, et al. Relationship between circulating FGF23 and total body atherosclerosis in the community. Nephrol Dial Transplant 2009;24(10):3125−31.

[166] Mirza MA, Larsson A, Lind L, Larsson TE. Circulating fibro-
      blast growth factor-23 is associated with vascular dysfunction
      in the community. Atherosclerosis 2009;205(2):385−90.
[167] Mirza MA, Larsson A, Melhus H, Lind L, Larsson TE. Serum
      intact FGF23 associate with left ventricular mass, hypertrophy
      and geometry in an elderly population. Atherosclerosis
      2009;207(2):546−51.
[168] Seiler S, Cremers B, Rebling NM, Hornof F, Jeken J, Kersting S,
      et al. The phosphatonin fibroblast growth factor 23 links
      calcium-phosphate metabolism with left-ventricular dysfunc-
      tion and atrial fibrillation. Eur Heart J 2011;32(21):2688−96.
[169] Roos M, Lutz J, Salmhofer H, Luppa P, Knauss A, Braun S, et al.
      Relation between plasma fibroblast growth factor-23, serum
      fetuin-A levels and coronary artery calcification evaluated by
      multislice computed tomography in patients with normal
      kidney function. Clin Endocrinol (Oxf) 2008;68(4):660−5.
[170] Taylor EN, Rimm EB, Stampfer MJ, Curhan GC. Plasma fibro-
      blast growth factor 23, parathyroid hormone, phosphorus, and
      risk of coronary heart disease. Am Heart J 2011;161(5):956−62.
[171] Kanaan N, Claes K, Devogelaer JP, Vanderschueren D,
      Depresseux G, Goffin E, et al. Fibroblast growth factor-23 and
      parathyroid hormone are associated with post-transplant bone
      mineral density loss. Clin J Am Soc Nephrol 2010;5(10):1887−92.
[172] Manghat P, Fraser WD, Wierzbicki AS, Fogelman I,
      Goldsmith DJ, Hampson G. Fibroblast growth factor-23 is
      associated with C-reactive protein, serum phosphate and bone
      mineral density in chronic kidney disease. Osteoporos Int
      2010;21(11):1853−61.
[173] Mirza MA, Karlsson MK, Mellstrom D, Orwoll E, Ohlsson C,
      Ljunggren O, et al. Serum fibroblast growth factor-23 (FGF-23) and
      fracture risk in elderly men. J Bone Miner Res 2011;26(4):857−64.
[174] Urena Torres P, Friedlander G, de Vernejoul MC, Silve C,
      Prie D. Bone mass does not correlate with the serum fibroblast
      growth factor 23 in hemodialysis patients. Kidney Int
      2008;73(1):102−7.
[175] Wesseling-Perry K, Pereira RC, Wang H, Elashoff RM, Sahney S,
      Gales B, et al. Relationship between plasma fibroblast growth
      factor-23 concentration and bone mineralization in children
      with renal failure on peritoneal dialysis. J Clin Endocrinol
      Metab 2009;94(2):511−7.
[176] Fliser D, Kollerits B, Neyer U, Ankerst DP, Lhotta K,
      Lingenhel A, et al. Fibroblast growth factor 23 (FGF23) predicts
      progression of chronic kidney disease: the Mild to Moderate
      Kidney Disease (MMKD) Study. J Am Soc Nephrol 2007;
      18(9):2600−8.
[177] Titan SM, Zatz R, Graciolli FG, dos Reis LM, Barros RT,
      Jorgetti V, et al. FGF-23 as a predictor of renal outcome in dia-
      betic nephropathy. Clin J Am Soc Nephrol 2011;6(2):241−7.
[178] Semba RD, Fink JC, Sun K, Cappola AR, Dalal M, Crasto C,
      et al. Serum fibroblast growth factor-23 and risk of incident
      chronic kidney disease in older community-dwelling women.
      Clin J Am Soc Nephrol 2012;7(1):85−91.
[179] Yu X, Ibrahimi OA, Goetz R, Zhang F, Davis SI, Garringer HJ,
      et al. Analysis of the biochemical mechanisms for the endocrine
      actions of fibroblast growth factor-23. Endocrinology
      2005;146(11):4647−56.

14

Bone Marrow Fat and Bone Mass

Masanobu Kawai[1], *Clifford J. Rosen*[2]

[1]Osaka Medical Center and Research Institute for Maternal and Child Health, Osaka, Japan
[2]Maine Medical Center Research Institute, Scarborough, ME, USA

INTRODUCTION

For a century adipocytes have been noted in the bone marrow of mammals. And although fat cells have been considered an integral part of the bone marrow micro-environment, few believed these cells were physiologically active. However, the developmental, mechanical, and physiological components of adipogenesis within the trabecular niche have recently become the focus of investigation by several groups. Coincident with that attention, significant progress has been made in understanding the differentiation programs of osteoblasts and adipocytes, as well as their common ancestor, the mesenchymal stem cell. This review will center on our current knowledge of the interaction between marrow fat and the skeleton. We will focus on mouse and human models, although our conclusions may extend to other vertebrates.

HISTORICAL VIGNETTE

Marrow adipocytes were recognized in pathologic human specimens as early as the 19th century as "large cells in the bone marrow," although their function was unknown. Neumann was the first to describe from autopsy samples that red marrow was replaced by marrow giant cells in the peripheral skeleton with age and then advanced the theorem that with advancing age, hematopoietic elements within the marrow are replaced by large yellow cells. Subsequently, from analyses of patients with arsenic toxicity, marrow "giant" cells were shown to have unique characteristics that resembled fat globules. In line with these observations, marrow adipocytes were recognized as a constant and unique feature of bone marrow aspirates and biopsies, and numerous studies identified the absence of marrow fat in some hematopoietic disorders or enhanced marrow adiposity in aplastic anemia due to chemicals or radiation. In 1936 Huggins and Blocksom reported that tail vertebrae from rodents were laden with marrow fat in contrast to more anterior vertebrae [1]. In 1971, Meunier et al. first reported that osteoporotic elderly women had abundant marrow fat, which was directly related to age and negatively correlated with trabecular bone volume [2]. Several reports followed which demonstrated that the increase in marrow adiposity was age dependent, but with gender, ethnic, and age variation. By the 1990s, MRI emerged as a means to image and quantitate marrow fat by spectroscopy [3]. Phenotyping mice for marrow adiposity has advanced recently with the use of high-field MRI and μCT with osmium staining. Future technological advances such as MRI with PET scanning promise to further define functional aspects of marrow adiposity.

MOLECULAR AND CELLULAR ASPECTS OF MARROW ADIPOGENESIS

Transcriptional Control of Adipogenesis

Adipogenesis is a complex and integrated process in which several transcription factors come into play in a context-specific manner [4–6]. The molecular and cellular mechanisms of adipocyte differentiation have been widely and extensively studied using *in vitro* and *in vivo* models. The initial step of adipogenesis is the lineage commitment of mesenchymal stem cells (MSCs) into preadipocytes. This occurs in the stromal vascular fraction of adipose depots and in the bone marrow. Following the expansion of preadipocytes, MSCs differentiate into mature adipocytes under the tight control of multiple transcription factors including C/EBPβ/δ and PPARγ. Among these, PPARγ, a nuclear receptor and transcription factor, plays a central role in adipogenesis as evidenced by the fact that the loss of *Pparg* in mouse embryonic fibroblasts leads to a complete absence of adipogenic capacity [7]. *In vitro*, multiple transcription factors and co-regulators have been implicated as modulators of the expression and function of PPARγ. For example, differentiation of 3T3-L1 cells, a well-recognized cell line that is used to recapitulate adipogenesis *in vitro*, is regulated by the integration of several transcription factors including the C/EBP family, C/EBPβ and δ. These factors stimulate *Pparg* transcription by directly binding to the promoter region [8]. Increased expression of *Pparg* activates the expression of another member of the C/EBP family, C/EBPα, which in turn enhances the expression of PPARγ. Partial loss of function of C/EBPα results in a mouse (A-Zip) with very little adipose tissue including virtually none in the bone marrow. Thus, the C/EBP family is critical for the induction of PPARγ *in vitro*. However, *in vivo* adipogenesis is much more complex and requires other transcriptional and cofactors for PPARγ regulation in part because PPARγ expression is maintained in adipose tissue of mice lacking C/EBPβ and/or δ [9].

The Central Role of Peroxisome Proliferator-activated Receptor-gamma (PPARγ)

Peroxisome proliferator-activated receptor-gamma (PPARγ) is a member of the PPAR family of transcriptional factors, which has multiple roles not only in cell fate determination, but in lipid biosynthesis, mitochondrial biogenesis, inflammation, neoplastic growth, and insulin sensitivity [10,11]. PPARγ is composed of four variants including PPARγ1 and 2, the two major forms of PPARγ protein, which are produced by differential usage of promoters and alternative splicing. PPARγ1 is widely expressed in many tissues including the liver, skeletal muscle, adipose tissue, and bone, while expression of PPARγ2, which possesses 30 additional amino acids in its N-terminus compared to PPARγ1, is restricted to adipogenic cells. Importantly, several lines of evidence demonstrate the existence of PPARγ2 in marrow stromal cells prior to their differentiation into adipocytes [10,12,13]. PPARγ dimerizes with the retinoic X receptor (RXR) alpha, and activates transcription of target genes, although a number of transcription factors and co-activators are also involved in the regulation of *Pparg* expression and function. As described earlier, the C/EBP family, C/EBPα, β, and δ, plays a pivotal role in adipogenesis in cooperation with PPARγ. PPARγ expression and function are also regulated by other transcription factors during adipogenesis including Srebp-1c, KLF5, KLF15, Zfp423, and early B cell factor (Ebf1), while KLF-2 and GATA2/3 negatively regulates PPARγ expression [4,14−18].

Naturally occurring substances such as fatty acids and metabolites of arachidonic acids are potential *in vivo* candidates for PPARγ liagnds [19,20]. 15-Deoxy-$\Delta^{12,14}$-prostaglandin J_2 (15d-PGJ2) is one such endogenous PPARγ ligand which is derived from arachidonic acid, although it still remains to be clarified whether 15d-PGJ2 is functional in terms of activating PPARγ *in vivo* [21,22]. In addition to these, a synthetic class of compounds, the thiazolidinediones (TZDs), are potent exogenous ligands for PPARγ and have been widely used in the treatment of diabetes [23−27].

PPARγ transcriptional activity is regulated by histone modification as well as ligand availability. In the absence of ligands, co-repressors such as NCoR and SMRT as well as histone deacetylases (HDAC) are recruited to the protein complex of PPARγ, thereby forcing PPARγ to be transcriptionally silent [28]. In contrast, when ligands are available, these proteins are dissociated from PPARγ protein complex machinery and co-activators such as CBP and histone acetyltransferase (HAT) are recruited. Another level of regulation is created by the histone methylation by histone methyltransferase. Non-canonical Wnt pathways activated by Wnt5a have been shown to suppress PPARγ transcriptional activation through the histone methyltransferase, SETDB1 (SET domain bifurcated 1) [29].

Posttranscriptional modifications of PPARγ are also important components in regulating PPARγ activity. PPARγ2 has been shown to be phosphorylated at serine 112 by secretory factors including EGF and PDGF, resulting in the impairment of PPARγ2 transcriptional activity [30−32]. On the other hand, phosphorylation at serine 273 by Cdk5 enhances adipogenesis and has been linked to greater fat deposition and suppression of adiponectin [33,34]. Agents that block Cdk5 phosphorylation including rosiglitazone have been demonstrated to enhance insulin sensitivity through this mechanism. Newer compounds that block Cdk5 phosphorylation but do not have transcriptional activity have recently been described as pure insulin sensitizers [33,34]. In addition to phosphorylation, sumoylation and ubiquitination confer a different level of posttranscriptional PPARγ regulation [35−37]. In sum the importance of this nuclear receptor and transcriptional factor for cellular metabolic fate cannot be overstated. Hence there are multiple layers of regulatory control over PPARγ activity.

PPARγ and the Skeleton

Osteoblasts and adipocytes share a common precursor (i.e. the mesenchymal stem cell, MSC), which also serves as a source of progenitors for marrow fibroblasts, chondrocytes, and supporting stroma for hematopoietic cells [38−40] (Fig. 14.1). Lineage

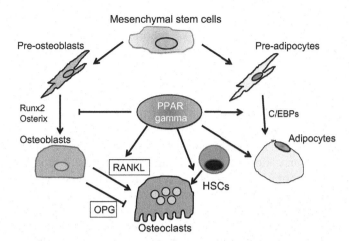

FIGURE 14.1 PPARγ regulates the cell fate decision of mesenchymal stem cells (MSCs) toward the adipogenic or osteogenic lineage. The role of PPARγ in osteoclast differentiation is still controversial and needs to be clarified. Marrow adipocytes produce a number of secretory factors and PPARγ regulates the expression of these genes. PPARγ: peroxisome proliferator-activated receptor-gamma. C/EBP: CCAAT enhancer binding protein. Runx2: runt-related transcription factor 2. Msx2: muscle segment homeobox homologue of 2. Please see color plate section.

allocation of marrow MSCs towards either adipocytes or osteoblasts is a finely tuned event in which lineage-specific transcription factors (such as Runx2 and Osterix for osteoblasts and PPARγ2 for adipocytes) play critical roles. Importantly, in some but not all situations lineage allocation of MSCs towards either of these cell types is considered to be mutually exclusive; i.e. activation of PPARγ leads to enhanced adipogenesis at the expense of osteoblastogenesis and is associated with reduced expression and function of osteogenic transcription factors such as Dlx5, Msx2, Runx2, and Osterix [41–44]. In line with this, suppression of PPARγ is reported to stimulate osteoblastogenesis and represses adipogenesis [45]. These observations are also consistent with the findings of aged mice models where marrow adiposity is increased and bone mass is reduced, associated with enhanced PPARγ2 expression [46]. Similarly, haploinsufficiency or a hypomorphic mutation of *Pparg* has been reported to have increased bone mass and reduced marrow adiposity associated with increased osteoblast number and bone formation [47,48]. In addition to the pivotal role of PPARγ in lineage allocation of MSCs, mounting evidence indicates the involvement of PPARγ in osteoclast differentiation as well. For example, PPARγ activation has been shown to activate bone resorption in part through enhancing osteoclast differentiation by recruitment of another co-activator of PPARγ, PGC-1beta [49–52]. Furthermore, the effect of PPARγ activation on osteoclastogenesis could be in part mediated by the increased expression of *Rankl* in an

age-dependent manner [53]; however, the exact role of PPARγ in osteoclastogenesis is still controversial and needs to be determined [54,55]. Additionally, we recently observed that conditional deletion of PPARγ in differentiated adipocytes using the aP2 promoter resulted in lipodystrophy by 26 weeks accompanied by high bone mass (Rosen CJ, personal observation). Interestingly, these mice exhibit increased osteoclast activity suggesting that the phenotypic effects of PPARγ are highly context specific with temporal effects from PPARγ deletion varying with the timing of inactivation.

DEVELOPMENT OF MARROW FAT

Marrow adipogenesis has recently gained attention among researchers because of its possible role as a modulator of physiological and pathological conditions. Marrow adipocytes have long been thought to result from a default pathway for MSCs during differentiation. In support of that tenet, the compositional ratio in bone marrow adipocytes relative to hematopoietic element changes with age. For example, in neonatal mammals, adipocytes are all but absent in the bone marrow and hematopoietic cells primarily occupy the marrow cavity at this stage. During pubertal growth, there is gradual but significant infiltration of marrow from the long bones with adipocytes. However, with advancing age, the number of adipocytes in the bone marrow increases dramatically, resulting in the appearance of fatty marrow. In humans, most of the femoral cavity is occupied by fat in the third decade of life, whereas in the vertebrae this does not occur until the 7th or 8th decade. Importantly, these age-related changes in marrow adiposity are associated with bone loss, although this does not necessarily imply cause and effect. On the other hand, marrow adipocytes are found in abundance in states such as aplastic or myelophthisic diseases, suggesting that adipogenesis could either be inhibitory to hematopoiesis or might occupy the marrow space in lieu of hematopoietic elements [56].

The process of marrow adipogenesis is likely governed by the same transcriptional cascades as observed in white adipocyte differentiation and hence PPARγ is certain to play a pivotal role. Streptozoticin-induced type 1 diabetic model mice exhibit massive development of marrow adiposity, which is antagonized by the treatment with the PPARγ inhibitor bisphenol A diglycidyl ether (BADGE) [57]. In the same vein, BADGE also suppresses the marrow adipogenesis following irradiation in mice [56]. Treatment with TZDs affects bone mass and marrow adiposity, further substantiating a role for PPARγ in marrow fat generation. These lines of evidence indicate that development of marrow adiposity is age specific and activation of PPARγ is likely central to the development of marrow adipocytes.

THE FUNCTION OF MARROW FAT

Some studies have suggested that marrow adipocytes, under most physiologically conditions, are metabolically inert. This process is often thought of as a default mechanism whereby MSCs enter the fat lineage because of their inability to differentiate into more complex cells such as osteoblasts or chondrocytes. Although this hypothesis can be considered tenable in light of several studies showing an inverse relationship between marrow fat and bone volume, there are mouse models to suggest this may not always be operative. Other studies suggest that marrow adipocytes may be self-promotive such that existing marrow adipocytes can induce differentiation of more MSCs into adipocytes, thereby preventing lineage allocation into other cell types [10,11]. Finally, we and others have shown that mouse adipocytes from certain depots can suppress osteoblastogenesis when co-cultured with bone marrow stromal cells, suggesting that these cells could be metabolically active and inhibit osteoblastogenesis through paracrine secretory factors (Rosen CJ, unpublished observation).

Marrow adipocyte infiltration is often associated with bone loss, but there is also evidence of a positive correlation between marrow adiposity and bone mass in human and animal models. For example, C3H/HeJ mouse exhibits high bone mass associated with increased marrow adiposity compared to C57BL/6J background [58]. In humans, marrow adiposity robustly increases during puberty when skeletal acquisition is maximized [59]. These indirect lines of evidence suggest that in physiological situations marrow adipocytes have a distinctly different role from adipocytes found in pathogenic conditions. In that same vein, leptin expression in the bone marrow increases at the time of puberty in mice when maximal bone mass is acquired and decreases with age, indicating that leptin could be one possible factor produced by marrow adipocytes that influences skeletal accrual (Rosen CJ, unpublished observation). In addition, mice with a global deletion of Ebf1 (an early B cell transcription factor) demonstrate a substantial increase in marrow adiposity that is accompanied by an increase in osteoblasts [60], suggesting that this nuclear factor may have a role in enhancing lineage allocation between adipocytes and osteoblasts. Thus, marrow adipocytes may be an important component of the bone marrow niche and establish a favorable skeletal

micro-environment for osteoblast differentiation. This could occur through the secretion of paracrine factors or by release of free fatty acids that might be utilized by osteoblasts.

Adipocytes in the bone marrow have been thought to be inhibitors of active hematopoiesis although further studies are required at different skeletal sites [56]. Interestingly, the appearance of adipogenesis in the femoral bone marrow after transplantation or injury may serve not as a true antagonist for hematopoiesis but rather as a "place-holder" to maintain hematopoietic progenitors in a stem cell state awaiting signals that permit entrance of those cells into their differentiation scheme. Alternatively, marrow adipogenesis may serve as a functional reservoir to re-establish the niche. For example, in C57BL6 mice that are lethally irradiated and then undergo marrow transplantation, the bone cavity fills with adipocytes between days 5 and 10 but those cells subsequently disappear 3 weeks after marrow transplantation. Moreover, in 1936 Huggins and Blocksom reported that when tail vertebrae that contain virtually all marrow fat and no red marrow are implanted into the peritoneal cavity there was a conversion of marrow adipocytes to hematopoietic marrow suggesting that temperature plays a key role in the switch from red to yellow marrow [1]. Indeed, this observation is very consistent with the distribution of marrow adipocytes in different skeletal sites with enhanced marrow adiposity noted in the extremities where the ambient temperature is lower than within the body cavity. Currently, the optimal temperature for hematopoiesis and osteogenesis within the marrow is not known.

Interestingly, expression analysis reveals the existence of genes involved in thermogenesis and lipid metabolism in marrow adipocytes, suggesting that marrow adipocytes could be metabolically active [61] (Rosen CJ, unpublished observation). In line with this, marrow adipocytes isolated from rabbit long bones are more responsive (i.e. increases in glycerol and fatty acid release) to external stimuli such as beta adrenergic and cyclic AMP analogs than adipocytes from gonadal or intra-abdominal depots (Rosen CJ, unpublished observation). Furthermore, comparative studies of fatty acid depots in the marrow, interscapular brown adipose tissue (BAT) and mesenteric sites using NMR spectroscopy reveal a saturated: unsaturated fatty acid ratio in the marrow identical to that seen in BAT. Similarly, mice treated with rosiglitazone have enhanced marrow adiposity that has spectroscopic characteristics identical to BAT. These observations indicate that marrow adipocytes may represent a metabolic tissue involved in the maintenance of the marrow micro-environment although further studies are needed (Fig. 14.2).

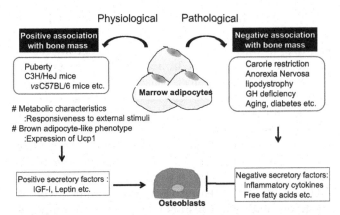

FIGURE 14.2 Marrow adipocytes produce a number of secretory factors. Such factors could have a significant role in osteoblast differentiation and/or function. In pathogenic conditions, these determinants could impact osteoblasts in a negative direction, whereas in physiological conditions these factors may have a different role from the one observed in the pathogenic conditions. There is also evidence that marrow fat is metabolically active and that genes which are characteristics to brown adipocytes are expressed in marrow adipocytes. Please see color plate section.

MOUSE MODELS TO STUDY MARROW ADIPOCYTES

Insulin Resistance Models

Clinical evidence demonstrates that type I diabetes is a significant risk factor for low bone mass and the increased incidence of fractures although the underlying mechanisms are not fully understood [62,63]. To understand the pathogenesis of low bone mass in diabetic patients, some animal models have been introduced and these have shown that accompanying insulin deficiency profoundly increases marrow adiposity. The two most commons strains are the spontaneous diabetic NOD mouse and C57BL6 mice in which diabetes is induced by streptozotocin [64,65]. In both of these models of type I diabetes, pro-adipocytic genes such as PPARγ and aP2 (FABP4) were found to be increased in long bones and this was correlated with decreased expression of osteocalcin [64,65]. Importantly, treatment with BADGE, a PPARγ antagonist, decreased the marrow adiposity observed in streptozotocin-induced diabetic models although skeletal loss was not reversed by the BADGE treatment. Thus, it is still unclear whether marrow adipocyte infiltration in diabetic patients plays a central role to the development of bone loss.

TZD-induced Mouse Models

Activation of PPARγ is associated with increased marrow adiposity as well as bone loss in rodent models although the effect of PPARγ agonists on increased marrow adiposity is strain and drug specific [66]. Troglitazone has been shown to increase marrow adiposity in the Apoe$^{-/-}$ strain, but no changes in bone mass were observed [67]. Darglitazone is 20 times more potent than rosiglitazone and 150 times more potent than pioglitazone [68]. A dose of darglitazone, 10 mg/kg/day, to 8-month-old male mice resulted in a profound decrease in both trabecular and cortical bone [49], but the effect of this TZD on marrow adiposity was not reported. Netoglitazone, a relatively weak TZD, was found to decrease whole body bone mineral content (BMC), but did not affect trabecular bone volume or whole body areal BMD in C57BL/6 mice, but this TZD also increased marrow adiposity [69]. Importantly, aging is a key factor determining susceptibility to TZD-induced bone loss because PPARγ has been shown to be activated with aging in the bone marrow. Consistent with these findings, rosiglitazone-induced bone loss is much more pronounced in older female C57BL/6J mice, and is associated with significant infiltration of the marrow with large adipocytes. Histomorphometric indices in these mice reveal a marked suppression in bone formation and increases in bone resorption consistent with a profound imbalance in bone remodeling. Not surprisingly, this effect is strain specific, such that some mice show only increased marrow adipogenesis but no bone loss (e.g. C3H/HeJ), while others display no skeletal or marrow effects from rosiglitazone [66].

Calorie Restriction

Not surprisingly, nutritional status is a pivotal factor regulating the number of marrow adipocytes. Contrary to peripheral fat depots, i.e. subcutaneous and abdominal fat depots, a diet containing excess amounts of fatty acid is not a strong inducer of marrow adipocytes. On the other hand, there is evidence that calorie restriction in young animals induces adipocytes in the bone marrow accompanied by decreased bone mass [70]. This effect appears to be time dependent as older mice on a 30% calorie restriction diet show enhanced bone mass but no evidence of increased marrow adiposity. In line with the findings observed in mouse models, patients with anorexia nervosa exhibit a massive infiltration of adipocytes in bone marrow despite minimal subcutaneous or peripheral fat, and a concomitant decrease in bone mass [71,72]. The remodeling changes are remarkable and include a reduction in bone formation and an increase in bone resorption. Induction of PPARγ could be in part responsible for the development of marrow adiposity, but the mechanism of how calorie restriction triggers the development of marrow adipocytes still remain to be elucidated. One possibility is that there is a systemic signal, either released centrally or locally, that triggers a hormonal response to induce marrow adipogenesis. One such candidate is the orixogenic hormone ghrelin which has also been shown to induce marrow adipogenesis in experimental animals [73].

Leptin-deficient Model

Leptin is a secretory factor produced by adipocytes that regulates body composition, fertility, appetite, and bone and energy metabolism. In addition, emerging evidence indicates the critical role of leptin in skeletal metabolism by relaying an adipokine signal at the hypothalamus [74–76]. The *ob/ob* (obese) strain of mice, first described in 1950 by Ingalls et al., carries a spontaneous non-sense mutation at codon 105 of the leptin gene that results in a complete loss of leptin protein [77,78]. As the name of this strain suggests, these mice are extremely obese: exhibiting profound hyperphagy, glucose intolerance, and hyperinsulinemia [78,79]. In the femur, *ob/ob* mice have increased marrow adipocytes and peripheral administration of leptin corrects the marrow adiposity phenotype seen in the femur of these mice [80–84]. Both long bones and axial skeleton of *ob/ob* mice show very high bone mass, despite absence of gonadal steroids and this is associated with decreased marrow adiposity [75,76,80], establishing the inverse relationship between marrow adiposity and bone mass in a compartment-specific manner.

IRS-1-deficient Mice

Insulin is a key factor in adipogenesis and fat storage. The IRKO mouse, which has global absence of the insulin receptor but in which expression of IR has been restored in pancreas, liver, and brain, but not muscle or fat, has extremely low numbers of marrow adipocytes, with normal trabecular BMD [64]. Similarly, we noted that in a spontaneous mutant, *small*, which has a homozygous recessive mutation in the intact IRS-1 molecule, there is a virtual absence of marrow fat despite very low bone mass during neonatal and adult life. As noted previously, bone loss, diabetes, and marrow adiposity have been described in several other mouse models all of which show reduced osteocalcin expression [65,85]. Furthermore, as was noted in *ob/ob* mice, the increase in marrow adipocytes appears limited to the calvaria and long bones and not the vertebrae [64].

Growth Hormone Deficiency

Growth hormone (GH) is produced and secreted from somatotrophs in the anterior pituitary and regulates linear growth, body composition, and lipid and glucose metabolism both in an IGF-I dependent and independent manner. GH is well known to induce lipolysis in adipose tissue and patients with GH deficiency have been shown to acquire more fat than normal controls, leading to the development of obesity-related metabolic complications. In bone, GH has been shown to have both direct effects on long bone growth and indirect effects via IGF-I. The *dw/dw* mutation is a spontaneous mutation that arose in the Lewis strain of rat. These rats are dwarfs as a result of GH deficiency, and have a profound increase in both adipocyte number and adipocyte size in the marrow of the long bones, compared to wild-type controls [86]. Treatment with GH results in a decrease in adipocyte number, whereas treatment with IGF-I results in a decrease in adipocyte volume [87]. Recently, Turner and colleagues demonstrated that acute pituitary insufficiency due to hypophysectomy resulted in significant marrow adiposity that can be reversed by GH, but not by IGF-I, estrogen, or cortisol [88]. Interestingly, LID mice, in which hepatic IGF-I is deleted, have very high GH levels and low IGF-I, but do not have marrow adiposity. On the other hand, *little* mice with a spontaneous mutation of the growth hormone releasing hormone receptor have significant marrow fat [88]. Thus, abnormalities in the GH–IGF-I axis are associated with marrow adipogenesis.

Inbred Strains

Inbred strains of mice are powerful tools for use in the study of the genetics of complex disease, since each mouse of a given strain represents essentially an identical twin of all other mice in that strain. As a result, phenotypic measures such as bone mineral density (BMD) or serum HDL levels remain relatively constant within a strain, but may vary greatly between strains (see http://www.jax.org/phenome). In a pilot study of marrow adipocyte numbers in the distal femur (immediately proximal to the growth plate) of four inbred strains of mice, we found that the number of marrow adipocytes per unit area varied greatly between strains (Table 14.1). Interestingly, BV/TV% was only found to be significantly correlated with marrow adipocyte number for the DBA/2J mice ($R = 0.78$, $p = 0.04$). Moreover, vBMD of the femur (which is principally a cortical

TABLE 14.1 Marrow Adiposity among Different Strains of Mice

Strain	Number of adipocytes/high-power field
C57BL/6J	31 +/− 4.8
C3H/HeJ	17.8 +/− 7.2
A/J	14 +/− 4.6
DBA/2J	30.6 +/− 9.9

Adapted from Rosen CJ et al. Crit Rev Eukaryot Gene Expr. 2009;19(2):109–24.

bone phenotype) did not correlate with marrow adipocyte number for any of the strains suggesting that the relationship between bone mass and marrow adiposity is not a simple inverse correlation.

Aging

In rodents and humans, aging is associated with a significant increase in marrow adiposity. C57BL6 is the most frequent strain studied, and in both males and females, mice older than 20 months accumulate marrow adipocytes in the distal femur and proximal tibia but not in the lumbar vertebrae. As noted this is associated with the age-related decline in trabecular bone mass but not with cortical bone density. Ovariectomy, a model of accelerated aging, also enhances adipocyte infiltration in the bone marrow and this is greater in older retired breeders than younger mice.

MARROW FAT IN HUMANS

Physiology

The physiologic role of adipocytes in human bone marrow is largely unknown. Marrow fat had long been regarded as "a filler" for space vacated by trabecular bone loss, which is often seen in aged people and patients with osteoporosis [89–92]. However, with an extensive revision of our understanding of fat tissue as an endocrine organ, a novel concept that marrow adipocytes possess similar metabolic characteristics as some peripheral or brown fat depots has emerged. Moreover, the juxtaposition of adipose tissue within the bone marrow milieu suggests that its presence may have consequences for the skeleton. Two theories are most prevalent as to the consequences of marrow adiposity. First, since the total bone marrow cavity is shared among adipose, bone, and hematopoietic tissues, fat overload would displace functional hematopoietic and/or osteogenic cells from the marrow cavity [93], therefore making it a negative determinant of bone mass. Second, a balanced bone marrow microenvironment including marrow adipocytes is essential for normal hematopoiesis and osteogenesis because of their strong energy needs [40,94]. Indeed, increased production of fat-related factors, such as fatty acids, could positively or negatively affect metabolism in the bone marrow depending on the nature of the fatty acid and the type of receptor activation such as the GPR 120 receptor on MSCs [95]. In addition, adipokines, steroids, and cytokines [96–98] can exert profound effects on neighboring marrow cells, sustaining hematopoietic and osteogenic processes [90,92,97,98]. Finally, if adipocytes generate heat as brown-like cells, this could

theoretically enhance or depress bone remodeling [61,99]. These possibilities require further testing but support the thesis that marrow adipocytes are a critical component of the bone marrow niche and influence the establishment of bone marrow environment.

Developmental of Marrow Fat in Humans

As described above, in newborns there is no marrow fat at any skeletal site; however, adipocyte number increases with age such that for individuals older than 30 years of age, most of the femoral cavity is occupied by adipose tissue. Indeed, recent studies have shown that in the appendicular skeleton of adults more than 70% of the marrow space is occupied by fat. This age-related increase in marrow adiposity is known to be associated with age-related bone loss and BMD, establishing the widely accepted tenet of the inverse correlation between these two parameters. This concept is largely true especially in the case of pathologic conditions including osteoporosis, drug use, and malnutrition. However, in physiological conditions this long-standing tenet may not be true. For example, the conversion from red to "yellow" marrow occurs around the time of peak bone acquisition, supporting the alternative hypothesis that marrow adipocytes create a favorable skeletal microenvironment for osteoblastogenesis, thereby maximizing bone accrual during puberty.

The development of marrow adipocytes is affected by the nutritional status. Despite the similarities in terms of sets of transcriptional machinery used in the development of marrow adipocytes as noted in white adipocyte development, the trigger for marrow adipocyte formation could be different from white adipose tissue. In fact, marrow adipocyte infiltration is often observed in the clinical conditions called "fat redistribution," in which marrow fat infiltration is associated with a decrease in peripheral adipose depot. For example, HIV-related lipodystrophy causes a significant decrease in peripheral adipose tissue whereas marrow adiposity is enhanced. In that same vein, states of malnutrition including anorexia nervosa lead to an increase in marrow adiposity while there is concurrent peripheral loss of adipose depots. Importantly, overnutrition is not a contributor to the development of marrow adiposity, suggesting that amount of peripheral fat depots is not correlated with marrow adiposity. In fact, in a recent work by Gilsanz and colleagues, adolescents and young adults had significant marrow adiposity in the appendicular skeleton, but this was not related to subcutaneous or visceral fat depots, nor with markers of cardiovascular risk [100]. However, this tenet has to be clarified and might be compartment specific because there is also evidence of a positive correlation between vertebral marrow adiposity and visceral fat mass in some scenarios [101].

The issue of whether fat is detrimental or agonistic to skeletal remodeling is not easily resolvable. Current methods including MRI with and without spectroscopy, CT, and histology do not provide functional information about the type of adipocyte and its role in the marrow. Recent work by Li et al. demonstrated that individuals with fractures, whether they were diabetic or not, had increased saturated fat relative to unsaturated fat, a pattern also seen in brown adipose tissue (see ASBMR Abstract FR0049 Patsch, 2011). These data plus evidence in experimental animals that brown-like adipogenic genes are expressed in the marrow of older animals raises the intriguing possibility that there is a dynamic around marrow adiposity such that white adipocytes could become "brown-like" under the influence of neurogenic, endocrine, or paracrine factors.

Clinical Implications

Aging

Age-related bone loss occurs universally in all mammals and unlike postmenopausal bone loss affects individuals regardless of sex steroid status. Because maintenance of bone homeostasis relies on the balance of bone remodeling, any factors which disturb this critical balance will lead to bone loss. The characteristic feature of age-related bone loss is the uncoupling of formation from resorption leading to a net loss of bone mass. The etiology of this uncoupling is multi-factorial and includes changes in endogenous gonadal steroids, increased reactive oxygen species, and a global decline in local growth factors that promote osteoblastic differentiation [2,102,103]. In addition, aging is also related to the alteration in lineage commitment of MSCs. For instance, it has been observed in humans that the number of MSCs committed to the adipocytic lineage increases with age, while those committed to the osteoblastic lineage decrease. There is increasing evidence of lineage allocation of MSC fate away from osteoblasts with aging and towards pre-adipocytes. This could result from increased activity of PPARg2, or the decreased expression of the TGF-β/BMP, Wnt/β-catenin, and IGF-I signaling pathways [46]. These changes could easily lead to reduced osteoblast differentiation, while the formation of new adipocytes is enhanced. In addition, an increase in marrow adipocytes would result in greater secretory factors which could be deleterious to bone formation, establishing a vicious loop which would accelerate bone loss. In addition to the alteration in cell fate determination, phenotypic changes of MSCs during the aging process could also be responsible for age-related bone loss. For example, impairment of cell proliferation and differentiation, as

well as chromosomal instabilities of MSCs, has been implicated in long-term cell culture models [104].

It has been reported that an increase in marrow adiposity is characterized not only by greater numbers of marrow adipocytes but also an increase in their size [93]. In a cross-sectional study of post-mortem iliac crest biopsies adipose tissue volume increased from 15 to 60% between 20 and 65 years old, while trabecular bone volume decreased from 26 to 16% [2]. More recently, Justesen et al. found that marrow adipose tissue increased from 40% at age 30 to 68% at 100 years old, while bone volume decreased to 12% [105]. Finally, in osteopenic bone it was observed that, in addition to the age-related inverse correlation between adipose and bone tissues, the hematopoietic tissue was replaced by fat [106]. Other conditions such as osteoporosis [2,105], immobilization [92,107,108], microgravity [109], ovariectomy [110], diabetes [111], or glucocorticoid treatment [112] also show an increase in the content of marrow adipose tissue and decreased bone volume.

TZDs

In the context of PPARγ activity, treatment of rodents or humans with rosiglitazone causes bone loss and structural fragility, in part due to impaired bone formation [113]. This phenotype resembles the process of aging in mammalian bone, which is also characterized by significant marrow adiposity, reduced trabecular bone volume fraction and increased bone resorption. Postmenopausal females tend to be the most sensitive to the bone loss by the thiazolidinediones [113]. In one report, older women lost more than 2% of their bone density after only 14 weeks of rosiglitazone treatment [113]. In several large randomized trials of rosiglitazone and pioglitazone, peripheral fractures were reported to be twice as likely in diabetic women treated with a TZD compared to those administered metformin, insulin, or sulfonylureas [114]. It still needs to be clarified whether TZDs can induce marrow adiposity in human populations as observed in rodent models, although in one prospective human study bone loss caused by TZDs is not associated with marrow fat infiltration [115]. Thus, it still remains unclear whether marrow adiposity occurs in humans as it does in mice after exposure to TZDs. However, biochemical markers of bone turnover in patients on TZDs reveal uncoupling with enhanced bone resorption and suppressed bone formation that are consistent with experimental findings in mice. Furthermore, the predisposition of postmenopausal women to the skeletal effects of TZDs suggest that an altered bone remodeling state due to greater rates of resorption than formation enhances the susceptibility to TZD-induced bone loss. Interestingly, the skeletal sites most frequently reported to fracture in diabetics are those that are predominantly cortical in nature rather than trabecular [114]. This would imply that drug-induced changes in metabolic factors such as adipokines may play a systemic role in TZD-induced bone loss, independent of changes in the trabecular compartment that is more directly related to enhanced marrow adiposity.

Other Clinical Scenarios

Thirty-five years ago Meunier reported that osteoporotic women had more marrow fat than controls [2]. Nearly a quarter of a century ago, Klibanski and colleagues noted an enhanced marrow fat signal in anorexic women who were osteoporotic (Klibanski, personal communication). Abella reported that on bone marrow biopsy, anorexia nervosa was associated with significant marrow adiposity [116]. Subsequently, Wehlri and colleagues noted by MRI that marrow fat in the vertebrae was inversely associated with bone mass [117]. Yeung et al. and Griffith et al. reported a similar negative correlation between marrow fat by spectroscopy and areal bone mass [3,118]. And very recently, this group reported that marrow adiposity was associated with reduced vascularity in the femoral head [119]. Hence, emerging evidence suggests that in human conditions, marrow fat may invade spaces previously occupied by trabecular bone. However, we do not know whether this is a primary or secondary event, or whether struggling osteoblasts require adjacent adipocytes for energy. Clinical scenarios provide some clues as to marrow fat function relative to bone.

Osteoporosis

Those who are suffering from osteoporosis, whether of primary or secondary origin, have more marrow adipocytes than age-matched controls. It has been shown that bone marrow stroma cells isolated from osteoporotic patients have enhanced adipogenic capacity either basally or during early cell differentiation compared to control subjects [38,98,120,121]. For instance, the proliferation rate and the mitogenic response to IGF-1 are significantly diminished, while the pERK/ERK ratio is increased in osteoporotic MSCs, compared with control MSCs [121,122]. In other cell types, activation of the MEK/ERK signaling pathway has been shown to enhance the activity of adipogenic transcription factors [123]. On the other hand, MSCs derived from osteoporotic donors have diminished alkaline phosphatase activity and less calcium deposition under osteogenic differentiation conditions, in agreement with their reduced capability to produce mature forming bone cells. In addition to the intrinsic characteristic of MSCs involved in cell commitment and differentiation, it is recognized that locally produced factors like leptin, estrogens, fatty acids, and

growth factors may be important in regulating neighboring osteoblasts. For example, in vitro studies confirmed that bone marrow MSCs were responsive to leptin, both through enhanced proliferation and differentiation into the osteoblastic lineage [124–126], as well as inhibition of MSCs into adipocytes [125,127].

After menopause, decreased endogenous estradiol enhances bone turnover. This is accompanied by a shift in the adipocyte to osteoblast ratio, favoring fat accumulation in the bone marrow [105,128]. A direct effect of estrogen on the skeleton has been underlined by developmental failure of bone in males with deficient estrogen activity [129,130]. The skeletal response to falling estrogen levels has also been demonstrated in vitro and in vivo. In the former, in human MSCs reciprocal estrogen regulation of osteogenic and adipogenic differentiation has been reported [131,132]. In the latter, bone biopsy samples from postmenopausal women revealed that estrogen replacement was associated with markedly reduced adipocytes compared to women without estrogen replacement (Khosla, personal communication). The observation that aromatase (the enzyme responsible for estrogen biosynthesis) and other enzymes implicated in sex metabolism are found in extra gonadal organs, including adipose and bone tissues [133–136], has strengthened the concept that locally generated androgens and estrogens can exert regulatory action on bone marrow cells. In fact, aromatase expression was found in MSCs [132], in osteoblasts, and osteoblast-like cells [133,134,137,138]. Studies during MSCs differentiation point to the potential importance of local estrogen production and action for osteogenic and adipogenic commitment [132,134], and as a negative regulator for adipogenesis [139,140]. All these observations support the hypothesis of a threshold estradiol level for normal skeletal remodeling [141,142], which could be attained by both appropriate endogenous aromatase activity and estrogenic precursors.

FUTURE DIRECTION

One of the most important questions to be answered is the function of adipose tissue within the marrow niche. Clearly, the infiltration of adipocytes is a dynamic process controlled at the progenitor level although not always at the expense of osteogenesis. As a corollary to the issue of function another question arises; i.e. if these adipocytes are "brown-like" do they generate heat, and is this important for optimal bone acquisition? In preliminary data from the Li laboratory at UCSF in B6 mice, the degree of saturation of marrow fat fell dramatically from 3 weeks of age to 16 weeks, an interval during and after peak bone acquisition. Similarly, one could ask whether the characteristics of marrow fat change with age; i.e. do aging mice and humans still have the capacity to generate "brown-like" adipocytes or is the marrow infiltration of aging purely a "filler" for empty marrow space. Regardless of the mechanism, the consequences of marrow adiposity as it relates to structural integrity still need to be defined before its magnitude can be defined as a risk factor for subsequent fractures. Finally, it is essential that we understand the afferent signals from the marrow and bone that influence the appearance of adipocytes. With newer cell and tissue functional studies, the possibilities of answering these questions are enhanced.

References

[1] Huggins C, Blocksom BH. Changes in bone marrow accompanying a local increase of temperature within physiological limits. J Exp Med 1936;1—26.

[2] Meunier P, Aaron J, Edouard C, Vignon G. Osteoporosis and the replacement of cell populations of the marrow by adipose tissue. A quantitative study of 84 iliac bone biopsies. Clin Orthop Relat Res 1971;80:147—54.

[3] Griffith JF, Yeung DK, Antonio GE, Wong SY, Kwok TC, Woo J, et al. Vertebral marrow fat content and diffusion and perfusion indexes in women with varying bone density: MR evaluation. Radiology 2006;241:831—8.

[4] Rosen ED, MacDougald OA. Adipocyte differentiation from the inside out. Nat Rev Mol Cell Biol 2006;7:885—96.

[5] Kawai M, Sousa KM, MacDougald OA, Rosen CJ. The many facets of PPARgamma: novel insights for the skeleton. Am J Physiol Endocrinol Metab 2010;299:E3—9.

[6] Rosen ED, Spiegelman BM. Molecular regulation of adipogenesis. Annu Rev Cell Dev Biol 2000;16:145—71.

[7] Kubota N, Terauchi Y, Miki H, Tamemoto H, Yamauchi T, Komeda K, et al. PPAR gamma mediates high-fat diet-induced adipocyte hypertrophy and insulin resistance. Mol Cell 1999;4:597—609.

[8] Darlington GJ, Ross SE, MacDougald OA. The role of C/EBP genes in adipocyte differentiation. J Biol Chem 1998;273:30057—60.

[9] Tanaka T, Yoshida N, Kishimoto T, Akira S. Defective adipocyte differentiation in mice lacking the C/EBPbeta and/or C/EBP-delta gene. EMBO J 1997;16:7432—43.

[10] Tontonoz P, Spiegelman BM. Fat and beyond: the diverse biology of PPARgamma. Annu Rev Biochem 2008;77:289—312.

[11] Kawai M, Rosen CJ. PPARgamma: a circadian transcription factor in adipogenesis and osteogenesis. Nat Rev Endocrinol 2010;6:629—36.

[12] Braissant O, Foufelle F, Scotto C, Dauca M, Wahli W. Differential expression of peroxisome proliferator-activated receptors (PPARs): tissue distribution of PPAR-alpha, -beta, and -gamma in the adult rat. Endocrinology 1996;137:354—66.

[13] Tontonoz P, Hu E, Graves RA, Budavari AI, Spiegelman BM. mPPAR gamma 2: tissue-specific regulator of an adipocyte enhancer. Genes Dev 1994;8:1224—34.

[14] Mori T, Sakaue H, Iguchi H, Gomi H, Okada Y, Takashima Y, et al. Role of Kruppel-like factor 15 (KLF15) in transcriptional regulation of adipogenesis. J Biol Chem 2005;280:12867—75.

[15] Oishi Y, Manabe I, Tobe K, Tsushima K, Shindo T, Fujiu K, et al. Kruppel-like transcription factor KLF5 is a key regulator of adipocyte differentiation. Cell Metab 2005;1:27—39.

[16] Gupta RK, Arany Z, Seale P, Mepani RJ, Ye L, Conroe HM, et al. Transcriptional control of preadipocyte determination by Zfp423. Nature 464:619—23.

[17] Banerjee SS, Feinberg MW, Watanabe M, Gray S, Haspel RL, Denkinger DJ, et al. The Kruppel-like factor KLF2 inhibits peroxisome proliferator-activated receptor-gamma expression and adipogenesis. J Biol Chem 2003;278:2581—4.

[18] Tong Q, Tsai J, Tan G, Dalgin G, Hotamisligil GS. Interaction between GATA and the C/EBP family of transcription factors is critical in GATA-mediated suppression of adipocyte differentiation. Mol Cell Biol 2005;25:706—15.

[19] Kawai M, Sousa KM, MacDougald OA, Rosen CJ. The many facets of PPARgamma: novel insights for the skeleton. Am J Physiol Endocrinol Metab 2010;299:E3—9.

[20] Kawai M, Rosen CJ. PPARgamma: a circadian transcription factor in adipogenesis and osteogenesis. Nat Rev Endocrinol 2010;6:629—36.

[21] Forman BM, Tontonoz P, Chen J, Brun RP, Spiegelman BM, Evans RM. 15-Deoxy-delta 12, 14-prostaglandin J2 is a ligand for the adipocyte determination factor PPAR gamma. Cell 1995;83:803—12.

[22] Bell-Parikh LC, Ide T, Lawson JA, McNamara P, Reilly M, FitzGerald GA. Biosynthesis of 15-deoxy-delta12,14-PGJ2 and the ligation of PPARgamma. J Clin Invest 2003;112:945—55.

[23] Ciaraldi TP, Gilmore A, Olefsky JM, Goldberg M, Heidenreich KA. In vitro studies on the action of CS-045, a new antidiabetic agent. Metabolism 1990;39:1056—62.

[24] Fujiwara T, Yoshioka S, Yoshioka T, Ushiyama I, Horikoshi H. Characterization of new oral antidiabetic agent CS-045. Studies in KK and ob/ob mice and Zucker fatty rats. Diabetes 1988;37:1549—58.

[25] Iwamoto Y, Kuzuya T, Matsuda A, Awata T, Kumakura S, Inooka G, et al. Effect of new oral antidiabetic agent CS-045 on glucose tolerance and insulin secretion in patients with NIDDM. Diabetes Care 1991;14:1083—6.

[26] Nolan JJ, Ludvik B, Beerdsen P, Joyce M, Olefsky J. Improvement in glucose tolerance and insulin resistance in obese subjects treated with troglitazone. N Engl J Med 1994;331:1188—93.

[27] Suter SL, Nolan JJ, Wallace P, Gumbiner B, Olefsky JM. Metabolic effects of new oral hypoglycemic agent CS-045 in NIDDM subjects. Diabetes Care 1992;15:193—203.

[28] Guan HP, Ishizuka T, Chui PC, Lehrke M, Lazar MA. Corepressors selectively control the transcriptional activity of PPARgamma in adipocytes. Genes Dev 2005;19:453—61.

[29] Takada I, Mihara M, Suzawa M, Ohtake F, Kobayashi S, Igarashi M, et al. A histone lysine methyltransferase activated by non-canonical Wnt signalling suppresses PPAR-gamma transactivation. Nat Cell Biol 2007;9:1273—85.

[30] Camp HS, Tafuri SR. Regulation of peroxisome proliferator-activated receptor gamma activity by mitogen-activated protein kinase. J Biol Chem 1997;272:10811—6.

[31] Hosooka T, Noguchi T, Kotani K, Nakamura T, Sakaue H, Inoue H, et al. Dok1 mediates high-fat diet-induced adipocyte hypertrophy and obesity through modulation of PPAR-gamma phosphorylation. Nat Med 2008;14:188—93.

[32] Hu E, Kim JB, Sarraf P, Spiegelman BM. Inhibition of adipogenesis through MAP kinase-mediated phosphorylation of PPARgamma. Science 1996;274:2100—3.

[33] Choi JH, Banks AS, Estall JL, Kajimura S, Bostrom P, Laznik D, et al. Anti-diabetic drugs inhibit obesity-linked phosphorylation of PPARgamma by Cdk5. Nature 2010;466:451—6.

[34] Choi JH, Banks AS, Kamenecka TM, Busby SA, Chalmers MJ, Kumar N, et al. Antidiabetic actions of a non-agonist

PPARgamma ligand blocking Cdk5-mediated phosphorylation. Nature 2011;477:477−81.

[35] Floyd ZE, Stephens JM. Interferon-gamma-mediated activation and ubiquitin-proteasome-dependent degradation of PPARgamma in adipocytes. J Biol Chem 2002;277:4062−8.

[36] Hauser S, Adelmant G, Sarraf P, Wright HM, Mueller E, Spiegelman BM. Degradation of the peroxisome proliferator-activated receptor gamma is linked to ligand-dependent activation. J Biol Chem 2000;275:18527−33.

[37] Yamashita D, Yamaguchi T, Shimizu M, Nakata N, Hirose F, Osumi T. The transactivating function of peroxisome proliferator-activated receptor gamma is negatively regulated by SUMO conjugation in the amino-terminal domain. Genes Cells 2004;9:1017−29.

[38] Bianco P, Riminucci M, Gronthos S, Robey PG. Bone marrow stromal stem cells: nature, biology, and potential applications. Stem Cells 2001;19:180−92.

[39] Jiang Y, Jahagirdar BN, Reinhardt RL, Schwartz RE, Keene CD, Ortiz-Gonzalez XR, et al. Pluripotency of mesenchymal stem cells derived from adult marrow. Nature 2002;418:41−9.

[40] Minguell JJ, Erices A, Conget P. Mesenchymal stem cells. Exp Biol Med (Maywood) 2001;226:507−20.

[41] Shockley KR, Lazarenko OP, Czernik PJ, Rosen CJ, Churchill GA, Lecka-Czernik B. PPARgamma2 nuclear receptor controls multiple regulatory pathways of osteoblast differentiation from marrow mesenchymal stem cells. J Cell Biochem 2009;106:232−46.

[42] Lecka-Czernik B, Gubrij I, Moerman EJ, Kajkenova O, Lipschitz DA, Manolagas SC, et al. Inhibition of Osf2/Cbfa1 expression and terminal osteoblast differentiation by PPARgamma2. J Cell Biochem 1999;74:357−71.

[43] Cheng SL, Shao JS, Charlton-Kachigian N, Loewy AP, Towler DA. MSX2 promotes osteogenesis and suppresses adipogenic differentiation of multipotent mesenchymal progenitors. J Biol Chem 2003;278:45969−77.

[44] Ichida F, Nishimura R, Hata K, Matsubara T, Ikeda F, Hisada K, et al. Reciprocal roles of MSX2 in regulation of osteoblast and adipocyte differentiation. J Biol Chem 2004;279:34015−22.

[45] Kang S, Bennett CN, Gerin I, Rapp LA, Hankenson KD, Macdougald OA. Wnt signaling stimulates osteoblastogenesis of mesenchymal precursors by suppressing CCAAT/enhancer-binding protein alpha and peroxisome proliferator-activated receptor gamma. J Biol Chem 2007;282:14515−24.

[46] Moerman EJ, Teng K, Lipschitz DA, Lecka-Czernik B. Aging activates adipogenic and suppresses osteogenic programs in mesenchymal marrow stroma/stem cells: the role of PPARgamma2 transcription factor and TGF-beta/BMP signaling pathways. Aging Cell 2004;3:379−89.

[47] Akune T, Ohba S, Kamekura S, Yamaguchi M, Chung UI, Kubota N, et al. PPARgamma insufficiency enhances osteogenesis through osteoblast formation from bone marrow progenitors. J Clin Invest 2004;113:846−55.

[48] Cock TA, Back J, Elefteriou F, Karsenty G, Kastner P, Chan S, Auwerx J. Enhanced bone formation in lipodystrophic PPARgamma(hyp/hyp) mice relocates haematopoiesis to the spleen. EMBO Rep 2004;5:1007−12.

[49] Li M, Pan LC, Simmons HA, Li Y, Healy DR, Robinson BS, et al. Surface-specific effects of a PPARgamma agonist, darglitazone, on bone in mice. Bone 2006;39:796−806.

[50] Sottile V, Seuwen K, Kneissel M. Enhanced marrow adipogenesis and bone resorption in estrogen-deprived rats treated with the PPARgamma agonist BRL49653 (rosiglitazone). Calcif Tissue Int 2004;75:329−37.

[51] Wan Y, Chong LW, Evans RM. PPAR-gamma regulates osteoclastogenesis in mice. Nat Med 2007;13:1496−503.

[52] Wei W, Wang X, Yang M, Smith LC, Dechow PC, Wan Y. PGC1beta mediates PPARgamma activation of osteoclastogenesis and rosiglitazone-induced bone loss. Cell Metab 11:503−16.

[53] Lazarenko OP, Rzonca SO, Hogue WR, Swain FL, Suva LJ, Lecka-Czernik B. Rosiglitazone induces decreases in bone mass and strength that are reminiscent of aged bone. Endocrinology 2007;148:2669−80.

[54] Bendixen AC, Shevde NK, Dienger KM, Willson TM, Funk CD, Pike JW. IL-4 inhibits osteoclast formation through a direct action on osteoclast precursors via peroxisome proliferator-activated receptor gamma 1. Proc Natl Acad Sci USA 2001;98:2443−8.

[55] Hounoki H, Sugiyama E, Mohamed SG, Shinoda K, Taki H, Abdel-Aziz HO, et al. Activation of peroxisome proliferator-activated receptor gamma inhibits TNF-alpha-mediated osteoclast differentiation in human peripheral monocytes in part via suppression of monocyte chemoattractant protein-1 expression. Bone 2008;42:765−74.

[56] Naveiras O, Nardi V, Wenzel PL, Hauschka PV, Fahey F, Daley GQ. Bone-marrow adipocytes as negative regulators of the haematopoietic microenvironment. Nature 2009;460: 259−63.

[57] Botolin S, McCabe LR. Inhibition of PPARgamma prevents type I diabetic bone marrow adiposity but not bone loss. J Cell Physiol 2006;209:967−76.

[58] Sheng MH, Baylink DJ, Beamer WG, Donahue LR, Rosen CJ, Lau KH, et al. Histomorphometric studies show that bone formation and bone mineral apposition rates are greater in C3H/HeJ (high-density) than C57BL/6J (low-density) mice during growth. Bone 1999;25:421−9.

[59] Kawai M, Rosen CJ. Insulin-like growth factor-I and bone: lessons from mice and men. Pediatr Nephrol 2009;24:1277−85.

[60] Horowitz MC, Bothwell AL, Hesslein DG, Pflugh DL, Schatz DG. B cells and osteoblast and osteoclast development. Immunol Rev 2005;208:141−53.

[61] Krings A, Rahman S, Huang S, Lu Y, Czernik PJ, Lecka-Czernik B. Bone marrow fat has brown adipose tissue characteristics, which are attenuated with aging and diabetes. Bone 2012 Feb;50(2):546−52. Epub 2011 Jun 24.

[62] Vestergaard P. Discrepancies in bone mineral density and fracture risk in patients with type 1 and type 2 diabetes—a meta-analysis. Osteoporos Int 2007;18:427−44.

[63] McCabe LR. Understanding the pathology and mechanisms of type I diabetic bone loss. J Cell Biochem 2007;102: 1343−57.

[64] Botolin S, Faugere MC, Malluche H, Orth M, Meyer R, McCabe LR. Increased bone adiposity and peroxisomal proliferator-activated receptor-gamma2 expression in type I diabetic mice. Endocrinology 2005;146:3622−31.

[65] Botolin S, McCabe LR. Bone loss and increased bone adiposity in spontaneous and pharmacologically induced diabetic mice. Endocrinology 2007;148:198−205.

[66] Ackert-Bicknell CL, Shockley KR, Horton LG, Lecka-Czernik B, Churchill GA, Rosen CJ. Strain-specific effects of rosiglitazone on bone mass, body composition, and serum insulin-like growth factor-I. Endocrinology 2009;150:1330−40.

[67] Tornvig L, Mosekilde LI, Justesen J, Falk E, Kassem M. Troglitazone treatment increases bone marrow adipose tissue volume but does not affect trabecular bone volume in mice. Calcif Tissue Int 2001;69:46−50.

[68] Aleo MD, Lundeen GR, Blackwell DK, Smith WM, Coleman GL, Stadnicki SW, et al. Mechanism and implications of brown adipose tissue proliferation in rats and monkeys treated with the thiazolidinedione darglitazone, a potent

peroxisome proliferator-activated receptor-gamma agonist. J Pharmacol Exp Ther 2003;305:1173—82.

[69] Lazarenko OP, Rzonca SO, Suva LJ, Lecka-Czernik B. Netoglitazone is a PPAR-gamma ligand with selective effects on bone and fat. Bone 2006;38:74—84.

[70] Devlin MJ, Cloutier AM, Thomas NA, Panus DA, Lotinun S, Pinz I, et al. Caloric restriction leads to high marrow adiposity and low bone mass in growing mice. J Bone Miner Res 2010;25:2078—88.

[71] Bredella MA, Fazeli PK, Miller KK, Misra M, Torriani M, Thomas BJ, et al. Increased bone marrow fat in anorexia nervosa. J Clin Endocrinol Metab 2009;94:2129—36.

[72] Fazeli PK, Bredella MA, Misra M, Meenaghan E, Rosen CJ, Clemmons DR, et al. Preadipocyte factor-1 is associated with marrow adiposity and bone mineral density in women with anorexia nervosa. J Clin Endocrinol Metab 2010;95:407—13.

[73] Thompson NM, Gill DA, Davies R, Loveridge N, Houston PA, Robinson IC, et al. Ghrelin and des-octanoyl ghrelin promote adipogenesis directly in vivo by a mechanism independent of the type 1a growth hormone secretagogue receptor. Endocrinology 2004;145:234—42.

[74] Elefteriou F, Ahn JD, Takeda S, Starbuck M, Yang X, Liu X, et al. Leptin regulation of bone resorption by the sympathetic nervous system and CART. Nature 2005;434:514—20.

[75] Takeda S, Elefteriou F, Levasseur R, Liu X, Zhao L, Parker KL, et al. Leptin regulates bone formation via the sympathetic nervous system. Cell 2002;111:305—17.

[76] Ducy P, Amling M, Takeda S, Priemel M, Schilling AF, Beil FT, et al. Leptin inhibits bone formation through a hypothalamic relay: a central control of bone mass. Cell 2000;100:197—207.

[77] Ingalls AM, Dickie MM, Snell GD. Obese, a new mutation in the house mouse. J Hered 1950;41:317—8.

[78] Zhang Y, Proenca R, Maffei M, Barone M, Leopold L, Friedman JM. Positional cloning of the mouse obese gene and its human homologue. Nature 1994;372:425—32.

[79] Charlton HM. Mouse mutants as models in endocrine research. Q J Exp Physiol 1984;69:655—76.

[80] Hamrick MW, Pennington C, Newton D, Xie D, Isales C. Leptin deficiency produces contrasting phenotypes in bones of the limb and spine. Bone 2004;34:376—83.

[81] Bartell SM, Rayalam S, Ambati S, Gaddam DR, Hartzell DL, Hamrick M, et al. Central (ICV) leptin injection increases bone formation, bone mineral density, muscle mass, serum IGF-1, and the expression of osteogenic genes in leptin-deficient ob/ob mice. J Bone Miner Res 2011;26:1710—20.

[82] Gryglewski RJ. Prostacyclin among prostanoids. Pharmacol Rep 2008;60:3—11.

[83] Iwaniec UT, Boghossian S, Trevisiol CH, Wronski TJ, Turner RT, Kalra SP. Hypothalamic leptin gene therapy prevents weight gain without long-term detrimental effects on bone in growing and skeletally mature female rats. J Bone Miner Res 2011;26:1506—16.

[84] Williams GA, Callon KE, Watson M, Costa JL, Ding Y, Dickinson M, et al. Skeletal phenotype of the leptin receptor-deficient db/db mouse. J Bone Miner Res 2011;26:1698—709.

[85] Martin LM, McCabe LR. Type I diabetic bone phenotype is location but not gender dependent. Histochem Cell Biol 2007;128:125—33.

[86] Charlton HM, Clark RG, Robinson IC, Goff AE, Cox BS, Bugnon C, et al. Growth hormone-deficient dwarfism in the rat: a new mutation. J Endocrinol 1988;119:51—8.

[87] Gevers EF, Loveridge N, Robinson IC. Bone marrow adipocytes: a neglected target tissue for growth hormone. Endocrinology 2002;143:4065—73.

[88] Menagh PJ, Turner RT, Jump DB, Wong CP, Lowry MB, Yakar S, et al. Growth hormone regulates the balance between bone formation and bone marrow adiposity. J Bone Miner Res 2010;25:757—68.

[89] Gimble JM. The function of adipocytes in the bone marrow stroma. New Biol 1990;2:304—12.

[90] Tavassoli M. Marrow adipose cells and hemopoiesis: an interpretative review. Exp Hematol 1984;12:139—46.

[91] Gimble JM, Robinson CE, Wu X, Kelly KA. The function of adipocytes in the bone marrow stroma: an update. Bone 1996;19:421—8.

[92] Payne MW, Uhthoff HK, Trudel G. Anemia of immobility: caused by adipocyte accumulation in bone marrow. Med Hypotheses 2007;69:778—86.

[93] Rozman C, Feliu E, Berga L, Reverter JC, Climent C, Ferran MJ. Age-related variations of fat tissue fraction in normal human bone marrow depend both on size and number of adipocytes: a stereological study. Exp Hematol 1989;17:34—7.

[94] Dazzi F, Ramasamy R, Glennie S, Jones SP, Roberts I. The role of mesenchymal stem cells in haemopoiesis. Blood Rev 2006;20:161—71.

[95] Cornish J, MacGibbon A, Lin JM, Watson M, Callon KE, Tong PC, et al. Modulation of osteoclastogenesis by fatty acids. Endocrinology 2008;149:5688—95.

[96] Aghaloo TL, Felsenfeld AL, Tetradis S. Osteonecrosis of the jaw in a patient on Denosumab. J Oral Maxillofac Surg 68:959—63.

[97] Gimble JM, Zvonic S, Floyd ZE, Kassem M, Nuttall ME. Playing with bone and fat. J Cell Biochem 2006;98:251—66.

[98] Nuttall ME, Gimble JM. Controlling the balance between osteoblastogenesis and adipogenesis and the consequent therapeutic implications. Curr Opin Pharmacol 2004;4:290—4.

[99] Lecka-Czernik B. Marrow fat metabolism is linked to the systemic energy metabolism. Bone 2012 Feb;50(2):534—9. Epub 2011 Jul 4. Review.

[100] Di Iorgi N, Mittelman SD, Gilsanz V. Differential effect of marrow adiposity and visceral and subcutaneous fat on cardiovascular risk in young, healthy adults. Int J Obes (Lond) 2008;32:1854—60.

[101] Bredella MA, Torriani M, Ghomi RH, Thomas BJ, Brick DJ, Gerweck AV, et al. Vertebral bone marrow fat is positively associated with visceral fat and inversely associated with IGF-1 in obese women. Obesity (Silver Spring) 2011;19:49—53.

[102] Manolagas SC. Cellular and molecular mechanisms of osteoporosis. Aging (Milano) 1998;10:182—90.

[103] Manolagas SC. From estrogen-centric to aging and oxidative stress: a revised perspective of the pathogenesis of osteoporosis. Endocr Rev 31:266—300.

[104] Wagner W, Bork S, Lepperdinger G, Joussen S, Ma N, Strunk D, et al. How to track cellular aging of mesenchymal stromal cells? Aging (Albany NY) 2010;2:224—30.

[105] Justesen J, Stenderup K, Ebbesen EN, Mosekilde L, Steiniche T, Kassem M. Adipocyte tissue volume in bone marrow is increased with aging and in patients with osteoporosis. Biogerontology 2001;2:165—71.

[106] Burkhardt R, Kettner G, Bohm W, Schmidmeier M, Schlag R, Frisch B, et al. Changes in trabecular bone, hematopoiesis and bone marrow vessels in aplastic anemia, primary osteoporosis, and old age: a comparative histomorphometric study. Bone 1987;8:157—64.

[107] Minaire P, Edouard C, Arlot M, Meunier PJ. Marrow changes in paraplegic patients. Calcif Tissue Int 1984;36:338—40.

[108] Belin de Chantemele E, Blanc S, Pellet N, Duvareille M, Ferretti G, Gauquelin-Koch G, et al. Does resistance exercise prevent body fluid changes after a 90-day bed rest? Eur J Appl Physiol 2004;92:555—64.

[109] LeBlanc A, Schneider V, Shackelford L, West S, Oganov V, Bakulin A, et al. Bone mineral and lean tissue loss after long

duration space flight. J Musculoskelet Neuronal Interact 2000; 1:157–60.

[110] Wronski TJ, Walsh CC, Ignaszewski LA. Histologic evidence for osteopenia and increased bone turnover in ovariectomized rats. Bone 1986;7:119–23.

[111] Forsen L, Meyer HE, Midthjell K, Edna TH. Diabetes mellitus and the incidence of hip fracture: results from the Nord-Trondelag Health Survey. Diabetologia 1999;42:920–5.

[112] Vande Berg BC, Malghem J, Lecouvet FE, Devogelaer JP, Maldague B, Houssiau FA. Fat conversion of femoral marrow in glucocorticoid-treated patients: a cross-sectional and longitudinal study with magnetic resonance imaging. Arthritis Rheum 1999 Jul;42(7):1405–11.

[113] Grey A, Bolland M, Gamble G, Wattie D, Horne A, Davidson J, Reid IR. The peroxisome proliferator-activated receptor-gamma agonist rosiglitazone decreases bone formation and bone mineral density in healthy postmenopausal women: a randomized, controlled trial. J Clin Endocrinol Metab 2007;92:1305–10.

[114] Habib ZA, Havstad SL, Wells K, Divine G, Pladevall M, Williams LK. Thiazolidinedione use and the longitudinal risk of fractures in patients with type 2 diabetes mellitus. J Clin Endocrinol Metab 95:592–600.

[115] Harslof T, Wamberg L, Moller L, Stodkilde-Jorgensen H, Ringgaard S, Pedersen SB, et al. Rosiglitazone decreases bone mass and bone marrow fat. J Clin Endocrinol Metab 2011; 96:1541–8.

[116] Abella E, Feliu E, Granada I, Milla F, Oriol A, Ribera JM, et al. Bone marrow changes in anorexia nervosa are correlated with the amount of weight loss and not with other clinical findings. Am J Clin Pathol 2002;118:582–8.

[117] Wehrli FW, Hopkins JA, Hwang SN, Song HK, Snyder PJ, Haddad JG. Cross-sectional study of osteopenia with quantitative MR imaging and bone densitometry. Radiology 2000;217:527–38.

[118] Yeung DK, Griffith JF, Antonio GE, Lee FK, Woo J, Leung PC. Osteoporosis is associated with increased marrow fat content and decreased marrow fat unsaturation: a proton MR spectroscopy study. J Magn Reson Imaging 2005;22:279–85.

[119] Griffith JF, Yeung DK, Tsang PH, Choi KC, Kwok TC, Ahuja AT, et al. Compromised bone marrow perfusion in osteoporosis. J Bone Miner Res 2008;23:1068–75.

[120] Gimble JM, Robinson CE, Wu X, Kelly KA, Rodriguez BR, Kliewer SA, et al. Peroxisome proliferator-activated receptor-gamma activation by thiazolidinediones induces adipogenesis in bone marrow stromal cells. Mol Pharmacol 1996; 50:1087–94.

[121] Rodriguez JP, Garat S, Gajardo H, Pino AM, Seitz G. Abnormal osteogenesis in osteoporotic patients is reflected by altered mesenchymal stem cells dynamics. J Cell Biochem 1999; 75:414–23.

[122] Rodriguez JP, Rios S, Fernandez M, Santibanez JF. Differential activation of ERK1,2 MAP kinase signaling pathway in mesenchymal stem cell from control and osteoporotic postmenopausal women. J Cell Biochem 2004;92:745–54.

[123] Prusty D, Park BH, Davis KE, Farmer SR. Activation of MEK/ERK signaling promotes adipogenesis by enhancing peroxisome proliferator-activated receptor gamma (PPARgamma) and C/EBPalpha gene expression during the differentiation of 3T3-L1 preadipocytes. J Biol Chem 2002;277:46226–32.

[124] Takahashi Y, Okimura Y, Mizuno I, Iida K, Takahashi T, Kaji H, et al. Leptin induces mitogen-activated protein kinase-dependent proliferation of C3H10T1/2 cells. J Biol Chem 1997;272: 12897–900.

[125] Thomas T, Gori F, Khosla S, Jensen MD, Burguera B, Riggs BL. Leptin acts on human marrow stromal cells to enhance differentiation to osteoblasts and to inhibit differentiation to adipocytes. Endocrinology 1999;140:1630–8.

[126] Reseland JE, Syversen U, Bakke I, Qvigstad G, Eide LG, Hjertner O, et al. Leptin is expressed in and secreted from primary cultures of human osteoblasts and promotes bone mineralization. J Bone Miner Res 2001;16:1426–33.

[127] Hess R, Pino AM, Rios S, Fernandez M, Rodriguez JP. High affinity leptin receptors are present in human mesenchymal stem cells (MSCs) derived from control and osteoporotic donors. J Cell Biochem 2005;94:50–7.

[128] Gambacciani M, Ciaponi M, Cappagli B, Piaggesi L, De Simone L, Orlandi R, et al. Body weight, body fat distribution, and hormonal replacement therapy in early postmenopausal women. J Clin Endocrinol Metab 1997;82:414–7.

[129] Smith EP, Boyd J, Frank GR, Takahashi H, Cohen RM, Specker B, et al. Estrogen resistance caused by a mutation in the estrogen-receptor gene in a man. N Engl J Med 1994; 331:1056–61.

[130] Morishima A, Grumbach MM, Simpson ER, Fisher C, Qin K. Aromatase deficiency in male and female siblings caused by a novel mutation and the physiological role of estrogens. J Clin Endocrinol Metab 1995;80:3689–98.

[131] Pino AM, Rodriguez JM, Rios S, Astudillo P, Leiva L, Seitz G, et al. Aromatase activity of human mesenchymal stem cells is stimulated by early differentiation, vitamin D and leptin. J Endocrinol 2006;191:715–25.

[132] Heim M, Frank O, Kampmann G, Sochocky N, Pennimpede T, Fuchs P, et al. The phytoestrogen genistein enhances osteogenesis and represses adipogenic differentiation of human primary bone marrow stromal cells. Endocrinology 2004; 145:848–59.

[133] Schweikert HU, Wolf L, Romalo G. Oestrogen formation from androstenedione in human bone. Clin Endocrinol (Oxf) 1995; 43:37–42.

[134] Janssen JM, Bland R, Hewison M, Coughtrie MW, Sharp S, Arts J, et al. Estradiol formation by human osteoblasts via multiple pathways: relation with osteoblast function. J Cell Biochem 1999;75:528–37.

[135] Compston J. Local biosynthesis of sex steroids in bone. J Clin Endocrinol Metab 2002;87:5398–400.

[136] Issa S, Schnabel D, Feix M, Wolf L, Schaefer HE, Russell DW, et al. Human osteoblast-like cells express predominantly steroid 5alpha-reductase type 1. J Clin Endocrinol Metab 2002; 87:5401–7.

[137] Tanaka S, Haji M, Nishi Y, Yanase T, Takayanagi R, Nawata H. Aromatase activity in human osteoblast-like osteosarcoma cell. Calcif Tissue Int 1993;52:107–9.

[138] Sasano H, Uzuki M, Sawai T, Nagura H, Matsunaga G, Kashimoto O, et al. Aromatase in human bone tissue. J Bone Miner Res 1997;12:1416–23.

[139] Heine PA, Taylor JA, Iwamoto GA, Lubahn DB, Cooke PS. Increased adipose tissue in male and female estrogen receptor-alpha knockout mice. Proc Natl Acad Sci USA 2000; 97:12729–34.

[140] Okazaki R, Inoue D, Shibata M, Saika M, Kido S, Ooka H, et al. Estrogen promotes early osteoblast differentiation and inhibits adipocyte differentiation in mouse bone marrow stromal cell lines that express estrogen receptor (ER) alpha or beta. Endocrinology 2002;143:2349–56.

[141] Riggs BL, Khosla S, Melton 3rd LJ. Sex steroids and the construction and conservation of the adult skeleton. Endocr Rev 2002;23:279–302.

[142] Gennari L, Nuti R, Bilezikian JP. Aromatase activity and bone homeostasis in men. J Clin Endocrinol Metab 2004;89: 5898–907.

15

Osteocalcin, Undercarboxylated Osteocalcin, and Glycemic Control in Human Subjects

Itamar Levinger [1], Jeffrey D. Zajac [2], Ego Seeman [2]

[1]Victoria University, Melbourne, Australia [2]University of Melbourne, Melbourne, Australia

OBESITY, DIABETES, AND LOW SERUM OSTEOCALCIN: CROSS-SECTIONAL STUDIES IN HUMAN SUBJECTS

Osteocalcin is an osteoblast-specific product that is secreted into the bone extracellular matrix and the general circulation. Osteocalcin is carboxylated in the osteoblasts on three glutamic acid residues and can be decarboxylated in resorption lacunae to become a hormone that reaches the general circulation where it can fulfill its endocrine functions. Studies in mice have shown that uncarboxylated osteocalcin (ucOC) increases insulin secretion and sensitivity. Although there are no studies examining whether there is a direct effect of ucOC on energy metabolism in human subjects, correlations between circulating osteocalcin (OC) and ucOC and measures of insulin sensitivity and glycemic control have been reported in several cross-sectional studies. The observations support the notion that products of the osteoblast, one of them being osteocalcin, modify insulin sensitivity, insulin secretion, and glycemic control in humans.

OC-deficient mice are obese and have glucose intolerance [1–3]. Accordingly, several groups of investigators have provided consistent evidence that obese subjects and patients with type 2 diabetes mellitus (T2DM) have lower circulating levels of OC and ucOC. For example, Foresta et al. [4] reported that overweight and obese individuals have a lower ucOC and ucOC/OC ratio. Kindblom et al. [5] reported that 153 diabetic elderly men (mean age 75.3) with T2DM had 21.7% lower circulating OC than 857 men without T2DM. Im et al. [6] reported 30% lower circulating OC levels in postmenopausal women with T2DM compared to postmenopausal non-diabetic women. Likewise, Oz et al. reported men and women in their 50s with diabetes ($n = 15$ and $n = 37$, respectively) had lower OC level

($\sim$42% and $\sim$50%, respectively) than those without diabetes ($n = 14$ and $n = 34$, respectively). Furthermore, Levinger et al. [7] reported that men with T2DM had 38% lower circulating levels of ucOC compared to non-diabetic men. Thus, patients with T2DM have lower circulating levels of OC and ucOC compared to individuals without T2DM. The question is whether there is a causal relationship between the lower OC and unOC and diabetes. This is a difficult question to address in humans.

Kindblom et al. [5] reported that circulating OC is inversely related to body mass index (BMI), fat mass, and plasma glucose ($p < 0.001$). Circulating OC explained 6.3% of the variance in plasma glucose. Multiple linear regression models adjusted for serum insulin and fat mass suggested that plasma OC was an independent negative predictor of plasma glucose [5]. Similarly, Im et al. [6] reported that postmenopausal women with OC in the highest quartile had a lower fasting glucose and hemoglobin A1c (HbA1c) levels than postmenopausal women with OC in the lowest quartile. OC was also negatively correlated with glucose, insulin, HbA1c, and insulin resistance.

Hwang et al. [8] reported that a higher serum ucOC was associated with improved glucose tolerance in 199 men aged 25–60 years (mean age, 47 years) and that the improved glucose tolerance may be related to enhanced β-cell function. More recently, the same group reported that circulating OC levels are lower in patients with T2DM compared to non-diabetics and that there is a correlation between OC and improved glucose tolerance, insulin sensitivity, and insulin secretion in 425 men and women aged 19–82 years (mean age, 53 years) [9]. Importantly, they reported that in humans, in contrast to animals, the increase in glucose tolerance, insulin sensitivity, and insulin secretion with increased levels of OC is independent of adiponectin levels [9].

Kanazawa et al. [10] reported that ucOC was negatively correlated with percent body fat, fasting glucose, and HbA1c in 180 men with T2DM. The same group [11] examined the correlation between OC and metabolic and cardiovascular risk factors in 179 men and 149 postmenopausal women with T2DM. After adjustment for age, BMI, and serum creatinine, OC was negatively correlated with glucose and HbA1c in men and women. In men, OC correlated with brachial–ankle pulse wave velocity and intima-media thickness after adjustment for systolic blood pressure, LDL cholesterol, HDL cholesterol, HbA1c, and the Brinkmann index. Others have also reported that OC is negatively correlated with premature myocardial infarction [12].

These data indicate that higher circulating OC and ucOC correlate with greater insulin sensitivity and lower circulating glucose levels. Higher BMI and percent body fat correlate with lower OC and ucOC levels. Bullo et al. [13] reported that OC and ucOC correlated with higher fasting insulin concentrations after adjustment for covariates. However, the correlation was observed only in individuals not taking oral antidiabetic drugs. Yeap et al. [14] reported that OC was negatively correlated with waist circumference, glucose, and triglyceride levels and insulin resistance. Men with metabolic syndrome had lower OC levels, elevated glucose, and triglyceride levels. Similarly, Saleem et al. [15] reported that OC levels were inversely correlated with BMI, fasting glucose, and insulin resistance and positively correlated with adiponectin after adjustment for age and sex. Thus, these cross-sectional studies suggest that elevated levels of OC and ucOC are associated with lower body fat and better glycemic control. Due to the cross-sectional nature of the studies causality cannot be determined.

OSTEOCALCIN AND GLYCEMIC CONTROL: INTERVENTIONAL STUDIES

To date, there is no study demonstrating ucOC (or OC) administration in humans regulates either insulin action or insulin secretion. We therefore examine the question of whether indirect interventions known to affect glycemic control also affect OC and ucOC levels. Kazanawa et al. [16] examined the effects of improved glycemic control using metformin, insulin, and sulfonylurea in 50 patients with poorly controlled T2DM. HbA1c decreased from 10 to 8.8%. Serum OC increased by 1.94 ng/ml ($p = 0.004$). UcOC also increased, but not significantly. The change in circulating OC, not ucOC, correlated with the change of HbA1c ($r = -0.3$, $p = 0.03$). Similarly, Sayinalp et al. [17] examined the effects of glycemic control in 27 men with poorly controlled T2DM (HbA1c >9%, fasting plasma glucose

>7.8 mmol/L). Improved glycemic control was accompanied by increased circulating OC and OC correlated negatively with HbA1c. Similarly, 8-week treatment with hypoglycemia agents in 59 patients with T2DM resulted in increased OC levels and reduced glucose variability [18]. Thus, changes in OC are related to changes in glycemic control and higher levels of OC are associated with improvements in serum glucose. However, the results of the above studies are difficult to interpret because of the use of insulin, metformin, sulfonylurea, and α-glucosidase inhibitor, medications that may affect OC and ucOC [7,10,11,16,19].

Bullo et al. [13] has examined whether the changes in OC and ucOC over 2 years were associated with insulin secretion and sensitivity in community-dwelling men aged 55–80 years. Increase in OC was associated with an increase in insulin secretion (b coefficient: 2.87; 95% CI: 0.23, 5.52; $p = 0.033$), and changes in ucOC were associated with an improvement in insulin resistance (HOMA-IR, b coefficient: 20.31; 95% CI: 20.60, 0.03; $p = 0.032$). Similarly, Pittas et al. [20] reported that in 380 older adults (mean age = 71 years, BMI = 26.9 kg/m^2, 5% with diabetes) OC was associated with baseline fasting plasma glucose, fasting insulin, insulin sensitivity, plasma high-sensitivity C-reactive protein, IL-6, and BMI and body fat. Furthermore, those in the highest tertiles of serum OC had lower fasting glucose than those in the lowest OC tertile ($p < 0.01$). Those with higher serum OC during follow-up had fewer rises in fasting plasma glucose after 3 years.

Shea et al. [21] also examined the correlation between OC and ucOC with insulin resistance at baseline ($n = 348$) and after 3 years ($n = 162$) in non-diabetic men and women (mean age 68 years). In contrast, they reported that lower circulating ucOC was not associated with higher insulin resistance. However, those in the lowest tertile of total OC and carboxylated OC at baseline had higher insulin resistance at baseline. The author concluded that in older adults, total OC and carboxylated OC, but not ucOC, were associated with lower insulin resistance.

Exercise (muscle contraction) is known to improve insulin sensitivity and glycemic control. Fernández-Real et al. [22] examined the relationship between OC, insulin sensitivity, and secretion in a cross-sectional study of 149 men (mean age = 50.2 years). They reported a linear relationship between circulating OC and insulin sensitivity and insulin secretion (Fig. 15.1). This correlation was more evident in lean men than those who were overweight. In the intervention studies, diet only led to a mean weight loss of 7.3% with modest increase in circulating OC. In the diet plus physical activity group, mean weight loss was 8.7%, but circulating OC increased. The increase in OC level was related to the reduction in visceral fat mass and increase in lean

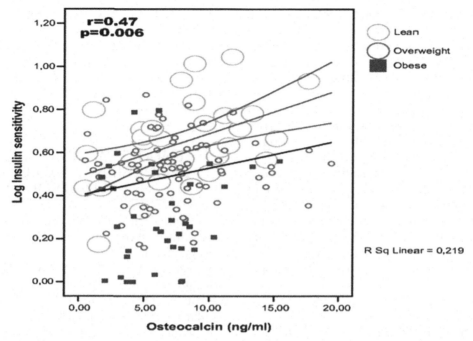

FIGURE 15.1 Linear relationship between circulating osteocalcin and insulin sensitivity in 149 men of the cross-sectional study (single line and correlation coefficient) and in lean men (95% confidence interval) for the mean and correlation coefficient in the upper left. *Adapted from Fernandez-Real et al. [22].*

mass and muscle strength. In addition, the OC level at the end of the activity intervention was related to increased insulin sensitivity ($r = 0.49$; $p = 0.03$) and negatively correlated with fasting triglycerides ($r = -0.54$; $p = 0.01$). The authors concluded that OC may participate in regulating insulin sensitivity in human subjects as it does in mice. Such a conservation of functions is expected since, to the best of our knowledge, no molecule identified as a hormone in rodents has been shown to have lost this function in humans.

Levinger et al. [7] examined whether the reduction in serum glucose level after acute aerobic and power exercise is related to change in ucOC in 28 middle-aged men with and without T2DM (mean age = 52.4 and mean BMI = $32.1\,\text{kg}\cdot\text{m}^{-2}$). At baseline, ucOC correlated negatively with glucose levels ($r = -0.53$, $p = 0.003$) and HbA1c ($r = -0.37$, $p = 0.035$). Both aerobic and power exercise increased OC and ucOC and reduced serum glucose levels. In patients with T2DM, the percentage change in OC and ucOC levels correlated with the percentage change in glucose levels post-exercise ($r = -0.51$, $p = 0.038$). The change in OC and ucOC levels from pre- to post-exercise were predictors for the change in glucose levels post-exercise, with slight superiority of ucOC.

Thus, these two studies suggest that exercise has an effect on circulating levels of OC and ucOC and that there is a correlation between the change in OC and ucOC and the improvements in glycemic control. Moreover, improvements in insulin sensitivity and glycemic

control with exercise may, at least in part, be mediated by OC and ucOC. How exercise influences OC and ucOC is not known and warrants further investigation.

INTERVENTIONAL STUDIES MANIPULATING VITAMIN K LEVELS

Another possible intervention is to alter circulating levels of ucOC by administration or deprivation of vitamin K and examine whether the increase or decrease in circulating levels of ucOC has an effect on glycemic control. Vitamin K is found in green leafy vegetables and is required for OC carboxylation [23]. Vitamin K supplementation increases carboxylation and lowers circulating ucOC [24] and, as such, vitamin K supplementation should increase insulin resistance and serum glucose levels. Kumar et al. [25] reported that 12 months of vitamin K_1 (phylloquinone) administration in postmenopausal women reduced ucOC by ~200% but there was no increase in insulin resistance. However, this study examined ucOC and glycemic control at rest, not after a meal or after glucose loading which may affect the results. Kumar et al. [25] suggested that the differing findings from studies in mice may be related to the deletion of OC genes in mice which led to abnormal ucOC level during development, whereas in humans the reduction in ucOC levels was induced later in life. As such, it may not have similar effects on insulin resistance. In addition, increases in hepatic insulin clearance may have masked the increase in insulin production by the pancreatic β cells, but there was no evidence to support this hypothesis. Nevertheless, these findings are inconsistent with the findings in mice and in some cross-sectional and interventional studies in humans.

Low circulating vitamin K should be associated with better glycemic control. However, in one study [26], men with low vitamin K intake had lower insulin response and higher plasma glucose 30 min after glucose loading. This and the findings from Kumar et al. do not support the hypothesis that ucOC is essential for glycemic control in humans. If OC also plays a role in insulin secretion and sensitivity in human subjects, it may explain why insulin resistance does not increase in the Kumar et al. [25] study. Further studies are needed to clarify the connection between vitamin K supplementation and deficiency, OC, ucOC, and glycemic control in humans.

WHAT IS THE ACTIVE FORM OF OSTEOCALCIN IN HUMANS?

In mice, ucOC, but not OC, participates in energy metabolism [1]. In the studies described above both OC and ucOC appear to be associated with increases in insulin sensitivity and glycemic control in humans. The active form of OC in humans is unknown, most likely because there are methodological limitations such as absence of specific commercially available assays used to detect ucOC. There are two main methods to analyze ucOC in humans, immunoassay after absorption of carboxylated OC on a hydroxyl-apatite column following the method described by Gundberg et al. [27] and electrochemiluminescence immunoassay (ELISA). The hydroxyl-apatite column is considered as the gold standard and it analyzes total OC, carboxylated OC, and ucOC in one analysis which enables assessment of the ucOC/OC ratio. This method is expensive. The electrochemiluminescence immunoassay is accurate between 0.39 and 50 ng/mL, covering the clinically important range. Assessment of reproducibility testing showed inter-assay CV = 1.5–5.9%. The electrochemiluminescence immunoassay for ucOC was validated against the hydroxyapatite binding assay [28]. The main limitations of the electrochemiluminescence immunoassay are that it is specific for ucOC and as such OC must be analyzed with a different assay so the ucOC/OC ratio cannot be determined. Importantly, the ELISA may overestimate ucOC levels as the antibody used may be attached to N-terminal fragments of OC [27]. To date, many studies have used the electrochemiluminescence immunoassay as it is more convenient and easier to perform compared to the hydroxyl-apatite binding method. Thus, development of valid, reliable,

and easy to use ELISA is needed to further explore the contribution of ucOC to energy metabolism. At this time it is difficult to determine which OC form is directly involved in increasing insulin sensitivity and glycemic control in humans, although it seems unlikely that the biology of osteocalcin would differ that much between mice and humans.

ENDOSTEAL SURFACE AREA, REMODELING, AND GLYCEMIC CONTROL

The cellular machinery of bone modeling and remodeling is the final common pathway mediating the effects of all genetic and environmental factors on the material composition and structure of bone and therefore bone strength [29]. Bone modeling may be formative or resorptive (not only formative) and is both the main cellular mechanism responsible for the change in bone size, shape, and architecture during growth in human subjects and the main mechanism responsible for growth and renewal of bone in rodent species throughout life. Modeling by bone formation (without prior resorption) or resorption (not followed by formation) occurs at different locations. Bone remodeling is responsible for renewal of osteonal bone in human subjects. Remodeling involves the resorption then deposition of a volume of bone matrix at the *same* location by teams of cells forming the basic multicellular unit (BMU).

Remodeling modifies the structure of bone by adding and removing bone upon the outer (periosteal) envelope and each of the three (intracortical, endocortical, and trabecular) contiguous components of its inner (endosteal) envelope. The mineralized bone matrix is that material "within" the periosteal envelope or surface and "outside" the three components of the inner envelope (Fig. 15.2).

OC is a bone formation marker and reflects, in part, the surface extent of bone remodeling. As bone modeling and remodeling throughout life are surface-dependent processes [30], we examined whether the structural configuration of bone, specifically its surface to volume ratio, is related to remodeling and to regulation of OC and ucOC and therefore regulation of blood glucose levels. Remodeling of bone matrix requires the surface to be initiated upon [31,32]. If signals arise from the osteoblasts of the bone remodeling unit, the greater the remodeling intensity, the greater the number of osteoblast cells. Bone matrix volume assembled with more surface is assembled with less mass and facilitates the need to maintain itself with fewer energy requirements while assembling a mechanically sound architecture. As such, it appears that during evolution the

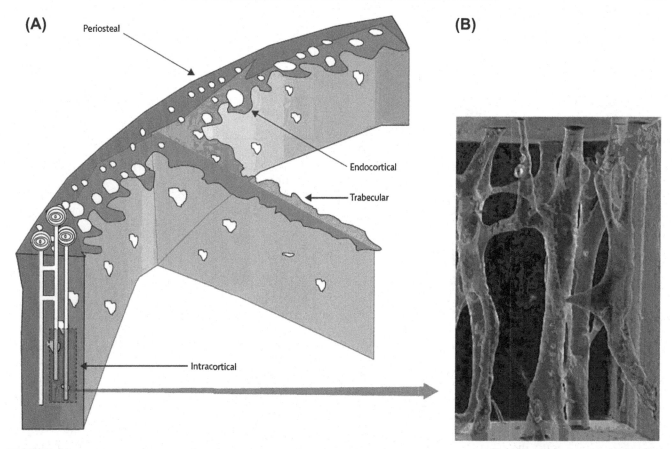

(A)

Periosteal

Endocortical

Trabecular

Intracortical

(B)

FIGURE 15.2   Structure of bone. (A) Cortical and trabecular bone, the periosteal (external) surface and the three (endocortical, trabecular, intracortical) contiguous components of the endosteal (internal) surface upon which matrix remodeling is initiated. **(B)** The intracortical surface formed by the lining of Haversian and Volkmann canals traverses the cortex. These canals are seen as pores in cross-section. Reconstructed with high-resolution quantitative CT. Please see color plate section. *Adapted from Zebaze et al. [31].*

skeleton has adapted to be strong and light, which may assist the body to conserve energy. On the other hand, the skeleton requires a constant supply of energy for modeling to allow growth and therefore ambulation and survival in the face of danger, and remodeling in order to prevent fractures (which in ancient times reduced the chance of survival) [33].

Bjornerem et al. [34] has examined the intracortical, endocortical, and trabecular bone surface area of the distal tibia and distal radius in 185 healthy female twin pairs aged 40 to 61 years using high-resolution peripheral quantitative computed tomography (HR-pQCT). They also examined the correlation between bone surface and markers of remodeling. They reported that intracortical surface area and intracortical porosity (surrogate of surface area) are correlated with remodeling markers such as OC, cross-linking telopeptides of type I bone collagen (CTX), and procollagen type 1 aminoterminal propeptide (P1NP) in both distal radius and distal tibia, while trabecular surface area was negatively correlated with those markers (Fig. 15.3). The authors concluded that the configuration of bone—and especially larger

intracortical and endocortical surface area—is likely to contribute to the intensity of remodeling; the larger the surface, the greater the accessibility of the bone matrix volume to being remodeled. However, the relationship between those bone surfaces and glycemic control was not studied.

No study has examined the connection between the intracortical, endocortical, and trabecular bone surface and glycemic control. It is accepted that patients with type 1 diabetes mellitus (T1DM) are characterized by lower BMD [35] and patients with T2DM have normal to high BMD [36] but the connection to surface area is unknown. Preliminary data from our research group (unpublished) suggests that in middle-aged men, porosity of the compact-appearing cortex of the tibia and radius, the transitional zone, and the fraction of the medullary cavity correlate with serum OC and ucOC (r ranging from 0.33 to 0.72, $p < 0.05$) [37]. Consequently, total, cortical, and trabecular vBMD correlated negatively with serum ucOC. Furthermore, circulating ucOC correlated negatively with serum glucose and HbA1c in this cohort. However, no detectable correlations where found between porosity of the compact-

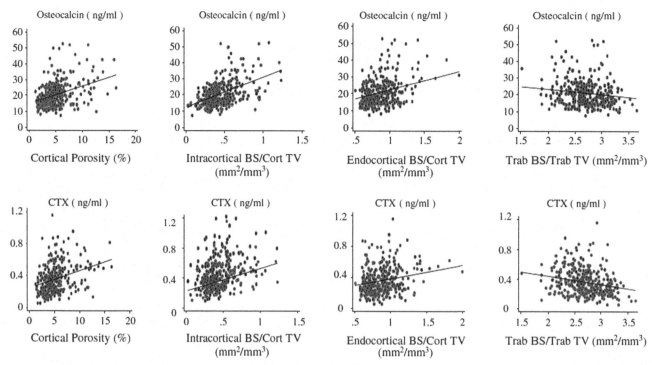

FIGURE 15.3   Bone remodeling markers osteocalcin and β-carboxyterminal cross-linking telopeptides of type I bone collagen (β-CTX) correlated directly with tibia intracortical and endocortical surface area/cortical tissue volume (TV) but inversely with trabecular surface area/ trabecular TV. *Adapted from Bjornerem et al. [34].*

appearing cortex of the tibia and radius, the transitional zone and the fraction of the medullary cavity and serum glucose or HbA1c. As such the preliminary data suggest that a larger bone surface area facilitates remodeling and may, indirectly, be related to glycemic control in humans. Nevertheless, future studies with a large cohort should be performed in order to investigate the contribution of bone surface area to glycemic control in humans. It is still not clear whether the intracortical, endocortical, and trabecular bone surface are directly related to insulin sensitivity and glycemic control but, if so, this provides opportunities for designing new pharmacological and non-pharmacological interventions to treat both bone diseases and T2DM. Further work is under way exploring these relationships.

OSTEOCALCIN AND GLYCEMIC CONTROL: CONCLUSIONS AND CLINICAL IMPLICATIONS

Animal models have shown that ucOC participates in energy metabolism. There is growing evidence in human subjects to support the hypothesis that higher levels of circulating ucOC are related to better glycemic control [33]. Daily injections of recombinant OC at 3 or 30 ng/g/day reduce blood glucose levels and improve glucose tolerance and insulin sensitivity in mice fed

a normal diet [38]. The improvement in blood glucose levels, glucose tolerance, and insulin sensitivity was related to the increase in β-cell mass and insulin secretion. Furthermore, daily injections of recombinant OC partially restored insulin sensitivity and glucose tolerance in mice fed a high-fat diet. Other benefits reported included higher number of skeletal muscle's mitochondria, increased energy expenditure, and protection from diet-induced obesity [38]. The authors concluded that daily injections of recombinant OC improve glycemic control as well as prevent the development of T2DM.

Whether ucOC plays a role in insulin secretion and sensitivity in humans and whether daily injection of ucOC treatment restores glycemic control in humans are unknown. If ucOC plays a role in glucose metabolism in humans it will provide avenues for designing new drugs that imitate these pathways for obese persons and patients with T2DM. Clearly, drugs which increase both insulin secretion and insulin sensitivity without weight gain would in many ways be the ideal agents for treating diabetes. Furthermore, targeting bone metabolism as a pathway to control whole body glucose homeostasis will be important as current therapies are limited in their specificity and effectiveness and may have a negative effect on bone health. Circulating ucOC is associated with increased insulin sensitivity and glycemic control in humans. Whether this association is causal will require prospective studies. There are neither longitudinal studies nor mechanistic studies to support the unOC hypothesis in humans. The mechanism by which ucOC may affect insulin sensitivity and secretion and glycemic control in humans is still largely unknown but it may resemble that in mice. If this regulatory mechanism of glucose metabolism occurs to a significant degree in humans it could have major effects on improving the treatment of T2DM. Thus, the exciting data in mice identifying a regulatory role of ucOC have not yet been definitively replicated in humans. However, preliminary reports suggest that it is likely there will be a similar effect in humans. The magnitude of this effect and whether it will be clinically significant still remain to be defined.

Acknowledgments

Dr. Itamar Levinger is a Heart Foundation Postdoctoral Research Fellow.

References

[1] Lee NK, Sowa H, Hinoi E, et al. Endocrine regulation of energy metabolism by the skeleton. Cell 2007;130:456–69.

[2] Clemens TL, Karsenty G. The osteoblast: an insulin target cell controlling glucose homeostasis. J Bone Miner Res 2011;26:677–80.

[3] Ferron M, Hinoi E, Karsenty G, Ducy P. Osteocalcin differentially regulates beta cell and adipocyte gene expression and affects the development of metabolic diseases in wild-type mice. Proc Natl Acad Sci USA 2008;105:5266–70.

[4] Foresta C, Strapazzon G, De Toni L, et al. Evidence for osteocalcin production by adipose tissue and its role in human metabolism. J Clin Endocrinol Metab 2010;95:3502–6.

[5] Kindblom JM, Ohlsson C, Ljunggren O, et al. Plasma osteocalcin is inversely related to fat mass and plasma glucose in elderly Swedish men. J Bone Miner Res 2009;24:785–91.

[6] Im JA, Yu BP, Jeon JY, Kim SH. Relationship between osteocalcin and glucose metabolism in postmenopausal women. Clinica Chim Acta. Int J Clin Chem 2008;396:66–9.

[7] Levinger I, Zebaze R, Jerums G, Hare DL, Selig S, Seeman E. The effect of acute exercise on undercarboxylated osteocalcin in obese men. Osteoporos Int 2011;22:1621–6.

[8] Hwang YC, Jeong IK, Ahn KJ, Chung HY. The uncarboxylated form of osteocalcin is associated with improved glucose tolerance and enhanced beta-cell function in middle-aged male subjects. Diabetes Metab Res Rev 2009;25:768–72.

[9] Hwang YC, Jeong IK, Ahn KJ, Chung HY. Circulating osteocalcin level is associated with improved glucose tolerance, insulin secretion and sensitivity independent of the plasma adiponectin level. Osteoporos Int 2012;23:1337–42.

[10] Kanazawa I, Yamaguchi T, Yamauchi M, et al. Serum undercarboxylated osteocalcin was inversely associated with plasma glucose level and fat mass in type 2 diabetes mellitus. Osteoporos Int 2011;22:187–94.

[11] Kanazawa I, Yamaguchi T, Yamamoto M, et al. Serum osteocalcin level is associated with glucose metabolism and atherosclerosis parameters in type 2 diabetes mellitus. J Clin Endocrinol Metab 2009;94:45–9.

[12] Goliasch G, Blessberger H, Azar D, et al. Markers of bone metabolism in premature myocardial infarction (</= 40 years of age). Bone 2011;48:622–6.

[13] Bullo M, Moreno-Navarrete JM, Fernandez-Real JM, Salas-Salvado J. Total and undercarboxylated osteocalcin predict changes in insulin sensitivity and beta cell function in elderly men at high cardiovascular risk. Am J Clin Nutr 2012;95:249–55.

[14] Yeap BB, Chubb SA, Flicker L, et al. Reduced serum total osteocalcin is associated with metabolic syndrome in older men via waist circumference, hyperglycemia, and triglyceride levels. European J Endocrinol/European Federation of Endocrine Societies 2010;163:265–72.

[15] Saleem U, Mosley Jr TH, Kullo IJ. Serum osteocalcin is associated with measures of insulin resistance, adipokine levels, and the presence of metabolic syndrome. Arterioscler Thromb Vasc Biol 2010;30:1474–8.

[16] Kanazawa I, Yamaguchi T, Yamauchi M, et al. Adiponectin is associated with changes in bone markers during glycemic control in type 2 diabetes mellitus. J Clin Endocrinol Metab 2009;94:3031–7.

[17] Sayinalp S, Gedik O, Koray Z. Increasing serum osteocalcin after glycemic control in diabetic men. Calcif Tissue Int 1995;57:422–5.

[18] Bao YQ, Zhou M, Zhou J, et al. Relationship between serum osteocalcin and glycaemic variability in Type 2 diabetes. Clin Exp Pharmacol Physiol 2011;38:50–4.

[19] Oz SG, Guven GS, Kilicarslan A, Calik N, Beyazit Y, Sozen T. Evaluation of bone metabolism and bone mass in patients with type-2 diabetes mellitus. J Natl Med Assoc 2006;98:1598–604.

[20] Pittas AG, Harris SS, Eliades M, Stark P, Dawson-Hughes B. Association between serum osteocalcin and markers of metabolic phenotype. J Clin Endocrinol Metab 2009;94:827–32.

[21] Shea MK, Gundberg CM, Meigs JB, et al. Gamma-carboxylation of osteocalcin and insulin resistance in older men and women. Am J Clin Nutr 2009;90:1230–5.

[22] Fernandez-Real JM, Izquierdo M, Ortega F, et al. The relationship of serum osteocalcin concentration to insulin secretion, sensitivity, and disposal with hypocaloric diet and resistance training. J Clin Endocrinol Metab 2009;94:237–45.

[23] Szulc P, Chapuy MC, Meunier PJ, Delmas PD. Serum undercarboxylated osteocalcin is a marker of the risk of hip fracture in elderly women. J Clin Invest 1993;91:1769–74.

[24] Binkley NC, Krueger DC, Engelke JA, Foley AL, Suttie JW. Vitamin K supplementation reduces serum concentrations of under-gamma-carboxylated osteocalcin in healthy young and elderly adults. Am J Clin Nutr 2000;72:1523–8.

[25] Kumar R, Binkley N, Vella A. Effect of phylloquinone supplementation on glucose homeostasis in humans. Am J Clin Nutr 2010;92:1528–32.

[26] Sakamoto N, Nishiike T, Iguchi H, Sakamoto K. Relationship between acute insulin response and vitamin K intake in healthy young male volunteers. Diabetes Nutr Metab 1999;12:37–41.

[27] Gundberg CM, Nieman SD, Abrams S, Rosen H. Vitamin K status and bone health: an analysis of methods for determination of undercarboxylated osteocalcin. J Clin Endocrinol Metab 1998;83:3258–66.

[28] Vergnaud P, Garnero P, Meunier PJ, Breart G, Kamihagi K, Delmas PD. Undercarboxylated osteocalcin measured with a specific immunoassay predicts hip fracture in elderly women: the EPIDOS Study. J Clin Endocrinol Metab 1997;82:719–24.

[29] Parfitt A. Skeletal heterogeneity and the purposes of bone remodelling: implications for the understanding of osteoporosis. In: Marcus R, Feldman D, Nelson D, Rosen C, editors. Osteoporosis. San Diego, CA: Academic; 2008. p. 71–89.

[30] Epker BN, Frost HM. A histological study of remodeling at the periosteal, haversian canal, cortical endosteal, and trabecular endosteal surfaces in human rib. Anatom Rec 1965;152:129–35.

[31] Zebaze RM, Ghasem-Zadeh A, Bohte A, et al. Intracortical remodelling and porosity in the distal radius and post-mortem femurs of women: a cross-sectional study. Lancet 2010;375: 1729–36.

[32] Parfitt A. The physiologic and clinical significance of bone histomorphometric data. In: Recker R, editor. Bone Histomorphometry Techniques and Interpretstion. Boca Raton: CRC Press; 1983. p. 142–223.

[33] Ducy P. The role of osteocalcin in the endocrine cross-talk between bone remodelling and energy metabolism. Diabetologia 2011;54:1291–7.

[34] Bjornerem A, Ghasem-Zadeh A, Bui M, et al. Remodeling markers are associated with larger intracortical surface area but smaller trabecular surface area: a twin study. Bone 2011;49:1125–30.

[35] Danielson KK, Elliott ME, LeCaire T, Binkley N, Palta M. Poor glycemic control is associated with low BMD detected in premenopausal women with type 1 diabetes. Osteoporos Int 2009;20:923–33.

[36] Dennison EM, Syddall HE. Aihie Sayer A, Craighead S, Phillips DI, Cooper C. Type 2 diabetes mellitus is associated with increased axial bone density in men and women from the Hertfordshire Cohort Study: evidence for an indirect effect of insulin resistance? Diabetologia 2004;47:1963–8.

[37] Levinger I, Zebaze R, Ghasem-Zadeh A, et al. Increased intracortical porosity is associated with higher serum undercarboxylated osteocalcin in middle-aged men. ANZBMS. Gold Coast; 2011.

[38] Ferron M, McKee MD, Levine RL, Ducy P, Karsenty G. Intermittent injections of osteocalcin improve glucose metabolism and prevent type 2 diabetes in mice. Bone 2012; 50:568–75.

16

Clinical Implications of Serotonin Regulation of Bone Mass

Elizabeth M. Haney, MD[1], *Chadi Calarge, MD*[2],
M. Michael Bliziotes, MD[1,3]

[1]Oregon Health & Science University, Portland, OR, USA [2]The University of Iowa, Iowa City, IA, USA
[3]Portland Veterans Affairs Medical Center, Portland, OR, USA

INTRODUCTION

Since the identification of a functional signaling system for the centrally acting neurotransmitter serotonin (5-hydroxytryptamine or 5-HT) in bone [1,2], evidence regarding the clinical implications of this system has accumulated. The discovery of a novel mechanism for regulating bone mass [3–5] stimulated additional interest in this area. However, the specific biochemical nature of serotonergic pathways and their direct and/or indirect effects on bone metabolism are still unclear. In other sections of this book, pre-clinical evidence for an effect of serotonin and altered serotonin signaling on bone metabolism is reviewed in detail. This chapter will focus on the current knowledge about clinical implications of the serotonin signaling systems in bone. It will build on the pre-clinical data from studies of individuals that have various perturbations of the serotonin signaling system, either by virtue of medications that block the serotonin transporter (selective serotonin reuptake inhibitors, or SSRIs), or disease states that are related to altered serotonin signaling (depression). It will also offer a perspective for how to begin incorporating this knowledge into clinical practice through screening, case finding, and population health.

SYNTHESIS AND FUNCTION OF SEROTONIN IN THE NERVOUS SYSTEM

Serotonin transporters (5-HTT or SERT) and receptors (5-HT$_{1-7}$) are located in the central, peripheral, and enteric nervous systems, and have been identified in several other peripheral tissues including bone. The function of both serotonin transporters and receptors appears to be similar in all locations, and medications that block the serotonin transporter are thought to effect central and peripheral 5-HTT with similar potency [1].

5-HT is synthesized from the essential amino acid tryptophan, in a two-step reaction that has tryptophan hydrozylase (TPH) as its rate-limiting step. TPH is encoded by two genes: *Tph-1* which is expressed in the periphery and *Tph-2* which is expressed in the brain. 5-HT does not freely cross the blood–brain barrier, making it possible for 5-HT to exert independent peripheral and central effects depending on the site of synthesis.

In the central nervous system (CNS), 5-HT is synthesized by *Tph2* in the raphe nuclei and is tightly regulated. The 5-HTT regulates 5-HT signaling by actively transporting 5-HT into neuronal cells at the presynaptic membrane (Fig. 16.1). Medications that block the 5-HTT, also known as selective serotonin reuptake inhibitors (SSRIs), increase the synaptic levels of 5-HT (potentiating 5-HT activity). SSRIs inhibit the 5-HTT both selectively and potently. They are first-line therapy for depression and widely used for treatment of several psychiatric and non-psychiatric conditions, including post-traumatic stress disorder, generalized anxiety disorder, and fibromyalgia.

In the periphery, 5-HT is synthesized primarily in the gastrointestinal tract through the action of *Tph-1*. Most (95%) of peripheral serotonin is stored in circulating platelets while the remainder is free in the plasma. 5-HT functions as a paracrine factor to stimulate peristalsis and mucus secretion in the gastrointestinal tract [6] and also has effects on the cardiovascular system via its peripheral action to stimulate blood vessel

Translational Endocrinology of Bone
DOI: http://dx.doi.org/10.1016/B978-0-12-415784-2.00016-6

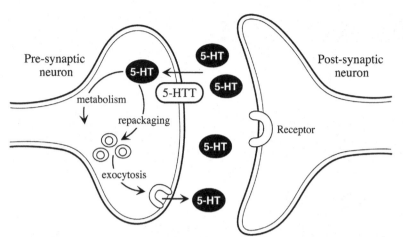

FIGURE 16.1 **5-HT signaling within the central nervous system.** 5-HT is synthesized by presynaptic neurons and stored in vesicles. 5-HT is released into the synaptic space, activates the post-synaptic receptors and stimulates the post-synaptic neuron. Membrane-bound 5-HT transporters (5-HTT) uptake released 5-HT to control the duration of 5-HT effects and recycle or degrade 5-HT. Inhibition of the 5-HTT prevents uptake of 5-HT resulting in its accumulation within the synaptic cleft and the prolonging of receptor activation.

constriction or dilation and smooth muscle hypertrophy and hyperplasia. 5-HT transporters and receptors are also present in osteoblasts, osteocytes, and osteoclasts. Activation of these receptors influences bone metabolism [1,7−9], demonstrating that this is a functional serotonergic signaling system in bone.

There are several theories for how 5-HT may interact with bone. Global inactivation of the 5-HTT leads to bone loss in mice [10]. Although osteoblasts, osteocytes, and osteoclasts all express Tph-1 at low levels [5,8] the functional source of 5-HT for bone cells is unclear. Yadav et al. demonstrated that the GI tract is the major source of skeletal 5-HT and that gut-derived 5-HT is a mediator for LRP-5 action on bone. Another group has been unable to demonstrate the same phenomenon, finding instead that peripheral 5HT synthesis does not affect bone mass [11]. On the other hand, several studies suggest that levels of circulating serotonin correlate with changes in bone mass [5,12−15]. Centrally, 5HT receptor activation inhibits the sympathetic nervous system (SNS) [16−18]. Inhibition of the sympathetic nervous system, in turn, promotes bone formation and reduces bone resorption [18].

These pre-clinical findings have raised concerns about the clinical effects that 5-HT might have on bone in humans. This is particularly the case given the widespread use of SSRIs. These medications act both centrally and peripherally, potentially impacting bone metabolism in complex ways. Thus, the remainder of this chapter will focus on clinical studies of SSRIs and bone outcomes.

STUDIES OF SEROTONIN INFLUENCE ON BONE IN HUMAN DEVELOPMENT

Prenatal SSRI Exposure

With as many as 18.4% of women suffering with depression during pregnancy and the prenatal use of

SSRIs quadrupling to 6.2% in recent years [19−21], concerns have arisen regarding the impact of prenatal SSRI exposure on skeletal development. This is particularly the case since SSRIs cross the maternal−fetal barrier and since the placenta is an important source of 5HT, modulating fetal development [22,23]. Moreover, nearly two-thirds of total body calcium and phosphorus in a term infant are accumulated in the third trimester. In fact, a number of studies have explored the potential effect of in utero SSRI exposure on skeletal birth defects; some of these have demonstrated an increased risk (e.g. cleft palate) [24−26]. In a recent study using quantitative ultrasound, 40 newborns exposed to SSRIs almost throughout the entire pregnancy showed a normal mid-left tibial bone speed of sound compared to gestational age-matched controls [27]. This was despite the fact that SSRI-exposed newborns had a smaller head circumference and marginally shorter height. While these initial findings are reassuring, quantitative ultrasound neither isolates trabecular from cortical bone nor characterizes bone microarchitecture. Moreover, longitudinal monitoring of bone mineralization in prenatally exposed children is critical since preclinical and clinical studies have implicated early-life SSRI exposure in downregulation of endogenous 5-HT signaling [28,29]. This, in turn, has been linked to exaggerated sympathetic nervous system activation that persists long after SSRI exposure had resolved [30]. Such sympathetic overactivation could reduce bone formation chronically, preventing eventual skeletal recovery which might occur if the exposure is limited to the postnatal period [31].

Child and Adolescent SSRI Exposure

Antidepressants, primarily SSRIs, are widely used in children and adolescents. For example, antidepressants were the third most commonly prescribed medications for US adolescents in 2007 and 2008, accounting for 4.8% of all prescriptions [32]. Therefore, establishing the long-term safety of these drugs is crucial.

In a case series of four adolescents (ages 11.6 to 13.7 years), longitudinal growth was found to be significantly hindered by treatment with SSRIs, recovering after medication discontinuation [33]. Moreover, in the one case where the SSRI (fluoxetine) was restarted, nearly 18 months after it had been discontinued, longitudinal growth was suppressed again [33]. Interestingly, the deleterious effect of SSRIs on growth could be observed in as little as 6 months with recovery of growth hormone secretion occurring within a month after discontinuing the medication.

In a multi-phase double-blind relapse prevention trial, Emslie et al. randomized youths with depression (mean age 12.7 years $\pm$ 2.6) to fluoxetine ($n = 109$) or placebo ($n = 110$) [34]. In the first 19-week phase of the study, patients randomized to fluoxetine lost 0.1 Z-score point in age–sex-adjusted height while those taking placebo gained 0.07 point. This between-group difference was statistically significant ($p = 0.001$) [35]. Interestingly, this decline in longitudinal growth was associated with a decrease in alkaline phosphatase which was significantly different from the placebo group (standardized difference $= 0.87$, $p < 0.001$) [35]. Bone-specific alkaline phosphatase, a marker of osteoid formation, comprises most of the circulating alkaline phosphatase in this age group [36]. That fluoxetine would reduce bone formation is consistent with findings from mice lacking the 5HT transporter as well as normal mice treated with fluoxetine, both models similarly showing reduced bone formation [37].

At the end of the first phase, those youths whose depression remitted on fluoxetine were re-randomized to placebo or to remain on the medicine while those who responded to placebo were maintained on it [34]. The subjects were followed for an additional 32 weeks. This design resulted in three groups: youths who remained on placebo throughout the initial and follow-up phases (P/P), those who were randomized to fluoxetine in both phases (F/F), and those who responded to fluoxetine and were then randomized to placebo in the second phase (F/P). When compared with the pre-study baseline, the F/F group continued to show a slight deficit in age–sex-adjusted height Z-score (-0.04 Z-score) while the P/P group showed a slight gain (Z-score 0.15). The difference did not reach statistical significance (effect size $= 0.46$, $p = 0.130$), likely due to the small sample size of 40 (after 65% of the original sample dropped out) (see authors' reply [38]).

One study used dual X-ray absorptiometry and peripheral quantitative computed tomography to evaluate the effect of SSRI use on bone density in 83 risperidone-treated boys, of whom 42 participants were taking fluoxetine, sertraline, citalopram, or escitalopram [39]. Equivalent daily doses were calculated based on a daily dose of 20 mg of fluoxetine. SSRI treatment was associated with lower lumbar bone mineral density (BMD) Z-score after adjustment for Tanner stage, age–sex-adjusted height and weight Z-scores, physical activity, total daily calcium intake, and prolactin. Similarly, SSRIs were associated with reduced trabecular volumetric BMD at the ultra-distal radius, after adjustment for Tanner stage, age–sex-adjusted height and body mass index Z-scores, and prolactin. Additional adjustment for depressive diagnosis strengthened this association. Interestingly, variants of the 5-HTT-linked polymorphic region of the 5-HTT gene moderated this association with carriers of the ls genotype being most vulnerable to the skeletal effects of SSRI treatment [40].

CLINICAL STUDIES DEMONSTRATING AN EFFECT OF SEROTONIN ON BONE IN ADULTS

Epidemiologic studies of adults taking SSRIs for various mental health conditions can offer insight into the effects on bone in the setting of chronically downregulated 5-HTT action in adults. Thus, several studies have explored the association between SSRI use and bone density, bone loss, and fractures as a way of understanding 5-HT influence on bone. These studies have varied with respect to their recruitment strategies, and this influences the conclusions that can be drawn from their results. Some studies recruited hospitalized psychiatric patients and compared them to healthy individuals; other cohorts were recruited to reflect the general population; and yet others use administrative databases (claims data, public health service records) to evaluate pharmaceutical records, claims in conjunction with bone-specific outcomes such as fractures. Studies that recruit participants from specialty clinics or hospital wards are less generalizable than those using population-based recruitment strategies. Population-based cohort studies tend to be very well characterized in terms of BMD measurements and fracture outcomes. As such, they are able to support conclusions regarding the mechanism of a potential effect of SSRIs on bone: namely contributing evidence that supports either a direct effect of SSRIs on bone density or an indirect effect through falls or depression on fracture rates. Despite these advantages population-based cohorts may lack specific pharmacy data to rigorously define the extent of SSRI use including dose and duration of use. Administrative database studies typically have more precise pharmacy data, but may have less-rigorous clinical outcome data and may be less able to adjust for confounders.

BONE DENSITY

There have now been several studies evaluating bone mineral density (BMD) among antidepressant users. These studies provide insight into whether any effect seen on fractures might be mediated through BMD. Typically, BMD evaluation is done in the setting of a population-based cohort study; therefore, these studies tend to be smaller than administrative database studies but have very well-characterized covariate information and may be either cross-sectional or longitudinal. Because studies of general antidepressant use are less able to illuminate the question of serotonin impact on bone, we present here only those cohort studies that have evaluated SSRIs separately from general antidepressant use.

Cross-sectional studies support an association between SSRIs and lower BMD in both men and women. Among men and women >age 50 in the Canadian Multicentre Osteoporosis Study (CaMOS) cohort ($n = 5008$), BMD was 4% lower at the hip for those taking SSRIs [41]. In men over age 65 enrolled in the Osteoporotic Fractures in Men (MrOS) cohort ($n = 5995$), BMD was 3.9% lower at the total hip and 5.9% lower at the lumbar spine [42]. While both these studies (CaMOS and MrOS) adjusted for depressive symptoms in addition to other potential confounders, Williams et al. attempted to further isolate the effect of SSRIs from any contribution from depression by limiting their study to 128 women with lifetime or current depression who were enrolled in the Geelong Osteoporosis Study. Even in this group, who all had clinically diagnosed depression, the SSRI users had 5.6% lower BMD at the femoral neck compared to non-users [43]. A limitiation of these studies is the difficulty in adjusting completely for a rigorous diagnosis of depression or the severity of depressive symptoms; and the generally low numbers of patients on SSRIs in these cohort studies. Overall, patients enrolled in cohort studies tend to be healthier and less depressed than the general population.

Longitudinal studies offer stronger evidence of causal associations, and the results for SSRIs and change in BMD have been mixed. Data from the Study of Osteoporotic Fractures demonstrates that SSRI users have at least 1.6-fold greater declines in BMD compared to those not taking SSRIs [44]. Results from and the Women's Health Initiative show no association between antidepressant use (not specifically SSRIs) and change in BMD [45].

FRACTURES

Prospective cohort studies also provide important data to inform the question of whether SSRI use contributes to fracture after adjusting for covariates. In the Osteoporotic Fractures in Men (MrOS) cohort, men taking SSRIs had an overall increased risk for non-spine fracture [46,47]. In the Study of Osteoporotic Fractures (SOF), women taking antidepressants (SSRIs and tricyclic antidepressants or TCAs) who were followed for 4.8 years on average ($n = 1256$) had a significantly elevated risk of hip and non-spine fracture (age adjusted RR 1.48 and 2.03, respectively). Adjustment for depression and other confounders attenuated this effect somewhat but the result was still significant for non-spine fracture and the RR just included 1 for hip fracture. Evaluating SSRIs and TCAs separately suggested that SSRI users were at higher risk of fracture than TCA users. SSRIs inhibit the 5-HT potently and specifically; TCAs inhibit both the 5-HT and the norepinephrine system, but are less specific and less potent at the 5-HT. In this study, the association between hip fracture and medication use was significant only for the TCA user group possibly because of low numbers in the SSRI user group ($n = 105$ SSRI users vs. 410 other antidepressant users; multivariate hazard ratio (HR) for hip fracture 1.83, 95% confidence interval (CI) 1.08–1.39 for TCA users; multivariate HR for hip fracture 1.54, 95% 0.62–23.82 for SSRI users) [48]. In the Canadian Multicentre Osteoporosis Study (CaMOS) cohort, older men and women taking SSRIs and followed for 5 years had higher rates of fracture compared to non-users (HR 2.1; 95% CI 1.3–3.4) [41]. Among men and women in Rotterdam age 55 and older, the risk of non-vertebral fracture was increased two-fold (HR 2.35 for current users compared to non-users, 95% CI 1.32–1.48) for both TCA and SSRI users [49]. The Women's Health Initiative reported increased risk of any fracture and non-clinical vertebral fracture for all antidepressant users, but did not separate SSRI users from other antidepressant users [45].

An association between antidepressants and increased risk of fracture is also supported by several large case–control studies using large administrative datasets from Denmark [50,51], the Netherlands [52,53], Canada [54,55], and the US [56,57]. While database studies can be problematic because of the inability to control for unmeasured variables (i.e. presence or severity of depressive symptoms), they add to the growing body of literature that support a contribution by SSRIs to fracture risk. Vestergaard demonstrated increased odds of hip and any fracture for users of either TCAs or SSRIs (adjusted OR 1.15–1.40 for all antidepressants; 95% CI 0.99–1.30 for TCAs (NS) and 1.08–1.62 for SSRIs across dosages) [51], as did Bolton (OR 1.45 for SSRI users, 95% CI 1.32–1.59) [54]. French at al. evaluated outpatient medication use among US veterans and found two-fold higher difference in the use of antidepressants overall (SSRIs and TCAs) among those with fracture compared to those without [58]. Evaluating multiple classes of medications using national prescription data from Denmark, Abrahamsen et al. identified SSRIs as one of several pharmacologic agents associated with fracture risk after 60 days of use (SSRI OR 1.7, 95% CI 1.6—1.9 for any fracture, OR 2.0, 95% CI 1.8—2.2 for hip fracture and 1.2, 95% CI 1.0—1.5 for spine fracture) [50].

Two studies have evaluated SSRI—fracture risk associations according to affinity at the 5-HTT [53,56]. Verdel et al. used the Dutch PHARMO RLS database to perform a case—control analysis of antidepressants and fractures. In this dataset with 16,717 cases of fracture and 61,517 controls, the risk of osteoporotic fracture was higher among SSRI users than TCA users, and specifically among users of high 5-HTT affinity antidepressants compared to low or medium affinity antidepressants [53]. Gagne et al. used Medicare claims data from two US states to examine whether variation in fracture risk among older adults could be attributed to differences in SSRI affinity for the 5-HTT [56]. In a propensity score-matched cohort of antidepressant users, SSRIs showed the highest association with composite (hip, humerus, pelvis, and wrist) fracture rate (HR 1.30, 95% CI 1.12—1.52) compared to secondary amine TCAs, followed by atypical antidepressants (HR 1.12, 95% CI 0.96—1.31) and tertiary amine TCAs (HR 1.01, 95% CI 0.87—1.18). Secondary amine TCAs are less serotonergic than tertiary amine TCAs. Rigorous methodology including use of validated algorithms to identify fractures from claims data, propensity matching within the cohort to account for confounding by indication, adjustment for other identified risk factures, and several sensitivity analyses support the validity of these findings. In a sensitivity analysis done according to duration of treatment at the time of incident fracture, they found that the fracture risk associated with SSRIs becomes evident within 90 days of starting the medication. To assess whether fracture incidence was related to sedating effect of the medication as a potential explanation for this effect (fracture related to falls due to sedation rather than changes in BMD), the investigators stratified by sedating potential and affinity for the 5-HTT. The highest fracture incidence occurred in the low-sedation, high-5-HTT stratum, corresponding to SSRIs; however, there were no other clear trends across the strata of 5-HTT affinity within the strata of medium or high sedating medications. Thus, there may be two different mechanisms contributing to fracture risk—one in the early stages of treatment and another as treatment progresses past 90 days [56].

CONSIDERATIONS FOR DETERMINATION OF CAUSALITY IN EPIDEMIOLOGIC STUDIES

Acceptance of causality requires a complementary set of studies that address several aspects of the associations in question. First is the question of biologic plausibility. The presence of functional serotonin transporters in bone cells forms the foundation for this plausibility [59]. The pre-clinical data demonstrating the existence of functional serotonin transporters and receptors [1,2], and the bone effects of inactivation of the serotonin transporter both *in vitro* and *in vivo* [7,8,37,60], provide further evidence for a biologically plausible mechanism through which serotonin can directly or indirectly influence bone metabolism.

A second consideration for causality is the question of consistency and strength of the demonstrated associations [59]. In the case of SSRIs, associations are shown in multiple studies with distinct populations and varied study designs. These associations hold across several different bone-specific outcomes: bone density, bone loss, and fractures. The associations are consistent after adjustment for confounding variables such as age, body mass index, lifestyle factors (alcohol, tobacco use), family history, and personal history of fractures. Two meta-analyses have concluded that SSRIs likely contribute independently to fracture risk [61,62].

Third, a demonstrated dose—response supports a causal association [59]. Ideally, studies will demonstrate dose and duration effects, thereby showing an increased risk for the negative outcome with increasing dose and/or duration of medication. In terms of the SSRIs, dose effect may be difficult to investigate because most have comparatively high affinity for the 5-HTT even at relatively low doses [63].

In examining studies of serotonin antagonism through SSRIs for evidence of dose effect, three studies provide varied results [41,51,54]. Among users of different classes of SSRI and TCA antidepressants, Vestergaard et al. demonstrated progressive increases in relative risk for any fracture, hip fracture, and spine fracture as the antidepressant dose increased across levels of defined daily dose (DDD): from <0.15 DDD; 0.15—0.75 DDD; and ≥0.75 DDD. In sub-analyses, increasing daily doses of TCAs showed progressive, but non-significant, increases in the RR of osteoporotic fractures, Colles' fractures, and spine fractures but not hip fracture; SSRIs showed increases in the RR of all categories of osteoporotic fracture across doses, but results were significant only for hip fracture. Other antidepressants showed no dose—response [51]. Bolton et al. also demonstrated a dose effect for SSRIs using the Manitoba dataset. Odds ratios for fracture among men and women over age 50 using SSRIs increased significantly across tertiles of SSRI dose ($p < 0.05$) [54]. The CaMOS study, a population-based cohort with pharmacy data, observed a dose-dependent effect for SSRIs: 1.5-fold increase in risk of fragility fracture for each unit increase in the daily dose of SSRI [36,41]. Other studies have not found a linear increase in risk with increasing dose [49].

Whether duration of SSRI use increases risk has been addressed using data from the CaMOS cohort: Richards et al. demonstrated higher fracture risk among men and women using SSRIs at baseline and 5 years later. Other studies suggest higher fracture risk within the first 15 days of treatment [60,64]. An analysis of men and women from the Rotterdam cohort failed to demonstrate a progressive increase in fractures with either increasing dose or increasing duration of SSRI treatment [44,49]. In the UK General Practice Research Database, the odds ratios (ORs) for fracture were highest for those with a first SSRI prescription given 0–14 days prior to the fracture compared with those prescriptions given 15–42 and ≥43 days before the fracture [64]. It is not anticipated that SSRIs could have an immediate effect on bone so as to contribute to risk for fracture directly within 2 weeks of initiation. Gagne et al. found an effect both within and after 90 days of treatment [56], and Abrahamsen found an effect of SSRIs on fracture after 60 days of treatment [50]. Therefore, one explanation is that SSRIs contribute to excess fracture risk through falls early in the course of treatment, and through a direct bone mechanism later in the course of treatment.

LIMITATIONS OF CURRENT STUDIES ON SSRIs' EFFECT ON BONE

Our interpretation of the epidemiologic studies of SSRIs in terms of their impact and potential causal association with bone loss and fracture is complicated by several methodologic issues. Confounding by indication can exist if a disease and its treatment both have potential to be associated with the outcome of interest [65]. In this case, depression has also been associated with low bone density in some [66–73] but not all [45,74–77] studies. Two meta-analyses also support an association between depression and low BMD [78,79]. Longitudinal studies in women have demonstrated mixed results. Using data from SOF (3977 women with Geriatic Depression Scale (GDS) scores <6 and 200 with GDS ≥6), Diem et al. found that depression is associated with higher rates of bone density loss at the total hip (loss of 0.69%/year among those with GDS <6 vs. 0.96%/year among those with GDS ≥6) [67]. However, using the very large WHI cohort, Spangler et al. found no association between depressive symptoms as measured by the Center for Epidemiologic Studies Depression Scale (CES-D), and changes in BMD [45]. Others have also observed mixed results for an association between depression and falls [77,80–83] and depression and fractures [45,72,75,77,80,83–85].

Therefore, the presence of depression/depressive symptoms in the people taking SSRIs has potential to bias results through confounding by indication. That

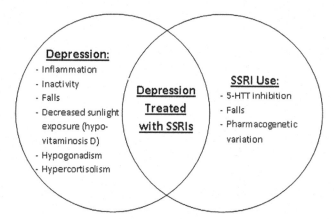

FIGURE 16.2   Overlapping risk factors for bone loss and fracture among those with depression and selective serotonin reuptake inhibitor (SSRI) use. Confounding by indication complicates the evaluation of 5-HT contributions to bone loss and fracture because SSRIs are used to treat depression, therefore most people on SSRIs will also have potential for increased fracture risk related to depression itself. Several mechanisms may contribute to increased fracture risk among people with depression and those treated with SSRIs. SSRI users may have persistent symptoms of depression, may be in remission from depression, or may be using SSRIs for a non-depressive condition.

is, within a particular study it can be difficult to determine whether the disease state (depression) or the treatment (SSRIs) is responsible for the effects seen. Depression and SSRIs have the potential to impact bone through distinct mechanistic pathways (Fig. 16.2). For instance, antagonism at the serotonin transporter as a result of SSRI use could cause reduced bone formation, increased bone resorption or both. Genetic differences in the serotonin transporter could modulate the skeletal response to SSRIs. Thus, SSRIs might lead to increased fractures through one of these direct cellular mechanisms, or through an indirect mechanism such as falls. In contrast, depression has potential to influence bone through separate pathways involving inflammation, physical inactivity, falls, decreased outdoor exposure (and therefore lower vitamin D levels), hypercortisolism, or hypogonadism. Theoretically, when a person has persistent depressive symptoms and is taking an SSRI, he/she could be at higher risk than those with only one risk factor (either depressive symptoms or SSRI use but not both) based on overlapping pathways. Those with depressive symptoms that are in remission after treatment with an SSRI, and those using SSRIs for non-depressive illness, may be at lower risk.

In terms of the studies that evaluate or best control for some of these other potential mechanisms, we look to the studies of SSRIs that use statistical adjustment to account for depressive symptoms, and other studies of SSRIs that evaluate outcomes such as falls and fractures. Most studies of SSRIs have used a standardized self-measure of depressive symptoms (SF-12 or SF-36, Center for Epidemiologic Studies 10-item Depression scale, Back Depression Inventory, Geriatric Depression Scale, and others). Williams et al. assessed all participants in their study with a structured clinical interview, a more rigorous method for diagnosing clinical depression, then adjusted for presence of either past or current depression that met DSM-IV diagnostic criteria when evaluating the impact of SSRIs on BMD [38]. Analyzing only those with lifetime history of depression, the SSRI users had 5.6% lower BMD at the femoral neck, 6.2% lower at the trochanter, and 4.4% lower at the mid-forearm ($p = 0.03$) than non-users [43].

Of concern remains the unclear association between SSRIs and fall risk. This open question continues to confound studies that are incompletely able to account for falls in the statistical analysis. On the one hand, some studies show an increase in falls among SSRI users, compared to other types of antidepressants, namely TCAs [5,81,86–88]. Other studies show equivalent or lower fall risk for SSRIs compared to TCAs [80,82]. Undermining the interpretation of these studies is the failure to clarify the dose of TCA medication, the indication for the antidepressant (TCAs are sometimes used for sleep), and the frailty of the individual patient. In geriatric practice, TCAs are generally avoided because of their side effect profile, and potential for drug–drug interactions [64]. If used at all, they are often given in doses well below those required to treat depression. In addition, SSRIs vary with respect to their inhibitory potency at the 5-HTT. Whether this variation among medications within a class is associated with variation in fall risk has not been studied. An Italian study of patients admitted to home care showed no increased risk for falls with any antidepressant or with SSRIs. This study had a particularly rigorous assessment of medications, self-reported falls within past 90 days, and was adjusted for depressive symptoms as assessed by the Minimum Data Set for Home Care (MDS-HC) [89]. Resolving these remaining questions about SSRIs and their potential contribution to bone loss, falls, and fractures will require additional mechanistic studies as well as further clinical studies that randomize patients to treatment with or without an SSRI and carefully measure and control for depressive symptoms.

IMPLICATIONS FOR SCREENING AND POPULATION HEALTH

The findings summarized above suggest a detrimental effect of SSRI use on bone health. Thus, it is reasonable for clinicians to be vigilant about detection of bone disease in patients who have perturbations in the serotonin system (either because of depression or due to pharmacologic influence on the transporters such as SSRIs). They might consider earlier testing of BMD by dual-energy x-ray absorptiometry (DXA) for patients on these medications as they do for patients taking corticosteroids, depomedroxyprogesterone, or anti-epileptic medications, among others [90].

One additional question is whether there are now adequate data in support of a causal role for SSRIs on bone loss and fracture to recommend bone density testing for patients on SSRIs. In other words, should patients taking SSRIs be systematically evaluated (screening or case finding). The US Preventive Services Task Force (USPSTF) recommendations contribute to screening guidelines across a variety of clinical disciplines and considers "screening" to be the process of detecting disease in those who are otherwise felt to be at average risk. In contrast, "case finding" is the detection of suspected disease based on clinical risk factors or symptoms. Ideally, a screening test should be able to detect disease before it becomes symptomatic, at a time in the disease course when effective treatments are available and acceptable to patients; and the disease must be one that has significant impact on health and well-being [87,91]. Using this approach, the USPSTF has considered and made recommendations on screening for osteoporosis in 2009, but they did not take up the question of new risk factors [92].

The question then becomes whether SSRIs should be considered as a secondary cause of osteoporosis. If so, clinicians would be prompted to evaluate for low bone density in those taking SSRIs, a case finding approach for detection of osteoporosis akin to what is done for glucocorticoid users. The National Osteoporosis Foundation (NOF) issued revised guidelines that suggest that early diagnostic testing and treatment should be considered for those patients with lifestyle characteristics that suggest increased risk for fracture [93]. Pertinent to this discussion, depression is included on the list of medical conditions that confer increased risk for both osteoporosis/fractures and falls; psychotropic medications are included with medications that cause oversedation as a medical risk factor for falls. SSRIs are not included on the NOF list of medications that cause or contribute to osteoporosis and fractures independently of sedation. It seems reasonable based on the current evidence that SSRIs might warrant inclusion on the list of medications that contribute directly to osteoporosis. Conservatively, one could certainly argue that patients taking SSRIs should have at least some discussion about bone health with their provider. Recommendations for measurement and replacement of vitamin D, supplementation with calcium, and recommendations for exercise also seem reasonable. It is too early to suggest that all SSRI users be tested with DXA (in the absence of other risk factors). That question would need to be addressed with clinical trials assessing whether screening with DXA improves outcomes over usual care—usual care in this case could include measuring/replacing vitamin D, supplementing with calcium and recommending exercise as described above, or doing nothing. Additional research should also strive to inform the essential risk—benefit discussions between patients and providers about medications.

CONCLUSION

The past decade has seen a tremendous growth in the field of neuroendocrine signaling in bone. Indeed, we are beginning to understand the specific mechanisms and clinical implications of neuroendocrine signaling, and questions in this area will define an important research agenda for years to come. Efforts to confirm the serotonergic effects on bone, the biochemical pathways utilized, and the feedback loops involved among bone, gut, and brain are under way. Additional work is needed in many areas that will inform the clinical implications of 5-HT signaling in bone—including how to counsel patients starting SSRIs and how to manage those with osteoporosis whose depressive disease requires use of an SSRI. An important clinical implication of the work on 5-HT signaling through LRP-5 is the potential for identifying novel therapeutic targets. This work will undoubtedly affect the way we consider serotonin and bone in the future.

References

[1] Bliziotes M, et al. Neurotransmitter action in osteoblasts: expression of a functional system for serotonin receptor activation and reuptake. Bone 2001;29(5):477—86.

[2] Westbroek I, et al. Expression of serotonin receptors in bone. J Biol Chem 2001;276(31):28961—8.

[3] Rosen CJ. Serotonin rising —the bone, brain, bowel connection 10.1056/NEJMp0810058. N Engl J Med 2009;360(10):957—9.

[4] Rosen CJ. Breaking into bone biology: serotonin's secrets. Nat Med 2009;15(2):145—6.

[5] Yadav VK, et al. Lrp5 Controls bone formation by inhibiting serotonin synthesis in the duodenum. Cell 2008;135(5):825—37.

[6] Gershon MD, Tack J. The serotonin signaling system: from basic understanding to drug development for functional GI disorders. Gastroenterology 2007;132(1):397—414.

[7] Battaglino R, et al. Serotonin regulates osteoclast differentiation through its transporter. J Bone Miner Res 2004;19(9):1420—31.

[8] Bliziotes MM, et al. Serotonin transporter and receptor expression in osteocytic MLO-Y4 cells. Bone 2006;39(6):1313—21.

[9] Gustafsson BI, et al. Serotonin and fluoxetine modulate bone cell function in vitro. J Cell Biochem 2006;98(1):139—51.

[10] Warden SJ, et al. Inhibition of the serotonin (5-hydroxytryptamine) transporter reduces bone accrual during growth. Endocrinology 2005;146(2):685—93.

[11] Cui Y, et al. Lrp5 functions in bone to regulate bone mass. Nat Med 17(6):684—91

[12] Frost M, et al. Patients with high-bone-mass phenotype owing to <I>Lrp5-T253I</I> mutation have low plasma levels of serotonin. J Bone Min Res 2010;25(3):673—5.

[13] Mödder UI, et al. Relation of serum serotonin levels to bone density and structural parameters in women. J Bone Min Res 2010;25(2):415—22.

[14] Saarinen A, et al. Low density lipoprotein receptor-related protein 5 (LRP5) mutations and osteoporosis, impaired glucose metabolism and hypercholesterolaemia. Clin Endocrinol 72(4):481—8

[15] Yadav VK, Ducy P. Lrp5 and bone formation. Ann NY Acad Sci 2010;1192(Skeletal Biology and Medicine):103—9.

[16] Bago M, Dean C. Sympathoinhibition from ventrolateral periaqueductal gray mediated by 5-HT$_{1A}$ receptors in the RVLM. Am J Physiol 2001;280:R976—84.

[17] Nalivaiko E, Sgoifo A. Central 5-HT receptors in cardiovascular control during stress. Neurosci Biobehav Rev 2009;33(2):95—106.

[18] Yadav VK, Karsenty G. Leptin-dependent co-regulation of bone and energy metabolism. Aging 2009;1(11):954—6.

[19] Andrade S, et al. Use of antidepressant medications during pregnancy. Am J Obstet Gynecol 2008;198(194):e1—5.

[20] Gavin N. Perinatal depression: a systematic review of prevalence and incidence. Obstet Gynecol 2005;106(5 Pt 1):1071—83.

[21] Widdowson E, Southgate D, Hey E. Fetal growth and body composition. Perinatal Nutrition. In: Lindblad BS, editors. New York: Academic Press; 1988.

[22] Bonnin A, et al. A transient placental source of serotonin for the fetal forebrain. Nature 2011;472(7343):347—50.

[23] Hendrick V, et al. Birth outcomes after prenatal exposure to antidepressant medication. Am J Obstet Gynecol 2003;188(3):812—5.

[24] Kornum JB, et al. Use of selective serotonin-reuptake inhibitors during early pregnancy and risk of congenital malformations: updated analysis. Clin Epidemiol 2010;2:29—36.

[25] Louik C, et al. First-trimester use of selective serotonin-reuptake inhibitors and the risk of birth defects. N Engl J Med 2007;356(26):2675—83.

[26] Pedersen L, et al. Selective serotonin reuptake inhibitors in pregnancy and congenital malformations: population based cohort study. BMJ 2009:339. b3569.

[27] Dubnov-Raz G, et al. Maternal use of selective serotonin reuptake inhibitors during pregnancy and neonatal bone density. Early Hum Develop 2011;88(3):191—4.

[28] Maciag D, et al. Neonatal antidepressant exposure has lasting effects on behavior and serotonin circuitry. Neuropsychopharmacology 2006;31(1):47—57.

[29] Pawluski JL, et al. Neonatal S100B protein levels after prenatal exposure to selective serotonin reuptake inhibitors. Pediatrics 2009;124(4):e662—70.

[30] Haskell SE, et al. Neonatal SSRI exposure increases sympathetic tone in adult mice (abstract). In: Pediatric Endocrine Society. Denver: Colorado; 2011.

[31] Gafni R, Baron J. Childhood bone mass acquisition and peak bone mass may not be important determinants of bone mass in late adulthood. Pediatrics 2007;119(Suppl. 2):S131—6.

[32] Gu Q, Dillon C, Burt V. NCHS data brief: prescription drug use continues to increase: U.S. Prescription Drug Data for 2007—2008. Statistics NCH. Hyattsville, MD: National Center for Health Statistics; 2010.

[33] Weintrob N, et al. Decreased growth during therapy with selective serotonin reuptake inhibitors 10.1001/archpedi.156.7.696. Arch Pediatr Adolesc Med 2002;156(7):696—701.

[34] Emslie GJ, et al. Fluoxetine for acute treatment of depression in children and adolescents: a placebo-controlled, randomized

clinical trial. J Am Acad Child & Adolesc Psychiatry 2002; 41(10):1205—15.

[35] Nilsson M, et al. Safety of subchronic treatment with fluoxetine for major depressive disorder in children and adolescents. J Child Adolesc Psychopharmacol 2004;14(3):412—7.

[36] Yang L, Grey V. Pediatric reference intervals for bone markers. Clin Biochem 2006;39(6):561—8.

[37] Warden SJ, et al. Neural regulation of bone and the skeletal effects of serotonin (5-hydroxytryptamine). Mol Cell Endocrinol 2005;242(1—2):1—9.

[38] Calarge C, Kuperman S. Fluoxetine for depression relapse prevention. J Am Acad Child & Adolesc Psychiatry 2005; 44(10):966—7. authors' reply 967—8.

[39] Calarge C, et al. A cross-sectional evaluation of the effect of risperidone and selective serotonin reuptake inhibitors on bone mineral density in boys. J Clin Psychiatry 2010;71: 338—47.

[40] Calarge C, et al. Variants of the serotonin transporter gene, selective serotonin reuptake inhibitors, and bone mineral density in risperidone-treated boys: a reanalysis of data from a cross-sectional study with emphasis on pharmacogenetics. J Clin Psychiatry 2011;72:1685—90.

[41] Richards JB, et al. The impact of selective serotonin reuptake inhibitors on the risk of fracture. Arch Intern Med 2007; 167(2):188—94.

[42] Haney EM, et al. Association of low bone mineral density with selective serotonin reuptake inhibitor use by older men. Arch Intern Med 2007;167(12):1246—51.

[43] Williams LJ, et al. Selective serotonin reuptake inhibitor use and bone mineral density in women with a history of depression. Int Clin Pscyhopharmacol 2008;23:84—7.

[44] Diem S, et al. Use of antidepressants and rates of hip bone loss in older women: the study of osteoporotic fractures. Arch Intern Med 2007;167(12):1240—5.

[45] Spangler L, et al. Depressive symptoms, bone loss, and fractures in postmenopausal women. J Gen Intern Med 2008;23(5): 567—74.

[46] Haney EM, et al. SSRI use is associated with increased risk of fracture among older men. JBMR 2007;22(Suppl. 1):s45.

[47] Lewis CE, et al. Predictors of non-spine fracture in elderly men: the MrOS Study. J Bone Min Res 2007;22(2):211—9.

[48] Ensrud KE, et al. Central nervous system active medications and risk for fractures in older women. Arch Intern Med 2003;163:949—57.

[49] Ziere G, et al. Selective serotonin reuptake inhibiting antidepressants are associated with an increased risk of nonvertebral fractures. J Clin Psychopharmacol 2008;28:411—7.

[50] Abrahamsen B, Brixen K. Mapping the prescriptiome to fractures in men—a national analysis of prescription history and fracture risk. Osteoporos Int 2009;20(4):585—97.

[51] Vestergaard P, Rejnmark L, Mosekilde L. Anxiolytics, sedatives, antidepressants, neuroleptics and the risk of fracture. Osteoporos Int 2006;17:807.

[52] van den Brand M, et al. Use of anti-depressants and the risk of fracture of the hip or femur. Osteoporos Int 2009;20(10): 1705—13.

[53] Verdel BM, et al. Use of antidepressant drugs and risk of osteoporotic and non-osteoporotic fractures. Bone 2010;47(3): 604—9.

[54] Bolton JM, et al. Fracture risk from psychotropic medications: a population-based analysis. J Clin Psychopharmacol 2008; 28(4):384—91.

[55] Liu B, et al. Use of selective serotonin-reuptake inhibitors or tricyclic antidepressants and risk of hip fractures in elderly people. Lancet 1998;351:1303—7.

[56] Gagne JJ, et al. Antidepressants and fracture risk in older adults: a comparative safety analysis. Clin Pharmacol Ther 2011;89(6):880—7.

[57] Ray WA, et al. Psychotropic drug use and the risk of hip fracture. N Engl J Med 1987;316(7):363—9.

[58] French DD, et al. Outpatient medications and hip fractures in the US: a national veterans study. Drugs & Aging 2005; 22(10):877—85.

[59] Hulley SB, et al. Designing clinical research. 2nd ed. Philadelphia, PA: Lippincott Williams & Wilkins; 2001.

[60] Warden SJ, et al. Serotonin (5-hydroxytryptamine) transporter inhibition causes bone loss in adult mice independently of estrogen deficiency. Menopause 2008;15(6): 1176—83.

[61] Eom C-S, et al. Use of selective serotonin reuptake inhibitors and risk of fracture: a systematic review and meta-analysis. J Bone Min Res 2012.

[62] Wu Q, et al. Selective serotonin reuptake inhibitor treatment and risk of fractures: a meta-analysis of cohort and case—control studies. Osteoporos Int 2012;23:365—75.

[63] Meyer JH, et al. Occupancy of serotonin transporters by paroxetine and citalopram during treatment of depression: a [11C]DASB PET imaging study. Am J Psychiatry 2001; 158(11):1843—9.

[64] Hubbard R, et al. Exposure to tricyclic and selective serotonin reuptake inhibitor antidepressants and the risk of hip fracture. Am J Epidemiol 2003;158(1):77—84.

[65] Psaty B, et al. Assessment and control for confounding by indication in observational studies. J Am Geriatr Soc 1997; 47(6):749—54.

[66] Coelho WS, Costa KC, Sola-Penna M. Serotonin stimulates mouse skeletal muscle 6-phosphofructo-1-kinase through tyrosine-phosphorylation of the enzyme altering its intracellular localization. Mol Gen Metab 2007;92(4): 364—70.

[67] Diem SJ, et al. Depressive symptoms and rates of bone loss at the hip in older women. J Am Geriatr Soc 2007;55:824—31.

[68] Eskandari F, et al. Low bone mass in premenopausal women with depression. Arch Int Med 2007;167(21):2329—36.

[69] Jacka FN, et al. Depression and bone mineral density in a community sample of perimenopausal women: Geelong Osteoporosis Study. Menopause 2005;12(1):88—91.

[70] Mussolino ME. Depression and hip fracture risk: the NHANES I Epidemiologic Follow-up Study. Public Health Reports 2005; 120(1):71—5.

[71] Robbins J, et al. The association of bone mineral density and depression in an older population. J Am Geriatr Soc 2001;49:732—6.

[72] Silverman SL, et al. Prevalence of depressive symptoms in postmenopausal women with low bone mineral density and/or prevalent vertebral fracture: results from the Multiple Outcomes of Raloxifene Evaluation (MORE) study. J Rheumatol 2007;34(1):140—4.

[73] Wong SYS, et al. Depression and bone mineral density: is there a relationship in elderly Asian men? Results from Mr. Os (Hong Kong). Osteoporos Int 2005;16:610—5.

[74] Reginster JY, et al. Depressive vulnerability is not an independent risk factor for osteoporosis in postmenopausal women. Maturitas 1999;33:133—7.

[75] Sogaard AJ, et al. Long-term mental distress, bone mineral density and non-vertebral fractures. The Tromso Study. Osteoporos Int 2005;16(8):887—97.

[76] Whooley MA, et al. Depressive symptoms and bone mineral density in older men. J Geriatr Psychiatry Neurol 2004; 17(2):88—92.

[77] Whooley MA, et al. Depression, falls, and risk of fracture in older women. Arch Intern Med 1999;159:484—90.

[78] Mezuk B, Eaton W, Golden S. Depression and osteoporosis: epidemiology and potential mediating pathways. Osteoporos Int 2008;19(1):1—12.

[79] Yimiya R, Bab I. Major depression is a risk factor for low bone mineral density: a meta-analysis. Biological Psychiatry 2009;66(5):423—32.

[80] Ensrud KE, et al. Central nervous system-active medications and risk for falls in older women. J Am Geriatr Soc 2002; 50:1629—37.

[81] Kerse N, et al. Falls, depression, and antidepressants in later life: a large primary care appraisal. PlosONE 2008;3(6): e2423.

[82] Thapa PB, et al. Antidepressants and the risk of falls among nursing home residents. N Engl J Med 1998;339(13):875—82.

[83] Whitson HE, et al. Depressive symptomatology and fracture risk in community-dwelling older men and women. Aging Clin Exp Res 2008;20:585—92.

[84] Forsen L, et al. Mental distress and risk of hip fracture. Do broken hearts lead to broken bones? J Epidemiol Comm Health 1999;53:343—7.

[85] Tolea MI, et al. Depressive symptoms as a risk factor for osteoporosis and fractures in older Mexican American women. Osteoporos Int 2007;18:315—22.

[86] French DD, et al. Drugs and falls in community-dwelling older people: a national veterans study. Clinical Therapeutics 2006;28(4):619—30.

[87] Hartikainen S, Lonnroos E, Louhivuori K. Medication as a risk factor for falls: critical systematic review. J Gerontol: MEDICAL SCIENCES 2007;62A(10):1172—81.

[88] Sterke CS, et al. The influence of drug use on fall incidents among nursing home residents: a systematic review doi: 10.1017/S104161020800714X. Int Psychogeriatr 2008;20(05): 890—910.

[89] Landi F, et al. Psychotropic medications and risk for falls among community-dwelling frail older people: an observational study. J Gerontol A Biol Sci Med Sci 2005;60(5):622—6.

[90] Chau K, Atkinson SA, Taylor VH. Are selective serotonin reuptake inhibitors a secondary cause of low bone density? J Osteoporos 2012. 2012: Article ID 323061, 7 pages.

[91] Harris RP, et al. Current methods of the U.S. Preventive Services Task Force: a review of the process. Am J Prevent Med 2001;3(Suppl. 1):21—35.

[92] U.S. Preventive Services Task Force, Screening for Osteoporosis: U.S. Preventive Services Task Force Recommendation Statement. Ann Int Med 154(5):356—64

[93] National Osteoporosis Foundation, Clinician's Guide to Prevention and Treatment of Osteoporosis. Washington, DC: BoneSource; 2009.

Significance of Organ Crosstalk in Insulin Resistance and Type 2 Diabetes

S. Bhatt, R.N. Kulkarni

Harvard Medical School, Boston, MA, USA

INTRODUCTION

Diabetes Mellitus—Classification

The current classification of diabetes mellitus (DM) was developed in 1997 by the American Diabetes Association (ADA) and the World Health Organization (WHO). Four distinct categories are recognized: [1] type 1 diabetes (T1D)—characterized by β-cell destruction that usually leads to absolute insulin deficiency; [2] type 2 diabetes (T2D)—which ranges from a predominant insulin resistance with relative insulin deficiency to a predominant secretory defect in pancreatic β-cells along with insulin resistance; [3] other specific DM types—including genetic β-cell function defects, exocrine pancreas diseases, endocrinopathies, drug or chemical-induced diabetes and infections and genetic syndromes associated with diabetes; and [4] gestational diabetes mellitus (GDM).

Pathogenesis of Type 2 Diabetes Mellitus

The world prevalence of T2D today is estimated to be 6.4% (285 million adults) and is expected to increase to >400 million people worldwide by the year 2030 [16]. The increasing incidence of T2D finds its origin in the global obesity epidemic worsened by physical inactivity and high-calorie diets. The links between excess calorie intake and diabetes has been extensively studied and although overfeeding almost universally leads to insulin resistance and frequently to obesity-related conditions (hypertension, cardiovascular disease, non-alcoholic fatty liver disease, polycystic ovarian syndrome), the incidence of T2D is evident in genetically predisposed individuals (with inherited secretory and glucose sensing defects in pancreatic β cells) whose pancreatic β cells fail to adapt over time to the nutrient overload (Fig. 17.1).

Glucose homeostasis is maintained by counter-regulatory actions of insulin, secreted by pancreatic islet β-cells, and glucagon, secreted by pancreatic islet alpha cells. While the primary role of insulin is to facilitate glucose uptake by peripheral tissues (muscle and bone—for use as energy/ATP source; adipose—converted to fatty acids for long-term storage; liver—converted to glycogen for short-term storage), glucagon acts via opposing mechanisms of stimulating glucose production by liver through increased gluconeogenesis (glucose synthesis) and glycogenolysis (breakdown of glycogen into glucose). Therefore, to maintain normoglycemia, hepatic glucose production and insulin-mediated glucose disposal act in concert [17,18].

In individuals with normal glucose tolerance, hepatic glucose production is counterbalanced by insulin-mediated glucose uptake by canonical insulin target tissues like liver, adipose, and muscle, and also non-canonical insulin target tissues such as β cells, brain, bone, vascular endothelium, etc. Upon glucose exposure (e.g. ingestion of a meal), endocrine and neural signals are transmitted from the gut to the endocrine pancreas, leading to an immediate decline in glucagon secretion by pancreatic α cells and a stimulation of insulin secretion by β cells leading to glucose uptake. This process occurs in two phases; in the first phase which takes approximately 10 minutes after a meal, β cells release stored insulin, resulting in a sharp rise in plasma insulin levels followed by a decline to near basal levels; the second phase lasts several hours, wherein β cells produce and release additional insulin [19–23].

When glucose tolerance is abnormal, patterns of insulin and glucagon secretion are disrupted. It has been estimated that glucagon is responsible for up to 75% of hepatic glucose production. When glucagon levels fail to decrease, hepatic glucose production remains elevated. When coupled with diminished glucose uptake

PATHOPHYSIOLOGY OF TYPE 2 DIABETES MELLITUS (T2D)

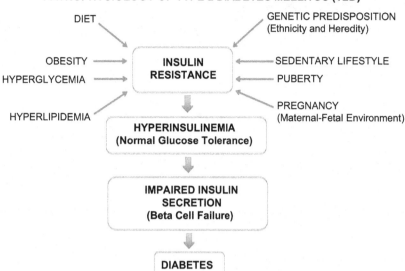

FIGURE 17.1   T2D results from a failure of the beta cell to compensate for the ambient insulin resistance leading to uncontrolled hyperglycemia.

by peripheral tissues due to defects in insulin secretion, the result is hyperglycemia, a potential cause for islet dysfunction and β-cell failure leading to diabetes. Understanding the underlying molecular mechanisms that lead to β-cell failure and identifying key players regulating the process will help unravel novel pathways for the identification of targets that can be used for pharmacological intervention in the treatment, prevention, or delay of the onset of this metabolic disorder [24,25].

Insulin Signaling Cascade

Insulin, a 51-amino acid peptide, is the key hormone responsible for maintaining glucose homeostasis. The action of insulin is initiated by binding to its cognate receptor and activation of the receptor's intrinsic protein tyrosine kinase activity, resulting in the phosphorylation of tyrosine residues located in the cytoplasmic face. The activated receptor, in turn, recruits and phosphorylates a panel of substrates, with insulin receptor substrate-1 (IRS1) and IRS2 being the prominent adapter proteins playing a major role in the coupling to the downstream kinases phosphatidylinositol 3-kinase (PI3K)—protein kinase B(PKB) and MAPK. Tyrosine phosphorylated IRS1/2 recruit the heterodimeric p85/p110 PI3K at the plasma membrane, where it produces the lipid second messenger PIP3, which, in turn, activates a serine/threonine phosphorylation cascade of PH domain-containing proteins. PIP3 targets include PDK1, the serine/threonine protein kinase B (PKB)/Akt, and the atypical protein kinase C, ζ, and λ isoforms [26—38].

Mechanistically, PDK1, Akt, and aPKCs, all of which contain a PH domain, are recruited at the plasma membrane by binding to PIP3; thereafter, PDK1

phosphorylates Akt and aPKCs on a threonine residue located in the activation loop of the catalytic domain, causing their activation. Major targets of activated Akt are GSK-3 and AS160. Upon Akt-mediated phosphorylation on Ser-9, GSK-3 is inactivated. This inactivation, parallel to protein phosphatase-1 (PP1) activation, relieves the inhibitory phosphorylation of glycogen synthase (GS), which becomes activated and promotes glycogen synthesis. Akt also regulates the insulin-stimulated translocation of the glucose transporter GLUT-4 at the plasma membrane, resulting in increased glucose uptake. This pathway involves an inhibitory phosphorylation of the RabGTPase activating protein AS160. Inhibition of AS160 favors the GTP-loaded state of Rab and relieves an inhibitory effect towards GLUT-4 translocation from intracellular compartments to the plasma membrane. In addition to the role of Akt in controlling GLUT-4 translocation, aPKCs act in parallel and can even substitute for Akt [39].

In a parallel pathway, activated IRS1/2 recruit Grb2, which associates to SOS and activates the ERK1/2 MAPK pathway (Fig. 17.2). Overall, alterations of the activation status of the proximal insulin signaling enzymes (IR, IRS1/2, PI3K), and downstream targets (PDK, Akt, and its targets GSK3B and AS160, aPKCs, and MAPK-family protein kinases) have been studied in canonical insulin target tissues such as muscle, liver, and adipose from insulin resistant, obese, and T2D subjects, and the underlying insulin resistance has been attributed to defects in one or more steps of the insulin signaling cascade [18,40,41].

A majority of the recent advances in the understanding of the molecular pathways underlying insulin signaling have been made possible by gene targeting

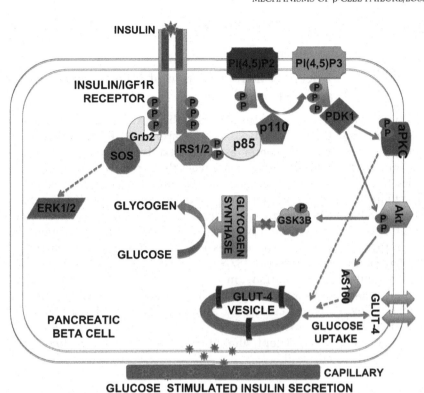

FIGURE 17.2 A typical schematic of the insulin signaling cascade involved in the regulation of glucose uptake and insulin secretion. Please see color plate section.

technology, wherein investigators have been able to create homozygous-null mutant mice to examine the effects of the total or partial lack of a particular gene product, overexpression of the native or mutant protein in the whole organism or in a cell-specific manner. To address this scientific question, many laboratories have been involved in generating tissue-specific monogenic and/or polygenic deletions, in addition to the previously studied global deletions of various genes that code for proteins with critical functions in regulating insulin and non-insulin-dependent glucose homeostasis [37,38,42–63]. The availability of these models has allowed investigators to attribute the resultant phenotype to reflect the physiological function of that particular gene product *in vivo*. Consequently, over the last decade, genetic engineering approaches have allowed the focus of research to extend beyond understanding the insulin signaling pathways not only in the classical insulin target tissues (muscle, liver, and adipose) [64], but also in non-classical cells types such as the islet cells, the neuronal cells, and the osteoblasts.

MECHANISMS OF β-CELL FAILURE/LOSS

Effects of Hyperglycemia

Blood glucose level is one of the determinants of the regulation of β-cell mass and function [65,66].

Transient increases in glucose levels within the physiological range induce insulin secretion and potentially beneficial signals. In contrast, glucotoxicity induced by prolonged hyperglycemia causes β-cell dysfunction and altered β-cell mass [67,68]. The effects of chronic hyperglycemia in β cells have been assessed in animal models and *in vitro* using insulinoma cells and isolated islets. In the setting of chronic exposure to hyperglycemia, rat islets exhibit basal insulin hypersecretion and defective glucose stimulated insulin secretion (GSIS) [69–71]. In animal models and humans, chronic hyperglycemia is associated with alterations in β-cell mass and function. The β cell has an incredible capacity to adapt and compensate for chronic hyperglycemia, as seen in the Zucker diabetic fatty (ZDF) rat, but ultimately, obesity, chronic hyperglycemia, and worsening insulin resistance lead to increased β-cell apoptosis [45,65,72–80].

Among the suggested mechanisms of glucotoxicity include mitochondrial dysfunction and production of reactive oxygen species (ROS), endoplasmic reticulum (ER) stress, and increased levels of intracellular calcium. Chronically increased glucose concentrations in the blood cause increased glucose metabolism through oxidative phosphorylation. This ultimately leads to mitochondrial dysfunction and increased production of ROS [81]. Several lines of evidence suggest that this is an important mechanism for the induction of β-cell dysfunction. β cells have a limited defense against excess ROS production due to low levels of ROX-detoxifying enzymes [82]. Consistent with this, markers of oxidative stress are significantly higher in the islets of type 2 diabetes compared with those from controls, and the levels of these markers correlate with the degree of impairment of GSIS [80]. Interestingly, overexpression of antioxidant enzymes in isolated islets resulting in decreased levels of ROS prevents islet dysfunction in conditions that mimic prolonged hyperglycemia. Also, improved β-cell function in db/db mice and ZDF rats treated with antioxidant agents such as n-acetylcysteine or aminoguanidine provide further evidence for the role of oxidative stress in the deleterious effects of chronic hyperglycemia [81,83]. A similar improvement in β-cell function was observed in isolated islets from diabetic patients treated with antioxidant agents [84]. Although the precise molecular mechanism(s) for the regulation of β-cell mass and function by ROS are not well understood, it is known that the generation of ROS will ultimately activate stress-induced pathways, including nuclear factor kB (NF-kB), c-Jun N-terminal kinase (JNK), and hexosamines. The activation of JNK signaling after induction of oxidative stress inhibits IRS1 signaling by phosphorylation of IRS1 on Ser^{307} [31], as does the nutrient-regulated mTOR/S6K signaling pathway. The biological and physiological effects of this feedback regulation are not clear, but modulation of mTOR/S6K could be implicated in the adaptive response of β cells to nutrient excess. However, there is no direct evidence suggesting that this mechanism is part of signaling events induced by glucotoxicity. In summary, there is some knowledge of the signaling pathways induced by chronic hyperglycemia; however, the downstream events and targets governing the effects of glucotoxicity have not been completely elucidated.

Effects of Hyperlipidemia

Dyslipidemia characterized by an increase in circulating free fatty acids (FFA) is one of the major abnormalities in the lipid profile of patients with diabetes. Experiments in humans suggest that elevation of FFA in healthy individuals has stimulatory effects on insulin secretion, but may contribute to progressive β-cell failure in some individuals with a genetic predisposition to diabetes [85,86]. In vitro experiments using isolated islets demonstrated toxic effects of fatty acids on insulin secretion and apoptosis [87]. It is noteworthy that several in vitro experiments have been performed using concomitant high glucose concentrations. The current evidence, therefore, suggests that the deleterious effects of lipids are observed predominantly in the presence of

high glucose, discussed in greater detail in the next section.

Effects of a Combination of Hyperglycemia and Hyperlipidemia

In the process of glucolipotoxicity, toxic actions of FFA on tissues become apparent in the context of hyperglycemia as described by Prentki et al. [88]. Studies in humans reveal that lipid infusion in type 2 diabetic patients causes impaired insulin secretion [89]. Long-term exposure of islets or insulin-secreting cells to increased levels of fatty acids is associated with inhibition of GSIS in vitro [90], impairment of insulin gene expression, and induction of cell death by apoptosis [87,89]. Notably, reducing plasma FFA concentrations in type 2 diabetics with the niacin derivative acipimox was associated with enhanced insulin sensitivity and improvement in oral glucose tolerance tests [68]. These and other findings support the concept that FFA alters β-cell function and survival.

Several mechanisms by which glucolipotoxicity impairs GSIS have been postulated. One of the proposed mechanisms for glucolipotoxicity is the inhibition of FFA oxidation by elevated glucose [88]. In the setting of hyperglycemia and elevated FFA, glucose metabolism results in elevated levels of malonyl CoA, a known inhibitor of carnitine palmitoyl transferase-1 (CPT1). The inhibition of CPT1 decreases fatty acid oxidation, which causes accumulation of elevated cytosolic long-chain acyl CoA esters, generation of ceramide and lipid partitioning [68]. Previous experiments have shown that long-chain acyl-CoA esters result in β-cell dysfunction. Studies also suggest that AMP-activated protein kinase (AMPK) activity may play a role in glucolipotoxicity. AMPK activation promotes fatty acid oxidation by phosphorylation and inhibition of acetyl-CoA carboxylase or via downregulation of the transcription factor sterol-regulatory-element-binding-protein-1c (SREBP1c) [82,91–93]. In addition to affecting insulin secretion, glucolipotoxicity can decrease insulin gene expression by alterations in Pdx1 and MafA binding to the insulin promoter, thereby causing β-cell dysfunction and eventually apoptosis.

Another possible mechanism by which FFA may impair β-cell function involves the expression of uncoupling protein-2 (UCP2), part of the UCP family of proteins, which act to regulate cellular ATP production [94,95]. Previous studies have shown that chronic exposure of islets or insulinoma cell lines to elevated FFA cause increased UCP2 expression and UCP−/− mice are protected from impaired β-cell function [96]. The mechanisms by which UCP2 may play a role in β-cell failure is yet undefined. Some studies have suggested increased UCP2 expression leading to increased ROS production as a possible mechanism, but this has not been reproduced nor have antioxidants been shown to cause any benefit in restoring impaired GSIS in lipid-exposed islets. Recently, the ATP-binding cassette transporter subfamily A member 1 (ABCA1), a mediator of reverse cholesterol efflux, was shown to be an important mediator of the effects of FFA on insulin secretion. Conditional deletion of ABCA1 results in increased cellular cholesterol content and impaired insulin secretion at the level of exocytosis [97].

As discussed above, multiple studies have shown that fatty acids can induce β-cell death by apoptosis and that this effect is potentiated by glucose [89]. Several mechanisms have been proposed to mediate fatty acid-induced apoptosis in β cells, including ceramide formation leading to altered lipid partitioning, and the generation of ROS. More recently, ER stress and the unfolded protein response, discussed in greater detail in the next section, have received experimental support [98,99]. In addition to these processes, apoptosis after fatty acid administration can result from the activation of the JNK pathway and decreased Akt signaling with subsequent activation of the Foxo-1-dependent gene expression [98]. While the exact mechanisms are not delineated, it is conceivable that the combination of elevated FFA and chronic hyperglycemia synergize to create a milieu conducive to β-cell dysfunction and failure (Fig. 17.3).

Endoplasmic Reticulum (ER) Stress

ER stress is an important contributor of β-cell failure in T2D and has been postulated to result from increased biosynthetic demand induced by chronic hyperglycemia, elevated FFA, and chronic overnutrition. Recent evidence suggests that ER stress links obesity with insulin resistance [100,101]. Studies in humans and rodent models provide evidence for ER stress in islets from type 2 diabetics by increased staining for ER chaperones and CHOP along with increased ER size. Additionally, in rodents, increased ER stress markers have been demonstrated in mouse islets from db/db mice [99,102,103]. Insulin-2 mutations in Akita mice induce accumulation of misfolded insulin and progressive β-cell loss caused by ER stress, demonstrating the importance of this pathway in β-cell survival. Taken together, these data suggest that ER stress is present in β cells and that this could be a common underlying mechanism for the two major pathophysiological events in T2D, insulin resistance and β-cell failure.

ER stress pathway is best understood in the context of the unfolded protein response (UPR), which alleviates ER stress, restores homeostasis, and prevents cell death by inducing a number of downstream responses such as: [1] decrease new protein influx into ER; [2] increase in

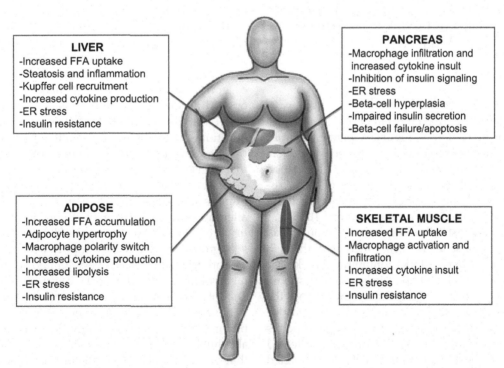

FIGURE 17.3 Mechanism of systemic insulin resistance and obesity induced β-cell failure. Please see color plate section.

the amount of ER chaperones to improve folding capacity; and [3] increase the cell's capacity to dispose misfolded proteins. The three primary modulators of UPR are: inositol requiring protein-1 alpha (IRE1-alpha), activating transcription factor 6 (ATF6), and protein kinase RNA (PRK)-like ER associated kinase (PERK) [104]. Under normal conditions these sensory proteins remain inactive via interaction with the ER chaperone BiP until activated by increased ER stress, eventually concluding with cell death [91,105−112].

The molecular mechanisms by which FFA and gluco-lipotoxicity-induced ER stress cause β-cell apoptosis are not clear. In addition to induction of CHOP, ER stress can induce apoptosis by induction of JNK, ATF-3 and inhibition of Bcl-2 and/or activation of proapoptotic members of the Bcl-2 family [113]. Mechanistically, activation of JNK could lead to suppression of IRS/Akt signaling through serine phosphorylation of IRS-1 in liver and β cells [114], which in turn reduces survival signals and ultimately leads to apoptosis. Recently, an important link between ER stress and IRS-2 signaling was revealed by transcriptional repression of the IRS-2 promoter by ATF3. While the exact mechanisms of ER stress-mediated apoptosis still need to be unraveled, there is ample evidence to suggest that cumulative damage from hyperglycemia, overnutrition and elevated FFA levels overwhelm the ER in β cells, resulting in activation of the UPR and eventually leading to apoptosis and β-cell failure.

INSULIN RESISTANCE—MULTIORGAN CROSSTALK OF INSULIN TARGET TISSUES

Canonical Insulin Target Tissues

Adipose, Liver, and Skeletal Muscle

The adipocyte is a dynamic endocrine organ and nutrient sensor that tightly regulates energy supply. When nutrient supply exceeds adipose tissue adaptation, adipocyte hypertrophy and other poorly understood factors set off a pathologic adipocyte−macrophage crosstalk [115−117]. Following this, the endoplasmic reticulum (ER) triggers the unfolded protein response (UPR) as a protective mechanism, leading to activation of an inflammatory response in fat cells, mediated through c-Jun N-terminal kinase (JNK), inhibitor kB kinase (IKK)/nuclear factor kB (NFkB), cyclic AMP response element binding protein H (CREBH, promoting the secretion of acute-phase proteins such as C-reactive protein), and production of reactive oxygen species (ROS) [118]. Furthermore, this metabolic stress is followed by the release of a host of adipokines (cytokines secreted by adipocytes) capable of causing local paracrine effects

(i.e. on macrophages) and more distal endocrine effects such as muscle and liver insulin resistance (i.e. tumor necrosis factor-α or TNF-α, interleukin-1, 6, and 8, resistin, monocyte chemoattractant protein-1 or MCP-1, plasminogen activator protein-1, visfatin, angiotensinogen, retinol-binding protein-4, serum amyloid A, transforming growth factor-β or TGF-β, and others) [119−124]. Infiltration of these activated macrophages promotes adipose tissue insulin resistance, excessive chronic release of FFA, and ectopic fat deposition ultimately resulting in adipocyte tissue hypoxia, and consequentially, muscle, liver, and pancreatic β-cell dysfunction [125−135].

How Excess FFAs in Adipose Tissue Relate to β-cell Dysfunction

There is a close interaction between FFA and glucose as sources of energy and triggers for insulin secretion. In the fasting state, fatty acids are the primary source of energy, not glucose. This is rapidly reversed upon feeding so that glucose becomes the major source of energy. Glucose is converted through glycolysis to pyruvate and enters the mitochondria to generate energy as ATP through the Krebs cycle. This promotes the formation of citrate, which when transported to the cytoplasm inhibits carnitine palmitoyltransferase-1, the transporter of long-chain fatty acyl-coenzyme As (CoAs) into the mitochondria. This is how malonyl-CoA acts as the "metabolic switch" for insulin secretion between periods of fasting and feeding [72,136]. This background may help in understanding how during times of metabolic excess, accumulation of FFA and lipotoxicity may lead to β-cell failure and T2D.

The concept of pancreatic β-cell lipotoxicity (i.e. chronic excess of fatty acids causing an activation of the NFkB pathway, formation of ROS, and lipid-induced β-cell apoptosis), proposed by Unger et al. [137], in islets of leptin-unresponsive Zucker diabetic fatty (ZDF) rats opened a new perspective on islet cell biology in T2D [133,138,139]. Although the ZDF rat model has been questioned as suboptimal given that their abnormal leptin signaling profoundly alters normal islet fatty acid metabolism, it is now well accepted that a sustained increase in fatty acids for approximately 24 to 48 h impairs glucose-stimulated insulin secretion (GSIS), alters insulin gene expression, and promotes apoptosis *in vitro* and *in vivo*. Pancreatic β cells are particularly susceptible to excess FFA supply because their ability to store triacylglycerol is very limited so that toxic lipid metabolites accumulate (e.g. ceramide, diacylglycerol, and others) and are shunted into harmful metabolic pathways [68]. It has been recently reported that a reduction in β-cell mass or triacylglycerol accumulation is not absolutely necessary for severe β-cell dysfunction but that there is increased glucose-responsive palmitate esterification and lipolysis in islets under lipotoxic conditions, associated with a marked depletion of insulin stores [140].

How Excess FFAs in Adipose Tissue Relate to Muscle Insulin Resistance

In striking similarity to the effect observed in other tissues such as β cells and hepatocytes, excessive FFAs promote the accumulation of intramyocellular lipids (IMCLs) and the formation of a variety of fat-derived potentially toxic lipid metabolites such as ceramide and diacylglycerol, which cause insulin resistance [128,141–145]. Accumulation of IMCLs is not believed to be the cause of insulin resistance, but rather an expression of reduced muscle lipid oxidation (Fig. 17.4).

In transgenic mice, overexpression of diacylglycerol acytransferase (DGAT1), the enzyme that catalyzes the final step in triglyceride synthesis, increases intramyocellular triglyceride content but is protective against lipotoxicity and insulin resistance by increasing mitochondrial fatty acid oxidation and reducing ceramide and DAG concentrations. Patients with T2D and lean subjects with a family history of diabetes (who are typically insulin resistant) have reduced mitochondrial oxidation capacity although the precise mechanisms continue to be subject to considerable debate.

How Excess FFAs in Adipose Tissue Relate to Hepatic Insulin Resistance

Fasting hyperglycemia in T2D is closely correlated to the rate of endogenous glucose production, of which more than 90% arises from glucose production by the liver [141,142]. The increase in endogenous glucose production in T2D is believed to be primarily due to excessive rates of hepatic gluconeogenesis, whereas glycogenolysis autoregulation is better preserved. There is ample evidence that increased plasma FFA concentrations cause hepatic insulin resistance, impair insulin signaling, and stimulate hepatic glucose production by driving both hepatic gluconeogenesis [146] and glycogenolysis [139]. In lean healthy subjects, induction of hepatic insulin resistance is fairly rapid following lipid infusion (within 2–4 h) and correlates closely with the increase in plasma FFA. Adaptation of FFA-induced hepatic insulin resistance in obesity, T2D, and other insulin-resistant states involves an increase in insulin secretion but also a reduction of hepatic insulin clearance that results in peripheral hyperinsulinemia [147–150]. In non-obese normal glucose-tolerant subjects with a family history of diabetes, the ability to adapt to this challenge is diminished and may contribute to the development of T2D [141,142]. One could speculate that over time this could accelerate the

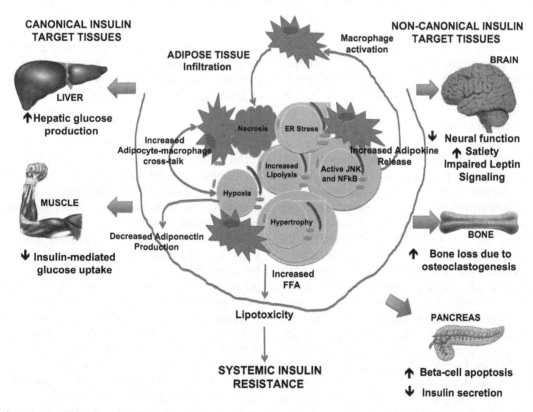

FIGURE 17.4 Multi-level organ crosstalk leading to systemic insulin resistance and obesity induced β-cell failure. Please see color plate section.

progression to T2D in genetically predisposed subjects, in the context of a lipotoxic environment. Taken together, these studies highlight the important role of FFAs on hepatic glucose homeostasis and insulin sensitivity.

NON-CANONICAL INSULIN TARGET TISSUES

Beta Cells, Brain, and Bone

Beta Cells as Endocrine Organs—Role in Insulin Production and Regulation of Glucose Homeostasis

The insulin producing β cells, along with glucagon producing α cells, somatostatin producing δ cells, pancreatic polypeptide producing cells, and ghrelin producing cells, form the microorgan islets of Langerhans. These islets, scattered within the exocrine pancreas and representing approximately 1–2% of total pancreatic volume (suggestive of about one million islets in the human pancreas), are highly vascularized by an extensive endothelial network and innervated by sympathetic, parasympathetic, and sensory nerves. In view of these multi-cellular/tissue connections, it is not surprising that multiple signals orchestrating from different tissues play a collective role in regulating proper functioning of beta cells under both basal and glucose-stimulated conditions. These signals include humoral factors (i.e. hormones, vitamins, nutrients, etc.) and nervous stimulation, as well as factors of intra-islet cell—cell communication (e.g. connexins, cadherins, ephrins). Whereas the paracrine effects of glucagon (stimulatory) and somatostatin (inhibitory) on insulin exocytosis by beta cells are well accepted [41], the auto-crine effect of secreted insulin on beta-cell function has been a matter of debate and still an active area of research. Unlike all other cell types, the pancreatic beta cell is unique in that it continuously secretes insulin: basal secretion under non-stimulatory conditions (e.g. low glucose concentration) and increased secretion under stimulatory conditions (e.g. high glucose concentration). Hence, the major argument that led to the conceptual disagreement, i.e. that beta cells cannot respond to insulin, was that beta cells are constantly exposed to insulin and that the respective signal-transduction pathways therefore should be already desensitized. The experimental disagreements rose from the report of all possible outcomes, like negative feedback, positive feedback, and no effect at all. Although historically insulin was exclusively discussed as a negative signal, recent data provide evidence for a positive role of insulin in cellular processes like gene regulation—both transcription and translation, Ca^{2+} flux, beta-cell proliferation as well as survival [51–54,151].

The relevance of insulin action in the β cells has recently been confirmed in humans [152–155]. Further studies and better understanding of multi-level tissue crosstalk will have to address the standing questions in the field of whether the observed insulin effect upon beta-cell function is caused directly by insulin or rather by factors originating from other cell types/tissues in response to the insulin stimulus.

Role of Bone in Regulating Insulin Sensitivity and Glucose Homeostasis

Bone is an endocrine organ that constantly destroys and regenerates itself through a process termed bone modeling during childhood and remodeling during adulthood. This is an energy-demanding process that allows longitudinal growth during childhood and the maintenance of a constant bone mass during adulthood [156–160]. The nuclear receptor peroxisome proliferator-activated receptor-gamma (PPARg) is a crucial cellular and metabolic switch that regulates many physiologic and disease processes including adipogenesis, lipid metabolism, insulin sensitivity, and inflammation. It is also important for bone homeostasis. As described in detail in the next section, thiazolidinediones (TZDs), such as rosiglitazone (Aandia—GlaxoSmithKline) and pioglitazone (Glustin—Takeda Pharmaceuticals), which are synthetic PPARg agonists, are widely used as drugs for treating insulin resistance and T2D; however, their long-term use increases the risk of fractures in patients with diabetes. Emerging evidence suggests that PPARg activation not only suppresses osteoblastogenesis (synthesis of osteoblasts or bone-forming cells), but also activates osteoclastogenesis (synthesis of osteoclasts or bone-resorbing cells), thereby decreasing bone formation while sustaining or increasing bone resorption [54,161–170].

Bone organogenesis is a complex process, involving differentiation and crosstalk of multiple cell types based on a cascade of transcriptional events in osteoblasts and osteoclasts [171–175]. Emerging evidence indicates a critical role of microRNA (miRNA)-mediated inhibition of cellular mRNA translation as a regulator of developmental osteogenic signaling pathways, osteoblast growth and differentiation, osteoclast-mediated bone resorption activity, and bone homeostasis in the adult skeleton [176–182]. Characterization of miRNAs that operate through tissue-specific transcription factors in osteoblast and osteoclast lineage cells has provided novel insights into the signaling pathways and regulatory networks controlling normal bone formation and turnover. Further investigation into this may not only enhance our understanding on how some of these pathways are controlled through signals received in paracrine fashion from other tissues but also highlight previously undiscovered cellular targets to prevent bone deterioration associated with diabetes and various other diseases [179,183,184].

The high cost associated with bone remodeling and the side effects of metabolic regulators like PPARg and others on skeletal homeostasis then raise the possibility that bone cells may have means of regulating the flow of energy supply/energy storage to fulfill their metabolic needs [185,186]. Furthermore, when energy is scarce one can logically conceive that there should be mechanisms to restrict bone growth. Studies designed to test these hypotheses have led to the identification of osteocalcin, a novel hormone secreted and activated by bone cells, which is at the core of the crosstalk between bone (re) modeling and glucose metabolism [187–194]. To identify putative bone-derived signals that could influence energy homeostasis, mutant mouse models lacking genes encoding osteoblast-specific secreted molecule were systematically analyzed for abnormalities in glucose handling or other metabolic dysregulations. This phenotypic screening identified mice deficient in osteocalcin, a small peptide hormone secreted specifically by osteoblasts that is present in the bone matrix and in the blood [195].

Interestingly, osteocalcin-deficient mice are hyperglycemic, hypoinsulinemic, have low beta cell mass, decreased insulin sensitivity, increased fat mass and decreased energy expenditure. Conversely, the subcutaneous infusion of recombinant osteocalcin into wild-type mice causes an increase in blood insulin levels, enhances glucose tolerance, and improves insulin sensitivity. From a mechanistic standpoint, islet perfusion assays showed that osteocalcin acts as an insulin secretagogue. Gene expression analyses of islets or cultured beta-cell lines further demonstrated that osteocalcin directly enhances the expression of the insulin genes as well as those encoding cyclin-dependent kinase 4 (Cdk4), cyclin D1 (Ccnd1), and D2 (Ccnd2). These findings explain the positive effect that osteocalcin has on both insulin production and beta cell proliferation. Likewise, *in vitro* and *ex vivo* analyses demonstrated that osteocalcin signals directly to adipocytes, where it promotes the expression of the gene encoding adiponectin [196–202]. Although a positive effect of osteocalcin on the expression of the genes for forkhead protein A2 (Foxa2) in the liver and of acyl-CoA dehydrogenase (Mcad) in muscle has been reported, it is not yet known whether it signals directly to these tissues. Likewise, more investigation into these pathways will need to be performed in order to unravel the mechanism of how osteocalcin enhances systemic insulin sensitivity and energy expenditure [160,203].

Role of Brain in Regulating Insulin Sensitivity and Glucose Homeostasis

An essential hallmark in the development of both obesity and diabetes is systemic insulin resistance (and insulin resistance within peripheral tissues like liver, muscle, β-cell and adipose tissue), which occurs through numerous pathways triggered by pathological conditions such as prolonged hyperglycemia, hyperinsulinemia, lipotoxicity, inflammation, oxidative stress, and adipokine overproduction and release [196,197,204]. Often all of these conditions can result from excessive calorie intake and a parallel reduction in energy expenditure, leading to a net positive energy status. Ultimately, this energy homeostasis is governed by the hypothalamus, which is evolutionarily conserved in vertebrates as a master regulator of critical biological processes such as energy balance, circadian rhythms, stress response, temperature control, osmotic regulation, and growth and metabolism. These responses are controlled by discrete nuclei within the hypothalamus, each expressing a heterogeneous population of neurons that have specialized functions [25,205–208].

While it is clear that the hypothalamus functions as the ultimate control center for energy homeostasis, and likely a primary underlying cause of pathology of obesity and diabetes, its heterogeneous nature makes a mechanistic analysis of the inner workings within the level of individual neurons incredibly difficult. To make matters complex it also receives inputs from other parts of the brain in order to regulate energy homeostasis [209–214]. To circumvent these problems researchers continue to develop a phenotypic array of hypothalamic neuronal cell lines and various transgenic rodent models with conditional perturbation of key genes in the insulin signaling pathway (e.g. insulin receptor, leptin receptor, IRS proteins, PI3K, Akt, etc.) [157–159], specifically in these neurons. Studies involving the neuron-specific deletion of insulin receptor or IRS-2, a key intracellular mediator of insulin signaling, provide intriguing evidence for the regulation of blood glucose levels by insulin, through its actions in the brain [215–218]. These mice display a mildly obese, hyperphagic, and insulin-resistant phenotype [219], establishing a requirement for neuronal insulin signaling in energy homeostasis and glucose metabolism. Furthermore, rescue of insulin receptor function selectively in liver and pancreatic β cells prevents the development of diabetes in insulin receptor-deficient mice when combined with concomitant expression of insulin receptor in brain [43]. Additionally, in rats, infusion of insulin into either the third ventricle or directly into mediobasal hypothalamus [in the area of the arcuate nucleus (ARC)] reduces hepatic gluconeogenesis by increasing liver insulin sensitivity [215]. Intrahypothalamic infusion also improves insulin sensitivity in mice. Similarly, increasing hypothalamic PI3K, a major intracellular mediator of insulin action, signaling by either IRS-2 (which links insulin receptors to PI3K) or the PI3K target, Akt, increases peripheral insulin

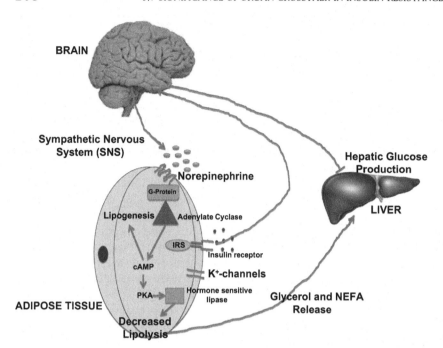

FIGURE 17.5 Role of brain-derived signals in regulating energy homeostasis and glucose metabolism. Please see color plate section.

sensitivity in rats with uncontrolled diabetes induced by streptozotocin (STZ) [220]. Taken together, these data implicate insulin signaling in the CNS for the regulation of both body weight and glucose metabolism [142,221].

The mechanism by which insulin action in the brain lowers plasma glucose levels appears to involve activation of ATP-sensitive potassium (K_{ATP}) channels on ARC neurons [215]. In addition to the ARC, the hypothalamic ventromedial nucleus (VMN) is implicated in the physiological control of both glucose metabolism and energy balance. In the 1980s Szabo and colleagues showed that microinjection of insulin into the VMN lowers blood glucose levels via an autonomic mechanism involving the vagus nerve. Subsequently, administration of leptin, a 167 amino acid long hormone and a polypeptide product of *ob* gene, into the VMN was shown to markedly increase glucose uptake into skeletal muscle and adipose tissue [222], further implicating VMN neurons in the control of peripheral insulin action. Consistent with these observations, conditional deletion of leptin signaling from these neurons established an essential role for leptin signaling for control of energy homeostasis in these cells.

Taken together, these observations support the hypothesis that, like the ARC, VMN neurons sense and integrate inputs from both hormonal (insulin, leptin, serotonin) and nutrient-related (glucose) signals to regulate autonomous outflow, energy intake, and peripheral insulin action via signal transduction mechanisms resembling those utilized by ARC neurons

[204,208,219,223−235]. However, how a signal from the hypothalamus mediates changes in peripheral insulin sensitivity remains an active area of investigation. One hypothesis proposes a key role for communication between hypothalamus and hindbrain areas that control autonomic outflow to the liver and other tissues via the vagus nerve. This hypothesis is supported by the observation that hepatic branch vagotomy attenuates the suppression of glucose production following intrahypothalamic infusion of insulin, FFAs, or a K^{ATP} channel opener, whereas there was no effect of selective vagal deafferentation. Whether additional mechanisms link hypothalamic nutrient and hormone sensing to the control of glucose metabolism in peripheral tissues is a key question that awaits further investigation (Fig. 17.5).

THERAPY FOR TYPE 2 DIABETES MELLITUS

Drugs Targeting β-cell Dysfunction

Agents that Increase or Preserve β-cell Mass (Table 17.1)

INCRETIN-BASED TREATMENTS

There is a growing body of evidence that the plasticity of the endocrine pancreas is a key factor in regulating glucose homeostasis. Indeed, the β-cell mass needs to adapt to insulin resistance that is either physiological, such as pregnancy, or pathophysiological, such as

TABLE 17.1 Agents that Increase or Preserve β-cell Mass

Stimulators of beta-cell proliferation and/or neogenesis	Inhibitors of beta-cell death/apoptosis
GLP-1	GLP-1
GIP	GIP
DPP-IV inhibitors	DPP-IV inhibitors
Insulin	Insulin
Epidermal growth factors/gastrin	Growth hormone
	Hepatocyte growth factor
TZDs	Insulin-like growth factors
Growth hormone	Parathyroid hormone-related peptide
Hepatocyte growth factor	
Human placental lactogen	
INGAP	
Insulin-like growth factors	
Parathyroid hormone-related peptide	
Prolactin	
Keratinocyte growth factor	
Betacellulin	

Abbreviations: GLP-1, glucagon like peptide-1; GIP, glucose-dependent insulinotropic polypeptide, DPP-IV, dipeptidyl-peptidase-IV; TZDs, thiazolidinediones; INGAP, islet neogenesis-associated protein.

obesity. A decrease in functional β-cell mass may be the main event partly responsible for the chronic hyperglycemia seen in diabetic patients. It is therefore logical to focus treatments to target pancreatic islet dysfunction [236]. Intestinal factors that are secreted in response to nutrients to enhance blood glucose lowering, known as incretins, are responsible for more than 50% of meal-related insulin secretion in healthy individuals. The well-studied incretins include glucose-dependent insulinotropic polypeptide (GIP) and glucagon-like peptide-1 (GLP-1) [237—242].

GLP-1 concentrations are often reduced in type 2 diabetes, but its biological potency is still retained, making it an attractive target for pharmacological intervention. GLP-1, a 30 amino acid polypeptide secreted from the L cell in the ileum and colon, potentiates glucose-dependent insulin secretion and glucagon suppression, slows gastric emptying, and reduces food intake with a long-term effect to help with weight loss. Besides its insulinotropic effect, GLP-1, through its Gs protein-coupled receptor, has also been shown to positively regulate β-cell mass by reducing apoptosis and increasing survival by regulating the expression of key genes involved in β-cell differentiation [243,244]. Double incretin (GIP and GLP-1) receptor knockout (DIRKO) mice, for example, have decreased islet numbers compared with their wild-type littermates. Although precise molecular mechanisms for the effects of GLP-1 on β-cell mass are yet to be clearly defined, data suggest the involvement of the protein kinase A (PKA)-dependent pathway. Consistent with these observations, *in vitro* studies have also reported that GLP-1 exposure of human islets prevents glucolipotoxicity [245]. In this study, the protective effect of GLP-1 was related to increased gene expression of anti-apoptotic proteins (Bcl2, IAP-2). Additionally, data also suggest that GLP-1 might independently promote glycogen accumulation in liver, increase glucose uptake, and lower circulating concentrations of triglycerides. Notably, only GLP-1, or its mimetics or enhancers, can be used for T2D treatment because β cells are resistant to GIP action, partly due to the downregulation of its pancreatic receptors in diabetic conditions [246—249] (Table 17.2).

Incretins are rapidly inactivated by dipeptidyl peptidase 4 (DPP-4), which cleaves the active peptide at the alanine residue that is penultimate to the N-terminus. DPP-4 is abundant, especially in plasma, on the surface of epithelial cells of the kidney, intestines, liver, and

TABLE 17.2 Incretins and Their Role in Glucose Metabolism

Incretin	Source	Biological actions	Effect of type 2 diabetes
GIP	Intestinal K cells in duodenum and jejunum	Potentiate glucose-stimulated insulin secretion Regulate fat metabolism Promote β-cell proliferation and survival	All functions severely impaired
GLP-1	Intestinal L cells in ileum and jejunum	Potentiate glucose-stimulated insulin secretion Suppress glucagon secretion and gluconeogenesis Slow gastric emptying Inhibit appetite and food intake Promote β-cell proliferation and survival Improve insulin receptor binding and insulin sensitivity Enhance glucose disposal	Normal functioning maintained but secretion reduced

Abbreviations: GLP-1, glucagon like peptide-1; GIP, glucose-dependent insulinotropic polypeptide.

Processing of Pro-glucagon in Intestinal L-Cells

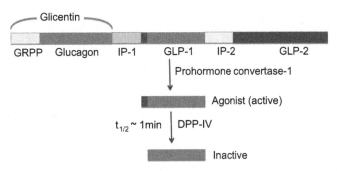

FIGURE 17.6 Biosynthesis and regulation of GLP-1. Please see color plate section.

pancreas, as well as on immune-cell leukocytes and endothelial cells lining vessels that drain from the intestinal mucosa, hence the rapid inactivation and short circulating half-life of incretins (<2 min for GLP-1 and 5–7 min for GIP). To extend the half-life, DPP-4-resistant GLP-1 analogs with GLP-1 receptor (GLP-1R) agonist properties have been developed (exenatide, liraglutide) [250,251]. Another strategy has been to increase endogenous GLP-1 by highly specific DPP-4 inhibitors (sitagliptin, vildagliptin, saxagliptin). Incretin mimetics and DPP-4 inhibitors hold promise not only for achieving glucose control, but also for potentially improving overall pancreatic islet function [252,253] (Fig. 17.6).

The incretin mimetic exenatide has proven useful as adjunct therapy to oral agents. This twice-daily injectable agent elicits significant HbA1c reduction and weight loss, with primarily minimal gastro-intestinal (GI) side effects. Data from animal models also suggest that exenatide ameliorates β-cell dysfunction, and potentially delays the requirement for exogenous insulin. The oral DPP-4 inhibitors offer signification reduction in glucose levels with neutral effects on weight and a favorable side-effect profile. Here, too, preclinical studies have demonstrated positive effects on β-cell function, with a potential to prevent disease progression. Early initiation of therapy that enhances β-cell/islet function may very well delay progression of diabetes, allowing patients to maintain target glucose levels longer on a single agent. However, the long-term effects of DPP-4 inhibitors and incretin mimetics on glycemic control, through long-term randomized and controlled studies in humans, have yet to be established. Many of these compounds have shown great promise in Phase 1 and 2 clinical trials and have Phase 3 trials in progress [240,254,255].

Non-incretin β-cell Stimulants

The phosphorylation of glucose by glucokinase after entry into β cell affects the rate of glucose metabolism and subsequent ATP production, which closes potassium-ATP channels and initiates insulin secretion. To enhance glucokinase action in β cells, several glucokinase activators have been developed, including piragliatin, compound 14, R1511, AZD1656, AZD6370, compound 6, and ID1101. Glucokinase activators increased insulin concentrations and reduced glucose concentrations in animal models of diabetes and patients with type 2 diabetes. These compounds, however, risk increasing triglyceride concentrations and causing hypoglycemia. This has prompted researchers to explore alternatives in the form of compounds that reduce oxidative stress and have been shown to reduce β-cell apoptosis in islets isolated from patients with type 2 diabetes; anti-inflammatory drugs such as IL-1R antagonists that have shown improved insulin secretion by β cells, leading to reduced hyperglycemia and fibrosis of islets, and enhanced islet vascularization with effects on β-cell mass and survival [256].

Drugs Targeting Alpha-cell Dysfunction

Patients with T2D usually have high fasting glucagon concentrations and impaired suppression of postprandial glucagon secretion (i.e. low insulin-to-glucagon ratio). Glucagon suppresses hepatic glycogen synthesis and stimulates glycogenolysis and gluconeogenesis. Thus, excess glucagon prevents normal suppression of hepatic glucose output, contributing to fasting and postprandial hyperglycemia in T2D. Incretin-based treatments (GLP-1R agonists and DPP-4 inhibitors) reduce glucagon secretion in a glucose-dependent manner (i.e. only in association with hyperglycemia), reducing postprandial glucose concentrations without compromising hypoglycemic counter-regulation.

Another mechanism to counter excess glucagon secretion is to block the glucagon receptor or its signaling post-hormone binding. Animal models with a null mutation of the glucagon receptor or reduced expression with antisense oligonucleotides show significant reduction in basal glycemia and improved glucose tolerance, but dramatic elevation in glucagon and alpha-cell hyperplasia might arise. Additionally, various peptide and non-peptide glucagon receptor antagonists have been assessed in animal models, but little evidence to date exists on their chronic efficacy [236].

Drugs Targeting Insulin Resistance: Metformin and Thiazolidinediones (TZDs)

T2D is a disease of deteriorating islet cell function on a background of insulin resistance. Diabetes may develop in insulin-resistant persons with inherited secretory and glucose-sensing defects in β cells. The pathogenesis of diabetes appears to involve a progressive decrease in β-cell mass, potentially triggered by abnormalities in adipocytokine release from intra-abdominal fat cells.

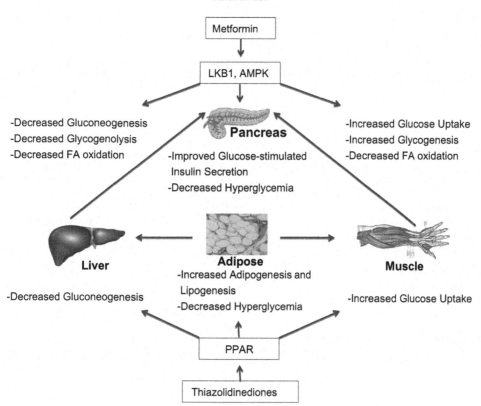

FIGURE 17.7 Treatment of insulin resistance—mechanism of action of metformin and thiazolidinedione. Please see color plate section.

Metformin and thiazolidinediones (TZDs) are used to treat insulin resistance, but their actions differ. Metformin reduces free fatty-acid efflux from fat cells, thereby suppressing hepatic glucose production, and indirectly improves peripheral insulin sensitivity and endothelial function [168–170,257–266]. TZDs improve peripheral insulin sensitivity by reducing circulating free fatty acids but also by suppressing adipocytokines, which increase insulin resistance. TZDs also improve endothelial function and may prevent or delay the onset of diabetes. Insulin is intrinsically anti-atherogenic but may mediate arterial inflammation in insulin-resistant patients. Unlike metformin, the TZDs suppress this inflammatory pathway and may indirectly help preserve β-cell function (Fig. 17.7).

PERSPECTIVE

In summary, we have reviewed recent advances in the field of insulin resistance with a focus on inter-organ crosstalk that is relevant for understanding the pathophysiology of T2D. While identification of proteins in the insulin and IGF-1 signaling pathways in the classical insulin target tissues continues to be a major focus of unraveling the defects that underlie T2D, additional work is necessary for systematically dissecting the crosstalk between these tissue and beta cells, brain, and bone. A better comprehension of how the crosstalk is able to maintain glucose homeostasis in the normal state will allow a greater perception of the defects that occur in the early stages of the disease and provide insights into progression of the defects leading to the overt pathophysiological state. It will also be important to appropriately consider other emerging areas including those related to epigenetics and microRNAs that impact each of the classical and non-classical insulin target organs for a global view of the disease.

Acknowledgments

The authors thank Kellianne Parlee for excellent assistance with the preparation of the manuscript and acknowledge support from NIH DK RO1 67536 and JDRF.

References

[1] Noble D, Mathur R, Dent T, Meads C, Greenhalgh T. Risk models and scores for type 2 diabetes: systematic review. BMJ 2011;343:d7163.

[2] Nolan CJ, Damm P, Prentki M. Type 2 diabetes across generations: from pathophysiology to prevention and management. Lancet 2011 July 9;378(9786):169–81.

[3] Weyer C, Bogardus C, Mott DM, Pratley RE. The natural history of insulin secretory dysfunction and insulin resistance in the

pathogenesis of type 2 diabetes mellitus. J Clin Invest 1999 September;104(6):787—94.

[4] Jetton TL, Lausier J, LaRock K, Trotman WE, Larmie B, Habibovic A, et al. Mechanisms of compensatory beta-cell growth in insulin-resistant rats: roles of Akt kinase. Diabetes 2005 August;54(8):2294—304.

[5] Kolb H, Eizirik DL. Resistance to type 2 diabetes mellitus: a matter of hormesis? Nat Rev Endocrinol 2011;8(3):183—92.

[6] Bluestone JA, Herold K, Eisenbarth G. Genetics, pathogenesis and clinical interventions in type 1 diabetes. Nature 2010 April 29;464(7293):1293—300.

[7] Buchanan TA. (How) can we prevent type 2 diabetes? Diabetes 2007 June;56(6):1502—7.

[8] DeFronzo RA, Tobin JD, Andres R. Glucose clamp technique: a method for quantifying insulin secretion and resistance. Am J Physiol 1979 September;237(3):E214—23.

[9] Bergman RN, Ider YZ, Bowden CR, Cobelli C. Quantitative estimation of insulin sensitivity. Am J Physiol 1979 June; 236(6):E667—77.

[10] Wallace TM, Levy JC, Matthews DR. Use and abuse of HOMA modeling. Diabetes Care 2004 June;27(6):1487—95.

[11] Quon MJ. QUICKI is a useful and accurate index of insulin sensitivity. J Clin Endocrinol Metab 2002 February;87(2): 949—51.

[12] Mari A, Pacini G, Murphy E, Ludvik B, Nolan JJ. A model-based method for assessing insulin sensitivity from the oral glucose tolerance test. Diabetes Care 2001 March;24(3): 539—48.

[13] Matsuda M, DeFronzo RA. Insulin sensitivity indices obtained from oral glucose tolerance testing: comparison with the euglycemic insulin clamp. Diabetes Care 1999 September; 22(9):1462—70.

[14] Mari A, Pacini G, Brazzale AR, Ahren B. Comparative evaluation of simple insulin sensitivity methods based on the oral glucose tolerance test. Diabetologia 2005 April;48(4):748—51.

[15] Virkamaki A, Ueki K, Kahn CR. Protein—protein interaction in insulin signaling and the molecular mechanisms of insulin resistance. J Clin Invest 1999 April;103(7):931—43.

[16] Shaw JE, Sicree RA, Zimmet PZ. Global estimates of the prevalence of diabetes for 2010 and 2030. Diabetes Res Clin Pract 2010 January;87(1):4—14.

[17] Leibiger IB, Leibiger B, Berggren PO. Insulin feedback action on pancreatic beta-cell function. FEBS Lett 2002 December 4;532(1—2):1—6.

[18] Miyake K, Ogawa W, Matsumoto M, Nakamura T, Sakaue H, Kasuga M. Hyperinsulinemia, glucose intolerance, and dyslipidemia induced by acute inhibition of phosphoinositide 3-kinase signaling in the liver. J Clin Invest 2002 November;110(10):1483—91.

[19] Ohara-Imaizumi M, Fujiwara T, Nakamichi Y, Okamura T, Akimoto Y, Kawai J, et al. Imaging analysis reveals mechanistic differences between first- and second-phase insulin exocytosis. J Cell Biol 2007 May 21;177(4):695—705.

[20] Aspinwall CA, Lakey JR, Kennedy RT. Insulin-stimulated insulin secretion in single pancreatic beta cells. J Biol Chem 1999 March 5;274(10):6360—5.

[21] Dobbins RL, Chester MW, Stevenson BE, Daniels MB, Stein DT, McGarry JD. A fatty acid- dependent step is critically important for both glucose- and non-glucose-stimulated insulin secretion. J Clin Invest 1998 June 1;101(11):2370—6.

[22] Roder ME, Porte Jr D, Schwartz RS, Kahn SE. Disproportionately elevated proinsulin levels reflect the degree of impaired B cell secretory capacity in patients with noninsulin-dependent diabetes mellitus. J Clin Endocrinol Metab 1998 February; 83(2):604—8.

[23] Garvey WT, Olefsky JM, Griffin J, et al. The effect of insulin treatment on insulin secretion and insulin action in type II diabetes mellitus. Diabetes 1985;34:222.

[24] Rhodes CJ. Type 2 diabetes—a matter of beta-cell life and death? Science 2005 January 21;307(5708):380—4.

[25] Kiba T, Tanaka K, Numata K, Hoshino M, Misugi K, Inoue S. Ventromedial hypothalamic lesion-induced vagal hyperactivity stimulates rat pancreatic cell proliferation. Gastroenterology 1996 March;110(3):885—93.

[26] Ueno M, Carvalheira JB, Tambascia RC, Bezerra RM, Amaral ME, Carneiro EM, et al. Regulation of insulin signalling by hyperinsulinaemia: role of IRS-1/2 serine phosphorylation and the mTOR/p70 S6K pathway. Diabetologia 2005 March; 48(3):506—18.

[27] Um SH, Frigerio F, Watanabe M, Picard F, Joaquin M, Sticker M, et al. Absence of S6K1 protects against age- and diet-induced obesity while enhancing insulin sensitivity. Nature 2004 September 9;431(7005):200—5.

[28] Tuttle RL, Gill NS, Pugh W, Lee JP, Koeberlein B, Furth EE, et al. Regulation of pancreatic beta-cell growth and survival by the serine/threonine protein kinase Akt1/PKBalpha. Nat Med 2001 October;7(10):1133—7.

[29] Bernal-Mizrachi E, Wen W, Stahlhut S, Welling CM, Permutt MA. Islet beta cell expression of constitutively active Akt1/PKB alpha induces striking hypertrophy, hyperplasia, and hyperinsulinemia. J Clin Invest 2001 December;108(11): 1631—8.

[30] Taniguchi CM, Emanuelli B, Kahn CR. Critical nodes in signalling pathways: insights into insulin action. Nat Rev Mol Cell Biol 2006 February;7(2):85—96.

[31] Aguirre V, Werner ED, Giraud J, Lee YH, Shoelson SE, White MF. Phosphorylation of Ser307 in insulin receptor substrate-1 blocks interactions with the insulin receptor and inhibits insulin action. J Biol Chem 2002 January 11;277(2): 1531—7.

[32] Rui L, Yuan M, Frantz D, Shoelson S, White MF. SOCS-1 and SOCS-3 block insulin signaling by ubiquitin-mediated degradation of IRS1 and IRS2. J Biol Chem 2002 November 1;277(44):42394—8.

[33] Saltiel AR, Kahn CR. Insulin signalling and the regulation of glucose and lipid metabolism. Nature 2001 December 13;414(6865):799—806.

[34] Carpentier JL, Paccaud JP, Gorden P, Rutter WJ, Orci L. Insulin-induced surface redistribution regulates internalization of the insulin receptor and requires its autophosphorylation. Proc Natl Acad Sci USA 1992 January 1;89(1):162—6.

[35] Accili D, Cama A, Barbetti F, Kadowaki H, Kadowaki T, Taylor SI. Insulin resistance due to mutations of the insulin receptor gene: an overview. J Endocrinol Invest 1992 December;15(11):857—64.

[36] Almind K, Bjorbaek C, Vestergaard H, Hansen T, Echwald SM, Pedersen O. Amino acid polymorphisms of insulin receptor substrate-1 in non-insulin-dependent diabetes mellitus. Lancet 1993;342(8875):828—32.

[37] Araki E, Lipes MA, Patti ME, Bruning JC, Haag III B, Johnson RS, et al. Alternative pathway of insulin signalling in mice with targeted disruption of the IRS-1 gene. Nature 1994 November 10;372(6502):186—90.

[38] Cho H, Mu J, Kim JK, Thorvaldsen JL, Chu Q, Crenshaw III EB, et al. Insulin resistance and a diabetes mellitus-like syndrome in mice lacking the protein kinase Akt2 (PKB beta). Science 2001 June 1;292(5522):1728—31.

[39] Abel ED, Peroni O, Kim JK, Kim YB, Boss O, Hadro E, et al. Adipose-selective targeting of the GLUT4 gene impairs insulin action in muscle and liver. Nature 2001;409:729—33.

[40] Fernandez AM, Kim JK, Yakar S, Dupont J, Hernandez-Sanchez C, Castle AL, et al. Functional inactivation of the IGF-I and insulin receptors in skeletal muscle causes type 2 diabetes. Genes Dev 2001 August 1;15(15):1926–34.

[41] Leibiger IB, Leibiger B, Berggren PO. Insulin signaling in the pancreatic beta-cell. Annu Rev Nutr 2008;28:233–51.

[42] Bluher M, Michael MD, Peroni OD, Ueki K, Carter N, Kahn BB, et al. Adipose tissue selective insulin receptor knockout protects against obesity and obesity-related glucose intolerance. Dev Cell 2002 July;3(1):25–38.

[43] Okamoto H, Nakae J, Kitamura T, Park BC, Dragatsis I, Accili D. Transgenic rescue of insulin receptor-deficient mice. J Clin Invest 2004 July;114(2):214–23.

[44] Kulkarni RN, Holzenberger M, Shih DQ, Ozcan U, Stoffel M, Magnuson MA, et al. Beta-cell-specific deletion of the Igf1 receptor leads to hyperinsulinemia and glucose intolerance but does not alter beta-cell mass. Nat Genet 2002 May;31(1):111–5.

[45] Martin BC, Warram JH, Krolewski AS, Bergman RN, Soeldner JS, Kahn CR. Role of glucose and insulin resistance in development of type 2 diabetes mellitus: results of a 25-year follow-up study. Lancet 1992 October 17;340(8825):925–9.

[46] Ueki K, Okada T, Hu J, Liew CW, Assmann A, Dahlgren GM, et al. Total insulin and IGF-I resistance in pancreatic beta cells causes overt diabetes. Nat Genet 2006 May;38(5):583–8.

[47] Hashimoto N, Kido Y, Uchida T, Asahara S, Shigeyama Y, Matsuda T, et al. Ablation of PDK1 in pancreatic beta cells induces diabetes as a result of loss of beta cell mass. Nat Genet 2006 May;38(5):589–93.

[48] Morioka T, Asilmaz E, Hu J, Dishinger JF, Kurpad AJ, Elias CF, et al. Disruption of leptin receptor expression in the pancreas directly affects beta cell growth and function in mice. J Clin Invest 2007 October;117(10):2860–8.

[49] Covey SD, Wideman RD, McDonald C, Unniappan S, Huynh F, Asadi A, et al. The pancreatic beta cell is a key site for mediating the effects of leptin on glucose homeostasis. Cell Metab 2006 October;4(4):291–302.

[50] Lewandoski M. Conditional control of gene expression in the mouse. Nat Rev Genet 2001 October;2(10):743–55.

[51] Kido Y, Burks DJ, Withers D, Bruning JC, Kahn CR, White MF, et al. Tissue-specific insulin resistance in mice with mutations in the insulin receptor, IRS-1, and IRS-2. J Clin Invest 2000 January;105(2):199–205.

[52] Kulkarni RN, Bruning JC, Winnay JN, Postic C, Magnuson MA, Kahn CR. Tissue-specific knockout of the insulin receptor in pancreatic β cells creates an insulin secretory defect similar to that in Type 2 diabetes. Cell 1999 February 5;96(3):329–39.

[53] Kulkarni RN. New insights into the roles of insulin/IGF-I in the development and maintenance of beta-cell mass. Rev Endocr Metab Disord 2005 August;6(3):199–210.

[54] Burant CF, Sreenan S, Hirano K, Tai TA, Lohmiller J, Lukens J, et al. Troglitazone action is independent of adipose tissue. J Clin Invest 1997 December 1;100(11):2900–8.

[55] Ross SR, Graves RA, Spiegelman BM. Targeted expression of a toxin gene to adipose tissue: transgenic mice resistant to obesity. Genes Dev 1993 July;7(7B):1318–24.

[56] Accili D, Drago J, Lee EJ, Johnson MD, Cool MH, Salvatore P, et al. Early neonatal death in mice homozygous for a null allele of the insulin receptor gene. Nat Genet 1996 January; 12(1):106–9.

[57] Bruning JC, Michael MD, Winnay JN, Hayashi T, Horsch D, Accili D, et al. A muscle-specific insulin receptor knockout exhibits features of the metabolic syndrome of NIDDM without altering glucose tolerance. Mol Cell 1998 November;2(5):559–69.

[58] Bruning JC, Winnay J, Bonner-Weir S, Taylor SI, Accili D, Kahn CR. Development of a novel polygenic model of NIDDM in mice heterozygous for IR and IRS-1 null alleles. Cell 1997 February 21;88(4):561–72.

[59] Joshi RL, Lamothe B, Cordonnier N, Mesbah K, Monthioux E, Jami J, et al. Targeted disruption of the insulin receptor gene in the mouse results in neonatal lethality. EMBO J 1996 April 1;15(7):1542–7.

[60] Otani K, Kulkarni RN, Baldwin AC, Krutzfeldt J, Ueki K, Stoffel M, et al. Reduced beta-cell mass and altered glucose sensing impair insulin-secretory function in betaIRKO mice. Am J Physiol Endocrinol Metab 2004 January;286(1):E41–9.

[61] Hennige AM, Burks DJ, Ozcan U, Kulkarni RN, Ye J, Park S, et al. Upregulation of insulin receptor substrate-2 in pancreatic beta cells prevents diabetes. J Clin Invest 2003 November; 112(10):1521–32.

[62] O'Rahilly S. Human genetics illuminates the paths to metabolic disease. Nature 2009 November 19;462(7271):307–14.

[63] Assmann A, Ueki K, Winnay JN, Kadowaki T, Kulkarni RN. Glucose effects on beta-cell growth and survival require activation of insulin receptors and insulin receptor substrate 2. Mol Cell Biol 2009 June;29(11):3219–28.

[64] van Haeften TW, Twickler TB. Insulin-like growth factors and pancreas beta cells. Eur J Clin Invest 2004 April;34(4):249–55.

[65] Chen C, Hosokawa H, Bumbalo LM, Leahy JL. Mechanism of compensatory hyperinsulinemia in normoglycemic insulin-resistant spontaneously hypertensive rats. Augmented enzymatic activity of glucokinase in beta-cells. J Clin Invest 1994 July;94(1):399–404.

[66] Srinivasan S, Bernal-Mizrachi E, Ohsugi M, Permutt MA. Glucose promotes pancreatic islet beta-cell survival through a PI 3-kinase/Akt-signaling pathway. Am J Physiol Endocrinol Metab 2002 October;283(4):E784–93.

[67] Poitout V, Robertson RP. Minireview: secondary beta-cell failure in type 2 diabetes—a convergence of glucotoxicity and lipotoxicity. Endocrinology 2002 February;143(2):339–42.

[68] Poitout V, Robertson RP. Glucolipotoxicity: fuel excess and beta-cell dysfunction. Endocr Rev 2008 May;29(3):351–66.

[69] Uchida T, Nakamura T, Hashimoto N, Matsuda T, Kotani K, Sakaue H, et al. Deletion of Cdkn1b ameliorates hyperglycemia by maintaining compensatory hyperinsulinemia in diabetic mice. Nat Med 2005 February;11(2):175–82.

[70] Porte Jr D. Clinical importance of insulin secretion and its interaction with insulin resistance in the treatment of type 2 diabetes mellitus and its complications. Diabetes Metab Res Rev 2001 May;17(3):181–8.

[71] Khaldi MZ, Guiot Y, Gilon P, Henquin JC, Jonas JC. Increased glucose sensitivity of both triggering and amplifying pathways of insulin secretion in rat islets cultured for 1 wk in high glucose. Am J Physiol Endocrinol Metab 2004 August;287(2):E207–17.

[72] Liu YQ, Jetton TL, Leahy JL. Beta-cell adaptation to insulin resistance. Increased pyruvate carboxylase and malate-pyruvate shuttle activity in islets of nondiabetic Zucker fatty rats. J Biol Chem 2002 October 18;277(42):39163–8.

[73] Okamoto H, Hribal ML, Lin HV, Bennett WR, Ward A, Accili D. Role of the forkhead protein FoxO1 in beta cell compensation to insulin resistance. J Clin Invest 2006 March;116(3):775–82.

[74] Jhala US, Canettieri G, Screaton RA, Kulkarni RN, Krajewski S, Reed J, et al. cAMP promotes pancreatic beta-cell survival via CREB-mediated induction of IRS2. Genes Dev 2003 July 1;17(13):1575–80.

[75] Donath MY, Ehses JA, Maedler K, Schumann DM, Ellingsgaard H, Eppler E, et al. Mechanisms of beta-cell death in type 2 diabetes. Diabetes 2005 December;54(Suppl. 2):S108–13.

[76] Bonner-Weir S, Deery D, Leahy JL, Weir GC. Compensatory growth of pancreatic beta-cells in adult rats after short-term glucose infusion. Diabetes 1989 January;38(1):49–53.

[77] Xu G, Stoffers DA, Habener JF, Bonner-Wier S. Exendin-4 stimulates both beta-cell replication and neogenesis, resulting in increased beta-cell mass and improved glucose tolerance in diabetic rats. Diabetes 1999;48:2270—6.

[78] Finegood DT, McArthur MD, Kojwang D, Thomas MJ, Topp BG, Leonard T, et al. Beta-cell mass dynamics in Zucker diabetic fatty rats. Rosiglitazone prevents the rise in net cell death. Diabetes 2001 May;50(5):1021—9.

[79] Butler AE, Janson J, Bonner-Weir S, Ritzel R, Rizza RA, Butler PC. Beta-cell deficit and increased beta-cell apoptosis in humans with type 2 diabetes. Diabetes 2003 January;52(1):102—10.

[80] Tanaka Y, Tran PO, Harmon J, Robertson RP. A role for gluta-thione peroxidase in protecting pancreatic beta cells against oxidative stress in a model of glucose toxicity. Proc Natl Acad Sci USA 2002 September 17;99(19):12363—8.

[81] Lowell BB, Shulman GI. Mitochondrial dysfunction and type 2 diabetes. Science 2005 January 21;307(5708):384—7.

[82] Prentki M, Nolan CJ. Islet beta cell failure in type 2 diabetes. J Clin Invest 2006 July;116(7):1802—12.

[83] Kaneto H, Kajimoto Y, Miyagawa J, Matsuoka T, Fujitani Y, Umayahara Y, et al. Beneficial effects of antioxidants in diabetes: possible protection of pancreatic beta-cells against glucose toxicity. Diabetes 1999 December;48(12):2398—406.

[84] Del GS, Lupi R, Marselli L, Masini M, Bugliani M, Sbrana S, et al. Functional and molecular defects of pancreatic islets in human type 2 diabetes. Diabetes 2005 March;54(3):727—35.

[85] Kashyap SR, Belfort R, Berria R, Suraamornkul S, Pratipranawatr T, Finlayson J, et al. Discordant effects of a chronic physiological increase in plasma FFA on insulin signaling in healthy subjects with or without a family history of type 2 diabetes. Am J Physiol Endocrinol Metab 2004 September;287(3):E537—46.

[86] Boden G, Shulman GI. Free fatty acids in obesity and type 2 diabetes: defining their role in the development of insulin resistance and beta-cell dysfunction. Eur J Clin Invest 2002 June;32(Suppl. 3):14—23.

[87] Shimabukuro M, Zhou YT, Levi M, Unger RH. Fatty acid-induced beta cell apoptosis: a link between obesity and dia-betes. Proc Natl Acad Sci USA 1998 March 3;95(5):2498—502.

[88] Prentki M, Joly E, El Assaad W, Roduit R. Malonyl-CoA signaling, lipid partitioning, and glucolipotoxicity: role in beta-cell adaptation and failure in the etiology of diabetes. Diabetes 2002 December;51(Suppl. 3):S405—13.

[89] El-Assaad W, Buteau J, Peyot ML, Nolan C, Roduit R, Hardy S, et al. Saturated fatty acids synergize with elevated glucose to cause pancreatic beta-cell death. Endocrinology 2003 September;144(9):4154—63.

[90] Itoh Y, Kawamata Y, Harada M, Kobayashi M, Fujii R, Fukusumi S, et al. Free fatty acids regulate insulin secretion from pancreatic beta cells through GPR40. Nature 2003 March 13;422(6928):173—6.

[91] Wang H, Kouri G, Wollheim CB. ER stress and SREBP-1 acti-vation are implicated in beta-cell glucolipotoxicity. J Cell Sci 2005 September 1;118(Pt 17):3905—15.

[92] Minokoshi Y, Kim YB, Peroni OD, Fryer LG, Muller C, Carling D, et al. Leptin stimulates fatty-acid oxidation by acti-vating AMP-activated protein kinase. Nature 2002 January 17;415(6869):339—43.

[93] Shimomura I, Hammer RE, Richardson JA, Ikemoto S, Bashmakov Y, Goldstein JL, et al. Insulin resistance and dia-betes mellitus in transgenic mice expressing nuclear SREBP-1c in adipose tissue: model for congenital generalized lipodys-trophy. Genes Dev 1998 October 15;12(20):3182—94.

[94] Enerback S, Jacobsson A, Simpson EM, Guerra C, Yamashita H, Harper ME, et al. Mice lacking mitochondrial uncoupling protein are cold-sensitive but not obese. Nature 1997 May 1; 387(6628):90—4.

[95] Kopecky J, Clarke G, Enerback S, Spiegelman B, Kozak LP. Expression of the mitochondrial uncoupling protein gene from the aP2 gene promoter prevents genetic obesity. J Clin Invest 1995 December;96(6):2914—23.

[96] Joseph JW, Koshkin V, Saleh MC, Sivitz WI, Zhang CY, Lowell BB, et al. Free fatty acid-induced beta-cell defects are dependent on uncoupling protein 2 expression. J Biol Chem 2004 December 3;279(49):51049—56.

[97] Brunham LR, Kruit JK, Pape TD, Timmins JM, Reuwer AQ, Vasanji Z, et al. Beta-cell ABCA1 influences insulin secretion, glucose homeostasis and response to thiazolidinedione treat-ment. Nat Med 2007 March;13(3):340—7.

[98] Kharroubi I, Ladriere L, Cardozo AK, Dogusan Z, Cnop M, Eizirik DL. Free fatty acids and cytokines induce pancreatic beta-cell apoptosis by different mechanisms: role of nuclear factor-kappaB and endoplasmic reticulum stress. Endocri-nology 2004 November;145(11):5087—96.

[99] Laybutt DR, Preston AM, Akerfeldt MC, Kench JG, Busch AK, Biankin AV, et al. Endoplasmic reticulum stress contributes to beta cell apoptosis in type 2 diabetes. Diabetologia 2007 April;50(4):752—63.

[100] Hotamisligil GS. Role of endoplasmic reticulum stress and c-Jun NH2-terminal kinase pathways in inflammation and origin of obesity and diabetes. Diabetes 2005 December;54(Suppl. 2): S73—8.

[101] Nakatani Y, Kaneto H, Kawamori D, Yoshiuchi K, Hatazaki M, Matsuoka TA, et al. Involvement of endoplasmic reticulum stress in insulin resistance and diabetes. J Biol Chem 2005 January 7;280(1):847—51.

[102] Huang CJ, Lin CY, Haataja L, Gurlo T, Butler AE, Rizza RA, et al. High expression rates of human islet amyloid polypeptide induce endoplasmic reticulum stress mediated beta-cell apoptosis, a characteristic of humans with type 2 but not type 1 diabetes. Diabetes 2007 August;56(8):2016—27.

[103] Marchetti P, Bugliani M, Lupi R, Marselli L, Masini M, Boggi U, et al. The endoplasmic reticulum in pancreatic beta cells of type 2 diabetes patients. Diabetologia 2007 December;50(12):2486—94.

[104] Kaufman RJ, Scheuner D, Schroder M, Shen X, Lee K, Liu CY, et al. The unfolded protein response in nutrient sensing and differentiation. Nat Rev Mol Cell Biol 2002 June;3(6):411—21.

[105] Wang J, Obici S, Morgan K, Barzilai N, Feng Z, Rossetti L. Overfeeding rapidly induces leptin and insulin resistance. Diabetes 2001 December;50(12):2786—91.

[106] Klionsky DJ, Emr SD. Autophagy as a regulated pathway of cellular degradation. Science 2000 December 1;290(5497): 1717—21.

[107] Bertolotti A, Zhang Y, Hendershot LM, Harding HP, Ron D. Dynamic interaction of BiP and ER stress transducers in the unfolded-protein response. Nat Cell Biol 2000 June;2(6):326—32.

[108] Lipson KL, Fonseca SG, Ishigaki S, Nguyen LX, Foss E, Bortell R, et al. Regulation of insulin biosynthesis in pancreatic beta cells by an endoplasmic reticulum-resident protein kinase IRE1. Cell Metab 2006 September;4(3):245—54.

[109] Lipson KL, Ghosh R, Urano F. The role of IRE1alpha in the degradation of insulin mRNA in pancreatic beta-cells. PLOS One 2008;3(2):e1648.

[110] Pirot P, Naamane N, Libert F, Magnusson NE, Orntoft TF, Cardozo AK, et al. Global profiling of genes modified by endoplasmic reticulum stress in pancreatic beta cells reveals the early degradation of insulin mRNAs. Diabetologia 2007 May;50(5):1006—14.

[111] Okada T, Yoshida H, Akazawa R, Negishi M, Mori K. Distinct roles of activating transcription factor 6 (ATF6) and

double-stranded RNA-activated protein kinase-like endoplasmic reticulum kinase (PERK) in transcription during the mammalian unfolded protein response. Biochem J 2002 September 1;366(Pt 2):585—94.

[112] Yamaguchi S, Ishihara H, Yamada T, Tamura A, Usui M, Tominaga R, et al. ATF4-mediated induction of 4E-BP1 contributes to pancreatic beta cell survival under endoplasmic reticulum stress. Cell Metab 2008 March;7(3):269—76.

[113] Eizirik DL, Cardozo AK, Cnop M. The role for endoplasmic reticulum stress in diabetes mellitus. Endocr Rev 2008 February;29(1):42—61.

[114] Ozcan U, Cao Q, Yilmaz E, Lee AH, Iwakoshi NN, Ozdelen E, et al. Endoplasmic reticulum stress links obesity, insulin action, and type 2 diabetes. Science 2004 October 15;306(5695):457—61.

[115] Rutkowski JM, Davis KE, Scherer PE. Mechanisms of obesity and related pathologies: the macro- and microcirculation of adipose tissue. FEBS J 2009 October;276(20):5738—46.

[116] Lumeng CN, Bodzin JL, Saltiel AR. Obesity induces a phenotypic switch in adipose tissue macrophage polarization. J Clin Invest 2007 January;117(1):175—84.

[117] Bergman RN, Kim SP, Catalano KJ, Hsu IR, Chiu JD, Kabir M, et al. Why visceral fat is bad: mechanisms of the metabolic syndrome. Obesity (Silver Spring) 2006 February;14(Suppl. 1): 16S—9S.

[118] Hotamisligil GS, Erbay E. Nutrient sensing and inflammation in metabolic diseases. Nat Rev Immunol 2008 December; 8(12):923—34.

[119] Hotamisligil GS, Arner P, Caro JF, Atkinson RL, Spiegelman BM. Increased adipose tissue expression of tumor necrosis factor-alpha in human obesity and insulin resistance. J Clin Invest 1995 May;95(5):2409—15.

[120] Kern PA, Saghizadeh M, Ong JM, Bosch RJ, Deem R, Simsolo RB. The expression of tumor necrosis factor in human adipose tissue. Regulation by obesity, weight loss, and relationship to lipoprotein lipase. J Clin Invest 1995 May;95(5):2111—9.

[121] Hotamisligil GS, Murray DL, Choy LN, Spiegelman BM. Tumor necrosis factor alpha inhibits signaling from the insulin receptor. Proc Natl Acad Sci USA 1994 May 24;91(11):4854—8.

[122] Uysal KT, Wiesbrock SM, Marino MW, Hotamisligil GS. Protection from obesity-induced insulin resistance in mice lacking TNF-alpha function. Nature 1997 October 9; 389(6651):610—4.

[123] Hotamisligil GS, Peraldi P, Budvari A, Ellis RW, White MF, Spiegelman BM. IRS-1 mediated inhibition of insulin receptor tyrosine kinase activity in TNF-α- and obesity-induced insulin resistance. Science 1996;271(5249):665—8.

[124] Asadullah K, Sterry W, Volk HD. Interleukin-10 therapy—review of a new approach. Pharmacol Rev 2003 June;55(2):241—69.

[125] Shoelson SE, Lee J, Goldfine AB. Inflammation and insulin resistance. J Clin Invest 2006 July;116(7):1793—801.

[126] Moitra J, Mason MM, Olive M, Krylov D, Gavrilova O, Marcus-Samuels B, et al. Life without white fat: a transgenic mouse. Genes Dev 1998 October 15;12(20):3168—81.

[127] Weisberg SP, McCann D, Desai M, Rosenbaum M, Leibel RL, Ferrante Jr AW. Obesity is associated with macrophage accumulation in adipose tissue. J Clin Invest 2003 December; 112(12):1796—808.

[128] Kim JK, Gimeno RE, Higashimori T, Kim HJ, Choi H, Punreddy S, et al. Inactivation of fatty acid transport protein 1 prevents fat-induced insulin resistance in skeletal muscle. J Clin Invest 2004 March;113(5):756—63.

[129] Maeda K, Cao H, Kono K, Gorgun CZ, Furuhashi M, Uysal KT, et al. Adipocyte/macrophage fatty acid binding proteins control integrated metabolic responses in obesity and diabetes. Cell Metab 2005 February;1(2):107—19.

[130] Greenfield JR, Campbell LV. Relationship between inflammation, insulin resistance and type 2 diabetes: "cause or effect"? Curr Diabetes Rev 2006 May;2(2):195—211.

[131] Hotamisligil GS. Inflammation and metabolic disorders. Nature 2006 December 14;444(7121):860—7.

[132] Nomiyama T, Perez-Tilve D, Ogawa D, Gizard F, Zhao Y, Heywood EB, et al. Osteopontin mediates obesity-induced adipose tissue macrophage infiltration and insulin resistance in mice. J Clin Invest 2007 October;117(10):2877—88.

[133] Santomauro AT, Boden G, Silva ME, Rocha DM, Santos RF, Ursich MJ, et al. Overnight lowering of free fatty acids with Acipimox improves insulin resistance and glucose tolerance in obese diabetic and nondiabetic subjects. Diabetes 1999 September;48(9):1836—41.

[134] Randle PJ, Garland PB, Hales CN, Newsholme FA. The glucose fatty-acid cycle: its role in insulin sensitivity and the metabolic disturbances of diabetes mellitus. Lancet 1963;1:785—9.

[135] Shulman GI. Cellular mechanisms of insulin resistance. J Clin Invest 2000 July;106(2):171—6.

[136] Furukawa S, Fujita T, Shimabukuro M, Iwaki M, Yamada Y, Nakajima Y, et al. Increased oxidative stress in obesity and its impact on metabolic syndrome. J Clin Invest 2004 December;114(12):1752—61.

[137] Unger RH, Zhou YT. Lipotoxicity of beta-cells in obesity and in other causes of fatty acid spillover. Diabetes 2001 February; 50(Suppl. 1):S118—21.

[138] Reaven GM, Hollenbeck C, Jeng CY, Wu MS, Chen YD. Measurement of plasma glucose, free fatty acid, lactate, and insulin for 24 h in patients with NIDDM. Diabetes 1988 August;37(8):1020—4.

[139] Boden G. Role of fatty acids in the pathogenesis of insulin resistance and NIDDM. Diabetes 1997;46(1):3—10.

[140] Delghingaro-Augusto V, Nolan CJ, Gupta D, Jetton TL, Latour MG, Peshavaria M, et al. Islet beta cell failure in the 60% pancreatectomised obese hyperlipidaemic Zucker fatty rat: severe dysfunction with altered glycerolipid metabolism without steatosis or a falling beta cell mass. Diabetologia 2009 June;52(6):1122—32.

[141] Cusi K. The epidemic of type 2 diabetes mellitus: its links to obesity, insulin resistance, and lipotoxicity. In: Regensteiner JG, Reusch JEB, Stewart KJ, Veves A, editors. Diabetes and exercise. Humana Press; 2009.

[142] Cusi K. Lessons learned from studying families genetically predisposed to type 2 diabetes mellitus. Curr Diab Rep 2009 June;9(3):200—7.

[143] Krebs M, Krssak M, Bernroider E, Anderwald C, Brehm A, Meyerspeer M, et al. Mechanism of amino acid-induced skeletal muscle insulin resistance in humans. Diabetes 2002 March;51(3):599—605.

[144] Levin N, Nelson C, Gurney A, Vandlen R, de Sauvage F. Decreased food intake does not completely account for adiposity reduction after ob protein infusion. Proc Natl Acad Sci USA 1996 February 20;93(4):1726—30.

[145] Sivitz WI, Fink BD, Donohoue PA. Fasting and leptin modulate adipose and muscle uncoupling protein: divergent effects between messenger ribonucleic acid and protein expression. Endocrinology 1999;140(4):1511—9.

[146] Roden M, Price TB, Perseghin G, Petersen KF, Rothman DL, Cline GW, et al. Mechanism of free fatty acid-induced insulin resistance in humans. J Clin Invest 1996 June 15; 97(12):2859—65.

[147] Xu H, Barnes GT, Yang Q, Tan G, Yang D, Chou CJ, et al. Chronic inflammation in fat plays a crucial role in the development of obesity-related insulin resistance. J Clin Invest 2003 December;112(12):1821—30.

[148] Kanda H, Tateya S, Tamori Y, Kotani K, Hiasa K, Kitazawa R, et al. MCP-1 contributes to macrophage infiltration into adipose tissue, insulin resistance, and hepatic steatosis in obesity. J Clin Invest 2006 June;116(6):1494−505.

[149] Steneberg P, Rubins N, Bartoov-Shifman R, Walker MD, Edlund H. The FFA receptor GPR40 links hyperinsulinemia, hepatic steatosis, and impaired glucose homeostasis in mouse. Cell Metab 2005 April;1(4):245−58.

[150] Smith BW, Adams LA. Nonalcoholic fatty liver disease and diabetes mellitus: pathogenesis and treatment. Nat Rev Endocrinol 2011;7(8):456−65.

[151] Assmann A, Hinault C, Kulkarni RN. Growth factor control of pancreatic islet regeneration and function. Pediatr Diabetes 2009 February;10(1):14−32.

[152] Halperin F, Lopez R, Manning R, Kahn CR, Kulkarni RN, Goldfine AB. Insulin augmentation of glucose-stimulated insulin secretion is impaired in insulin-resistant humans. Diabetes 2012 February;61(2):301−9.

[153] Lopez X, Cypess A, Manning R, O'Shea S, Kulkarni RN, Goldfine AB. Exogenous insulin enhances glucose-stimulated insulin response in healthy humans independent of changes in free Fatty acids. J Clin Endocrinol Metab 2011 December; 96(12):3811−21.

[154] Bouche C, Lopez X, Fleischman A, Cypess AM, O'Shea S, Stefanovski D, et al. Insulin enhances glucose-stimulated insulin secretion in healthy humans. Proc Natl Acad Sci USA 2010 March 9;107(10):4770−5.

[155] Kawamori D, Kulkarni RN. Insulin modulation of glucagon secretion: the role of insulin and other factors in the regulation of glucagon secretion. Islets 2009 November;1(3):276−9.

[156] Elefteriou F, Takeda S, Ebihara K, Magre J, Patano N, Kim CA, et al. Serum leptin level is a regulator of bone mass. Proc Natl Acad Sci USA 2004 March 2;101(9):3258−63.

[157] Fu L, Patel MS, Bradley A, Wagner EF, Karsenty G. The molecular clock mediates leptin-regulated bone formation. Cell 2005 September 9;122(5):803−15.

[158] Karsenty G. Convergence between bone and energy homeostases: leptin regulation of bone mass. Cell Metab 2006 November;4(5):341−8.

[159] Takeda S, Elefteriou F, Levasseur R, Liu X, Zhao L, Parker KL, et al. Leptin regulates bone formation via the sympathetic nervous system. Cell 2002 November 1;111(3):305−17.

[160] Reid IR. Leptin deficiency—lessons in regional differences in the regulation of bone mass. Bone 2004 March;34(3):369−71.

[161] Ahmed LA, Joakimsen RM, Berntsen GK, Fonnebo V, Schirmer H. Diabetes mellitus and the risk of non-vertebral fractures: the Tromso study. Osteoporos Int 2006;17(4):495−500.

[162] Grey A. Skeletal consequences of thiazolidinedione therapy. Osteoporos Int 2008 February;19(2):129−37.

[163] Rzonca SO, Suva LJ, Gaddy D, Montague DC, Lecka-Czernik B. Bone is a target for the antidiabetic compound rosiglitazone. Endocrinology 2004 January;145(1):401−6.

[164] Wan Y, Chong LW, Evans RM. PPAR-gamma regulates osteoclastogenesis in mice. Nat Med 2007 December;13(12): 1496−503.

[165] Vestergaard P. Discrepancies in bone mineral density and fracture risk in patients with type 1 and type 2 diabetes—a meta-analysis. Osteoporos Int 2007 April;18(4):427−44.

[166] Motoshima H, Wu X, Sinha MK, Hardy VE, Rosato EL, Barbot DJ, et al. Differential regulation of adiponectin secretion from cultured human omental and subcutaneous adipocytes: effects of insulin and rosiglitazone. J Clin Endocrinol Metab 2002 December;87(12):5662−7.

[167] Azen SP, Peters RK, Berkowitz K, Kjos S, Xiang A, Buchanan TA. TRIPOD (TRoglitazone In the Prevention Of

Diabetes): a randomized, placebo-controlled trial of troglitazone in women with prior gestational diabetes mellitus. Control Clin Trials 1998 April;19(2):217−31.

[168] Reginato MJ, Lazar MA. Mechanisms by which thiazolidinediones enhance insulin action. Trends Endocrinol Metab 1999 December;10(1):9−13.

[169] Antonucci T, Whitcomb R, McLain R, Lockwood D, Norris RM. Impaired glucose tolerance is normalized by treatment with the thiazolidinedione troglitazone. Diabetes Care 1997 February;20(2):188−93.

[170] Petersen KF, Krssak M, Inzucchi S, Cline GW, Dufour S, Shulman GI. Mechanism of troglitazone action in type 2 diabetes. Diabetes 2000 May;49(5):827−31.

[171] Schiavi SC. Bone talk. Nat Genet 2006 November;38(11):1230−1.

[172] Yamaguchi M, Weitzmann MN, Murata T. Exogenous regucalcin stimulates osteoclastogenesis and suppresses osteoblastogenesis through NF-kappaB activation. Mol Cell Biochem 2012 January;359(1−2):193−203.

[173] Kobayashi T, Kronenberg H. Minireview: transcriptional regulation in development of bone. Endocrinology 2005 March;146(3):1012−7.

[174] Hassan MQ, Tare R, Lee SH, Mandeville M, Weiner B, Montecino M, et al. HOXA10 controls osteoblastogenesis by directly activating bone regulatory and phenotypic genes. Mol Cell Biol 2007 May;27(9):3337−52.

[175] Albers J, Schulze J, Beil FT, Gebauer M, Baranowsky A, Keller J, et al. Control of bone formation by the serpentine receptor Frizzled-9. J Cell Biol 2011 March 21;192(6):1057−72.

[176] Kapinas K, Delany AM. MicroRNA biogenesis and regulation of bone remodeling. Arthritis Res Ther 2011;13(3):220.

[177] Sugatani T, Hruska KA. Impaired micro-RNA pathways diminish osteoclast differentiation and function. J Biol Chem 2009 February 13;284(7):4667−78.

[178] Taipaleenmaki H, Bjerre HL, Chen L, Kauppinen S, Kassem M. Mechanisms in endocrinology: Micro-RNAs: targets for enhancing osteoblast differentiation and bone formation. Eur J Endocrinol 2012 March;166(3):359−71.

[179] Lian JB, Stein GS, van Wijnen AJ, Stein JL, Hassan MQ, Gaur T, et al. MicroRNA control of bone formation and homeostasis. Nat Rev Endocrinol 2012 April;8(4):212−27.

[180] Kapinas K, Kessler C, Ricks T, Gronowicz G, Delany AM. miR-29 modulates Wnt signaling in human osteoblasts through a positive feedback loop. J Biol Chem 2010 August 13; 285(33):25221−31.

[181] Kapinas K, Kessler CB, Delany AM. miR-29 suppression of osteonectin in osteoblasts: regulation during differentiation and by canonical Wnt signaling. J Cell Biochem 2009 September 1;108(1):216−24.

[182] Krishnan V, Bryant HU, MacDougald OA. Regulation of bone mass by Wnt signaling. J Clin Invest 2006 May;116(5):1202−9.

[183] Kantharidis P, Wang B, Carew RM, Lan HY. Diabetes complications: the microRNA perspective. Diabetes 2011 July;60(7):1832−7.

[184] Fernandez-Valverde SL, Taft RJ, Mattick JS. MicroRNAs in beta-cell biology, insulin resistance, diabetes and its complications. Diabetes 2011 July;60(7):1825−31.

[185] Akune T, Ohba S, Kamekura S, Yamaguchi M, Chung UI, Kubota N, et al. PPARgamma insufficiency enhances osteogenesis through osteoblast formation from bone marrow progenitors. J Clin Invest 2004 March;113(6):846−55.

[186] Kintscher U, Law RE. PPARgamma-mediated insulin sensitization: the importance of fat versus muscle. Am J Physiol Endocrinol Metab 2005 February;288(2):E287−91.

[187] Lee NK, Karsenty G. Reciprocal regulation of bone and energy metabolism. Trends Endocrinol Metab 2008 July;19(5):161−6.

[188] Lee NK, Sowa H, Hinoi E, Ferron M, Ahn JD, Confavreux C, et al. Endocrine regulation of energy metabolism by the skeleton. Cell 2007 August 10;130(3):456–69.

[189] Karsenty G, Ferron M. The contribution of bone to whole-organism physiology. Nature 2012 January 19;481(7381):314–20.

[190] Karsenty G, Oury F. Biology without walls: the novel endocrinology of bone. Annu Rev Physiol 2012;74:87–105.

[191] Clemens TL, Karsenty G. The osteoblast: an insulin target cell controlling glucose homeostasis. J Bone Miner Res 2011 April; 26(4):677–80.

[192] Karsenty G, Oury F. The central regulation of bone mass, the first link between bone remodeling and energy metabolism. J Clin Endocrinol Metab 2010 November;95(11):4795–801.

[193] Ferron M, Wei J, Yoshizawa T, Del FA, DePinho RA, Teti A, et al. Insulin signaling in osteoblasts integrates bone remodeling and energy metabolism. Cell 2010 July 23;142(2):296–308.

[194] Hinoi E, Gao N, Jung DY, Yadav V, Yoshizawa T, Kajimura D, et al. An Osteoblast-dependent mechanism contributes to the leptin regulation of insulin secretion. Ann NY Acad Sci 2009 September;1173(Suppl. 1):E20–30.

[195] Ferron M, Hinoi E, Karsenty G, Ducy P. Osteocalcin differentially regulates beta cell and adipocyte gene expression and affects the development of metabolic diseases in wild-type mice. Proc Natl Acad Sci USA 2008 April 1;105(13):5266–70.

[196] Yamauchi T, Kamon J, Waki H, Terauchi Y, Kubota N, Hara K, et al. The fat-derived hormone adiponectin reverses insulin resistance associated with both lipoatrophy and obesity. Nat Med 2001 August;7(8):941–6.

[197] Hivert MF, Sullivan LM, Fox CS, Nathan DM, D'Agostino RB, Sr Wilson PW, et al. Associations of adiponectin, resistin, and tumor necrosis factor-alpha with insulin resistance. J Clin Endocrinol Metab 2008 August;93(8):3165–72.

[198] Kadowaki T, Yamauchi T, Kubota N, Hara K, Ueki K, Tobe K. Adiponectin and adiponectin receptors in insulin resistance, diabetes, and the metabolic syndrome. J Clin Invest 2006 July;116(7):1784–92.

[199] Shinoda Y, Yamaguchi M, Ogata N, Akune T, Kubota N, Yamauchi T, et al. Regulation of bone formation by adiponectin through autocrine/paracrine and endocrine pathways. J Cell Biochem 2006 September 1;99(1):196–208.

[200] Ealey KN, Kaludjerovic J, Archer MC, Ward WE. Adiponectin is a negative regulator of bone mineral and bone strength in growing mice. Exp Biol Med (Maywood) 2008 December; 233(12):1546–53.

[201] Richards JB, Valdes AM, Burling K, Perks UC, Spector TD. Serum adiponectin and bone mineral density in women. J Clin Endocrinol Metab 2007 April;92(4):1517–23.

[202] Williams GA, Wang Y, Callon KE, Watson M, Lin JM, Lam JB, et al. In vitro and in vivo effects of adiponectin on bone. Endocrinology 2009 August;150(8):3603–10.

[203] Thrailkill KM, Lumpkin Jr CK, Bunn RC, Kemp SF, Fowlkes JL. Is insulin an anabolic agent in bone? Dissecting the diabetic bone for clues. Am J Physiol Endocrinol Metab 2005 November;289(5):E735–45.

[204] Bjorbaek C, Kahn BB. Leptin signaling in the central nervous system and the periphery. Recent Prog Horm Res 2004;59:305–31.

[205] Ducy P, Amling M, Takeda S, Priemel M, Schilling AF, Beil FT, et al. Leptin inhibits bone formation through a hypothalamic relay: a central control of bone mass. Cell 2000 January 21;100(2):197–207.

[206] Elefteriou F, Ahn JD, Takeda S, Starbuck M, Yang X, Liu X, et al. Leptin regulation of bone resorption by the sympathetic nervous system and CART. Nature 2005 March 24; 434(7032):514–20.

[207] Abizaid A, Horvath TL. Brain circuits regulating energy homeostasis. Regul Pept 2008 August 7;149(1–3):3–10.

[208] Farooqi IS, Matarese G, Lord GM, Keogh JM, Lawrence E, Agwu C, et al. Beneficial effects of leptin on obesity, T cell hyporesponsiveness, and neuroendocrine/metabolic dysfunction of human congenital leptin deficiency. J Clin Invest 2002 October;110(8):1093–103.

[209] Marty N, Dallaporta M, Thorens B. Brain glucose sensing, counterregulation, and energy homeostasis. Physiology (Bethesda) 2007 August;22:241–51.

[210] Thorens B. Brain glucose sensing and neural regulation of insulin and glucagon secretion. Diabetes Obes Metab 2011 October;13(Suppl. 1):82–8.

[211] Levin BE, Sherwin RS. Peripheral glucose homeostasis: does brain insulin matter? J Clin Invest 2011 September;121(9): 3392–5.

[212] Havel PJ. Peripheral signals conveying metabolic information to the brain: short-term and long-term regulation of food intake and energy homeostasis. Exp Biol Med (Maywood) 2001 December;226(11):963–77.

[213] Fry M, Hoyda TD, Ferguson AV. Making sense of it: roles of the sensory circumventricular organs in feeding and regulation of energy homeostasis. Exp Biol Med (Maywood) 2007 January; 232(1):14–26.

[214] Ivanov TR, Lawrence CB, Stanley PJ, Luckman SM. Evaluation of neuromedin U actions in energy homeostasis and pituitary function. Endocrinology 2002 October;143(10):3813–21.

[215] Obici S, Zhang BB, Karkanias G, Rossetti L. Hypothalamic insulin signaling is required for inhibition of glucose production. Nat Med 2002 December;8(12):1376–82.

[216] Coll AP, Farooqi IS, O'Rahilly S. The hormonal control of food intake. Cell 2007 April 20;129(2):251–62.

[217] Plum L, Schubert M, Bruning JC. The role of insulin receptor signaling in the brain. Trends Endocrinol Metab 2005 March;16(2):59–65.

[218] Baskin DG, Figlewicz Lattemann D, Seely RJ, Woods SC, Porte Jr D, Schwartz MW. Insulin and leptin: dual adiposity signals to the brain for the regulation of food intake and body weight. Brain Res 1999;848(1–2):114–23.

[219] Bruning JC, Gautam D, Burks DJ, Gillette J, Schubert M, Orban PC, et al. Role of brain insulin receptor in control of body weight and reproduction. Science 2000;289:2122–5.

[220] Withers DJ, Gutierrez JS, Towery H, Burks DJ, Ren JM, Previs S, et al. Disruption of IRS-2 causes type 2 diabetes in mice. Nature 1998 February 26;391(6670):900–4.

[221] Cota D, Proulx K, Smith KA, Kozma SC, Thomas G, Woods SC, et al. Hypothalamic mTOR signaling regulates food intake. Science 2006 May 12;312(5775):927–30.

[222] Morton GJ, Gelling RW, Niswender KD, Morrison CD, Rhodes CJ, Schwartz MW. Leptin regulates insulin sensitivity via phosphatidylinositol-3-OH kinase signaling in mediobasal hypothalamic neurons. Cell Metab 2005 December;2(6):411–20.

[223] De Souza CT, Araujo EP, Bordin S, Ashimine R, Zollner RL, Boschero AC, et al. Consumption of a fat-rich diet activates a proinflammatory response and induces insulin resistance in the hypothalamus. Endocrinology 2005 October;146(10):4192–9.

[224] Plum L, Belgardt BF, Bruning JC. Central insulin action in energy and glucose homeostasis. J Clin Invest 2006 July; 116(7):1761–6.

[225] Koishi R, Ando Y, Ono M, Shimamura M, Yasumo H, Fujiwara T, et al. Angptl3 regulates lipid metabolism in mice. Nat Genet 2002 February;30(2):151–7.

[226] Oike Y, Akao M, Yasunaga K, Yamauchi T, Morisada T, Ito Y, et al. Angiopoietin-related growth factor antagonizes obesity and insulin resistance. Nat Med 2005 April;11(4):400–8.

[227] Ahima RS, Lazar MA. Adipokines and the peripheral and neural control of energy balance. Mol Endocrinol 2008 May;22(5):1023−31.

[228] Niswender KD, Baskin DG, Schwartz MW. Insulin and its evolving partnership with leptin in the hypothalamic control of energy homeostasis. Trends Endocrinol Metab 2004 October;15(8):362−9.

[229] Choudhury AI, Heffron H, Smith MA, Al-Qassab H, Xu AW, Selman C, et al. The role of insulin receptor substrate 2 in hypothalamic and beta cell function. J Clin Invest 2005 April;115(4):940−50.

[230] Cowley MA, Smart JL, Rubinstein M, Cerdan MG, Diano S, Horvath TL, et al. Leptin activates anorexigenic POMC neurons through a neural network in the arcuate nucleus. Nature 2001 May 24;411(6836):480−4.

[231] Spanswick D, Smith MA, Groppi VE, Logan SD, Ashford ML. Leptin inhibits hypothalamic neurons by activation of ATP-sensitive potassium channels. Nature 1997 December 4;390(6659):521−5.

[232] Gavrilova O, Marcus-Samuels B, Graham D, Kim JK, Shulman GI, Castle AL, et al. Surgical implantation of adipose tissue reverses diabetes in lipoatrophic mice. J Clin Invest 2000 February;105(3):271−8.

[233] Colombo C, Cutson JJ, Yamauchi T, Vinson C, Kadowaki T, Gavrilova O, et al. Transplantation of adipose tissue lacking leptin is unable to reverse the metabolic abnormalities associated with lipoatrophy. Diabetes 2002 September;51(9):2727−33.

[234] Shimomura I, Hammer RE, Ikemoto S, Brown MS, Goldstein JL. Leptin reverses insulin resistance and diabetes mellitus in mice with congenital lipodystrophy. Nature 1999 September 2;401(6748):73−6.

[235] Gavrilova O, Marcus-Samuels B, Leon LR, Vinson C, Reitman ML. Leptin and diabetes in lipoatrophic mice. Nature 2000;403(6772):850−1.

[236] Tahrani AA, Bailey CJ, Del PS, Barnett AH. Management of type 2 diabetes: new and future developments in treatment. Lancet 2011 July 9;378(9786):182−97.

[237] Drucker DJ. The biology of incretin hormones. Cell Metab 2006 March;3(3):153−65.

[238] Holst JJ, Gromada J. Role of incretin hormones in the regulation of insulin secretion in diabetic and nondiabetic humans. Am J Physiol Endocrinol Metab 2004 August;287(2):E199−206.

[239] Baggio LL, Drucker DJ. Biology of incretins: GLP-1 and GIP. Gastroenterology 2007 May;132(6):2131−57.

[240] Meier JJ, Nauck MA. Is the diminished incretin effect in type 2 diabetes just an epi-phenomenon of impaired beta-cell function? Diabetes 2010 May;59(5):1117−25.

[241] Seino Y, Fukushima M, Yabe D. GIP and GLP-1, the two incretin hormones: similarities and differences. J Diabetes Invest 2010;1(1−2):8−83.

[242] Verdich C, Toubro S, Buemann B, Lysgard MJ, Juul HJ, Astrup A. The role of postprandial releases of insulin and incretin hormones in meal-induced satiety—effect of obesity and weight reduction. Int J Obes Relat Metab Disord 2001 August;25(8):1206−14.

[243] Trumper A, Trumper K, Trusheim H, Arnold R, Goke B, Horsch D. Glucose-dependent insulinotropic polypeptide is a growth factor for beta (INS-1) cells by pleiotropic signaling. Mol Endocrinol 2001 September;15(9):1559−70.

[244] Buteau J, Foist S, Joly E, Prentki M. Glucagon-like peptide 1 induces pancreatic beta-cell proliferation via transactivation of the epidermal growth factor receptor. Diabetes 2003;52:124−32.

[245] Farilla L, Bulotta A, Hirshberg B, Li CS, Khoury N, Noushmehr H, et al. Glucagon-like peptide 1 inhibits cell apoptosis and improves glucose responsiveness of freshly isolated human islets. Endocrinology 2003 December; 144(12):5149−58.

[246] Perfetti R, Zhou J, Doyle ME, Egan JM. Glucagon-like peptide-1 induces cell proliferation and pancreatic-duodenum homeobox-1 expression and increases endocrine cell mass in the pancreas of old, glucose-intolerant rats. Endocrinology 2000 December; 141(12):4600−5.

[247] Stoffers DA, Kieffer TJ, Hussain MA, Drucker DJ, Bonner-Weir S, Habener JF, et al. Insulinotropic glucagon-like peptide 1 agonists stimulate expression of homeodomain protein IDX-1 and increase islet size in mouse pancreas. Diabetes 2000 May;49(5):741−8.

[248] De Leon DD, Deng S, Madani R, Ahima RS, Drucker DJ, Stoffers DA. Role of endogenous glucagon-like peptide-1 in islet regeneration after partial pancreatectomy. Diabetes 2003 February;52(2):365−71.

[249] Tourrel C, Bailbe D, Meile MJ, Kergoat M, Portha B. Glucagon-like peptide-1 and exendin-4 stimulate beta-cell neogenesis in streptozotocin-treated newborn rats resulting in persistently improved glucose homeostasis at adult age. Diabetes 2001 July;50(7):1562−70.

[250] Fehse F, Trautmann M, Holst JJ, Halseth AE, Nanayakkara N, Nielsen LL, et al. Exenatide augments first- and second-phase insulin secretion in response to intravenous glucose in subjects with type 2 diabetes. J Clin Endocrinol Metab 2005 November; 90(11):5991−7.

[251] Vilsboll T, Krarup T, Madsbad S, Holst JJ. Defective amplification of the late phase insulin response to glucose by GIP in obese Type II diabetic patients. Diabetologia 2002 August; 45(8):1111−9.

[252] Kieffer TJ, McIntosh CH, Pederson RA. Degradation of glucose-dependent insulinotropic polypeptide and truncated glucagon-like peptide 1 in vitro and in vivo by dipeptidyl peptidase IV. Endocrinology 1995 August;136(8):3585−96.

[253] Deacon CF, Johnsen AH, Holst JJ. Degradation of glucagon-like peptide-1 by human plasma in vitro yields an N-terminally truncated peptide that is a major endogenous metabolite in vivo. J Clin Endocrinol Metab 1995 March; 80(3):952−7.

[254] Winzell MS, Ahren B. G-protein-coupled receptors and islet function—implications for treatment of type 2 diabetes. Pharmacol Ther 2007 December;116(3):437−48.

[255] Chang AM, Jakobsen G, Sturis J, Smith MJ, Bloem CJ, An B, et al. The GLP-1 derivative NN2211 restores beta-cell sensitivity to glucose in type 2 diabetic patients after a single dose. Diabetes 2003 July;52(7):1786−91.

[256] Feve B, Bastard JP. The role of interleukins in insulin resistance and type 2 diabetes mellitus. Nat Rev Endocrinol 2009 June;5(6):305−11.

[257] Knowler WC, Barrett-Connor E, Fowler SE, Hamman RF, Lachin JM, Walker EA, et al. Reduction in the incidence of type 2 diabetes with lifestyle intervention or metformin. N Engl J Med 2002 February 7;346(6):393−403.

[258] Kitabchi AE, Temprosa M, Knowler WC, Kahn SE, Fowler SE, Haffner SM, et al. Role of insulin secretion and sensitivity in the evolution of type 2 diabetes in the diabetes prevention program: effects of lifestyle intervention and metformin. Diabetes 2005 August;54(8):2404−14.

[259] Inzucchi SE, Maggs DG, Spollett GR, Page SL, Rife FS, Walton V, et al. Efficacy and metabolic effects of metformin and troglitazone in type II diabetes mellitus. N Engl J Med 1998 March 26;338(13):867−72.

[260] Kim YB, Ciaraldi TP, Kong A, Kim D, Chu N, Mohideen P, et al. Troglitazone but not metformin restores insulin-stimulated phosphoinositide 3-kinase activity and increases p110beta

protein levels in skeletal muscle of type 2 diabetic subjects. Diabetes 2002 February;51(2):443—8.

[261] Karlsson HK, Hallsten K, Bjornholm M, Tsuchida H, Chibalin AV, Virtanen KA, et al. Effects of metformin and rosiglitazone treatment on insulin signaling and glucose uptake in patients with newly diagnosed type 2 diabetes: a randomized controlled study. Diabetes 2005 May;54(5):1459—67.

[262] Bailey CJ, Turner RC. Metformin. N Engl J Med 1996 February 29;334(9):574—9.

[263] Stumvoll M, Nurjhan N, Perriello G, Dailey G, Gerich JE. Metabolic effects of metformin in non-insulin-dependent diabetes mellitus. N Engl J Med 1995 August 31;333(9):550—4.

[264] Dunn CJ, Peters Metformin DH. A review of its pharmacological properties and therapeutic use in non-insulin-dependent diabetes mellitus. Drugs 1995 May;49(5):721—49.

[265] Matthaei S, Hamann A, Klein HH, Benecke H, Kreymann G, Flier JS, et al. Association of Metformin's effect to increase insulin-stimulated glucose transport with potentiation of insulin-induced translocation of glucose transporters from intracellular pool to plasma membrane in rat adipocytes. Diabetes 1991;40:850—7.

[266] Fantus IG, Brosseau R. Mechanism of action of metformin: insulin receptor and postreceptor effects in vitro and in vivo. J Clin Endocrinol Metab 1986 October;63(4):898—905.

Index

Page numbers with "f" denote figures; "t" tables.

Color Plates

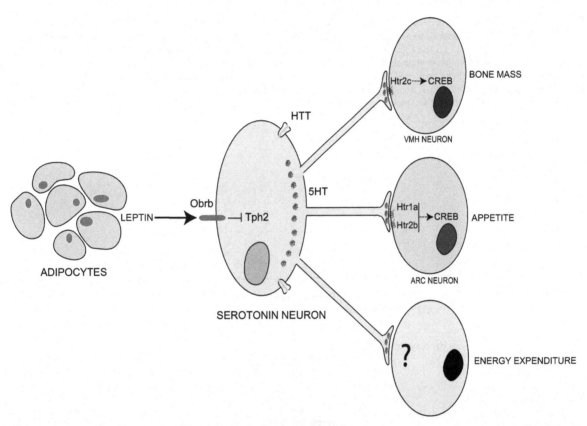

FIGURE 5.1 **Serotonin-dependent neuronal relay in the leptin regulation of bone mass, appetite, and energy expenditure.** Leptin inhibits synthesis and release of brain-derived serotonin, among other neuronal relays, which favors bone mass accrual and appetite through its action on ventromedial and arcuate hypothalamic neurons. VMH, ventromedial hypothalamus; ARC, arcuate; HTT, 5-hydroxytryptamine transporter. Structures not to scale.

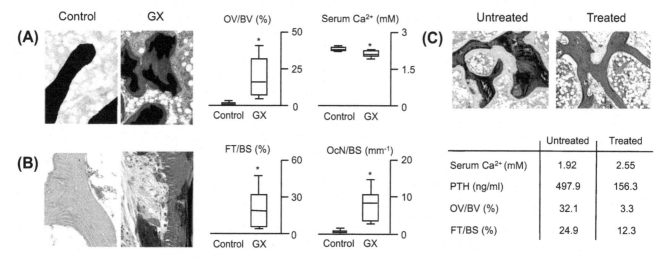

FIGURE 6.1   **Osteomalacia in gastrectomized patients. (A)** von Kossa/van Gieson staining of sections from non-decalcified bone biopsies derived from gastrectomized (GX) patients revealed a pathological enrichment of osteoid. Quantification of the osteoid volume per bone volume (OV/BV) and serum calcium is given on the right. Boxes include data from the 25th to 75th percentile. $n = 12$ individuals per group. *$p < 0.05$ compared to the control group. **(B)** Goldner staining revealed fibroosteoclasia in the GX patients. Quantification of fibrous tissue per bone surface (FT/BS) and osteoclast number per bone surface (OcN/BS) is given on the right. $n = 12$ individuals per group. *$p < 0.005$ compared to the control group. **(C)** Goldner staining of sections from non-decalcified bone biopsies derived from one patient before supplementation with calcium and vitamin D3 (untreated) and 1 year thereafter (treated). Quantification of serum calcium, PTH, OV/BV, and FT/BS is given below.

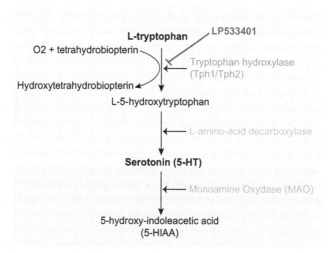

FIGURE 7.1   **Mechanism of serotonin biosynthesis (yellow box) and degradation (gray box).** Enzymes are in blue. LP533401 (in red) inhibits Tph activity, and thereby serotonin production, by preventing binding of its tetrahydrobiopterin cofactor.

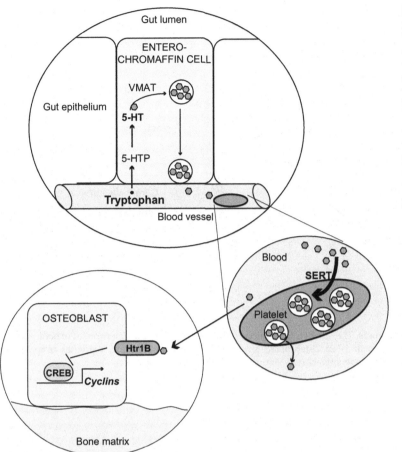

FIGURE 7.2 Schematic representation of the functional link between gut-derived serotonin and bone formation. Serotonin is synthesized in enterochromaffin cells located within the gut epithelium via the enzymatic transformation of tryptophan (see Fig. 7.1 for details). Following its association within the VMAT transporter it is stored in secretory granules before being released into the general circulation where most (95%) of it is absorbed by platelets through the SERT transporter. The remaining amount of circulating serotonin can reach bone and bind to osteoblasts that express the Htr1b receptor. This binding triggers a signaling cascade that results in the decreased expression and activity of the transcription factor CREB. As a result expression of *Cyclins* is lowered and osteoblast proliferation is decreased.

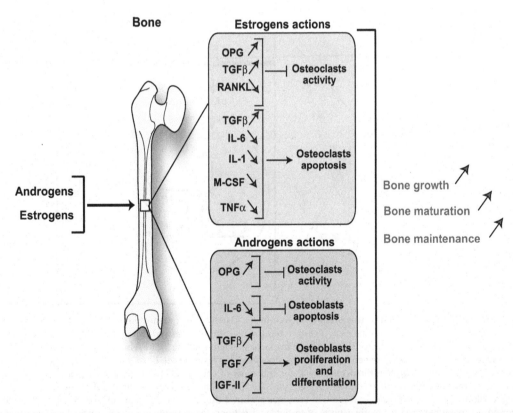

FIGURE 11.1 **Molecular mediators of sex steroid hormone action on bone cells.** Sex steroid hormones secreted by gonads play a crucial role during skeletal growth, maturation, and maintenance in both men and women. This figure summarizes the major targets of estrogens and androgens in bone cells. Their activation or repression is associated with effects on apoptosis and/or proliferation of osteoblasts and/or osteoclasts.

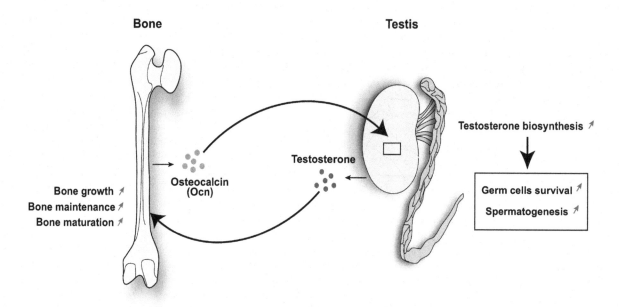

FIGURE 11.2 **Mutual dependence between bone and gonads.** The sex steroid hormone testosterone is a crucial determinant of bone growth during puberty, maturation, and maintenance of bone mass accrual. Osteocalcin, an osteoblast-derived hormone, regulates testosterone production by Leydig cells. Testosterone in testis favors spermatogenesis, sexual maturity, and germ cell survival.

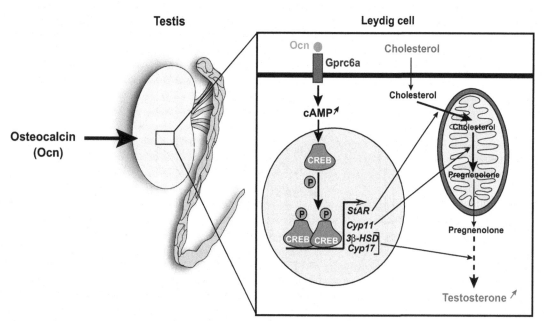

FIGURE 11.3 **Bone endocrine regulation of testosterone biosynthesis.** Osteocalcin, an osteoblast-derived hormone, regulates testosterone production in testis. Following osteocalcin binding to a G-couple receptor (Gprc6a) expressed in Leydig cells, cAMP production is increased leading to the activation of the transcription factor CREB (cAMP response element binding). CREB binds to the promoter regions and activates the expression of several genes encoding for the enzymes that are necessary for testosterone biosynthesis, such as *StAR*, *Cyp11a*, *3β-HSD*, and *Cyp17*. Steroidogenic acute regulatory protein (StAR) is crucial for transport of cholesterol to mitochondria where biosynthesis of steroids is initiated. *Cyp11a* encodes the cholesterol side-chain cleavage enzyme (P450scc) that catalyzes the first and rate-limiting step, which converts cholesterol to pregnenolone. *3β-HSD* and *Cyp17* encode two enzymes required during the conversion of pregnenolone to testosterone. Testosterone is a sex steroid hormone required for many aspects of testicular functions, for example germ cell survival and spermatogenesis.

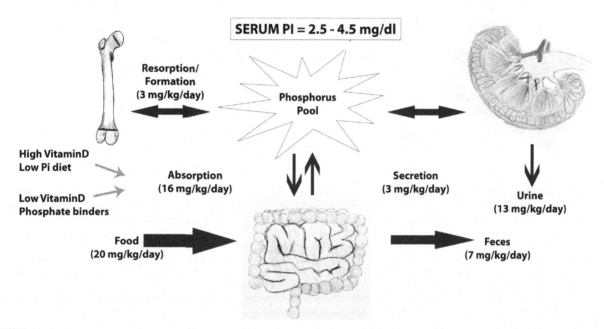

SERUM PI = 2.5 - 4.5 mg/dl

Resorption/
Formation
(3 mg/kg/day)

Phosphorus
Pool

High VitaminD
Low Pi diet

Low VitaminD
Phosphate binders

Absorption
(16 mg/kg/day)

Secretion
(3 mg/kg/day)

Urine
(13 mg/kg/day)

Food
(20 mg/kg/day)

Feces
(7 mg/kg/day)

FIGURE 12.1   **Phosphate homeostasis.** The human body has 15–20 M of phosphate under healthy conditions. The amount of phosphate is a balance between intake and excretion in the intestines and kidneys. The level of phosphate in the serum is 2.5–4.5 mg/dl and this level is maintained by the constant interchange of phosphate between the serum and bone. The skeleton contains the bulk of the phosphate in the body, accounting for 80–90% of the total amount. Phosphate is transferred between bone and serum at a rate of about 3 mg per kilogram of body weight per day (3 mg/kg/day) as bone forms and is reabsorbed to balance bone strength and serum phosphate levels. Phosphate is abundant in the diet, with the average adult ingesting about 20 mg per kg of body weight. The intestine absorbs 55–80% of this intake. Around 16 mg/kg/day are absorbed in the proximal intestine while the digestive process eliminates 3 mg/kg/day. Approximately 7 mg/kg/day phosphate is excreted in the feces. The kidneys contribute to phosphate balance by regulating how much phosphate is excreted in the urine or reabsorbed into the serum. Under normal conditions, approximately 13 mg/kg/day, the equivalent of the amount taken in by the intestines, is excreted in the urine.

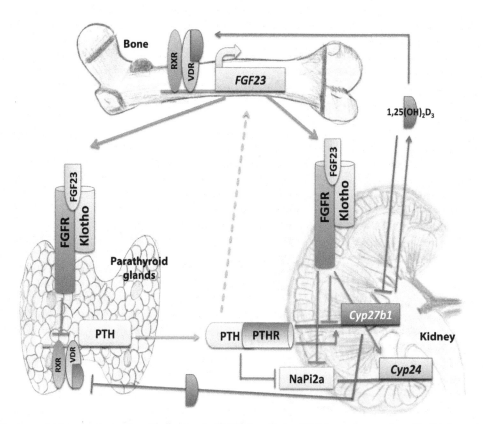

FIGURE 12.2 The bone, kidney, and parathyroid gland axis. FGF23 from bone, PTH from the parathyroid glands, and vitamin D from the kidneys regulate phosphate serum levels and each other. PTH is produced in the parathyroid glands and targets the kidney to increase phosphate wasting by downregulating the sodium transporter, NaPi2a. It also increases the production of active vitamin D by upregulating Cyp27b1 which converts 25(OH) vitamin D to its active form ($1,25(OH)_2D_3$). $1,25(OH)_2D_3$ downregulates PTH production in a negative feedback loop to regulate PTH activity. $1,25(OH)_2D_3$ stimulates FGF23 production in the bone which also targets the kidney to reduce NaPi2a activities, thereby increasing urinary phosphate wasting. In addition, FGF23 suppresses active vitamin D production in the kidney by downregulating Cyp27b1 and upregulating Cyp24, a hydroxylase that catabolizes $1,25(OH)_2D_3$. This forms a second negative feedback loop in the phosphate regulatory network. Finally, PTH and FGF23 mutually regulate each other to form the third feedback loop. PTH stimulates FGF23 production in bone while FGF23 suppresses PTH in the parathyroid glands. Klotho is an important member of the network since it is required for FGF23 binding and signaling. Presence of Klotho in the parathyroid glands and kidneys allows FGF23 to specifically target these organs to maintain physiologic phosphate balance.

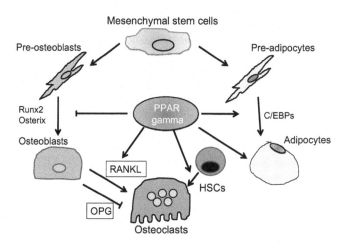

FIGURE 14.1 PPARγ regulates the cell fate decision of mesenchymal stem cells (MSCs) toward the adipogenic or osteogenic lineage. The role of PPARγ in osteoclast differentiation is still controversial and needs to be clarified. Marrow adipocytes produce a number of secretory factors and PPARγ regulates the expression of these genes. PPARγ: peroxisome proliferator-activated receptor-gamma. C/EBP: CCAAT enhancer binding protein. Runx2: runt-related transcription factor 2. Msx2: muscle segment homeobox homologue of 2.

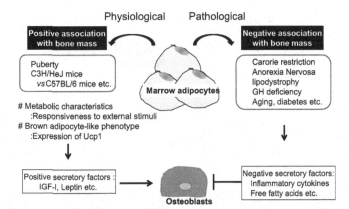

FIGURE 14.2 **Marrow adipocytes produce a number of secretory factors.** Such factors could have a significant role in osteoblast differentiation and/or function. In pathogenic conditions, these determinants could impact osteoblasts in a negative direction, whereas in physiological conditions these factors may have a different role from the one observed in the pathogenic conditions. There is also evidence that marrow fat is metabolically active and that genes which are characteristics to brown adipocytes are expressed in marrow adipocytes.

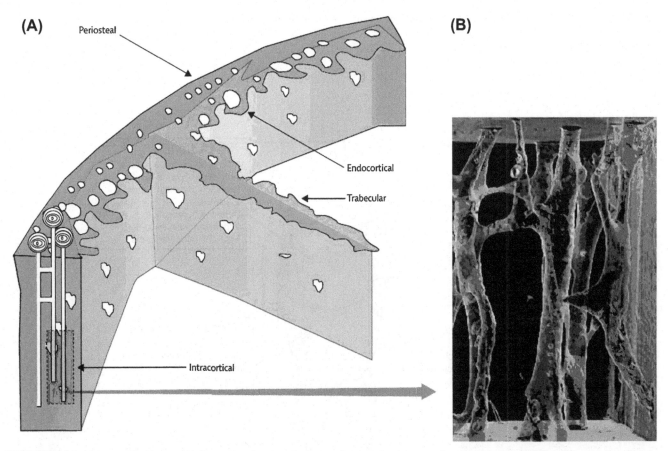

FIGURE 15.2 **Structure of bone.** **(A)** Cortical and trabecular bone, the periosteal (external) surface and the three (endocortical, trabecular, intracortical) contiguous components of the endosteal (internal) surface upon which matrix remodeling is initiated. **(B)** The intracortical surface formed by the lining of Haversian and Volkmann canals traverses the cortex. These canals are seen as pores in cross-section. Reconstructed with high-resolution quantitative CT. *Adapted from Zebaze et al. [31].*

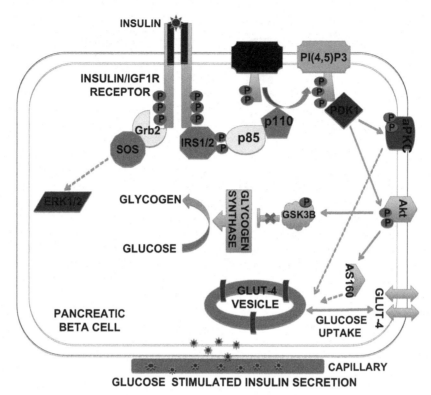

FIGURE 17.2   A typical schematic of the insulin signaling cascade involved in the regulation of glucose uptake and insulin secretion.

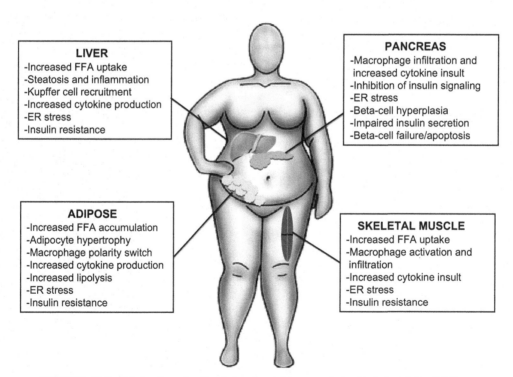

FIGURE 17.3   Mechanism of systemic insulin resistance and obesity induced β-cell failure.

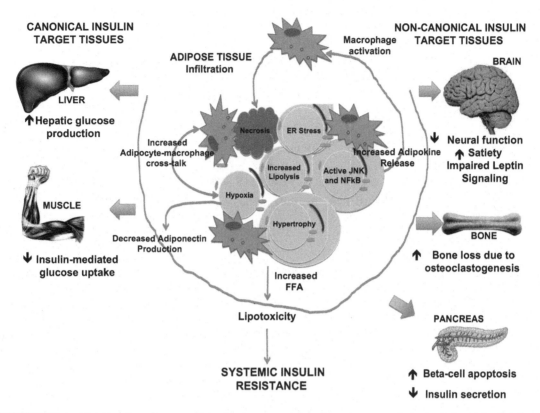

FIGURE 17.4 Multi-level organ crosstalk leading to systemic insulin resistance and obesity induced β-cell failure.

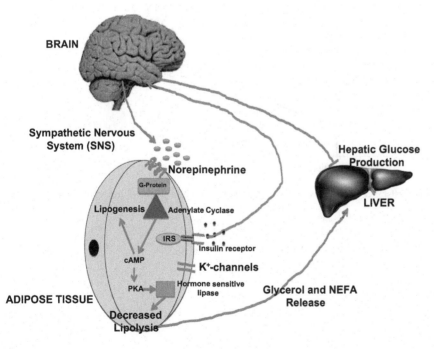

FIGURE 17.5 Role of brain-derived signals in regulating energy homeostasis and glucose metabolism.

Processing of Pro-glucagon in Intestinal L-Cells

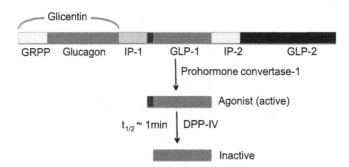

FIGURE 17.6   Biosynthesis and regulation of GLP-1.

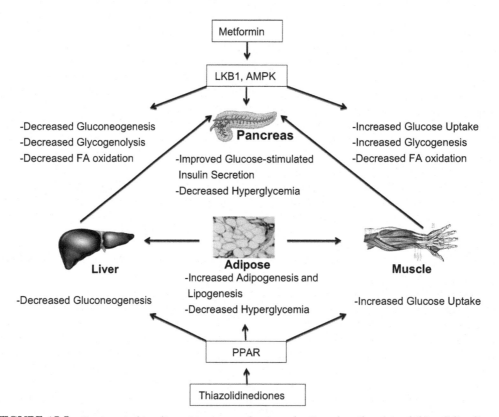

FIGURE 17.7   Treatment of insulin resistance—mechanism of action of metformin and thiazolidinedione.

Printed in the United States
By Bookmasters